Evidence-Based Cardiology

BENJAMIN A. STEINBERG, MD, MHS

Division of Cardiovascular Medicine
Department of Medicine
Duke University Medical Center
Durham, North Carolina

CHRISTOPHER P. CANNON, MD

Professor of Medicine
Harvard Medical School
Cardiovascular Division
Brigham and Women's Hospital
Executive Director, Cardiometabolic Trials
Harvard Clinical Research Institute
Boston, Massachusetts

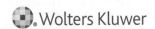 Wolters Kluwer

Philadelphia • Baltimore • New York • London
Buenos Aires • Hong Kong • Sydney • Tokyo

Acquisitions Editor: Julie Goolsby
Product Development Editor: Andrea Vosburgh
Editorial Assistant: Brian Convery
Marketing Manager: Stephanie Kindlick
Production Project Manager: Priscilla Crater
Design Coordinator: Holly McLaughlin
Manufacturing Coordinator: Beth Welsh
Prepress Vendor: SPi Global

4th edition

Library of Congress Cataloging-in-Publication Data
Cannon, Christopher P., author, editor.
  Evidence-based cardiology / editors, Benjamin A. Steinberg, Christopher P. Cannon. — Fourth edition.
     p. ; cm.
  Authors' names reversed on the previous edition.
  Includes bibliographical references and index.
  ISBN 978-1-4511-9330-5
  I. Steinberg, Benjamin A., author, editor. II. Title.
  [DNLM: 1. Heart Diseases—therapy—Abstracts. 2. Heart Diseases—therapy—Handbooks. 3. Evidence-Based Medicine—methods—Abstracts. 4. Evidence-Based Medicine—methods—Handbooks. 5. Heart Diseases—diagnosis—Abstracts. 6. Heart Diseases—diagnosis—Handbooks. 7. Randomized Controlled Trials as Topic—Abstracts. 8. Randomized Controlled Trials as Topic—Handbooks. WG 39]
  RC669.15
  616.1'2—dc23
                                                                            2015008648

Contributors

Christopher P. Cannon, MD
Professor of Medicine
Harvard Medical School
Cardiovascular Division
Brigham and Women's Hospital
Executive Director,
    Cardiometabolic Trials
Harvard Clinical Research
    Institute
Boston, Massachusetts

Justin M. Dunn, MD, MPH
Interventional Cardiology Fellow
Department of Cardiovascular
    Medicine
Cleveland Clinic
Cleveland, Ohio

Alexander C. Fanaroff, MD
Resident in Internal Medicine
Department of Internal Medicine
Duke University
Durham, North Carolina

**Matthew W. Sherwood, MD,
MHS**
Interventional Cardiology Fellow
Duke University Hospital
Durham, North Carolina

**Benjamin A. Steinberg, MD,
MHS**
Division of Cardiovascular
    Medicine
Department of Medicine
Duke University Medical Center
Durham, North Carolina

Preface

In the field of cardiology, perhaps more than any other field of medicine, advances in diagnosis and management of patients are guided by data from large clinical trials. This has been heralded as the era of "evidence-based medicine." Over the past 15 years, across now four editions, it has been exciting to keep updating *Evidence-Based Cardiology* with the large number of major trials evaluating pharmacologic agents and diagnostic and therapeutic procedures in the literature. Since the publication of the last edition, there have been many new trials and lots of guideline updates to incorporated into this fourth edition.

The two primary goals of *Evidence-Based Cardiology* remain the systematic summarization of major trial data and placing the information from these annotated studies in context. The results of major randomized trials in six major topic areas are presented in a systematic fashion, including the design, study population, treatment regimen, and results; some older trials have been eliminated to limit the book length. Meta-analyses, review articles, and nonrandomized and less important trials have abbreviated summaries. Importantly, the chapter overviews preceding the annotated references have been expanded with particular attention to discussing relevant ACC/AHA Practice Guidelines.

Chapter 1 focuses on preventive cardiology, particularly lipid and diet management, but also each of the multiple risk factors for coronary artery disease; in the fourth edition, the new statin trials and the updated (albeit controversial) 2013 ACC/AHA Cholesterol Guideline are reviewed. There is also increased material on other emerging coronary heart disease risk factors and assessment measures, including the new atherosclerotic cardiovascular disease (ASCVD) risk calculator and calcium scoring. Chapter 2 focuses on revascularization procedures, primarily coronary artery stenting and bypass surgery. New material includes data on drug-eluting stents and distal embolic protection devices, and transcatheter aortic valve replacement (TAVR). Chapters 3 and 4 cover the wealth of data on acute coronary syndromes. New material includes trial data on potent antiplatelet agents, as well as various strategies combining different antithrombotic agents. Chapter 5 focuses on the pharmacologic management of heart failure, with new pharmacologic agents that reduce mortality, and new trials of cardiac resynchronization therapy for CHF. Chapter 6 has been expanded to include the many new anticoagulant options for stroke prevention in atrial fibrillation, as well as new data on pacemakers and ventricular arrhythmias and implantable cardioverter–defibrillators (ICDs).

We wish to acknowledge the coauthors of Chapters 1, 2, 3, and 4 (Alexander C. Fanaroff, Justin M. Dunn, and Matthew W. Sherwood), who provided extensive assistance in revising, updating, and expanding these chapters. We hope that this updated guide can be helpful in keeping you up to date on new trial data and how it impacts the clinical care of your patients.

Christopher P. Cannon, MD and Benjamin A. Steinberg, MD, MHS

Contents

CHAPTER 2 Coronary Revascularization and Percutaneous Procedures   110

Christopher P. Cannon, Benjamin A. Steinberg, and Justin M. Dunn

CHAPTER 3 Unstable Angina/Non–ST Elevation MI 215

Christopher P. Cannon, Benjamin A. Steinberg,
and Matthew W. Sherwood

EPIDEMIOLOGY 215

PATHOPHYSIOLOGY 215

CHAPTER 4 ST Elevation Myocardial Infarction   266

Christopher P. Cannon, Benjamin A. Steinberg,
and Justin M. Dunn

CHAPTER 5 **Heart Failure**   374

Benjamin A. Steinberg and Christopher P. Cannon

CHAPTER 6 Arrhythmias   428

Benjamin A. Steinberg and Christopher P. Cannon

Preventive Cardiology: Risk Factors for Coronary Artery Disease and Primary and Secondary Prevention

Christopher P. Cannon, Benjamin A. Steinberg, and Alexander C. Fanaroff

CHOLESTEROL AND LIPIDS

Epidemiology

An estimated 98.9 million Americans have elevated total cholesterol (TC) levels, and historically, nearly one in five adults in the United States has been eligible for cholesterol-lowering therapy. A 10% decrease in TC is associated with an approximately 10% to 15% lower coronary heart disease (CHD) mortality rate and an approximately 20% decrease in the risk of myocardial infarction (MI). When TC levels are reduced by lifestyle modification (e.g., diet, exercise) and/or pharmacologic intervention, more benefit is derived in younger individuals, and the full benefits of a sustained decrease are not achieved for at least 5 years. Cardiac risk tables have been created to estimate the risk of CHD death at various cholesterol levels and in combination with other major cardiac risk factors. Prior guidelines have used modified Framingham Risk Score tables to estimate the 10-year CHD risk; however, more recently, newer Pooled Cohort Equation has been emphasized to incorporate broader populations (**Table 1.1**).

Low-density lipoprotein (LDL) has been shown in several studies, including the Framingham Heart Study (FHS), Multiple Risk Factor Intervention Trial (MRFIT), and Lipid Research Clinics (LRC) trial, to be a stronger predictor of CHD than TC. In fact, for every 30-mg/dL rise in LDL above 40 mg/dL, relative risk for coronary artery disease (CAD) increases by 30% (*Circulation* 2004;110:227). Moreover, LDL lowering with various pharmacologic agents has been shown to reduce cardiovascular mortality. As a result, LDL levels have been and continue to be the primary focus of the guideline-recommended management for elevated cholesterol to reduce cardiovascular risk. The most recent ACC/AHA Guidelines, however, have put more emphasis on use of statin therapy than on the actual amount of LDL reduction.

Table 1.1	The 2014 Atherosclerotic Cardiovascular Disease Risk Estimator

Components (http://tools.cardiosource.org/ASCVD-Risk-Estimator/)

Gender	Systolic blood pressure	HDL cholesterol
Age	Treatment for HTN	Total cholesterol
Race		
Smoker		
Diabetes		

The latest guidelines employed a risk-based approach (14) with an online risk calculator, which includes the components above. Lipid-lowering therapy, either standard or high dose, is then based on the calculated risk (see **Fig. 1.2**).

High levels of high-density lipoproteins (HDLs) are associated with a decreased risk of CHD mortality; a 1% lower HDL is associated with a 2% to 3% higher CHD risk (16). Therefore, low HDL (<40 mg/dL) has been considered an indicator of increased risk, whereas a level of 60 mg/dL or greater is a negative cardiac risk factor. Furthermore, low HDL is one of five diagnostic criteria for the metabolic syndrome (see page 15) (*Circulation* 2005;112:2735). Importantly, though many drugs have been shown to increase HDL levels, pharmacologic increase in HDL has not been shown to reduce cardiovascular events. Non-HDL cholesterol levels also have been demonstrated to be predictors of cardiovascular disease (CVD) (17).

Growing evidence indicates that high triglyceride (TG) levels are a modest independent predictor of increased CHD mortality (24). One analysis of studies with nearly 60,000 participants found that even after adjustment for multiple cardiac risk factors, high TG levels are associated with significant 14% and 37% increases in cardiovascular risk in men and women, respectively. Obesity, physical inactivity, glucose intolerance, hypothyroidism, and the use of β-blockers, estrogen, and diuretics are associated with an increased risk of hypertriglyceridemia. While TG levels of <150 mg/dL have been considered desirable, the latest guidelines acknowledge the lack of robust evidence of improvement in clinical outcomes when treating to a specific TG target. Levels of >500 mg/dL should prompt evaluation for secondary hyperlipidemia, however. Additionally, hypertriglyceridemia joins low HDL among the five clinical criteria for diagnosis of the metabolic syndrome (see page xx).

Lipoprotein(a) [Lp(a)], which is structurally similar to LDL except for the addition of a single apolipoprotein(a) molecule, is a weak independent risk factor for CHD. Although individual studies have yielded conflicting results (23,24,26,27), a meta-analysis of 27 studies with at least 1 year of follow-up data found a 1.6-fold higher risk among those in top third of Lp(a) levels compared with those in the bottom third (26). However, levels are difficult to measure, and various measurement and storage techniques have been used in different studies. Nevertheless, agents are in development with the goal of reducing cardiovascular risk through lowering Lp(a) (83).

ACC/AHA Guidelines

The latest ACC/AHA guidelines marked a dramatic shift in the approach to the treatment of blood cholesterol for the prevention of CVD (14). Whereas prior NCEP guidelines set distinct treatment goals for lipid levels, the latest round of guidelines (now published by the ACC/AHA) acknowledges that the most robust clinical trials did not test strategies of *treatment goals*. That is, they were trials of medication versus placebo, or different doses of medication, and did not test the benefit of titrating doses to lipid levels. Thus, the new guidelines panel revised the overall approach to emphasize appropriate risk stratification and the identification of patient populations who have been shown to benefit from pharmacotherapy for hyperlipidemia (at either standard or high doses). The guidelines continue the primary emphasis on healthy lifestyle habits as the foundation of CVD prevention. They recommend assessment of 10-year cardiovascular risk every 4 to 6 years in patients aged 40 to 75, without known atherosclerotic CVD or diabetes, and with LDL 70 to 189 mg/dL. Like NCEP III, however, they do implicitly consider diabetes a disease equivalent for the purpose of risk stratification. Other high-risk disorders (peripheral vascular disease, symptomatic carotid disease, and abdominal aortic aneurysm) are also included in the recommendations for treatment. For the remainder of patients, a revised risk calculator, using Pooled Cohort Equations (see http://my.americanheart.org/cvriskcalculator and http://www.cardiosource.org/science-andquality/practice-guidelines-and-quality-standards/2013-prevention-guideline-tools.aspx), was developed in place of the Framingham Risk Score to estimate 10-year risk and a cutoff of 7.5% was selected, above which statin therapy should be considered. A summary of the latest ACC/AHA guidelines is shown in **Figure 1.1**.

Drugs

BILE RESINS (E.G., CHOLESTYRAMINE, COLESTIPOL)

These agents lower lipid levels by binding and blocking the reabsorption of bile acids. They typically decrease LDL cholesterol by 15% to 30%, increase HDL by 3% to 5%, and possibly increase TG levels. Compliance is often problematic because of their poor taste and gastrointestinal side effects, such as abdominal fullness, bloating, flatulence, and constipation. Numerous drug interactions also are found, and use is associated with an increased risk of gallstones. In the Lipid Research Clinic Coronary Primary Prevention Trial (29), cholestyramine use in 3,806 men with a mean TC of 291 mg/dL and LDL of 215 mg/dL resulted in 17% fewer MIs and a 19% reduction in CHD death and MI over the 7.4-year follow-up period. However, the all-cause mortality rate was not significantly different. The Familial Atherosclerosis Treatment Study (FATS) (41) and a National Heart, Lung, and Blood Institute Study were angiographic studies that

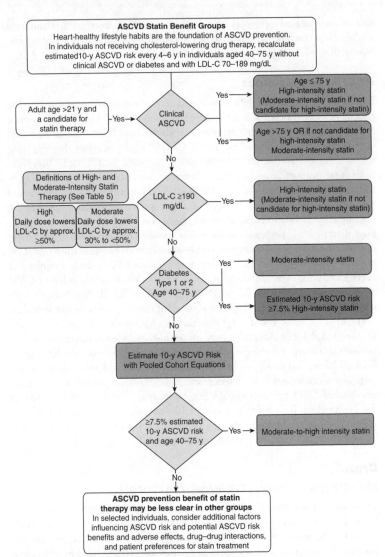

ASCVD Statin Benefit Groups
Heart-healthy lifestyle habits are the foundation of ASCVD prevention.
In individuals not receiving cholesterol-lowering drug therapy, recalculate
estimated 10-y ASCVD risk every 4–6 y in individuals aged 40–75 y without
clinical ASCVD or diabetes and with LDL-C 70–189 mg/dL

Adult age >21 y and a candidate for statin therapy —Yes→ Clinical ASCVD

Yes → Age ≤ 75 y High-intensity statin (Moderate-intensity statin if not candidate for high-intensity statin)

Yes → Age >75 y OR if not candidate for high-intensity statin Moderate-intensity statin

No

Definitions of High- and Moderate-Intensity Statin Therapy (See Table 5)

| High Daily dose lowers LDL-C by approx. ≥50% | Moderate Daily dose lowers LDL-C by approx. 30% to <50% |

LDL-C ≥190 mg/dL —Yes→ High-intensity statin (Moderate-intensity statin if not candidate for high-intensity statin)

No

Diabetes Type 1 or 2 Age 40–75 y

Yes → Moderate-intensity statin

Yes → Estimated 10-y ASCVD risk ≥7.5% High-intensity statin

No

Estimate 10-y ASCVD Risk with Pooled Cohort Equations

≥7.5% estimated 10-y ASCVD risk and age 40–75 y —Yes→ Moderate-to-high intensity statin

No

ASCVD prevention benefit of statin therapy may be less clear in other groups
In selected individuals, consider additional factors influencing ASCVD risk and potential ASCVD risk benefits and adverse effects, drug–drug interactions, and patient preferences for statin treatment

Figure 1.1 • Major recommendations for statin therapy for ASCVD prevention.
(From Stone NJ, et al. 2013 ACC/AHA Guideline on the treatment of blood cholesterol to reduce atherosclerotic cardiovascular risk in adults: a report of the American College of Cardiology/American Heart Association Task Force on Practice Guidelines. *Circulation* 2014;129:S1–S45.)

both showed beneficial lipid-lowering effects and better angiographic outcomes in colestipol-treated patients.

However, while these agents were pivotal in helping to prove the "lipid hypothesis"—that cholesterol was key to cardiovascular events and that lowering cholesterol levels would improve clinical outcomes—they have largely fallen by the wayside in clinical practice, owing to their side effect profile, interactions, and the development of more effective and better-tolerated alternatives.

FIBRIC ACID DERIVATIVES (E.G., GEMFIBROZIL, FENOFIBRATE)

These agents (e.g., gemfibrozil, fenofibrate) typically increase HDL levels by 10% to 15%, decrease TGs by 20% to 50%, and have a minimal effect on LDL levels. They are usually well tolerated. The Helsinki Heart Study (30) evaluated the effect of gemfibrozil in 4,081 asymptomatic hypercholesterolemic men. At 5-year follow-up, gemfibrozil use was associated with 34% fewer cardiac events and a 26% lower CHD mortality rate. However, the overall mortality rate was not significantly different because of more deaths due to accidents, violence, and intracranial hemorrhage in the gemfibrozil group. The Veterans Administration HDL Intervention Trial (VA-HIT), which was a secondary prevention trial of 2,531 patients, found that gemfibrozil was associated with a nonsignificant 10% mortality reduction and 20% reduction in the incidence of CAD-related death and MI (45).

In the 10,000-patient Fenofibrate Intervention and Event Lowering in Diabetes (FIELD) trial, those randomized to fenofibrate (vs. placebo) seemed to have improved clinical outcomes over their counterparts (56). Unfortunately, many more patients in the fenofibrate group than the placebo group initiated statin therapy (see below) during the follow-up period, thus clouding the results. Investigators from the ACCORD (Action to Control Cardiovascular Risk in Diabetes) study group added fenofibrate or placebo to the regimens of 5,518 patients with type 2 diabetes already on simvastatin. At 4.7 years, there was no difference in the primary outcome of cardiovascular death, MI, or stroke. However, based on subgroup analyses, the data do not rule out fenofibrate use for hypertriglyceridemia or low HDL.

CHOLESTEROL ABSORPTION INHIBITORS

This class of agents works by inhibiting the intestinal absorption of dietary and biliary cholesterol by blocking the passage across the intestinal wall. Ezetimibe use results in moderate LDL reduction when used as monotherapy (18% in one study; see *Clin Ther* 2001;23:1209). More important, its effects appear additive to those provided by the statins (35,36). In one randomized study of 769 patients not at LDL goal at baseline, 72% taking ezetimibe and a statin achieved LDL goal compared with 19% taking statin alone. Coadministration is well tolerated (33,40). However, further research into the *clinical* benefits of ezetimibe added to statins is still ongoing. In a study of 720 patients with familial hypercholesterolemia, the Ezetimibe and Simvastatin in Hypercholesterolemia Enhances Atherosclerosis Regression (ENHANCE) investigators randomized the group to 80 mg of simvastatin plus either 10-mg ezetimibe or placebo (37). They found no significant difference in changes to carotid artery intima–media thickness, the primary outcome, as a surrogate for improvement in atherosclerotic disease. The recently completed, landmark IMPROVE-IT trial (39), powered to assess ezetimibe's efficacy for prevention of clinical events when added to a statin, demonstrated significant clinical benefit of the addition of ezetimibe to statin therapy in high-risk patients. The trial broadened the scope of lipid therapies available with evidence for improvement in clinical outcomes.

3-HYDROXY-3-METHYLGLUTARYL-COENZYME A REDUCTASE INHIBITORS (STATINS)

These drugs have, for many years now, served as the foundation of lipid management for the prevention of CVD. They inhibit the rate-limiting step of cholesterol synthesis in the liver and typically decrease LDL by 20% to 60%, increase HDL by 5% to 15%, and decrease TGs by 10% to 20%. All except pravastatin and pitavastatin are metabolized by the cytochrome P450 system. Side effects of the statins are uncommon (occurring in approximately 1% to 2% of patients) and include mild gastrointestinal intolerance, increased liver function test values, and myositis (rare and usually with concurrent niacin, cyclosporine, gemfibrozil, or erythromycin). Historically, titration of statin to a target LDL goal was emphasized; however, this is now in debate. Modern population-based surveys show improvement in control of LDL, but 23% to 33% of statin-treated high-risk patients still have LDL cholesterol > 100 mg/dL, and 74% to 80% have LDL > 70 mg/dL (*J Am Heart Assoc* 2012;1:e0001800).

The major mechanism of statins is to lower LDL levels, and in turn decreased cholesterol content in atherosclerotic lesions, leading to more stable fibrous cap and other plaque stabilization effects (see *Circulation* 2001;103:926). Several additional mechanisms of action beyond lowering LDL ("pleiotropism") are proposed by which these agents achieve significant reductions in CHD and overall mortality:

1. Restoration of endothelium-dependent vasodilatation: A small study found that initiation early after acute coronary syndromes (ACSs) (10.4 ± 0.7 days) rapidly improved endothelial function after 6 weeks of therapy.
2. Inhibition of thrombus formation (see the later section on "Early Statin Initiation Trials").
3. Anti-inflammatory effects: Statins significantly reduce CRP levels.

A meta-analysis of 59 randomized controlled trials found that several classes of lipid agents lower cholesterol, but only the statins significantly reduced CHD-related and all-cause mortality [34% and 25% RR reductions (RRRs), respectively] (60). In another meta-analysis of only statin trials (3), statin-treated patients had a 22% lower overall mortality rate, a 28% lower cardiovascular mortality rate, and 29% fewer strokes. Per 1 mmol/L (39 mg/dL) reduction in on-treatment LDL, statins reduce cardiovascular events by 20% (61); this relative risk reduction is even greater in patients at low risk of coronary events (62).

Another analysis found that the effect of these agents widens with time; mortality is 7% in the first 2 years and 25% by 5 years on treatment.

Additional, in-depth analysis of the PROVE IT-TIMI 22 trial (see below) highlighted many potential pleiotropic phenomena observed specifically in patients with ACSs and frequently independent of the cholesterol-lowering effect (64). These include effects on endothelial activation/function, mitigation of the coagulation cascade, and favorable effects on markers of inflammation.

Primary Prevention Trials

The West of Scotland Coronary Prevention Study (WOSCOPS) (31) was a randomized, placebo-controlled trial of 6,595 patients with an average TC of 272 mg/dL. At 5 years, the pravastatin group had 29% fewer nonfatal MIs ($p < 0.001$), a 32% lower cardiovascular mortality rate ($p = 0.033$), and a 22% lower overall mortality rate ($p = 0.051$). The atorvastatin versus placebo arm of the Anglo-Scandinavian Cardiac Outcomes Trial (ASCOT) (10,305 patients) was stopped in October 2002 because the atorvastatin group had a significant 36% reduction in nonfatal MI and fatal CHD compared with those with placebo (1.9% vs. 3.0%, $p = 0.0005$) (33).

More contemporary primary prevention trials include the Collaborative AtoRvastatin Diabetes Study (CARDS) (32), which enrolled 2,838 patients with type 2 diabetes mellitus, but no previously documented CVD; they were randomized to either atorvastatin 10 mg daily or placebo. The trial was stopped early after a 37% relative risk reduction for the primary end point of ACS, coronary revascularization, or stroke was demonstrated in the intervention group. Additionally, one of the latest primary prevention trials to open a new door for primary prevention of atherosclerosis is the Justification for the Use of Statins in Prevention: an Intervention Trial Evaluating Rosuvastatin (JUPITER) study (34). The JUPITER investigators randomly assigned nearly 18,000 apparently healthy adults with LDL cholesterol levels of <130 mg/dL and high-sensitivity CRP of 2.0 mg/L or higher to rosuvastatin 20 mg daily or placebo. They demonstrated an impressive 44% reduction in cardiovascular events with rosuvastatin versus placebo ($p < 0.00001$), highlighting another potential risk stratification step for patients without documented CVD: the use of CRP.

Additionally, several primary prevention studies have been done to look at atherosclerotic burden in patients taking statins, using vascular ultrasound [either carotid or coronary intravascular ultrasound (IVUS)] to assess primary end points. Both the ASTEROID study (a study to evaluate the effect of rosuvastatin on IVUS-derived coronary atheroma burden) (JAMA 2006;295: 1556–1565) and the METEOR trial (measuring effects on intima–media thickness: an evaluation of rosuvastatin) (JAMA 2007;297:1344–1353) assessed plaque burdens in patients taking rosuvastatin. Both demonstrated decreased plaque burden in the respective vascular sites, and the ASTEROID trial even demonstrated regression of such disease with the use of high-dose rosuvastatin, indicating that the improvements in cardiovascular events are accompanied by improvements in measured atherosclerosis.

Secondary Prevention Trials

The Scandinavian Simvastatin Survival Study (4S) (42) was a randomized, placebo-controlled trial enrolling 4,444 patients with an elevated TC (≥213 mg/dL) and a history of CAD. At 5.4-year follow-up, the use of simvastatin, 40 mg/day, was associated with a 25% lower TC, a 35% lower LDL, a 42% lower CHD mortality rate, and a highly significant 30% relative reduction in lower overall mortality rate ($p = 0.0003$). Simvastatin patients also underwent 34% fewer coronary revascularization procedures and had fewer fatal and nonfatal cerebrovascular events.

The Cholesterol and Recurrent Events (CARE) trial (43) examined the use of pravastatin (40 mg/day) in patients with normal or mildly elevated TC (<240 mg/dL). At 5 years, pravastatin was associated with 24% fewer cardiac deaths and nonfatal MIs ($p = 0.003$). If the baseline LDL level was <125 mg/dL, only diabetic patients had a significant benefit.

The Long-term Intervention with Pravastatin in Ischemic Disease (LIPID) trial (44) enrolled more than 9,000 patients with known CAD and average TC levels (155 to 271 mg/dL). Pravastatin (40 mg/day) was associated with a 24% RRR in CHD mortality ($p < 0.001$), 22% RRR in overall mortality rate ($p < 0.001$), 19% RRR in strokes ($p = 0.048$), and 20% RRR in revascularization procedures ($p < 0.001$). Thus, both the LIPID and CARE trials provide compelling data to support aggressive lipid lowering with statins in CAD patients with normal TC levels.

Two of the largest, contemporary, secondary prevention trials are the TNT (Treating to New Targets) and the IDEAL (Incremental Decrease in End Points Through Aggressive Lipid Lowering) trials (51,52). Both enrolled patients with stable CAD (10,001 in TNT; 8,888 in IDEAL), randomized them to high- or standard-dose statins (10- vs. 80-mg atorvastatin in TNT, 20-mg simvastatin vs. 80-mg atorvastatin in IDEAL), and followed them for roughly 5 years for clinical end points. The TNT trial resulted in a 2.2% absolute reduction ($p < 0.001$) in the primary outcome (composite of cardiovascular death, nonfatal MI, resuscitation from cardiac arrest, or any stroke). In the IDEAL trial, patients in the high-dose statin group (atorvastatin 80 mg) did experience fewer primary end point events (coronary death, nonfatal MI, or cardiac arrest resuscitation), but the hazard ratio of 0.89 for the high-dose group did not meet statistical significance ($p = 0.07$). However, when measured based on the end points of any number of similar trials, including TNT, the IDEAL results prove consistent with the clinical benefit.

Additional trials of medical therapy, compared to invasive procedures for secondary prevention, are described in detail in Chapter 2.

Combined Primary and Secondary Prevention Trials

In the HPS (54), which randomized 20,536 patients with CAD, diabetes, or other occlusive arterial disease to simvastatin, 40 mg/day, or placebo, the statin group had a significantly lower all-cause mortality (12.9% vs. 14.7%; $p = 0.003$). Significant benefit also was observed among those with an initial LDL <3 mmol (116 mg/dL).

In the PROspective Study of Pravastatin in the Elderly at Risk (PROSPER) study, 5,804 patients aged 70 to 82 years with vascular disease or risk factors were randomized to pravastatin, 40 mg/day, or placebo, and the pravastatin group had a 24% relative reduction in CHD death. This large study provides strong evidence that the benefits associated with statin therapy extend to older patients.

Early Statin Initiation Trials

Several studies have examined the early initiation of statins after acute coronary events. In the Myocardial Ischemia Reduction with Aggressive Cholesterol Lowering (MIRACL) study (50), 3,086 patients with unstable angina or non–ST elevation MI (UA/NSTEMI) were enrolled, and atorvastatin, 80 mg/day, was found to have a significant 15% relative reduction in the composite primary end point compared with placebo, primarily because of fewer recurrent ischemic events (14.8% vs. 17.4%; $p = 0.048$). This benefit occurred regardless of LDL level or the percentage by which LDL was lowered, suggesting the presence of non–lipid-lowering, pleiotropic effects.

The PROVE IT-TIMI 22 trial randomized 4,162 patients hospitalized for ACS to either 40 mg of pravastatin daily ("standard" therapy) or 80 mg of atorvastatin daily ("intensive" therapy), with the primary end point being a composite of death, MI, rehospitalization for unstable angina, revascularization, or stroke at a mean follow-up of 24 months (51). After 2 years of mean follow-up, 26.3% of patients in the standard therapy group experienced an event versus 22.4% in the intensive therapy, a significant 16% reduction in the hazard ratio in favor of intensive therapy in patients hospitalized for ACS ($p = 0.005$). This benefit appeared to emerge within 30 days.

In the "Z" phase of the Aggrastat to Zocor (A to Z) trial, 4,497 patients with ACS were randomized to simvastatin 40 mg daily for 1 month and then 80 mg daily ("early high-dose" group) versus placebo for 4 months and then 20-mg simvastatin ("late standard dosing") (52). They were followed for up to 24 months for the development of a composite primary end point of cardiovascular death, nonfatal MI, readmission for ACS, or stroke. Despite a 2.3% absolute risk reduction in the primary end point favoring the early high-dose group, this result did not meet statistical significance ($p = 0.14$), though the overall trends in the trial confirmed the findings of other studies, such as PROVE IT-TIMI 22 and TNT. When these two trials are combined with the results from TNT and IDEAL (see *J Am Coll Cardiol* 2006;48:438–445), the evidence for intensive lipid-lowering therapy in patients with CAD is robust. Initiation of statin therapy before hospital discharge, in addition to providing probable non–lipid-lowering benefits, results in higher use rates. In the Cardiac Hospitalization Atherosclerosis Management Program (CHAMP) study, statin use increased from 6% to 86% when started in the hospital, and 58% reached their LDL goal (<100 mg/dL) versus 6% (see *Am J Cardiol* 2001;87:219).

Though some have raised concerns that statin versus placebo and also high-dose statin versus standard-dose statin therapy increase risk of new-onset diabetes mellitus, several meta-analyses have noted that the risk–benefit ratio continues to favor intensive lipid lowering in secondary prevention; over a year of treatment, approximately three vascular events are prevented for each new case of diabetes mellitus (68).

RAISING HDL CHOLESTEROL
Niacin

Niacin is a B vitamin that inhibits the mobilization of free FAs from peripheral tissues, with a resulting decrease in hepatic synthesis of TGs and secretion of very low density lipoproteins (VLDLs). Niacin typically decreases LDL by 10% to 25%, increases HDL by 15% to 35%, decreases TGs by 20% to 50%, and decreases Lp(a). A common side effect is flushing, which is often controllable by daily ASA use. A long-acting formulation of niacin and a combination pill including the prostaglandin D2 receptor inhibitor laropiprant both appear to reduce flushing. Other side effects of niacin include hyperglycemia, increased uric acid levels, increased liver function tests, exacerbation of peptic ulcer disease, and rhabdomyolysis (rare). In the historic Coronary Drug Project (40), a randomized trial enrolling more than 8,000 men with prior MI, the use of niacin, 3 g/day, was associated with a 27% lower nonfatal MI rate at 5-year follow-up and a significant 11% reduction in overall mortality at 15 years. Other trials evaluating the use of niacin in combination with other agents [e.g., CLAS, FATS, HDL-Atherosclerosis Treatment Study (HATS) (41,46)] also showed significant favorable changes in lipid levels and reduced rates of CHD mortality.

However, in two large recent randomized double-blind, placebo-controlled trials involving statin-treated patients, both extended-release niacin and a niacin–lapropitant combination pill have failed to reduce cardiovascular mortality. The Atherothrombosis Intervention in Metabolic Syndrome with Low HDL/High Triglycerides: Impact on Global Health Outcomes (AIM-HIGH) study (70) randomized 3,414 patients with known stable vascular disease to extended-release niacin, 1,500 to 2,000 mg/day, or matching placebo containing 50-mg niacin to induce flushing and conceal treatment class. Despite favorable changes in lipid profile, the use of niacin did not reduce the incidence of clinical events; at 3-year follow-up, 16.4% of patients randomized to niacin had a cardiovascular event, compared to 16.2% of patients randomized to placebo.

Similarly, in the randomized, placebo-controlled Treatment of HDL to Reduce the Incidence of Vascular Events (HPS2-THRIVE) study (71) involving 42,424 statin-treated patients with stable vascular disease, treatment with an extended-release niacin–lapropitant combination pill failed to reduce major vascular events at 3.9-year follow-up. The trial was terminated prematurely due to an excess of adverse events and treatment discontinuation in the niacin–lapropitant group. Though neither trial showed a reduction in cardiovascular events, some have argued that both trials enrolled patients with LDL already lowered, in whom niacin would not necessarily have been indicated, and still see a role for niacin in statin-intolerant patients (see *N Engl J Med* 2011;365:2318–2330 and *J Am Coll Cardiol* 2012;59:2058–2064). Others have argued that the beneficial effects of niacin may be confined to patients with low HDL and high triglycerides. Regardless, these two trials, together enrolling over 45,000 patients, indicate that extended-release niacin probably does not have a role in the routine management of patients already treated with statins.

Cholesterol Ester Transfer Protein Inhibitors

Low HDL cholesterol remains a risk factor for CVD, and alternative therapies targeted to raising HDL have been aggressively pursued. One class has been the cholesterol ester transfer protein (CETP) inhibitors, which have been demonstrated to significantly raise HDL levels. The first agent to make it to phase three trials, torcetrapib, was abandoned when these trials demonstrated increased mortality in the active treatment arm (75,76); the putative mechanism was the drug's tendency to increase BP significantly, through mechanisms not well understood. Dalcetrapib is another CETP inhibitor that also increased HDL levels but did not significantly increase blood pressure in preclinical testing. However, in dal-OUTCOMES (77), a randomized, double-blind, placebo-controlled trial enrolling 15,871 statin-treated patients within 6 months after ACS, dalcetrapib, 600 mg/day, did not reduce the incidence of a composite of major vascular events or cardiac death, despite a 31% to 40% on-treatment increase in HDL and no substantial effect on blood pressure. Despite the failure of dalcetrapib and torcetrapib to reduce cardiovascular events, development of anacetrapib and evacetrapib continues. In phase II trials, these agents have been demonstrated to raise HDL levels with greater potency than dalcetrapib while also producing substantial decreases in LDL (78,79). Their effect on clinical end points remains to be determined.

DIET AND VITAMINS

The nutrient composition of the therapeutic lifestyle changes diet includes the following: saturated fat, 5% to 6% of total calories; total fat, 25% to 35% of calories; fiber, 20 to 30 g/day; and cholesterol, <200 mg/day. Fiber has minimal impact on cholesterol, and approximately 25% of compliant patients have no response; the average response is a reduction in TC of only 10% to 15%.

In the Cambridge Heart Antioxidant Study (CHAOS) (91), a randomized study of 2,002 CAD patients, vitamin E supplementation was associated with a significantly lower incidence of cardiovascular death and MI. However, in further studies, investigators found no benefit associated with vitamin E supplementation (92,93), and a meta-analysis of high-dose supplementation demonstrated *increased* mortality in those taking vitamin E (105).

Special Diets

1. Fish and omega-3 fatty acid (FA) consumption: In a study of 852 Dutch men, the mortality rate was more than 50% lower among those consuming over 30 g of fish per day (the equivalent of one or two servings per week). In the 2,033-patient randomized Diet and Reinfarction trial, the group advised to increase omega-3 fatty acid intake via fish consumption or fish oil supplementation had a 29% lower mortality compared to a no-advice control group. In the 11,324-patient GISSI-Prevenzione trial, supplementation with 850 mg of omega-3 fatty acid decreased sudden death by 45% and all-cause mortality by

20%, even in those receiving standard therapy [e.g., aspirin (ASA), statins]. Evidence also exists that increased fish intake results in a reduced risk of ischemic stroke (see JAMA 2002;288:3130). Several subsequent studies have supported the use of polyunsaturated fatty acid (PUFA) supplementation, however to a varying degree (101–103,107).

Based on these and other data, the American Heart Association (AHA) issued recommendations that persons with documented CHD should consume about 1 g of omega-3 fatty acids per day (109). In those unable to eat sufficient amounts of fish to meet this requirement, it recommends daily supplementation with 1-g fish oil capsules that contain 180 mg of eicosapentaenoic acid and 120 mg of docosahexaenoic acid. In individuals with high TG levels, higher amounts (2 to 4 g/day) should be considered. However, a 2012 systematic review of the data on long- and short-chain omega-3 fatty acid supplementation failed to identify a benefit in mortality or CVD (107), noting that the positive results of early studies have not been replicated by several large modern randomized controlled trials.

2. High fiber: An analysis of 21,930 patients showed the risk of CHD death to be inversely related to fiber intake, with the quintile of subjects consuming the most fiber (34.8 g/day) having a 31% reduction in their risk of CHD death compared to the quintile consuming the least fiber (16.1 g/day) (111). A Nurses' Health Study (NHS) analysis also found a significant association between fiber intake and CHD events. A 10-g/day increase in daily fiber intake was associated with a multivariate RR for CHD events of 0.81 [95% confidence interval (CI), 0.66 to 0.99]. This benefit has not been demonstrated with fiber supplementation, or in clinical trials where subjects were instructed to increase their fiber intake.

3. Mediterranean (includes more bread, fruit, and margarine and less meat, butter, and cream): The randomized 605-patient Lyon Heart Study investigated the Mediterranean diet in secondary prevention, finding a 73% reduction in death and MI at 2.3-year follow-up and a significant 56% all-cause mortality reduction at 3.8-year follow-up (114). More recently, a large, randomized controlled trial found a significant benefit of the Mediterranean diet in a high-risk primary prevention population: the 7,447-patient Primary Prevention of Cardiovascular Disease with a Mediterranean Diet (PREDIMED) demonstrated a 30% relative risk reduction in major adverse cardiac events with a Mediterranean diet supplemented with either nuts or extra-virgin olive oil (117).

Continuing research into the effects of various diets on weight loss and CVD has yielded varied results. However, there have been some clear messages. The 2005 OmniHeart randomized trial tested three diets low in saturated fat, but enhanced with (a) carbohydrates, (b) protein, or (c) monounsaturated fat (115). While all three diets demonstrated improved blood pressure (BP) and LDL cholesterol compared to baseline, both the diets enriched in protein and the one enriched with monounsaturated fat demonstrated further improvement of such markers. In their 2005 comparison of four "fad" diets (the Atkins, Ornish, Weight Watchers, and Zone diets), Dansinger et al. found that all four could favorably affect weight and cardiometabolic risk factors—provided patients were able to stick with them long enough (116). In a secondary, observational, analysis of 31,546 patients enrolled in modern secondary prevention trials, subjects eating a healthier diet were at lower risk of major adverse cardiac events than were those eating a less healthy diet (113). The bottom line has been that diet *can* affect weight and cardiovascular health—and it is more important to find a diet that the patient can stick with than to pick and choose the right ingredients. However, with the data from the PREDIMED trial, the Mediterranean diet is now the one proven for cardiovascular prevention.

Alcohol

Several observational studies have shown that moderate alcohol consumption (e.g., one to two drinks per day) is associated with a significantly lower rate of CHD and overall mortality (118,119). A Physicians' Health Study (PHS) analysis reported adjusted relative mortality risks of 0.79 and 0.84 in those consuming one and two drinks per day, respectively. Another study of 38,000 male health professionals found that consumption of alcohol at least 3 to 4 days per week was associated with a >30% lower rate of MI (119); neither the type of beverage nor the proportion consumed with meals substantially altered this association.

Mechanisms for the benefits of alcohol appear to include increased HDL levels, antiplatelet effects, and improved insulin resistance. Because of the significant health risks associated with more substantial alcohol consumption, many physicians hesitate to recommend alcohol consumption as a means to reduce cardiovascular risk. Indeed, several reports have actually demonstrated that binge drinking impairs endothelial function (see *J Am Coll Cardiol* 2013;62: 201–207). AHA Nutrition Committee recommendations acknowledge the data supporting alcohol's protective effects; however, they do not recommend alcohol solely for CVD prevention. Instead, they recommend that the risks and benefits be weighed, and support its consumption at a maximum of two drinks per day for men and one drink daily for women (see *Circulation* 2006;114:82–96).

LIFESTYLE FACTORS

Obesity

Approximately two in three US adults are overweight or obese (133), compared with one in four in the early 1960s. Another measure, BMI (weight/body surface area), is often used (desirable, 18.0 to 24.9 kg/m²; overweight, 25 to 30 kg/m²; obese, >30 kg/m²); however, its shortcomings have also been identified—it can be difficult to distinguish adipose obesity from lean muscle mass (see *Eur Heart J* 2007;28:2087–2093).

Several studies have shown that obesity reduces life expectancy markedly, especially among younger adults (134,135). Nearly 300,000 deaths per year have been attributed to obesity, and it is the leading preventable cause of morbidity and mortality in the United States. Data from the National Health Service (NHS) show that even modest weight gains over a period of 18 years result in significantly higher risks of CHD death and nonfatal MI; RRs ranged from 1.25 for a 5- to 7.9-kg gain to 2.65 for a 20-kg gain (131). Prospective but nonrandomized data have demonstrated that durable weight loss brought about by bariatric surgery is significantly associated with reductions in overall mortality, cardiovascular events, and cardiovascular mortality (138,140). Several new trials have shown the effects of multifaceted lifestyle interventions (e.g., Look AHEAD, 174), and new medications have been studied and approved, including lorcaserin, phentermine/topiramate, and naltrexone/bupropion (141–143).

Exercise

Favorable effects associated with exercise include weight loss and favorable alteration of lipoprotein profiles, especially HDL levels (see *N Engl J Med* 2002;347:1483). Observational studies have shown that individuals with low fitness levels have a 25% to 100% increased mortality risk. One meta-analysis showed a nearly twofold risk of CHD death among individuals in sedentary (vs. active) occupations.

Studies have shown increasing benefit with increasing intensity and frequency of exercise. An analysis of MRFIT subjects showed a 27% lower CAD mortality rate among subjects with moderate versus less-active physical activity (144). Another study found that running (aerobic) was better than lifting weights (typically more anaerobic) (150). However, in a study of endothelium function following exercise in patients with recent MI, all forms of exercise resulted in favorable changes (aerobic, resistance, resistance plus aerobic). Of note, these changes disappeared with cessation of training at 1 month (see *Circulation* 2009;119:1601–1608).

Although high-intensity, aerobic exercise appears to be best, doing less is better than no activity, as evidenced in one study of over 40,000 postmenopausal Iowa women that found substantial benefits associated with walking (148). An NHS analysis of more than 72,000 women found brisk walking (more than 3 hours a week) associated with a 35% reduction in coronary events (149). Walking also reduces body weight and body fat (see *JAMA* 2003;289:323). Contemporary data have even demonstrated that regular exercise, even *without* significant weight loss, still can reduce cardiovascular risk (see *Arch Intern Med* 2008;168:884–890). In a meta-analysis, 150 hours per week of moderate exercise reduced the incidence of CAD by 14% (151).

Formal exercise testing can also provide a more accurate risk assessment. In the Lipid Research Clinics Mortality Follow-up Study, the least-fit quartile on a standard treadmill test had a greater than eightfold risk of CAD mortality compared with the fittest quartile. In another study of 6,213 men, peak exercise capacity was the strongest predictor of death in those with and without CVD [every 1 metabolic equivalent of the task (MET) increase correlated with a 12% improvement in survival].

Other studies have shown that exertion can be a trigger of acute MI, with a markedly increased RR of MI (>100 times) in the 1 hour after heavy exertion in those who exercise infrequently (no more than once per week) (145,146); however, a more recent analysis of high- and moderate-intensity exercise in cardiac rehabilitation centers failed to demonstrate an excess of cardiovascular events with supervised high-intensity exercise (147). Thus, although exercise is protective, the initiation of any exercise program should generally be preceded by evaluation or consultation with a physician and initiated gradually, ideally in a controlled setting.

Smoking

Current smoking is associated with an approximately threefold increased risk of MI and an approximately twofold increased risk of CHD-related death (153–157). Smoking in combination with another major cardiac risk factor [e.g., hypertension (HTN), diabetes, hypercholesterolemia] results in an approximately 20-fold increase in death and MI (153). Among those who quit smoking, the risk gradually returns to baseline after several years (154), whereas resumption of smoking after quitting following ACS increases 1-year mortality threefold. Passive or secondhand smoke exposure results in an average 20% to 25% increase in CHD mortality (156–158), and frequent or heavy exposure can result in a nearly twofold increased risk (see *Circulation* 1997;95:2374–2379). In fact, several follow-up studies of smoking bans implemented in public areas have identified measurable declines in coronary disease incidence in these areas (159,160). Financial incentives have also been found to be effective in some scenarios, for assistance in smoking cessation (see also *N Engl J Med* 2009;360:699–709).

Additional pharmacologic therapies to aid in smoking cessation continue to be developed. In addition to the use of well-known antidepressant, bupropion, as a smoking cessation aid, a newer agent, varenicline, has proved even more effective (161). An alpha-4beta-2 nicotinic acetylcholine receptor partial agonist, varenicline is approved to aid in smoking cessation and many have found it very effective. Importantly, varenicline also appears safe in patients with known CVD (162).

METABOLIC SYNDROME

This disorder has received increasing attention and was recognized as a major problem in the NCEP III report. The syndrome is defined as the presence of three or more of the following: (a) abdominal obesity (waist circumference more than 40 inches in men and more than 35 inches in women); (b) TGs, 150 mg/dL or more; (c) HDL, <40 mg/dL (men) or <50 mg/dL (women) (or on pharmacologic treatment for hypertriglyceridemia); (d) systolic BP more than 129 or diastolic BP more than 84 mm Hg (or on pharmacologic treatment for HTN); and (e) fasting glucose more than 99 mg/dL (or on pharmacologic treatment for elevated glucose). In the National Health and Nutrition Examination Survey (NHANES) III survey, the prevalence of the metabolic syndrome was more than 20% (168); this has increased to 34% in NHANES 2003 to 2006 data (see *Circulation* 2013;127(1):e6–e245). A Finnish study found those with the syndrome had a three- to fourfold increased risk of CHD death, (169) but other studies have shown that patients with metabolic syndrome, in the absence of diabetes, did not appear to have an increased risk (170). A recent meta-analysis of 87 studies found that the metabolic syndrome was associated with significant 2.35- and 1.58-fold increased risks of CVD and all-cause mortality, respectively, (172) but it was unclear whether the metabolic syndrome carried risk in excess of its component metabolic derangements.

DIABETES

The Centers for Disease Control and Prevention estimate that 18.8 million individuals in the United States have diagnosed diabetes mellitus and an additional 7 million are undiagnosed in 2010; more than 95% have type 2 diabetes mellitus, formerly known as non–insulin-dependent diabetes mellitus. Additionally, the organization estimates that as many as 79 million Americans may have prediabetes, a state of glucose intolerance thought to precede the development of diabetes. The significant decline in CHD mortality seen in the general population in the last several decades did not occur in diabetes (164), and 77% of US hospital stays for diabetics are attributable to CVD. Type 2 diabetes is associated with approximately two- and threefold increased risks of CHD death in men and women, respectively. The risks of death from MI and CHD are as high in diabetics without prior MIs as in nondiabetics with prior MIs (163,165), though newer data have suggested that only patients with long-standing diabetes truly have the same risk of future MI as do patients with known CHD. Though guidelines consider diabetes a CHD risk equivalent and formerly recommended that all diabetics older than 30 years take ASA (≥81 mg daily), newer guidelines only recommend the use of aspirin in diabetics with a 10-year risk of CHD of at least 10%. Diabetics also have an approximately twofold increased risk of stroke.

Patients with diabetes frequently have other modifiable risk factors, including HTN and obesity. Addressing these risk factors [e.g., by exercise, dietary modification, or pharmacologic agent(s)] is essential to reducing an individual's cardiac risk. Prior studies have indicated that BP control significantly reduces the incidence of both macrovascular and microvascular (e.g., retinopathy) complications (215); the most recent Joint National Committee (JNC) 8 Guidelines recommend <140/90 mm Hg. Of note, the ACCORD trial found no benefit of targeting a systolic BP < 120 mm Hg as compared with the more standard approach of <140 mm Hg (220), but did demonstrate a surfeit of excess risk. A subsequent meta-analysis of five randomized controlled trials demonstrated similar findings (221).

Intensive glycemic control of individuals with type 1 diabetes in the Diabetes Control and Complications Trial (DCCT) resulted in a 34% reduction in LDL levels and a 41% reduction in major cardiovascular and peripheral vascular events (see *N Engl J Med* 1993;329:977). However, the ACCORD and ADVANCE (Action in Diabetes and Vascular Disease: Preterax and Diamicron Modified Release Controlled Evaluation) trials tested the hypothesis that strict glycemic control could improve clinical cardiovascular outcomes.

ACCORD (175) randomized 10,251 patients with type 2 diabetes to either standard therapy targeting a hemoglobin A1c (HbA1c) of 7% to 7.9% or intensive therapy, targeting A1c <6%. The trial was discontinued prematurely when an excess rate of death was identified in the intensive glycemic control arm after a mean of 3.5 years of follow-up. At 5-year follow-up, excess death in the intensive therapy group persisted despite relaxation of this group's glycemic control. The ADVANCE trial (176) randomized 11,140 patients with type 2 diabetes to either standard care or intensive glycemic control (goal A1c, <6.5%) and followed for a mean of 5 years for both macrovascular and microvascular cardiovascular outcomes. While the trial met its primary end point (a composite of macro- and microvascular events), this was predominantly driven by a decreased incidence of nephropathy, without statistically significant effects on major adverse cardiovascular events (MACE) (death, MI, stroke, heart failure). The ORIGIN trial (179), which randomized 12,537 patients with diabetes or prediabetes and a high risk of cardiovascular events to insulin provision or placebo, also failed to demonstrate a reduction in cardiovascular events, despite succeeding in reducing fasting glucose to <95 mg/dL. Clinical trials involving other new oral antidiabetic agents (rosiglitazone, saxagliptin, alogliptin) also have failed to demonstrate reductions in cardiovascular events, though these agents do appear to be safe in patients with CHD.

Subsequent analyses of ACCORD and ADVANCE demonstrated a significant excess risk of hypoglycemia in the strict control groups and a significantly increased risk of major cardiovascular events in those patients with hypoglycemic events. Though a causal link between hypoglycemia and cardiovascular events in patients targeted for intensive glycemic control has not been proven, this remains a leading hypothesis (180). It is unclear whether using agents with less risk of causing hypoglycemia (specifically, metformin) would have changed the results of ACCORD and ADVANCE.

In the STENO-2 study, comprehensive intensive therapy, consisting of behavioral modification and drug therapy, which targeted all the previously mentioned areas (hyperglycemia, HTN, dyslipidemia, microalbuminuria), reduced the risk of cardiovascular and microvascular events by about 50% compared with conventional therapy (173). This small study emphasizes the benefits of comprehensive risk factor modification in diabetic patients. The 5,154-patient Look AHEAD trial (174) randomized overweight or obese patients with type 2 diabetes to usual care along with an intensive lifestyle intervention promoting weight loss or to usual care alone, which included evidence-based drug therapy. Subjects were followed for a median of 9.6 years for a composite outcome of death from cardiovascular causes or major cardiovascular events. Despite greater weight loss and improvement in cardiac risk factors in the intensive intervention group (at both 1-year follow-up and study end), there was no difference in cardiovascular events between the two groups. Though this intervention aimed at weight loss failed to improve mortality, it did improve surrogate end points, and does not challenge STENO-2's conclusions that intensive risk factor modification (including drug therapy) can reduce mortality.

HYPERTENSION

Epidemiology

Approximately 78 million Americans have hypertension, and an additional 60 to 70 million have prehypertension. Hypertension occurs in the absence of other cardiac risk factors in 20%. From ages 30 to 65 years, systolic blood pressure (SBP) and diastolic blood pressure (DBP) increase by approximately 20 and 10 mm Hg, respectively. According to the American Heart Association's 2014 statistical update (1), 75% of adults with hypertension receive treatment, but only 53% of those receiving treatment (or roughly 40% of all adults with HTN) have adequate control, and nearly 20% remain unaware of their hypertension. Still, awareness of hypertension and control have generally improved over time; a Framingham Heart Study analysis (187) showing the age-adjusted prevalence of stage 2 HTN (SBP ≥ 160 mm Hg or DBP ≥ 100 mm Hg) declined significantly from 1950 to 1989 (men, 18.5% to 9.2%; women, 28.0% to 7.7%), largely due to more frequent treatment of these patients with antihypertensive agents. However, another Framingham analysis found that the lifetime risk of developing hypertension is 90% or higher (188), and one in eight patients with hypertension has resistant hypertension (BP above goal despite 3 or more antihypertensive medications), according to a 2013 study (186). However, even the diagnosis of prehypertension (SBP, 120 to 140; or DBP, 80 to 90) carries a 36% increased risk of CAD (233).

Etiology

Approximately 90% to 95% of cases have no known cause (essential hypertension). Secondary causes include renal parenchymal disease (2% to 5%), renovascular hypertension (approximately 1%), primary aldosteronism (adrenal adenoma, 60%; bilateral hyperplasia, 40%), Cushing syndrome, pheochromocytoma, coarctation of aorta, numerous drugs [e.g., glucocorticoids, anabolic steroids, nonsteroidal anti-inflammatory drugs (NSAIDs) (227), alcohol, oral contraceptives, cocaine, cyclosporine, sympathomimetics, tricyclic antidepressants, and amphetamines], hyperparathyroidism, and acromegaly.

Diagnosis

Unless BP is markedly elevated, it should be measured on three separate occasions before initiating therapy. Previously, the Joint National Committee (JNC 7) classification staged hypertension as follows (183):

- Prehypertension: SBP, 120 to 139 mm Hg; DBP, 80 to 89 mm Hg
- Stage I hypertension: SBP, 140 to 159 mm Hg; DBP, 90 to 99 mm Hg
- Stage II: SBP ≥ 160 mm Hg; DBP ≥ 100 mm Hg

However, in the most recent JNC 8 (184), targets are more discretely defined, without categories, and more consistent across populations, as guided by the evidence (or lack thereof; **Fig. 1.2**).

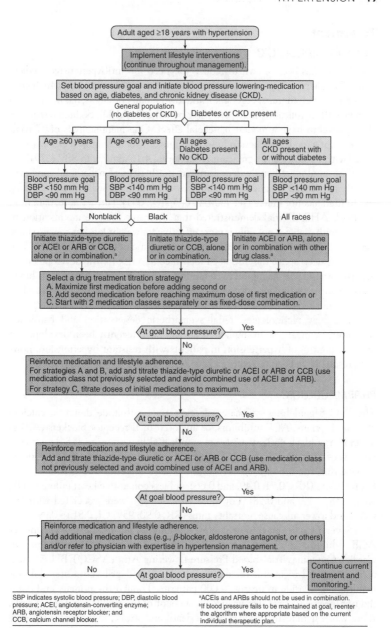

Figure 1.2 • 2014 hypertension guideline management algorithm. (From James PA, et al. 2014 evidence-based guideline for the management of high blood pressure in adults: report from the panel members appointed to the Eighth Joint National Committee (JNC 8). JAMA 2014;311(5):507–520.)

Treatment

NONPHARMACOLOGIC

Weight loss has been shown to reduce the need for antihypertensive medications. The Dietary Approaches to Stop Hypertension (DASH) diet, which consists of a diet rich in fruits, vegetables, and low-fat dairy products, has been shown to reduce BP significantly in hypertensive patients (189,190). Sodium restriction also appears to have a modest beneficial effect. One meta-analysis of 37 trials showed that a modest reduction in sodium intake over at least 4 weeks was associated with a statistically significant reduction of 4.18 mm Hg in SBP (229).

One randomized study demonstrated the benefit of behavioral modification that included weight loss, sodium reduction, increased physical activity, and limited alcohol intake (see *JAMA* 2003;289:2083). Furthermore, data from the Look AHEAD trial demonstrated that intensive lifestyle modification in patients with diabetes not only is more effective for weight loss but can also have significant impact on cardiovascular risk markers, including lipids and BP (174). Untreated sleep apnea has also been identified as a risk for the development of hypertension (191), but studies attempting to demonstrate reduction in blood pressure with continuous positive airway pressure (CPAP) treatment have had mixed results (192,193).

Two new technologies, renal sympathetic denervation and baroreflex activation by means of an implanted device, have recently been developed to improve control of hypertension in patients with resistant hypertension; however, results have been mixed (225,226).

PHARMACOLOGIC

The JNC 8 guidelines advocate selecting among thiazide diuretics, calcium channel blockers, ACE inhibitors, or angiotensin II receptor blockers (ARBs) for most nonblack patients with uncomplicated hypertension (184). A meta-analysis of 18 randomized trials enrolling a total of more than 48,000 patients showed that the use of β-blockers and low-dose diuretics was associated with fewer strokes (RRs, 0.71, 0.49, and 0.66) and less congestive heart failure (CHF; RRs, 0.58, 0.17, and 0.58). Low-dose diuretics also were associated with less CAD and lower all-cause mortality rates (RR, 0.90; 95% CI, 0.81 to 0.99).

Several studies have now compared diuretics and β-blockers with newer ACE inhibitors and calcium channel blockers. The Anglo-Scandinavian Cardiac Outcomes Trial-Blood Pressure Lowering Arm (ASCOT-BPLA) megatrial compared regiments of amlodipine plus perindopril versus atenolol plus bendroflumethiazide in nearly 20,000 patients. Though the primary end point did not meet statistical significance on account of the trial being stopped early, there was a significantly higher rate of death and stroke, individually, favoring the amlodipine arm (196). Additional analyses did not find this effect mitigated by tachycardia (see *J Am Coll Cardiol* 2009;54:1154–1161).

The Avoiding Cardiovascular Events through Combination Therapy in Patients Living with Systolic Hypertension (ACCOMPLISH) trial randomized

11,506 patients with hypertension and at high risk for cardiovascular events to either benazepril plus amlodipine or benazepril plus hydrochlorothiazide (197). The primary end point was the composite of death from cardiovascular causes, nonfatal MI, nonfatal stroke, hospitalization for angina, resuscitation after sudden cardiac arrest, or coronary revascularization. The trial was stopped prematurely, after a mean follow-up of 36 months, when a significant absolute reduction in the primary end point of 2.2% was observed (relative risk 19.6%) favoring the ACE inhibitor and calcium channel blocker combination.

In order to test the hypothesis of dual renin–angiotensin–aldosterone system blockade, investigators for the ONTARGET trial randomized over 25,000 high-risk patients to ramipril, telmisartan, or both (206). While there was no benefit to dual therapy for the primary end point of cardiovascular death, MI, stroke, or CHF hospitalization, there was a significant excess of adverse events in the combination therapy group. A meta-analysis of 33 randomized controlled trials found similar results (207), providing a clear signal that dual ACEI/ARB therapy is unlikely to provide substantial clinical benefit over one or the other. Moreover, a meta-analysis including 20 large contemporary clinical trials of renin–angiotensin–aldosterone system inhibitors in hypertensive patients found a 10% relative reduction in all-cause mortality ($p = 0.004$) with ACE inhibitors, but no corresponding significant reduction in mortality with ARBs (203).

The JNC 8 guidelines do provide for the consideration of different agents in specific types of patients or conditions, though less strictly than previous versions (184). The use of ACE inhibitors should still be considered in individuals with diabetes, and/or chronic kidney disease, where they have been shown to help preserve renal function (216–218). However, there is less emphasis on patients with left ventricular dysfunction with or without prior ACS, those with prior stroke, or those with high coronary disease risk. The treatment of patients 60 years or older still represents a challenge.

The Antihypertensive and Lipid-Lowering Treatment to Prevent Heart Attack Trial (ALLHAT) enrolled 33,357 participants aged 55 years or older with hypertension and at least one other CHD risk factor (211). Patients received the diuretic chlorthalidone, 12.5 to 25 mg/day; amlodipine, 2.5 to 10 mg/day; or lisinopril, 10 to 40 mg/day; the fourth arm (doxazosin) was stopped early because of increased cardiovascular events and CHF hospitalizations. At a mean follow-up of 4.9 years, no significant differences were found between the three remaining treatment groups in the incidence of fatal CHD or nonfatal MI (overall rate, 8.9%). Certain secondary outcomes occurred less often with the chlorthalidone group compared with the amlodipine group (HF) and lisinopril group (combined CVD, stroke, and HF). Although some criticisms of this important study exist (see comments in annotated summary, page 90), the results suggest that in patients in whom cardiovascular events are the greater risk, a thiazide-type diuretic is the preferred first agent.

The second Australian National Blood Pressure Study (ANBP-2) enrolled 6,083 elderly Caucasian subjects. Patients received any ACE inhibitor or diuretic in an open-label fashion. The ACE inhibitor group had a significantly lower incidence of death or any cardiovascular event, but this benefit was restricted to men (HR 0.83

vs. HR 1.00 in women). This study is methodologically weaker than ALLHAT, but its results suggest Caucasian men may benefit more from ACE inhibitor therapy.

TARGET BLOOD PRESSURE

The Hypertension Optimal Treatment (HOT) study (210) randomized 18,790 patients to target DBP levels of 90 mm Hg or less, 85 mm Hg or less, or 80 mm Hg or less. The incidence of major events did not differ between the three groups. However, the power to detect such a difference was less than planned for two reasons: (a) actual mean BPs were approximately 2 mm Hg apart instead of 5 mm Hg apart and (b) only 724 major cardiovascular events occurred over a period of 3.8 years versus the projected 1,100 over a period of 2.5 years. Thus, the trial was not adequately powered to determine whether a target DBP of approximately 80 mm Hg results in the fewest major events. Nevertheless, significantly fewer cardiovascular events and deaths were found among diabetic patients assigned to a target DBP of 80 mm Hg or less compared with 90 mm Hg or less ($p = 0.005$; $p = 0.016$). In the African American Study of Kidney (AASK) Disease and Hypertension Study, tighter BP control (mean, 128/78 mm Hg) was associated with an 18% lower incidence of cardiovascular mortality and hospitalizations compared with looser BP control (mean, 141/85 mm Hg).

NONMODIFIABLE RISK FACTORS

Family History

A family history of disorders appears most important in those otherwise at low risk. One analysis of 45,317 physicians showed that if a parent had an MI before age 70 years, the RRs of cardiac death, percutaneous transluminal coronary angioplasty (PTCA), and revascularization procedures were approximately twofold higher, whereas a study of 21,004 Swedish twins showed that the risk of CHD death was as high as eightfold greater if the other monozygous twin died of CHD before age 55 years (see N Engl J Med 1994;330:1041–1046). A cohort analysis of more than 20,000 individuals found that approximately 15% of CHD cases were attributable to family history, independent of other known risk factors (235).

Age

Advancing age is associated with a gradual deterioration in cardiovascular function (e.g., diastolic function, BP regulation) and increasing risks of CHD death (234). Historically, guidelines have considered age of 45 years or older in men and 55 years or older in women a CAD risk factor.

Gender

Atherosclerotic-related events are more common in men. This gender disparity is largely owing to a later onset of symptomatic CAD in women (approximately 10 years), which is likely related to the protective effects of estrogen.

Genetic Markers

Since the publication of the human genome in 2003, genetic and genomic research has rapidly proliferated. Overall, 30 different genetic loci have been associated with MI and CAD (239). While these loci have helped elucidate novel pathways in the pathogenesis of atherosclerosis and ACSs, they have not added substantially to traditional risk prediction models, and a recent AHA policy statement did not recommend genetic testing (240).

HORMONAL STATUS AND HORMONAL THERAPY

Estrogen replacement therapy in postmenopausal women results in an approximately 15% to 20% reduction in LDL and 15% to 20% elevation in HDL levels. Significant epidemiologic data suggested that estrogen replacement was associated with significantly lower CHD mortality (88,89), though breast cancer rates are 10% to 30% higher, and endometrial cancer occurs up to six times more often.

However, in contrast to the epidemiologic data, the first large prospective, randomized trial [Heart and Estrogen/Progestin Replacement Study (HERS)] showed that a combination of estrogen and progestin in 2,763 women with a CHD event in the preceding 6 months did not result in a significant reduction in cardiovascular death and MI [relative hazard (RH), 0.99] (95); the hormone group had more events in year 1 but fewer events in years 4 and 5.

The subsequent Women's Health Initiative, which randomized 16,608 postmenopausal women to estrogen and progestin or placebo, was terminated early (at 5.2 years of follow-up) (96). The hormone group had significantly higher rates of CHD (hazard ratio, 1.29), breast cancer (HR, 1.26), and stroke (HR, 1.41), with similar overall mortality rates. Based on these data, the overall risk–benefit profile for estrogen and progestin therapy does not meet the requirements for a clearly safe and efficacious intervention for primary prevention.

Raloxifene is a selective estrogen modulator used for treatment of osteoporosis. In the Multiple Outcomes of Raloxifene Evaluation (MORE) trial, 7,705 osteoporotic postmenopausal women were randomized to raloxifene, 60 mg/day; raloxifene, 120 mg/day; or placebo (97). At 4-year follow-up, no significant differences were found between the treatment groups in coronary and cerebrovascular events. However, among the 1,035 women with increased cardiovascular risk at baseline, those assigned to raloxifene (either dose) had a significantly lower risk of cardiovascular events compared with placebo (RR, 0.60; 95% CI, 0.38 to 0.95). Confirmation in a trial with evaluation of cardiovascular outcomes as the primary objective was required—the Raloxifene Use for The Heart (RUTH) trial randomized 10,101 postmenopausal women with CAD or multiple risk factors for CHD to 60 mg of raloxifene daily or placebo and followed them for a median of 5.6 years. The trial had two primary outcomes: (a) a composite of death from coronary causes, MI, or hospitalization for ACS and (b) invasive breast cancer. The results demonstrated no significant difference in coronary events between the two groups, but did show that raloxifene reduced the risk of invasive breast cancer.

INFLAMMATION

C-Reactive Protein

C-reactive protein is an acute-phase reactant produced by the liver in response to interleukin 6 (IL-6). A high-sensitivity assay (hsCRP) has allowed accurate measurement at the low levels (<10 mg/L) that predict CHD risk. Numerous studies have shown that elevated hsCRP levels are strongly associated with an increased risk of cardiovascular events. CRP also may be more than a marker of CHD risk, as some research suggests it impairs endothelial vasoreactivity and promotes atherosclerosis (see *Circulation* 2000;102:1000, 2165).

In nested case–control studies of WHS and Women's Health Initiative participants (244), the highest hsCRP levels were associated with a more than fourfold higher risk of cardiovascular events and twofold increased risk of CHD, respectively; individuals in the highest quartile of hsCRP had increased rates of stroke (RR, 1.9), MI (RR, 2.9), and peripheral vascular disease (RR, 4.1). In the PHS, high levels of CRP were associated with increased risk of MI (adjusted RR, 1.5), and those in the highest quartiles of both CRP and TC had a fivefold higher risk (241). Another analysis of both PHS and WHS participants found that those in the highest quintiles of CRP *and* TC/HDL had an eight- to ninefold increased risk of major events (see *Circulation* 2001;103:1813).

CRP also has predictive value in those with known CAD. In the CARE study, those in the highest quintile of CRP levels had nearly a twofold increased risk of recurrent events (see *Circulation* 1998;98:839–844). An analysis of prospective European studies of patients with stable and unstable angina found a 45% increase in nonfatal MI and sudden cardiac death (SCD) in those with increased CRP levels. In patients with ACS, high CRP levels are predictive of worse prognosis (246). In the initial evaluation of such patients, hsCRP measurement provides additional prognostic information to other markers (see *Circulation* 2002;105:1760) and may prove useful in those with normal troponin levels.

hsCRP may even be a stronger predictor of first cardiovascular events than is LDL cholesterol. An analysis of the 27,939 WHS participants found that both baseline LDL and hsCRP levels had a strong linear relation with the incidence of cardiovascular events, although the two were minimally correlated ($r = 0.08$) (245). The adjusted RRs of first cardiovascular events according to increasing quintiles of CRP, as compared with women in the lowest quintile, were 1.4, 1.6, 2.0, and 2.3 ($p < 0.001$), compared with corresponding RRs in increasing quintiles of LDL of 0.9, 1.1, 1.3, and 1.5 ($p < 0.001$). Because 46% of major events occurred among those with LDL <130 mg/dL, CRP may be particularly helpful in identifying patients at high CHD risk among those with low LDL levels.

CRP levels appear to be effectively lowered by statins. The PRINCE trial enrolled 2,884 patients (including 1,182 with known CVD off statins for at least 12 weeks) (see *JAMA* 2001;286:64–70). In the primary prevention cohort, pravastatin reduced hsCRP by 16.9% compared with no change with placebo. In the open-labeled CVD cohort (all received statin therapy), a similar 14.3% reduction in hsCRP was found. An analysis of AFCAPS/TexCAPS participants found that lovastatin decreased CRP levels by 14% during the course of the study ($p < 0.001$) (242). Several studies have shown that statins lower hsCRP within weeks of therapy initiation, an effect independent of their effect on LDL cholesterol (see *Circulation* 2001;103:1191; 2002;106:1447). Prospective studies to evaluate whether CRP lowering by statins reduces major events are ongoing; however, secondary analyses of several major statin trials have demonstrated that neither baseline CRP nor baseline LDL modifies the statin-mediated relative risk reductions in cardiovascular events (243), and CRP lowering while on statin treatment has not been shown to correlate with decreased risk of subsequent cardiovascular events.

Subsequently, the FDA moved to include hsCRP in a package label to guide pharmacologic lipid-lowering therapy. Based on data from the JUPITER trial (34), rosuvastatin is indicated in patients who met entry criteria for this trial: those with normal LDL cholesterol, but increased risk of cardiovascular events based on elevated CRP, age, and at least one other CVD risk factor. It was suggested that as many as 21% of Americans ineligible for statin therapy under prior NCEP guidelines would meet entry criteria for JUPITER (see *Am J Cardiol* 2010;105:77–81).

Homocysteine and B Vitamins

Hyperhomocysteinemia appears to be a modest independent risk factor for CHD, CVD, and PVD. Most studies have confirmed that high homocysteine levels are associated with an increased CHD mortality rate (253,254); however, other studies have shown no association (95). A meta-analysis found that in prospective studies, a 25% lower homocysteine level was associated with an 11% lower risk of ischemic heart disease (IHD) and 19% lower stroke risk (250); analysis of 5,569 AFCAPS/TexCAPS participants found that higher baseline homocysteine levels were associated with increased risk of future acute coronary events; however, in contrast to findings in this trial for CRP, homocysteine levels did not help to define low LDL subgroups with different responses to statin therapy (255). Furthermore, homocysteine levels in elderly persons without known CHD predicted cardiovascular mortality better than the Framingham Risk Score (see *BMJ* 2009;338:a3083).

Two studies reported that folic acid fortification and multivitamin use are associated with lower homocysteine levels (252). However, eight trials (enrolling over 37,000 subjects) of homocysteine as a therapeutic target, mostly involving B vitamins, have yielded disappointing results—lowering homocysteine does not prevent events. These trials included NORVIT (256), HOPE 2 (257), a VA study of homocysteine lowering (258), WENBIT (260), SEARCH (261), and FAVOR (259) (see also *JAMA* 2008;299(17):2027–2036; *JAMA* 2008;300(7):795–804).

Lipoprotein-Associated Phospholipase A2

Lipoprotein-associated phospholipase A_2 (Lp-PLA$_2$) is an enzyme produced predominantly by macrophages and monocytes and is also known as platelet-activating factor acetylhydrolase (PAF-AH). Its action is to convert oxidized LDL within the plaque into two inflammatory compounds: free fatty acids and lysoPC (see *Eur Heart J* 2009;30:2930–2938). While its exact involvement in atherosclerosis is not yet clear, its levels were found to correlate closely with future coronary, as well as cerebrovascular events, in observational and case–cohort studies (see *Circulation* 2004;110:1903–1908; *Circulation* 2005;111:570–575). Additional data from a large collaborative study support the significant association between CHD and Lp-PLA$_2$ activity and mass, comparable to that of blood pressure or non-HDL cholesterol (see *Lancet* 2010;375:1536–1544). Darapladib, a selective inhibitor of LP-PLA$_2$, reduces serum IL-6 and CRP (265); two large trials powered to detect clinical end points both failed to demonstrate any benefit (see *N Engl J Med* 2014 370(18):1702–1711 [STABILITY] and *JAMA* 2014 312(10):1006–1015 [SOLID-TIMI 52]).

Infections and Cardiovascular Disease

Historical studies demonstrated an increased risk of CAD in individuals who are seropositive for certain infectious agents, and this led to clinical trials of antimicrobial treatment to prevent CVD. However, in patients with stable CAD, the azithromycin for the secondary prevention of coronary events (ACES) trial did not demonstrate benefit of 600 mg of azithromycin in 4,012 patients over 1 year (269). The larger Weekly Intervention with Zithromax for Atherosclerosis and its Related Disorders (WIZARD) trial (267), which enrolled more than 7,000 post-MI patients with elevated *Chlamydophila pneumoniae* titers, showed no significant benefit from short-term treatment with azithromycin versus placebo at 2 years' follow-up.

To test whether longer-term antibiotic treatment could reduce coronary events, the antibiotic arm of the PROVE IT-TIMI 22 trial randomized 4,162 patients presenting with ACS to gatifloxacin or placebo over a mean treatment duration of 2 years (10 days per month of therapy) (268). After 2 years of follow-up, there was no significant difference in the rates of the primary end point, a composite of death from all causes, MI, documented unstable angina requiring rehospitalization, revascularization (performed at least 30 days after randomization), and stroke. This study effectively ended the concept that bacterial infection was a modifiable risk factor for recurrent cardiovascular events (see *N Engl J Med* 2005;352:1637–1645).

In contrast, there is clear epidemiologic evidence that chronic infection with the human immunodeficiency virus (HIV) is associated with increased risk of MI (270,271). While some of this excess risk stems from the adverse metabolic effects of several antiretroviral agents, there also appears to be a contribution from the inflammatory effect of chronic inflammation. Despite the contribution from chronic inflammation, control of HIV with antiretroviral agents does not reduce the risk of MI (272,273). The optimal primary and secondary prevention strategies in HIV patients remain unknown.

ANTIPLATELET DRUGS FOR PRIMARY AND SECONDARY PREVENTION

Aspirin

PRIMARY PREVENTION TRIALS

Several trials of aspirin for primary prevention have been conducted. The PHS found that ASA-treated patients (325 mg every other day) had 44% fewer non-fatal MIs and a nonsignificant 4% reduction in cardiovascular deaths (277). This study was stopped prematurely because of concerns about the high stroke rate (RR, 2.1). In 39,876 healthy women, Ridker and colleagues demonstrated a nonsignificant reduction in MI, stroke, or cardiovascular death (RR 0.91, $p = 0.013$) and a significant reduction in stroke ($p = 0.009$), with a noted increase in hemorrhagic stroke (RR 1.24, $p = 0.031$) (279).

Ultimately, the evidence from many of the trials was combined in a meta-analysis involving over 90,000 patients free of CVD—over 50,000 women and 40,000 men. The meta-analysis demonstrated that aspirin used in primary prevention reduced the risk of cardiovascular events in both men and women, but that the primary driver of cardiovascular events was MI in men and stroke in women (286). Largely on the basis of this meta-analysis, the U.S. Preventive Services Task Force (USPSTF) encouraged the use of aspirin for primary prevention in men aged 45 to 79 (when the reduction in MI outweighs the risk of bleeding) and women aged 55 to 79 (when the benefit of stroke reduction outweighs the risk of bleeding). However, the task force found insufficient data to make recommendations for patients 80 years old and greater (see *Ann Intern Med* 2009;150:396–404). In the ATT Collaboration, the Framingham Risk Score was useful in identifying patients at very low risk who had very little benefit, whereas patients above a 5% to 10% risk did have a clinical benefit (**Fig. 1.3**) (287). Subsequent meta-analyses have been less enthusiastic about the benefit of aspirin in primary prevention; one found that the number needed to treat (NNT) with aspirin to prevent one cardiovascular event was 120, while the NNT to cause one significant bleeding event was 73 (288). The American Diabetes Association, which had previously recommended that all individuals with diabetes older than 30 years receive ASA, revised their guidelines to recommend that only diabetic patients with Framingham Risk Score predicting a 10% 10-year risk or greater should take aspirin (see *Diabetes Care* 2010;33:1395–1402).

SECONDARY PREVENTION TRIALS

Aspirin for secondary prevention of CVD has been studied in depth and resulted in several meta-analyses. One meta-analysis of low-dose (<325 mg/day) aspirin in secondary prevention found a significant 18% reduction in all-cause mortality, 20% reduction in stroke, and 30% reduction in MI with low-dose aspirin compared to placebo (288).

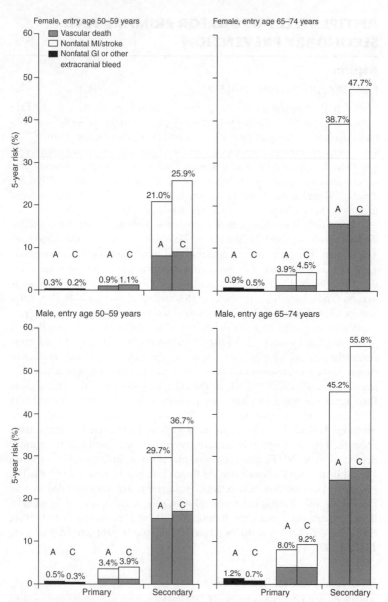

Figure 1.3 • Risk of 5-year events by age and sex in met-analysis of aspirin (A) versus control (C). (From Antithrombotic Trialists' (ATT) Collaboration. Aspirin in the primary and secondary prevention of vascular disease: collaborative meta-analysis of individual participant data from randomised trials. *Lancet* 2009;373:1849–1860.)

The Antithrombotic Trialists' Collaboration landmark meta-analysis examined 287 randomized studies with 135,000 patients in comparisons of antiplatelet therapy versus control and 77,000 in comparisons of different antiplatelet regimens (285). Among high-risk patients (e.g., acute MI, acute stroke, previous stroke or transient ischemic attack, peripheral arterial disease, atrial fibrillation), antiplatelet therapy reduced the incidence of serious vascular events (nonfatal MI or stroke, vascular death) by approximately one-fourth, nonfatal MI by approximately one-third, nonfatal stroke by approximately one-fourth, and vascular mortality by approximately one-sixth (all $p < 0.00001$). In each of the high-risk categories, the absolute benefits outweighed the absolute risks of major extracranial bleeding.

Though preparations are approved at up to 1,300 mg/day, another meta-analysis of including a range of aspirin doses for the prevention of CVD demonstrated little benefit to doses higher than 75 to 81 mg/day and an increased risk of hemorrhage, specifically GI bleeding, at higher doses (see JAMA 2007;297:2018–2024).

Clopidogrel

The Clopidogrel versus Aspirin in Patients at Risk of Ischaemic Events (CAPRIE) trial randomized more than 19,000 patients with a recent MI, ischemic stroke, or PAD to clopidogrel, 75 mg once daily, or ASA, 325 mg once daily (280). Overall, clopidogrel was associated with a significantly lower incidence in the primary composite end point, consisting of ischemic stroke, MI, or vascular death (5.32% vs. 5.83%/year; $p = 0.043$). Another analysis of all enrolled patients showed a statistically significant 19.2% reduction in the MI event rate ($p = 0.008$) (see Am J Cardiol 2002;90:760). Based on these data, the use of clopidogrel in all patients with recent MI or stroke or documented peripheral arterial disease appears to result in a small but significant reduced risk of subsequent MI, stroke, or CV death. Furthermore, the subsequent results of the CURE, CREDO, COMMIT, and CLARITY-TIMI 28 studies (see Chapters 2 through 4) confirmed the benefits of clopidogrel for secondary prevention in PCI patients, and across the spectrum of ACS. The results of TRITON-TIMI 38 and PLATO (see Chapters 2 through 4) have proven the efficacy of the newer P2Y12/ADP receptor antagonists prasugrel and ticagrelor in the secondary prevention of CVD following ACS. Most recently, data from the Prevention of Cardiovascular Events in Patients with Prior Heart Attack Using Ticagrelor Compared to Placebo on a Background of Aspirin–Thrombolysis in Myocardial Infarction 54 (PEGASUS-TIMI 54) trial have also supported the use of ticagrelor in the secondary prevention population (see N Engl J Med. 2015 May 7;372(19):1791–1800).

In those with history of stroke or peripheral arterial disease or at high risk for CHD events, the combination of clopidogrel and ASA was evaluated in the Clopidogrel for High Atherothrombotic Risk and Ischemic Stabilization, Management, and Avoidance (CHARISMA) trial (282). A total of 15,603 patients either with known CVD (cardiac, cerebrovascular, or peripheral) or with multiple cardiovascular risk factors were enrolled and randomized to 75 mg of clopidogrel or placebo over a median follow-up period of 28 months. When taken together, the trial failed to meet its primary end point, a composite of stroke, MI, or cardiovascular death at 28 months (6.8% in the clopidogrel group vs. 7.3% in the placebo group). However, in the group with known CVD, clopidogrel proved statistically beneficial (6.9% in the clopidogrel group vs. 7.9% in the placebo group), reaffirming the findings of the CAPRIE study (as this was the "CAPRIE-like" cohort). Therefore, dual antiplatelet therapy with aspirin and a P2Y12 receptor antagonist (such as clopidogrel) has been recommended for secondary prevention following ACS, for a duration of at least 1 year.

REFERENCES

General Articles

1. Go, AS, et al. Heart disease and stroke statistics—2014 update: a report from the American Heart Association. *Circulation* 2014;129(3):e28–e292.

The most recent update to the American Heart Association's annual CVD statistics.

2. Pearson TA, et al. AHA Guidelines for primary prevention of cardiovascular disease and stroke: 2002 update: consensus panel guide to comprehensive risk reduction for adult patients without coronary or other atherosclerotic vascular diseases: American Heart Association Science Advisory and Coordinating Committee. *Circulation* 2002;106:388–391.

3. Smith SC, et al. AHA/ACCF secondary prevention and risk reduction therapy for patients with coronary and other atherosclerotic vascular disease: 2011 update: a guideline from the American Heart Association and American College of Cardiology Foundation. *Circulation* 2011;124:2458–2473.

4. Mosca L, et al. Effectiveness-based guidelines for the prevention of cardiovascular disease in women—2011 update: a guideline from the American Heart Association. *Circulation* 2011;123:1243–1252.

5. Goff, DC, Jr, et al. 2013 ACC/AHA guideline on the assessment of cardiovascular risk: A report of the American College of Cardiology/American Heart Association Task Force on Practice Guidelines. *Circulation* 2013;129:S49–S73. doi: 10.1161/01. cir.0000437741.48606.98

6. Yusuf S, et al. Effect of potentially modifiable risk factors associated with myocardial infarction in 52 countries (the INTERHEART study): case-control study. *Lancet* 2004;364:937–952.

This very large international case–control study of acute MI assessed the relationship of smoking, HTN, diabetes, waist-to-hip ratio, dietary patterns, physical activity, alcohol consumption, blood lipids, and psychosocial factors to MI incidence. The investigators concluded that these modifiable risk factors could account for 90% of the risk of MI in these populations.

7. Bhatt D, et al.; for the REACH Registry Investigators. International prevalence, recognition, and treatment of cardiovascular risk factors in outpatients with atherothrombosis. *JAMA* 2006;295:180–189.

8. Steg PG, et al. for the REACH Registry Investigators. One-year cardiovascular event rates in outpatients with atherothrombosis. *JAMA* 2007;297:1197–1206.

The REduction of Atherothrombosis for Continued Health (REACH) Registry represents a unique look at over 50,000 outpatients with CVD or significant risk factors. These manuscripts examine the contemporary diagnosis and management of such patients, as well as their event rates. The results are stratified by vascular bed of disease (coronary, cerebral, peripheral, or risk factors only), with patients diagnosed with atherothrombosis of multiple vascular beds having escalating 1-year event rates.

9. Ford ES, et al. Explaining the decrease in U.S. deaths from coronary disease, 1980–2000. N Engl J Med 2007;356:2388–2398.

The authors examine the rates of CVD mortality in the United States among adults aged 25 to 84 from 1980 to 2000, finding a drop from 542.9 to 266.8 deaths per 100,000 population in men and from 263.3 to 134.4 deaths per 100,000 women. They attribute these declines to both improved medical and surgical treatments (primary and second-ary preventive therapies for MI, revascularization, treatments for heart failure, and other therapies) as well as a decline in risk factors (reductions in TC, BP, smoking prevalence, and physical inactivity), with both contributing roughly equally to the improvement. Unfortunately, they found part of these gains offset by an increase in population-wide body mass index, boosting cardiovascular mortality.

10. Berry JD, et al. Lifetime risks of cardiovascular disease. N Engl J Med 2012;366:321–329.

This meta-analysis of 18 cohort studies involving 257,384 black and white men and women used four major risk factors—TC, blood pressure, smoking status, and diabetes—to group patients into five risk strata. Those participants with optimal risk factor profiles (zero of the four risk factors) had substantially lower risks of CVD through age 80 than did patients with two or more risk factors (4.7% vs. 29.6% in men, 6.4% vs. 20.5% in women). These relationships held regardless of race.

11. Wilkins JT, et al. Lifetime risk and years lived free of total cardiovascular disease. JAMA 2012;308:1795–1801.

The investigators pooled data from 5 large NHLBI-funded cohorts to generate 905,115 person-years of data involving 15.175 individuals free of CVD at the time of entry into their cohort. Using these data, they generated models for lifetime risk of CVD based on risk factors and age. In general, risk of CVD was high, with residual lifetime risk through age 85 exceeding 40% for a 55-year-old man without risk factors and exceeding 30% for a 55-year-old woman without risk factors. Risk of CVD increased with an increasing number of risk factors.

Lipids and Cholesterol

GUIDELINES

12. NCEP Guidelines. Expert panel on detection, evaluation, and treatment of high blood cholesterol in adults: executive summary of the third report of the National Cholesterol Education Program (NCEP) expert panel on detection, evaluation, and treatment of high blood cholesterol in adults (Adult Treatment Panel III). JAMA 2001;285:2486–2497.

These prior guidelines focused on LDL cholesterol goals and cut points for therapeutic lifestyle changes and drug therapy. High-risk groups were identified by using a modified Framingham point score. Attention also was given to TG levels, non-HDL levels, and the metabolic syndrome.

13. Grundy SM, et al. Implications of recent clinical trials for the National Cholesterol Education Program Adult Treatment Panel III guidelines. Circulation 2004;110:227–239.

This update to the 2001 guidelines highlighted the evidence from high-dose statin trials (viz., HPS, ALLHAT, ASCOT-LLA, PROVE IT-TIMI 22), reviewing their implications on clinical practice. Importantly, the panel offered a new optional therapeutic target of LDL < 70 mg/dL in the highest-risk patients.

14. Stone, NJ, et al. 2013 ACC/AHA guideline on the treatment of blood cholesterol to reduce atherosclerotic cardiovascular risk in adults: a report of the American College of Cardiology/American Heart Association Task Force on Practice Guidelines. *Circulation* 2014;129:S1–S45. doi: 10.1161/01.cir.0000437738.63853.7a

This update of the guidelines was the first time the lipid guidelines were written by the ACC/AHA and represented a dramatic shift in approach. The task force could not identify strong enough evidence to advocate distinct treatment targets for LDL cholesterol (or any other lipids). Instead, they reviewed the evidence and based recommendations on the questions studied in clinical trials. This resulted in the identification of patient groups who should be treated with a statin, at standard or high dose, but without titration to resulting LDL levels.

EPIDEMIOLOGY

15. Martin MJ, et al. Multiple risk factor intervention trial (MRFIT): serum cholesterol, blood pressure and mortality: implications from a cohort of 361,662 men. *Lancet* 1986;2:933–939.

This analysis of 6-year follow-up data showed that cardiovascular mortality correlated with cholesterol levels. Increased cardiovascular mortality risk was seen with TC levels as low as 181 mg/dL. RR was 3.8 for cholesterol levels above the 85th percentile (>253 mg/dL).

16. Gordon DJ, et al. High-density lipoprotein cholesterol and cardiovascular disease: four prospective American studies. *Circulation* 1989;79:8–15.

This analysis examined data from the Framingham Heart Study, Lipid Research Clinics Prevalence Mortality Follow-up Study (LRCF), Coronary Primary Prevention Trial (CPPT), and MRFIT. A 1-mg/dL (0.026 mM) increase in HDL was associated with a significant CHD risk reduction of 2% in men (FHS, CPPT, and MRFIT) and 3% in women (FHS). In LRCF, in which only fatal outcomes were documented, a 1-mg/dL increase in HDL was associated with significant 3.7% (men) and 4.7% (women) decreases in cardiovascular mortality rates.

17. Cui Y, et al. Non-high-density lipoprotein cholesterol level as a predictor of cardiovascular disease mortality. *Arch Intern Med* 2001;161:1413–1419.

This study analyzed data on 2,406 men and 2,056 women aged 40 to 64 years from the Lipid Research Clinics Program Follow-up Study. At follow-up (average, 19 years), baseline levels of HDL and non–HDL cholesterol were strong predictors of CVD death in both sexes, whereas LDL level was a slightly weaker CVD predictor. Increases of 30 mg/dL in non–HDL and LDL levels corresponded to increases in CVD risk of 19% and 15%, respectively, in men and 11% and 8%, respectively, in women.

18. Ridker PM, et al. Non-HDL cholesterol, apolipoproteins A-I and B100, standard lipid measures, lipid ratios, and CRP as risk factors for cardiovascular disease in women. *JAMA* 2005;294:326–333.

This analysis of the WHS looked at several lipid markers to identify those with strong prognostic importance: TC, LDL, HDL, non–HDL cholesterol, apolipoproteins A-I and B100, high-sensitivity CRP, and the ratios of TC to HDL, LDL to HDL, apolipoprotein B100 to apolipoprotein A-I, and apolipoprotein B100 to HDL. They concluded that non–HDL cholesterol and the ratio of TC to HDL could be equally useful to apolipoprotein fractions and that hsCRP added prognostic significance to all lipid markers, after controlling for major clinical risk factors.

19. Ference BA, et al. Effect of long-term exposure to lower low-density lipoprotein cholesterol beginning early in life on the risk of coronary heart disease: a Mendelian randomization analysis. *J Am Coll Cardiol* 2012;60:2631–2639.

In a meta-analysis of 312,321 patients with genetic polymorphisms that produce lower LDL, the authors found that lifelong exposure to lower LDL levels via genetic polymorphism reduced the incidence of CAD by 54.5% (95% CI, 48.8% to 59.5%) per 38.7 mg/dL (1 mmol/L) LDL reduction. This per unit reduction is approximately threefold greater than demonstrated in trials of statin started later in life and has been cited by some as proof of principle that LDL-lowering therapy should be initiated at an earlier age in order to capture all of its potential benefits (see *J Am Coll Cardiol* 2012;60:2640–2642).

20. Boekholdt SM, et al. Association of LDL cholesterol, non-HDL cholesterol, and apolipoprotein B levels with risk of cardiovascular events among patients treated with statins: a meta-analysis. **JAMA** 2012;307:1302–1309.

In this meta-analysis of 38,153 patients treated with statins for at least 1 year in 8 randomized placebo-controlled clinical trials, investigators calculated the hazard ratios for major cardiovascular events (fatal or nonfatal MI, fatal or nonfatal stroke, fatal events from other CVD, or hospitalization for unstable angina) with on-treatment levels of various lipid levels. Higher on-treatment levels of LDL, non-HDL cholesterol, and apolipoprotein B were all associated with a greater risk of cardiovascular events, but the association was stronger for non-HDL cholesterol (HR, 1.16 per 1 SD increase; 95% CI, 1.12 to 1.19) than apolipoprotein B (HR, 1.14 per 1 SD increase) and LDL (HR, 1.13 per 1 SD increase).

21. Michos ED, et al. Prevalence of low low-density lipoprotein cholesterol with elevated high sensitivity C-reactive protein in the U.S.: implications of the JUPITER (justification for the use of statins in primary prevention: an intervention trial evaluating rosuvastatin) study. **J Am Coll Cardiol** 2009;53:931–935.

Using data from the NHANES, the investigators estimated the number of patients qualifying for statin therapy under current guidelines, and those who might additionally qualify were the guidelines to be broadened based on the results of the JUPITER study (broadly, patients with LDL <130 mg/dL and hsCRP > 2 mg/L). They estimated that an additional 6.5 million American patients would be eligible for statin therapy as primary prevention for CVD.

22. Carroll MD, et al. Trends in lipids and lipoproteins in US adults, 1988-2010. **JAMA** 2012;308:1545–1554.

The investigators use three US cross-sectional surveys (NHANES, 1988 to 1994, 1999 to 2002, and 2007 to 2010) to calculate changes in mean lipid parameters over time. Between the first and third survey periods, mean TC decreased from 206 to 196 mg/dL, mean LDL decreased from 129 to 116 mg/dL, and mean HDL increased from 50.7 to 52.5 mg/dL. The prevalence of treatment with lipid-lowering drugs increased from 3.4% in the first survey to 15.5% in the last survey, but mean lipid profiles were similar in those subjects taking and not taking lipid-lowering drugs. The study was not designed to explain these changes, but the authors speculate that decreases in *trans*-fatty acid consumption, cigarette smoking, and carbohydrate consumption may be responsible in the absence of data demonstrating increased exercise, decreased saturated fat intake, or reduction in obesity.

23. Criqui MH, et al. Plasma triglyceride level and mortality from coronary heart disease. **N Engl J Med** 1993;328:1220–1225.

This study analyzed 7,505 patients in the Lipid Research Clinics Follow-up trial. The 12-year incidence of coronary death in both men and women increased with TG levels. However, after adjustment for potential covariates, this association was no longer statistically significant.

24. Jeppensen J, et al. Triglyceride concentration and ischemic heart disease. **Circulation** 1998;97:1029–1036.

This study of 2,906 Copenhagen Male Study participants initially free of CVD found that high fasting TG level is an independent risk factor for IHD. At 8-year follow-up, the risk factor–adjusted RRs of IHD were 1.5 (95% CI, 1.0 to 2.3; $p = 0.05$) and 2.2 (95% CI, 1.4 to 3.4; $p < 0.001$) for middle and higher thirds of TG levels. A clear gradient of risk was found with increasing TG levels within each level of HDL, including high HDL.

25. Miller M, et al.; PROVE IT-TIMI 22 Investigators. Impact of triglyceride levels beyond low-density lipoprotein cholesterol after acute coronary syndrome in the PROVE IT-TIMI 22 trial. J Am Coll Cardiol 2008;51:724–730.

This *post hoc* analysis of the PROVE IT-TIMI 22 study looked at the prognostic significance of TG levels, measured while on intensive statin therapy with LDL levels of <70 mg/dL. Through both univariate and multivariable analyses, a TG level of <150 mg/dL on treatment with statins was associated with a significant reduction in death, MI, or recurrent ACS. This was a robust finding that persisted after adjustment for LDL levels, non-HDL levels, CRP, and other covariates.

26. Danesh J, et al. Lipoprotein(a) and coronary heart disease: meta-analysis of prospective studies. Circulation 2000;102:1082–1085.

This meta-analysis examined 27 prospective studies with at least 1 year of follow-up (mean, 10). Comparison of individuals in the top third of baseline plasma Lp(a) measurements with those in the bottom third resulted in a combined risk ratio of CHD death or nonfatal MI of 1.6 (95% CI, 1.4 to 1.8; 2 p < 0.00001). The findings were similar when the analyses were restricted to the 18 studies of general populations (combined RR, 1.7; 95% CI, 1.4 to 1.9; 2 p < 0.00001).

27. Schaefer EJ, et al. Lipid Research Clinics Coronary Primary Prevention Trial (LRC-CPPT). Lipoprotein(a) levels and risk of coronary heart disease in men. JAMA 1994;271:999–1003.

This study enrolled 3,806 men aged 35 to 59 years with TC >265 mg/dL and LDL >190 mg/dL and randomized them to either cholestyramine or placebo. Lp(a) was measured in serum obtained (and frozen) before randomization from 233 patients who manifested CHD during the study (7 to 10 years' follow-up) as well as from 390 CHD-free controls. Baseline Lp(a) levels were 21% higher in patients who ultimately manifested CHD (adjusted p < 0.01).

28. Martin SS, et al. Comparison of a novel method vs the Friedewald equation for estimating low-density lipoprotein cholesterol levels from the standard lipid profile. JAMA 2013;310(19):2061–2068.

The authors compared the classic calculation of LDL, using the Friedewald equation, to a novel equation that used an adjustable factor for TGs:VLDL ratio. In over 1 million participants in the NHANES survey, they demonstrated improved risk classification over the Friedewald equation, when compared to direct LDL measurement.

PRIMARY PREVENTION
Early Trials
29. Lipid Research Clinics Coronary Primary Prevention Trial (LRC-CPPT) results: reduction in incidence of CHD. JAMA 1984;251:351–364.

Design: Prospective, randomized, double-blind, placebo-controlled, multicenter study. Primary end point was CHD-related death and nonfatal MI. The average follow-up was 7.4 years.

Purpose: To evaluate the effects of cholestyramine on cholesterol levels and major cardiac events in hypercholesterolemic men at high risk of CHD events.

Population: 3,806 men aged 35 to 59 years with TC > 265 mg/dL and LDL > 190 mg/dL.

Treatment: Cholestyramine (24 g/day) or placebo.

Results: Cholestyramine use was associated with 9% lower TC and 13% lower LDL. Cholestyramine group had a 19% reduction in CHD-related death and MI (8.1% vs. 9.8%, p < 0.05).

30. Frick MH, et al. Helsinki Heart Study: primary-prevention trial with gemfibrozil in middle-aged men with dyslipidemia. N Engl J Med 1987;317:1237–1245.

Design: Prospective, randomized, double-blind, placebo-controlled, multicenter study. Primary end point was cardiac death and MI. The follow-up period was 5 years.

Purpose: To investigate the effect of gemfibrozil on the incidence of CHD in asymptomatic middle-aged men at high risk because of elevated lipid levels.

Population: 4,081 men aged 40 to 55 years with non-HDL cholesterol level of ≥200 mg/dL.

Treatment: Gemfibrozil, 600 mg twice daily, or placebo.

Results: Gemfibrozil initially increased HDL levels by more than 10%, followed by a small decline over time. TC and LDL levels were decreased by 11% and 10%, respectively, and remained consistent throughout the trial. The gemfibrozil group had 34% fewer cardiac events (7.3 vs. 41.4/1,000; $p < 0.02$); the decline in incidence became evident in the second year. No significant mortality difference was detected between groups (2.19% vs. 2.07%).

Statins in Primary Prevention

31. Shepherd J, et al. West of Scotland Coronary Prevention Study Group (WOSCOPS): prevention of coronary heart disease with pravastatin in men with hypercholesterolemia. N Engl J Med 1995;333:1301–1307.

Design: Prospective, randomized, double-blind, multicenter trial. Primary end point was death from CHD and nonfatal MI. The average follow-up period was 4.9 years.

Purpose: To evaluate the effectiveness of an HMG-CoA reductase inhibitor in preventing events in men with moderate hypercholesterolemia and no history of MI.

Population: 6,544 men aged 45 to 64 years with TC ≥252 mg/dL (mean, 272) and no history of MI.

Treatment: Pravastatin, 40 mg once daily, or placebo.

Results: The pravastatin group had 20% lower TC, 26% lower LDL, 31% fewer coronary events (nonfatal MI, death from CHD; $p < 0.001$), 32% lower cardiovascular mortality ($p = 0.033$), and a nearly significant 22% reduction in overall mortality ($p = 0.051$). The reduction in coronary events was independent of baseline cholesterol level.

32. Colhoun HM, et al.; on behalf of the CARDS investigators. Primary prevention of cardiovascular disease with atorvastatin in type 2 diabetes in the Collaborative Atorvastatin Diabetes Study (CARDS): multicentre randomised placebo-controlled trial. Lancet 2004;364:685–696.

Design: Prospective, randomized, double-blind, multicenter study in the United Kingdom and Ireland. Composite primary end point was time to first acute CHD event, coronary revascularization, or stroke.

Purpose: To compare atorvastatin (10 mg daily) with placebo for the prevention of first major cardiovascular events in patients with diabetes but without clinically evident atherosclerosis.

Population: 2,838 patients aged 40 to 75 with type 2 diabetes, no known CVD, LD ≤ 4.14 mmol/L (160 mg/dL), fasting TG ≤ 6.78 mmol/L (600 mg/dL), and at least one of the following risk factors: retinopathy, albuminuria, current smoking, or HTN.

Exclusion Criteria: HbA1c of 12% or more, elevated creatinine.

Treatment: Atorvastatin 10 mg daily, or placebo.

Results: The trial was stopped 2 years short of the anticipated duration, at the second interim analysis, after a median follow-up of 3.9 years. Atorvastatin was associated with an RRR of 37% in the composite primary end point ($p = 0.001$). This yielded an NNT of 37 to prevent one primary event over 4 years. There was a nonsignificant reduction in death from any cause ($p = 0.059$).

33. Sever PS, et al.; for the ASCOT Investigators. Prevention of coronary and stroke events with atorvastatin in hypertensive patients who have average or lower-than-average cholesterol concentrations in the Anglo-Scandinavian Cardiac Outcomes Trial-Lipid Lowering Arm (ASCOT-LAA): a multicenter randomized controlled trial. *Lancet* 2003;361:1149–1158.

Design: Prospective, randomized, double-blind, multicenter trial. Primary end point was nonfatal MI and fatal CHD. Median follow-up was 3.3 years; the trial was stopped early).

Purpose: To assess the benefits of cholesterol lowering in primary prevention of CHD in hypertensive patients with normal cholesterol levels.

Population: 10,342 of 19,342 total ASCOT patients with TC ≤ 250 mg/dL; all were aged 40 to 79 years and with at least three other cardiac risk factors in addition to HTN.

Exclusion Criteria: Included prior MI, currently treated angina, CVA in past 3 months, and heart failure.

Treatment: Atorvastatin 10 mg or placebo.

Results: The atorvastatin group had 36% fewer primary events compared to placebo (1.9% vs. 3.0%, hazard ratio, 0.64, $p = 0.0005$). This benefit emerged in the first year of follow-up. There were 13% fewer deaths in the atorvastatin group ($p = 0.16$).

Comments: The rest of the trial, which compares amlodipine ± perindopril with atenolol ± bendrofluazide for treating HTN, is reported below (196).

34. Ridker PM, et al.; for the JUPITER Study Group. Rosuvastatin to prevent vascular events in men and women with elevated C-reactive protein. *N Engl J Med* 2008;359:2195–2207.

Design: Prospective, randomized, double-blind, multicenter study. Composite primary end point of MI, stroke, arterial revascularization, hospitalization for unstable angina, or death from cardiovascular causes. Median follow-up was 1.9 years; the trial was stopped early.

Purpose: To compare rosuvastatin (20 mg daily) with placebo for the primary prevention of first major cardiovascular events in apparently healthy men and women with LDL at goal (<130 mg/dL), but elevated hsCRP.

Population: 17,802 men (50 years and older) and women (60 years and older), with no known history of CVD, and LDL cholesterol < 130 mg/dL with hsCRP ≥ 2 mg/L.

Exclusion Criteria: Previous or current lipid-lowering therapy, underlying systemic inflammatory conditions, and current immunosuppressant agents.

Treatment: Rosuvastatin 20 mg daily, or placebo.

Results: The trial was stopped after a median of 1.9 years of follow-up. In the rosuvastatin group, LDL was reduced by 50% and hsCRP by 37%. There was a hazard reduction of 44% for the primary end point in the rosuvastatin group (absolute event rates 0.77 and 1.36 per 100 person-years in the rosuvastatin and placebo groups, respectively; $p < 0.00001$). Each component of the primary end point demonstrated strong reductions, with the end point driven by clinically adverse events: HR was 0.46 for any MI ($p < 0.0002$), 0.52 for any stroke ($p = 0.002$), 0.54 for arterial revascularization ($p < 0.0001$), 0.59 for hospitalization for unstable angina ($p = 0.09$), and 0.80 for death from any cause ($p = 0.02$).

Comments: Importantly, this was a study of using hsCRP to identify an additional population that might benefit from statin therapy, *not* a trial of hsCRP as a *therapeutic goal* of statin therapy. The FDA granted an indication for treatment with rosuvastatin for this patient population, based on this study.

Combination Therapy in the Statin Era

35. Dujovne CA, et al. Ezetimibe Study Group: efficacy and safety of a potent new selective cholesterol absorption inhibitor, ezetimibe, in patients with primary hypercholesterolemia. *Am J Cardiol* 2002;90:1092–1097.

Design: Prospective, randomized, double-blind, placebo-controlled, multicenter trial. Primary end point was the percentage reduction in direct plasma LDL at 12 weeks.

Purpose: To evaluate the safety and efficacy of the new cholesterol absorption inhibitor ezetimibe.

Population: 892 patients with primary hypercholesterolemia.

Exclusion Criteria: MI, CABG surgery, or PTCA in previous 6 months; CHF (NYHA Class III or IV); unstable angina; impaired renal function; hepatobiliary disease.

Treatment: After 2 weeks or more on an NCEP Step I or stricter diet and a 4- to 8-week single-blind placebo lead-in, those with LDL between 130 and 250 mg/dL and TGs $\geq$ 350 mg/dL were randomized in 3:1 fashion to ezetimibe, 10 mg, or placebo each morning for 12 weeks.

Results: Ezetimibe significantly decreased LDL levels by 17%, compared with a 0.4% increase with placebo ($p < 0.01$). The LDL-lowering effect occurred early (2 weeks) and persisted throughout the 12-week treatment period. Ezetimibe also significantly improved calculated LDL, apolipoprotein B, TC, TGs, and HDL ($p < 0.01$). Ezetimibe was well tolerated: compared with placebo, no differences were seen in laboratory parameters, or GI, liver, or muscle side effects.

36. Davidson MH, et al. Ezetimibe coadministered with simvastatin in patients with primary hypercholesterolemia. *J Am Coll Cardiol* 2002;40:2125–2134.

After dietary stabilization, a 2- to 12-week washout period, and a 4-week, single-blind, placebo lead-in period, 591 patients with baseline LDL between 145 and 250 mg/dL and TGs $\geq$ 350 mg were randomized to 1 of 10 treatments administered daily for 12 consecutive weeks: ezetimibe, 10 mg; simvastatin, 10, 20, 40, or 80 mg; ezetimibe, 10 mg plus simvastatin 10, 20, 40, or 80 mg; or placebo. Ezetimibe plus simvastatin resulted in LDL reductions of 44% to 57%, TG reductions of 20% to 28%, and HDL increases of 8% to 11%, depending on the simvastatin dose. Compared with simvastatin alone, ezetimibe and simvastatin significantly improved LDL (13.8% incremental reduction; $p < 0.01$), HDL (2.4% increase; $p = 0.03$), and TG (7.5% reduction; $p < 0.01$). Coadministration of ezetimibe with simvastatin was well tolerated and comparable with that of simvastatin alone.

37. Kastelein JJP, et al.; for the ENHANCE Investigators. Simvastatin with or without ezetimibe in familial hypercholesterolemia. *N Engl J Med* 2008;358:1431–1443.

Design: Prospective, randomized, double-blind, multicenter trial. Primary end point was the change in the mean carotid artery intima–media thickness at 24 months.

Purpose: To assess the effect on progression of atherosclerosis with the addition of ezetimibe to simvastatin in patients with familial hypercholesterolemia.

Population: A total of 720 men and women, ages 30 to 75 (average 46), with familial hypercholesterolemia and LDL cholesterol > 210 mg/dL off lipid-lowering therapy.

Exclusion Criteria: Severe carotid artery disease or previous carotid revascularization, homozygous familial hypercholesterolemia, severe heart failure, arrhythmia, or recent cardiovascular event.

Treatment: Simvastatin, 80 mg/day, plus ezetimibe, 10 mg/day, or simvastatin, 80 mg/day, plus placebo.

Results: Despite a significant reduction in mean LDL level in the simvastatin–ezetimibe group compared to the simvastatin alone group (192.7 mg/dL vs. 141.3 mg/dL; $p < 0.01$), there was no significant change in carotid artery intima–media thickness (0.0058 mm in simvastatin only vs. 0.0111 mm in simvastatin plus ezetimibe, $p = 0.29$).

38. The ACCORD Study Group. Effects of combination lipid therapy in type 2 diabetes. N Engl J Med 2010;362:1563–1574.

Design: Multicenter, randomized, placebo-controlled trial. Primary end point was cardiovascular death, MI, or stroke at mean follow-up of 4.7 years.

Purpose: To assess the impact of fenofibrate for cardiovascular prevention, as supplemental therapy to a statin.

Population: 5,518 patients with type 2 diabetes mellitus.

Treatment: Simvastatin, plus either fenofibrate or placebo.

Results: Annual rates of the primary end point were 2.2% and 2.4% in the fenofibrate and placebo groups, respectively ($p = 0.32$). However, prespecified subgroup analyses did show heterogeneity of these effects, particularly according to sex, and possibly those with hypertriglyceridemia and low HDL cholesterol.

39. Cannon CP, et al.; The IMProved Reduction of Outcomes: Vytorin Efficacy International Trial (IMPROVE-IT) Investigators. Comparison of ezetimibe/simvastatin versus simvastatin monotherapy on cardiovascular outcomes in patients with acute coronary syndromes. Am Heart J 2008;156(5):826–832.

This randomized trial assigned 18,144 patients at high risk following ACS to either ezetimibe/simvastatin 10/40 mg or simvastatin monotherapy 40 mg, with subsequent titration of simvastatin to LDL <79 mg/dL. The primary end point was a composite of cardiovascular death, MI, coronary revascularization (more than 30 days postrandomization), or rehospitalization for unstable angina at mean follow-up of 6 years. Preliminary results presented at the American Heart Association Scientific Sessions demonstrated a significant reduction in the primary end point in the ezetimibe arm (32.7% vs. 34.7%, HR 0.94, 95% CI, 0.89 to 0.99; $p = 0.016$). Among components of the primary composite end point, MI (13.1% vs. 14.8%, $p = 0.002$), stroke (4.2% vs. 4.8%, $p = 0.05$), and ischemic stroke (3.4% vs. 4.1%, $p = 0.008$) were also significantly reduced with ezetimibe. There were no significant differences in all-cause or cardiovascular mortality.

SECONDARY PREVENTION

Placebo-Controlled Trials

40. Coronary Drug Project. Coronary Drug Project Research Group: clofibrate and niacin in coronary heart disease. JAMA 1975;231:360–381.

Design: Prospective, randomized, multicenter study. Primary end point was all-cause mortality. Mean follow-up was 74 months.

Purpose: To evaluate the effects of clofibrate and niacin on cholesterol levels and major cardiac events.

Population: 8,341 men aged 30 to 64 years with ECG-documented prior MI.

Treatment: Clofibrate, 1.8 g/day, niacin, 3 g/day, or placebo.

Results: The clofibrate group had a nonsignificant 6% decrease in TC and 7% fewer MIs; niacin group had a 10% decrease in TC, 26% lower TGs, and a significant decrease in nonfatal MIs (but not fatal MIs).

Comments: At 15-year follow-up, the niacin group had a significant 11% mortality reduction compared with placebo (52.0% vs. 58.2%; $p = 0.0004$).

41. Brown G, et al.; Familial Atherosclerosis Treatment Study (FATS). Regression of coronary artery disease as a result of intensive lipid-lowering therapy in men with high levels of apolipoprotein B. N Engl J Med 1990;323:1289–1298.

This prospective, randomized, double-blind, placebo-controlled (or colestipol-controlled), multicenter study enrolled 146 men with documented CAD and family history of CAD. Patients were assigned to (a) lovastatin, 20 mg twice daily, and colestipol, 5 mg three times daily, for 10 days initially and then increased to 20 g three times daily; (b) niacin, 125 mg twice daily initially, gradually increased to 1 g four times daily at 2 months, and colestipol; or (c) placebo plus colestipol only if LDL was elevated. At 2.5 years' follow-up, group c (conventional therapy) had minimal changes in LDL and HDL (–7% and +5%, respectively), whereas the changes were substantial in the treatment groups: colestipol and lovastatin, –46% and +15%, and niacin and colestipol, –32% and +43%. Lesion progression in one of nine proximal coronary segments was seen in 46% of the conventional group, compared with 21% and 25% in treatment groups a and b, respectively. Lesion regression was more frequently observed in the treatment groups (32% and 39% vs. 11%). Clinical events (death, MI, revascularization for worsening symptoms) occurred significantly less often in the treatment groups (6.5% and 4.2% vs. 19.2%).

42. Scandinavian Simvastatin Survival Study Group (4S). Randomised trial of cholesterol lowering in 4444 patients with coronary heart disease: the 4S. *Lancet* 1994;344:1383–1389.

Design: Prospective, randomized, double-blind, placebo-controlled, multicenter study. Primary end point was all-cause mortality. Median follow-up period was 5.4 years.

Purpose: To evaluate whether simvastatin would improve survival of patients with CHD.

Population: 4,444 patients aged 35 to 70 years with angina pectoris or previous MI (≥6 months earlier) and TC between 5.5 and 8.0 mmol/L (213 and 309 mg/dL).

Exclusion Criteria: Unstable angina, secondary hypercholesterolemia, planned CABG, or angioplasty.

Treatment: Simvastatin, 20 to 40 mg once daily, or placebo.

Results: At the end of the follow-up period, the simvastatin group had 25% lower TC, 35% lower LDL, and 8% higher HDL levels; simvastatin-treated patients had a significant 30% RRR in overall mortality (8.2% vs. 11.5%; $p = 0.0003$) as well as 39% fewer nonfatal MIs (7.4% vs. 12.1%), 41% fewer IHD deaths (5.0% vs. 8.5%), and 34% fewer coronary revascularization procedures (11.3% vs. 17.2%). A 35% risk reduction was even noted among patients in the lowest quartile of baseline LDL. Cost analysis showed that simvastatin-treated patients had 34% fewer cardiovascular-related hospital days and that there was $3,872 savings/patient.

43. Sacks FM, et al. Cholesterol and Recurrent Events (CARE): the effect of pravastatin on coronary events after MI in patients with average cholesterol levels. *N Engl J Med* 1996;335:1001–1009.

Design: Prospective, randomized, double-blind, placebo-controlled, multicenter study. Primary end point was CHD death and nonfatal MI. Median follow-up period was 5 years.

Purpose: To study the effectiveness in a typical population of lowering LDL levels to prevent coronary events after MI.

Population: 4,159 patients with MI within the prior 3 to 20 months, TC < 240 mg/dL (mean, 209) and LDL between 115 and 174 mg/dL (mean, 139).

Exclusion Criteria: EF < 25%; fasting glucose > 220 mg/dL; symptomatic HF.

Treatment: Pravastatin, 40 mg once daily, or placebo.

Results: The pravastatin group had 24% fewer cardiac deaths and nonfatal MIs (10.2% vs. 13.2%; $p = 0.003$), 26% lower rate of CABG surgery (7.5% vs. 10%; $p = 0.005$), 23% lower rate of balloon angioplasty (8.3% vs. 10.5%; $p = 0.03$), 31% fewer strokes ($p = 0.03$), and a nonsignificant reduction in mortality ($p = 0.10$). The reduction in primary events was restricted to those with a baseline LDL ≥ 125 mg/dL (150 to 175 mg/dL, 35% reduction; 125 to 150 mg/dL, 26% reduction; < 125 mg/dL, 3% *increase*). Subsequent analysis found pravastatin use associated with a 32% reduction in stroke ($p = 0.03$) and 27% reduction in stroke or TIA ($p = 0.02$). Another subsequent analysis found that among those with baseline LDL < 125 mg/dL, only diabetics had a significant reduction in primary events (see *Circulation* 2002;105:1424).

44. The Long-term Intervention with Pravastatin in Ischaemic Disease (LIPID) Study Group. Prevention of cardiovascular events and death with pravastatin in patients with coronary heart disease and a broad range of initial cholesterol levels. N Engl J Med 1998;339:1349–1357.

Design: Prospective, randomized, double-blind, placebo-controlled, multicenter study. Primary end point was cardiovascular mortality. Mean follow-up period was 6.1 years.

Purpose: To evaluate the effects of lipid-lowering therapy on overall mortality in patients with a history of CAD and average cholesterol levels.

Population: 9,014 patients aged 31 to 75 years with MI or unstable angina within 3 to 36 months before study entry and an initial TC of 155 to 271 mg/dL.

Exclusion Criteria: Renal or hepatic disease, use of cholesterol-lowering medications, and significant medical or surgical event in prior 3 months.

Treatment: Pravastatin, 40 mg daily, or placebo.

Results: The pravastatin group had significant reduction in death from CHD, 6.4% versus 8.3% (RRR, 24%; $p < 0.001$). Pravastatin patients also had a lower overall mortality rate (11.0% vs. 14.1%; RRR, 22%; $p < 0.001$), fewer MIs (7.4% vs. 10.3%; RRR, 29%; $p < 0.001$), fewer strokes (3.7% vs. 4.5%; RRR, 19%; $p = 0.048$), and less revascularization (13% vs. 15.7%; RRR, 20%; $p < 0.001$). No significant adverse effects were reported with pravastatin.

45. Rubins HB, et al. Gemfibrozil for the secondary prevention of coronary heart disease in men with low levels of high-density lipoprotein cholesterol. Veterans Affairs HDL Cholesterol Intervention Trial (VA-HIT) Study Group. N Engl J Med 1999;341:410–418.

Design: Prospective, randomized, placebo-controlled, double-blind, multicenter study. Primary outcome was a combined incidence of CHD death or nonfatal MI. Mean follow-up was 5.1 years.

Purpose: To evaluate whether increasing HDL cholesterol levels and lowering TG levels would reduce major cardiac events in men with low HDL and LDL cholesterol.

Population: 2,531 men, aged 74 years, with CHD, HDL $\geq$ 40 mg/dL, LDL $\leq$ 140 mg/dL, and TG $\leq$ 300 mg/dL.

Treatment: Gemfibrozil, 1,200 mg once daily, or placebo.

Results: Gemfibrozil therapy did not significantly reduce LDL levels, but did increase HDL by 6% and decrease TG levels by 31% at 1 year. The gemfibrozil group had a significant reduction in CHD-related death or MI (17.3% vs. 21.7%; RRR, 22%; $p = 0.006$). A nonsignificant 10% reduction was noted in all-cause mortality (15.7% vs. 17.4%; $p = 0.23$).

46. Brown BG, et al.; HATS (HDL-Atherosclerosis Treatment Study). Simvastatin and niacin, antioxidant vitamins, or the combination for the prevention of coronary disease. N Engl J Med 2001;345:1583–1592.

Design: Prospective, randomized, double-blind, placebo-controlled trial. Primary end point was mean change per patient in the most severe coronary stenosis from initial to final arteriogram. Primary clinical end point was the occurrence of a first cardiovascular event (death, MI, stroke, or revascularization). Follow-up was 3 years.

Purpose: To determine whether lipid-lowering and antioxidant therapy provide independent and additive benefits for patients with CAD and low HDL levels.

Population: 160 patients with coronary disease (prior MI, coronary interventions, or confirmed angina), low HDL (men, < 35 mg/dL; women, $\leq$ 40 mg/dL), and normal LDL ($\leq$145 mg/dL).

Exclusion Criteria: Previous CABG, severe HTN, and uncontrolled diabetes.

Treatment: Simvastatin plus niacin, simvastatin–niacin plus antioxidants, antioxidant vitamins, or placebos. Placebo niacin was 50 mg active drug to provoke flushing without altering lipids.

Results: In the simvastatin–niacin group, LDL decreased by 42% and HDL increased by 26%; the levels were unchanged in the antioxidant vitamin and placebo groups. The protective increase in HDL with simvastatin plus niacin was attenuated by concurrent therapy with antioxidants. The average stenosis progressed by 3.9% with placebos, 1.8% with antioxidants, and 0.7% with simvastatin–niacin plus antioxidants ($p = 0.004$) and regressed by 0.4% with simvastatin–niacin alone ($p < 0.001$). This study was not powered to evaluate clinical events, but they did observe that the incidence of the composite clinical end point was significantly lower in the simvastatin–niacin–alone group compared with the placebo group (3% vs. 24%; $p = 0.003$); the incidence was an intermediate 14% in simvastatin–niacin plus antioxidants group.

Intensive- Versus Standard-Dose Statin Regimens in Stable CAD

47. LaRosa JC; for the Treating to New Targets (TNT) Investigators. **Intensive lipid lowering with atorvastatin in patients with stable coronary disease.** N Engl J Med 2005;352:1425–1435.

Design: Prospective, randomized, active-controlled, double-blind, multicenter study. Primary outcome was a combined incidence of CHD death, nonfatal MI unrelated to a procedure, resuscitation after cardiac arrest, or any stroke at a median of 4.9 years of follow-up.

Purpose: To examine the effects of lowering LDL cholesterol below 100 mg/dL in patients with stable CHD.

Population: A total of 10,001 patients, ages 35 to 75, with clinically evident CHD (a history of MI, a diagnosis of angina with objective evidence of CHD, or previous coronary revascularization) and LDL < 130 mg/dL.

Treatment: Atorvastatin, 10 mg daily, or 80 mg daily.

Results: Patients receiving atorvastatin 80 mg daily had average LDL cholesterol levels of 77 mg/dL versus 101 mg/dL in the group receiving 10 mg daily. Primary events occurred in 8.7% of patients receiving 80-mg atorvastatin versus 10.9% in the 10-mg group (22% relative reduction, $p < 0.001$). Overall mortality was similar in the two groups; however, there was a significantly higher incidence of liver enzyme elevation in the high-dose group (1.2% vs. 0.2%, $p < 0.001$).

48. Pedersen TR, et al.; for the Incremental Decrease in End Points Through Aggressive Lipid Lowering (IDEAL) Study Group. **High-dose atorvastatin vs. usual-dose simvastatin for secondary prevention after myocardial infarction: the IDEAL Study: a randomized controlled trial.** JAMA 2005;294:2437–2445.

Design: Prospective, randomized, active-controlled, double-blind, multicenter study. Primary outcome was a combined incidence of CHD death, nonfatal MI, or resuscitation after cardiac arrest. Median follow-up was 4.8 years.

Purpose: To compare high-dose atorvastatin versus standard-dose simvastatin for secondary CVD prevention in patients with a previous MI.

Population: A total of 8,888 patients, 80 years or younger, with a history of acute MI.

Treatment: Atorvastatin, 80 mg daily, or simvastatin, 20 mg daily.

Results: Patients receiving atorvastatin had an average LDL of 81 mg/dL versus 104 mg/dL in the group receiving simvastatin. Primary events occurred in 9.3% of patients receiving atorvastatin versus 10.4% in the simvastatin group (HR, 11%, $p = 0.07$). There was a significant reduction in nonfatal MI in the atorvastatin group (7.2% vs. 6.0%, $p = 0.02$); however, there were no significant differences in the risk of overall or cause-specific mortality.

49. Nicholls SJ, et al. Effect of two intensive statin regimens on progression of coronary disease. N Engl J Med 2011;365:2078–2087.

In this cohort study, 1,039 patients with CHD underwent coronary angiography with intravascular ultrasonography at baseline and after 104 weeks of treatment with either atorvastatin, 80 mg daily, or rosuvastatin, 40 mg daily; percent atheroma volume in a given segment of coronary artery was measured before and after treatment. Both maximal statin treatment regimens decreased percent atheroma volume, by 0.99% with atorvastatin and by 1.22% with rosuvastatin.

Early Statin Initiation in ACS

50. Schwartz GG, et al.; for the Myocardial Ischemia Reduction with Aggressive Cholesterol Lowering (MIRACL) study investigators. Effects of atorvastatin on early recurrent ischemic events in acute coronary syndromes: the MIRACL study: a randomized controlled trial. JAMA 2001;285:1711–1718.

Design: Prospective, randomized, double-blind, placebo-controlled, multicenter trial. Primary end point was death, MI, cardiac arrest with resuscitation, or recurrent symptomatic ischemia with objective evidence requiring emergency hospitalization. Follow-up was 4 months.

Purpose: To evaluate the efficacy of early initiation of lipid-lowering therapy with atorvastatin in ACS patients.

Population: 3,086 conservatively managed patients with UA/NSTEMI. Patients had the following: (a) chest pain for longer than 15 minutes at rest or with minimal exertion within 24 hours, and a change from a previous pattern of angina; (b) new or dynamic ST- or T-wave changes, or new wall motion abnormality, or positive noninvasive test; and (c) troponin or CK-MB greater than two times ULN for NSTEMI.

Exclusion Criteria: TC > 270 mg/dL, Q-wave MI within 4 weeks, CABG within 3 months, PCI within 6 months, left bundle branch block (LBBB) or paced rhythm, lipid-lowering drugs other than niacin at doses <500 mg daily, vitamin E (unless <400 IU daily), liver dysfunction, and insulin-dependent diabetes.

Treatment: Randomization within 24 to 96 hours after MI to high-dose atorvastatin (80 mg/day), or matching placebo.

Results: The atorvastatin group had a significant 15% relative reduction in the composite primary end point compared with placebo (14.8% vs. 17.4%; $p = 0.048$), primarily because of fewer recurrent ischemic events with objective evidence (RR, 0.74; $p = 0.02$). No differences were found between the groups in death, MI, or cardiac arrest. Stroke was significantly decreased in the atorvastatin group (RR, 0.41; $p = 0.02$). Lipid levels were decreased by approximately 40% with atorvastatin, but findings were not coupled to degree of lipid lowering. Only 3% had an increase in liver function tests to more than three times normal, and no cases of rhabdomyolysis were observed.

51. Cannon CP, et al.; for the Pravastatin or Atorvastatin Evaluation and Infection Therapy—Thrombolysis in Myocardial Infarction 22 (PROVE-IT TIMI 22) Investigators. Intensive versus moderate lipid lowering with statins after acute coronary syndromes. N Engl J Med 2004;350:1495–1504.

Design: Prospective, randomized, active-controlled, multicenter trial. Primary end point was a composite of death from any cause, MI, documented unstable angina requiring rehospitalization, revascularization (at least 30 days after randomization), and stroke.

Purpose: To establish the *noninferiority* of pravastatin, compared with atorvastatin, with respect to the primary end point over a mean follow-up time of 24 months.

Population: 4,162 men and women over the age of 18 hospitalized for an ACS within the previous 10 days. Enrollment was completed after any revascularization procedure and included patients naive to lipid-lowering therapy (if TC < 240 mg/dL) or those already on lipid-lowering agents (if TC < 200 mg/dL).

Treatment: Pravastatin, 40 mg daily (standard therapy), or atorvastatin, 80 mg daily (intensive therapy).

Results: Mean LDL values were 95 and 62 mg/dL in the standard and intensive therapy groups, respectively ($p < 0.001$). There was a significantly lower rate of the primary event in the intensive therapy group (22.4%) versus the standard therapy group (26.3%), with a 16% hazard reduction ($p = 0.005$).

Comments: This groundbreaking trial helped establish that lower is better for LDL cholesterol.

52. De Lemos JA, et al.; for the A to Z Investigators. Early vs. a delayed conservative simvastatin strategy in patients with acute coronary syndromes. JAMA 2004;292:1307–1316.

Design: Prospective, randomized, double-blind, active-controlled, multicenter trial. Primary end point was a composite of cardiovascular death, nonfatal MI, readmission for ACS, or stroke, over a median of 721 days of follow-up.

Purpose: To assess the advantage of early, intensive initiation of statin therapy in patients with ACS.

Population: 4,497 patients, aged 21 to 80 years, with acute MI (ST or non–ST elevation), with TC ≤ 250 mg/dL, who were not already on statin therapy.

Treatment: Simvastatin, 40 mg daily for 1 month and then 80 mg daily thereafter (intensive group), or placebo for 4 months followed by simvastatin 20 mg daily.

Results: Median LDL cholesterol levels at 8 months were 63 and 77 mg/dL in the intensive and standard therapy groups, respectively. 14.4% of patients in the intensive therapy group and 16.7% of those in the standard therapy group experienced a primary event (HR, 0.89, $p = 0.14$). There was a significant decline in cardiovascular death (4.1% vs. 5.4% favoring intensive therapy, $p = 0.05$), but no statistically significant differences in the remaining end points. Rates of myopathy were significantly higher in the intensive therapy group (9 patients vs. 1 patient in the standard therapy group, $p = 0.02$).

Comments: While this trial did not meet its primary end point, all the trends were consistent with previous and concomitant trials. Additionally, the difference in LDL between the two groups in A to Z was less than that in other trials, so when the trial is assessed based on the degree of lipid lowering, it appears to be consistent with similar trials.

53. Patti G, et al. Atorvastatin pretreatment improves outcomes in patients with acute coronary syndromes undergoing early percutaneous coronary intervention: results of the ARMYDA-ACS randomized trial. J Am Coll Cardiol 2007;49:1272–1278.

Design: Prospective, randomized, double-blind, placebo-controlled, multicenter trial. Primary end point was a composite of death, MI, or unplanned revascularization at 30 days.

Purpose: To determine the advantage, if any, of early, aggressive statin therapy in the setting of PCI for NSTEMI.

Population: 171 patients with NSTEMI undergoing revascularization, who were statin naive.

Treatment: Atorvastatin (80 mg 12 hours before PCI and 40 mg preprocedure), or placebo. All patients received long-term atorvastatin therapy (40 mg daily).

Results: A primary end point event occurred in 5% of patients in the atorvastatin group and 17% of those in the placebo group ($p = 0.01$), driven predominantly by a decreased incidence of recurrent MI. There was also a statistically significant reduction in incidence of postprocedure CK-MB elevation (7% vs. 27%, $p = 0.001$, respectively).

COMBINED PRIMARY AND SECONDARY PREVENTION TRIALS

54. Heart Protection Study (HPS) Collaborative Group. MRC/BHF Heart Protection Study of cholesterol lowering with simvastatin in 20,536 high-risk individuals: a randomised placebo-controlled trial. *Lancet* 2002;360:7–22.

Design: Prospective, randomized, double-blind, placebo-controlled, multicenter trial. Primary end point was mortality and fatal or nonfatal vascular events (for subcategory analyses).

Purpose: To determine whether reducing LDL may reduce the development of vascular disease, irrespective of initial cholesterol concentrations.

Population: 20,536 UK men and women with coronary disease, other occlusive arterial disease, diabetes, or HTN in men older than 65 years.

Exclusion Criteria: Chronic liver disease, impaired renal function, inflammatory muscle disease, and severe heart failure.

Treatment: Simvastatin, 40 mg daily (average compliance, 85%), or matching placebo (average nonstudy statin use, 17%).

Results: The simvastatin group had a significant reduction in all-cause mortality compared with the placebo group (12.9% vs. 14.7%; $p = 0.0003$), because of a highly significant 18% relative reduction in coronary death rate (5.7% vs. 6.9%; $p = 0.0005$), a marginally significant reduction in other vascular deaths (1.9% vs. 2.2%; $p = 0.07$), and a nonsignificant reduction in nonvascular deaths (5.3% vs. 5.6%; $p = 0.4$). Simvastatin was also associated with lower rates of nonfatal MI or coronary death (8.7% vs. 11.8%; $p < 0.0001$), nonfatal or fatal stroke (4.3% vs. 5.7%; $p < 0.0001$), and coronary or noncoronary revascularization (9.1% vs. 11.7%; $p < 0.0001$). The reductions in major events were not significant in the first year, but were then highly significant for each subsequent year. The proportional reduction in the event rate was similar (and significant) in all subcategories, including those with cerebrovascular disease, peripheral arterial disease, diabetes, those either younger than or older than 70 years at entry, and even those who had an initial LDL < 116 mg/dL (3 mmol/L) or TC < 193 mg/dL (5 mmol/L). The annual excess risk of myopathy with this regimen was only about 0.01%. No significant adverse effects on cancer incidence were found.

Comments: This landmark study demonstrated that adding simvastatin safely provides substantial benefits for high-risk patients, regardless of their initial cholesterol concentrations. After making allowance for noncompliance, actual use of this regimen would likely decrease major event rates by about one-third.

55. ALLHAT-LLT (ALLHAT Lipid Lowering Trial): The ALLHAT officers and coordinators for the ALLHAT Collaborative Research Group. Major outcomes in moderately hypercholesterolemic, hypertensive patients randomized to pravastatin versus usual care. *JAMA* 2002;288:2998–3007.

Design: Prospective, randomized, active-controlled, multicenter trial. Primary end point was all-cause mortality. Secondary outcomes included combined nonfatal MI or fatal CHD (CHD events), cause-specific mortality, and cancer. Mean follow-up was 4.8 years.

Purpose: To determine whether pravastatin compared with usual care reduces all-cause mortality in older, moderately hypercholesterolemic, hypertensive participants with at least one additional CHD risk factor.

Population: 10,355 individuals aged 55 years or older, with LDL of 120 to 189 mg/dL (100 to 129 mg/dL if known CHD) and TG < 350 mg/dL. During the trial, 32% of usual-care participants with and 29% without CHD started taking lipid-lowering drugs.

Treatment: Pravastatin, 40 mg/day, or usual care.

Results: At year 4, the pravastatin group had 17% lower TC levels compared with an 8% reduction with usual care. Among those who had LDL assessed, levels were reduced by 28% with pravastatin versus 11% with usual care. All-cause mortality was similar for the two groups (14.9% with pravastatin vs. 15.3% with usual care; $p = 0.88$). A nonsignificant 9% relative reduction was noted in 6-year CHD event rates in the pravastatin group (9.3% vs. 10.4%; RR, 0.91; $p = 0.16$).

Comments: The lack of a significant difference between the usual-care group and those randomized to receive a statin may be explained by the inclusion of statins in the usual-care group for secondary prevention.

56. Keech A; for the FIELD study investigators. **Effects of long-term fenofibrate therapy on cardiovascular events in 9795 people with type 2 diabetes mellitus (the FIELD study): randomised controlled trial.** *Lancet* 2005;366:1849–1861.

Design: Prospective, randomized, placebo-controlled, double-blind, multicenter study. Primary outcome was a combined incidence of CHD death or nonfatal MI.

Purpose: To evaluate the effect of fenofibrate therapy on cardiovascular outcomes in patients with type 2 diabetes and dyslipidemia.

Population: A total of 9,795 patients, ages 50 to 75, with type 2 diabetes mellitus and with a TC concentration of 3.0 to 6.5 mmol/L (116 to 251 mg/dL) and a total cholesterol–HDL cholesterol ratio of 4.0 or more, or plasma TG of 1.0 to 5.0 mmol/L (89 to 443 mg/dL).

Treatment: Fenofibrate, 200 mg daily, or placebo.

Results: In the fenofibrate group, 5.2% experienced a primary event versus 5.9% of patients taking placebo (relative reduction of 11%, $p = 0.16$). There was a significant reduction in the risk of nonfatal MI in the fenofibrate group (24%, $p = 0.010$) and a nonsignificant trend toward increased CHD mortality (19%, $p = 0.22$).

Comments: In the placebo group, more patients began other lipid-lowering therapy (predominantly statins) during the trial than in the fenofibrate group (17% vs. 8%, $p < 0.0001$), making interpretation of the results difficult.

PRIMARY AND SECONDARY PREVENTION TRIALS IN PATIENTS WITH COMORBIDITIES

57. Fellström BC, et al.; for the AURORA Study Group. **Rosuvastatin and cardiovascular events in patients undergoing hemodialysis.** *N Engl J Med* 2009;360: 1395–1407.

Design: Prospective, randomized, placebo-controlled, double-blind, multicenter international study. Primary outcome was a combined incidence of cardiovascular death, nonfatal stroke, and nonfatal MI. Median follow-up was 3.8 years.

Purpose: To assess the efficacy of rosuvastatin in the primary and secondary prevention of cardiovascular events in subjects with end-stage renal disease in hemodialysis.

Population: 2,776 patients, ages 50 to 80, with end-stage renal disease on maintenance hemodialysis. 40% of subjects had known CVD, and the mean LDL at trial entry was 100 mg/dL.

Treatment: Rosuvastatin, 10 mg/day, or placebo

Results: At 3 months, mean LDL was nearly 40 mg/dL lower in the rosuvastatin group than the placebo group ($p < 0.001$); this difference converged somewhat over the course of the study but remained >30 mg/dL. CRP, which was elevated at baseline, was also reduced by 11.5% in the rosuvastatin group compared to no change in the placebo group ($p < 0.001$). Despite this difference in LDL and CRP, the primary end point occurred in similar numbers of patients assigned to each group (9.2 events per 100 patient-years with rosuvastatin vs. 9.5 events per 100 patient-years with placebo; HR, 0.96; 95% CI, 0.84 to 1.11; $p = 0.59$). There was no association between rosuvastatin treatment and any of the components of the primary end point.

58. Kjekshus J, et al.; for the CORONA Group. Rosuvastatin in older patients with systolic heart failure. N Engl J Med 2007;357(22):2248–2261.

Design: Prospective, randomized, placebo-controlled, double-blind, multicenter international study. Primary outcome was a combined incidence of cardiovascular death, nonfatal stroke, and nonfatal MI. Median follow-up was 32.8 months.

Purpose: To assess the efficacy of rosuvastatin in the secondary prevention of cardiovascular events in subjects with ischemic, systolic congestive heart failure.

Population: 5,011 patients, ≥60 years old, with ischemic cardiomyopathy and NYHA Class II, III, or IV symptoms. Mean LDL cholesterol at trial entry was 3.56 mmol/L (138 mg/dL).

Treatment: Rosuvastatin, 10 mg/day, or placebo.

Results: Mean LDL was 45% lower in the rosuvastatin group than the placebo group ($p < 0.001$), and CRP was 37.1% lower ($p < 0.001$). Despite this difference in LDL and CRP, there was no significant difference in the incidence of the primary end point in the two groups, though there was a trend toward a reduction in the rosuvastatin group (HR, 0.92; 95% CI, 0.83 to 1.02; $p = 0.12$). There was a significant reduction in cardiovascular hospitalizations in the rosuvastatin group (2,193 hospitalizations vs. 2,564; $p < 0.001$).

59. GISSI-HF Investigators. Effect of rosuvastatin in patients with chronic heart failure (the GISSI-HF trial): a randomised, double-blind, placebo-controlled trial. Lancet 2008;372:1231–1239.

Design: Prospective, randomized, placebo-controlled, double-blind, multicenter study. Coprimary outcomes were time to death and time to death or cardiovascular hospital admission. Median follow-up was 3.9 years.

Purpose: To assess the efficacy of rosuvastatin in the primary and secondary prevention of cardiovascular events in subjects with congestive heart failure.

Population: 4,574 patients, ≥ 18 years old, with congestive heart failure and NYHA Class II, III, or IV symptoms. Mean age was 68 years, and mean LVEF was 33%; only 10% of patients had LVEF > 40%. CHF was due to ischemic cardiomyopathy in only 40% of patients.

Treatment: Rosuvastatin, 10 mg/day, or placebo.

Results: There was no significant difference in the incidence of either primary end point in the two groups: 29% of patients died in the rosuvastatin group compared to 28% in the placebo group (adjusted HR, 1.00; 95.5% CI, 0.90 to 1.22; $p = 0.943$); 57% of patients died or were hospitalized in the rosuvastatin group compared to 56% in the placebo group (adjusted HR, 1.01; 99% CI, 0.91 to 1.11; $p = 0.903$). In subset analyses, there was no significant difference in the risk of the primary outcome in patients with ischemic cardiomyopathy (HR 1.03) or TC > 4.97 mmol/L (192 mg/dL) (HR 1.00).

Comment: The results of these trials have demonstrated that the beneficial effect of statins seen in secondary prevention and high-risk primary prevention trials may not apply to patients with advanced disease processes such as end-stage renal disease and significant congestive heart failure (see Lancet 2009;9645:1195–1196). The reason for this discrepancy is unclear; however, these data are reflected in the revised trial-based approach to the guidelines (see JAMA 2013;310:1123–1124).

META-ANALYSES AND NONCHOLESTEROL EFFECTS OF STATINS

60. Bucher HC, et al. Systematic review of the risk and benefit of different cholesterol-lowering interventions. Arterioscler Thromb Vasc Biol 1999;19:187–195.

This analysis of 59 randomized controlled trials with 85,431 participants included 13 statin trials, 12 fibrate trials, 8 bile resin trials, 8 hormone trials, 2 niacin trials, 3 n-3 fatty acid trials, and 16 dietary intervention studies. Only statins showed a significant reduction in CHD-related mortality (RRR, 0.66; 95% CI, 0.54 to 0.79) and all-cause mortality rates (RRR, 0.75; 95% CI, 0.65 to 0.86). A meta-regression analysis showed that the variability of results across trials was largely explained by the magnitude of cholesterol reduction.

61. Baigent C, et al. Efficacy and safety of cholesterol lowering treatment: prospective meta-analysis of data from 90,056 participants in 14 randomised trials of statins. *Lancet* 2005;366:1267–1278.

This landmark compilation of 14 trials of statins in CVD, both primary and secondary prevention studies, included 90,056 patients, accruing 8,186 deaths, 14,348 major adverse vascular events, and 5,103 new diagnoses of cancer. Analyses were performed *per unit reduction in LDL*, demonstrating impressive 20% reduction in events per 1 mmol/L (39 mg/dL) reduction, with the absolute events rates related to individual patient characteristics.

62. Cholesterol Treatment Trialists' Collaborators. The effects of lowering LDL cholesterol with statin therapy in people at low risk of vascular disease: meta-analysis of individual data from 27 randomised trials. *Lancet* 2012;380:581–590.

In this meta-analysis, investigators combined data from 22 trials comparing statin to placebo and 5 trials comparing high- to low-dose statin, and stratified participants by 5-year vascular event risk at the time of trial entry. As above, analyses were performed per unit reduction in LDL, demonstrating at least a 19% relative risk reduction for participants at each strata of risk. The benefits were especially pronounced in those participants at the lowest risk of CVD (5-year risk < 5% or 5% to 10%), in whom a 1 mmol/L (39 mg/dL) reduction in LDL produced relative risk reductions of 38% and 31% for major vascular events. Based on these relative risk reductions, the authors calculate that in these low-risk patients (most of whom would not be candidates for statin therapy under current guidelines), a reduction in LDL cholesterol by 1 mmol/L would prevent 11 vascular events per 1,000 patients treated for 5 years and suggest that guidelines for lipid therapy should be revisited.

63. Cannon CP, et al. Meta-analysis of cardiovascular outcomes trials comparing intensive versus moderate statin therapy. *J Am Coll Cardiol* 2006;48(3):438–445.

This analysis of the four major trials (PROVE IT-TIMI 22, A to Z, TNT, IDEAL), totaling 27,548 patients over roughly 4 years' follow-up, demonstrated a significant 16% odds reduction in death or MI, 18% reduction in stroke, and a *trend* (though not significant) in reduced cardiovascular mortality for patients taking high-dose statins as compared with those on standard doses (including various doses of pravastatin, simvastatin, and atorvastatin). An updated meta-analysis (see *Eur Heart J* 2011;32:1409–1415) found similar results, but noted that in a subset analysis of patients with ACS, high-dose statins *did* reduce all-cause mortality (RR, 0.75; 95% CI, 0.61 to 0.91; $p = 0.005$) and cardiovascular mortality (RR, 0.74; 95% CI, 0.59 to 0.94; $p = 0.013$).

64. Ray K, et al. The potential relevance of the multiple lipid-independent (pleiotropic) effects of statins in the management of acute coronary syndromes. *J Am Coll Cardiol* 2005;46:1425–1433.

The culmination of a journal supplement devoted to the many lessons from the PROVE IT-TIMI 22 trial, this review highlights the evidence for, potential mechanisms of, and clinical consequences of the many biochemical effects of statins (independent of the LDL-lowering capacity) in CVD.

65. Sattar, N, et al. Statins and risk of incident diabetes: a collaborative meta-analysis of randomised statin trials. *Lancet* 2010;375(9716):735–742.

Thirteen statin trials of more than 1,000 patients each were identified and combined to assess the incident risk of diabetes in patients receiving statins versus those not. In a total population of 91,140, they identified a 9% increased risk of incident diabetes. This risk tracked with older age patients, but was consistent across trials and independent of LDL levels. The investigators estimate a single additional case of diabetes for every 225 patients treated with statin therapy for 4 years.

66. Ray, KK, et al. Statins and all-cause mortality in high-risk primary prevention: a meta-analysis of 11 randomized controlled trials involving 65,229 participants. *Arch Intern Med* 2010;170(12):1024–1031.

The authors sought to identify the mortality benefit, if any, to statins in high-risk patients without manifest CVD. They combined 11 trials with 65,229 patients totaling 244,000 person-years and 2,793 deaths. Statins were not associated with a significant reduction in all-cause mortality in this population (risk ration 0.91, 95% CI, 0.83 to 1.01).

67. Hackam DG, et al. Statins and intracerebral hemorrhage: collaborative systematic review and meta-analysis. *Circulation* 2011;124:2233–2242.

In this meta-analysis of 19 observational studies and 23 randomized trials involving 248,391 patients, the authors failed to find an association between statin treatment and the incidence of intracerebral hemorrhage.

68. Priess D, et al. Risk of incident diabetes with intensive-dose compared with moderate-dose statin therapy. *JAMA* 2011;305:2556–2664.

This meta-analysis of 5 statin trials comparing moderate-dose to intensive-dose statin therapy (all such trials involving more than 1,000 patients and more than 1-year follow-up) included 32,752 subjects. Over a weighted mean follow-up of 4.9 years, the OR for new-onset diabetes with intensive- versus moderate-dose statin was 1.12 (95% CI, 1.04 to 1.22) and the OR for cardiovascular events with intensive- versus moderate-dose statin was 0.84 (95% CI, 0.75 to 0.94). The NNT with intensive-dose statin for 1 year to prevent one cardiovascular event was 155, and the NNT with intensive-dose statin for 1 year to cause one case of diabetes mellitus was 498.

69. Ridker PM, et al. Cardiovascular benefits and diabetes risks of statin therapy in primary prevention: an analysis from the JUPITER trial. *Lancet* 2012;380: 565–571.

This analysis of the JUPITER trial attempted to determine whether the cardiovascular and mortality benefit of rosuvastatin exceeded the risk of new-onset diabetes. The investigators divided participants into 2 groups: those at high risk of incident diabetes mellitus (those with metabolic syndrome, impaired fasting glucose, obesity, or prediabetes) and those at lower risk. In individuals at low risk of new-onset diabetes mellitus, rosuvastatin reduced the incidence of the trial's primary outcome (a composite of MI, stroke, unstable angina, arterial revascularization, or cardiovascular death) by 52% (95% CI, 32% to 67%; $p = 0.0001$) and did not have an appreciable effect on the incidence of diabetes mellitus. Even in those patients at high risk for the development of new-onset diabetes mellitus, 134 vascular events were avoided for every 54 new cases of diabetes mellitus.

HDL-RAISING THERAPIES

Niacin

70. AIM-HIGH Investigators. Niacin in patients with low HDL cholesterol levels receiving intensive statin therapy. *N Engl J Med* 2011;365:2255–2267.

Design: Randomized, double-blind, placebo-controlled, multicenter study. The primary end point was the first event of a composite of cardiovascular death, nonfatal MI, stroke, hospitalization for ACS, or symptom-driven cerebral or coronary revascularization. Mean follow-up was 3 years before the trial was stopped due to lack of efficacy.

Purpose: To evaluate the effectiveness of extended-release niacin in the secondary prevention of cardiovascular events in patients at goal on LDL-lowering therapy.

Population: 3,414 patients with established vascular disease (stable CAD, cerebrovascular disease, or peripheral vascular disease) treated with simvastatin plus ezetimibe to maintain LDL cholesterol levels between 40 and 80 mg/dL.

Intervention: Extended-release niacin, 1,500 to 2000 mg daily, or matching placebo containing 50-mg niacin to produce flushing and blind patients and study personnel to treatment class.

Results: Niacin effectively increased HDL (from 35 to 42 mg/dL) and lowered TGs, but there was no difference in clinical events between the two groups: 16.4% of patients in the niacin group reached the primary end point compared to 16.2% of patients in the placebo group.

Comment: Though this trial and the HPS2-THRIVE randomized trial failed to show a clinical benefit with the addition of niacin to a statin-based regimen, some have argued that both trials evaluated extended-release niacin, and the cardiovascular benefits of niacin may be limited to the immediate release form.

71. HPS2-THRIVE Collaborative Group. HPS2-THRIVE randomized placebo-controlled trial in 25,673 high-risk patients of ER niacin/laropiprant: trial design, prespecified muscle and liver outcomes, and reasons for stopping study treatment. *Eur Heart J* 2013;34:1279–1291.

Design: Randomized, double-blind, placebo-controlled, multicenter study. The primary end point was the time to first major vascular event—a composite of cardiovascular death, arterial revascularization, stroke, or nonfatal MI. Mean follow-up was 3.9 years before the trial was stopped due to excessive risk of side effects and treatment discontinuation in the niacin group.

Purpose: To evaluate the effectiveness of extended-release niacin plus lapropitant, a prostaglandin D2 receptor inhibitor, in the secondary prevention of cardiovascular events.

Population: 42,424 patients with stable CAD, cerebrovascular disease, or peripheral vascular disease treated with simvastatin with or without ezetimibe to maintain TC levels < 3.5 mmol/L (135 mg/dL).

Intervention: Extended-release niacin 1 g plus 20-mg lapropitant daily, escalating to extended-release niacin 2 g plus 40-mg lapropitant daily during the prerandomization phase, or matching placebo.

Results: At 3.9-year follow-up, 25.4% of patients randomized to niacin/lapropitant had stopped study treatment due to side effects, compared to 16.9% randomized to placebo. In combination with simvastatin with or without ezetimibe, extended-release niacin plus lapropitant increased the risk of treatment stoppage due to adverse reaction involving the skin (5.4% vs. 1.2%; $p < 0.0001$), gastrointestinal tract (3.9% vs. 1.7%; $p < 0.0001$), and musculoskeletal system (1.8% vs. 1.0%; $p < 0.0001$). Definite myopathy was increased 4.4-fold (95% CI, 2.6 to 7.5; $p < 0.0001$) in the group taking extended-release niacin plus lapropitant. The efficacy results were published separately (see below).

72. Landray MJ, et al.; HPS2-THRIVE Collaborative Group. Effects of extended-release niacin with laropiprant in high-risk patients. *N Engl J Med* 2014;371(3): 203–212.

This separate publication subsequently detailed the efficacy outcomes of the HPS2-THRIVE trial. Extended-release niacin–laropiprant led to an average 10 mg/dL lower LDL cholesterol level and an average 6 mg/dL higher HDL cholesterol level, compared to placebo. However, there was no significant difference in major vascular events (13.2% for niacin–laropiprant vs. 13.7% for placebo; rate ratio, 0.96; 95% CI, 0.90 to 1.03; $p = 0.29$).

CETP Inhibitors

73. Chapman MJ, et al. Cholesterol ester transfer protein: at the heart of the action of lipid-modulating therapy with statins, fibrates, niacin, and cholesteryl ester transfer protein inhibitors. *Eur Heart J* 2010;31:149–164.

This review describes the mechanism by which CETP contributes to dyslipidemia and presents data regarding the elevation of CETP in clinical states related to the metabolic syndrome. It notes the CETP-modulating effects of existing classes of lipid-modifying medications and compares these effects to the direct CETP inhibitors.

74. Kastelein JJP, et al.; for the RADIANCE Investigators. Effect of torcetrapib on carotid atherosclerosis in familial hypercholesterolemia. *N Engl J Med* 2007;356:1620–1630.

Design: Prospective, randomized, double-blind, placebo-controlled, multicenter trial. Primary end point was a measure of increase in maximum carotid intima–media thickness, as assessed by ultrasonography, at baseline and at 2 years of follow-up.

Purpose: This was an early clinical trial of HDL-increasing therapy with torcetrapib, a novel CETP inhibitor, using carotid intima–media thickness as a surrogate clinical end point.

Population: 850 patients with heterozygous familial hypercholesterolemia.

Treatment: Atorvastatin monotherapy versus atorvastatin with torcetrapib 60 mg daily.

Results: There was a significant difference in HDL levels between the two groups, 52.4 mg/dL in the atorvastatin monotherapy group versus 81.5 mg/dL in the combination therapy group. However, there was no significant difference in progression of carotid intima–media thickness in the two groups, 0.0053 mm per year in the atorvastatin monotherapy group versus 0.0047 mm per year in the torcetrapib–atorvastatin group ($p = 0.87$).

Comment: As confirmed in later studies, there was a significantly higher increase in SBP in the group receiving torcetrapib (1.3 mm Hg in the atorvastatin-only group and 4.1 mm Hg in the torcetrapib–atorvastatin group, $p < 0.001$).

75. Nissen SE, et al.; for the ILLUSTRATE Investigators. Effect of torcetrapib on the progression of coronary atherosclerosis. *N Engl J Med* 2007;356:1304–1316.

Design: Prospective, randomized, double-blind, placebo-controlled, multicenter trial. Primary end point was percent atheroma volume as measured by intravascular ultrasonography at baseline and after 2 years of follow-up.

Purpose: To assess the effect of torcetrapib on progression of coronary atherosclerosis, as measured by intravascular coronary ultrasound.

Population: 1,188 patients with known CAD.

Treatment: Torcetrapib 60 mg daily, or placebo; all patients were on atorvastatin therapy to target LDL < 100 mg/dL.

Results: Patients taking torcetrapib had significantly higher HDL levels, by nearly 60%, and lower LDL levels (by 20%). The percent atheroma volume increased in both groups, by 0.19% in the placebo group versus 0.12% in the torcetrapib group ($p = 0.72$).

Comment: Once again, torcetrapib was associated with a significant rise in blood pressure.

76. Barter PJ, et al.; for the ILLUMINATE Investigators. Effects of torcetrapib in patients at high risk for coronary events. *N Engl J Med* 2007;357:2109–2122.

Design: Prospective, randomized, double-blind, placebo-controlled, multicenter trial. Primary end point was a composite of death from CHD, nonfatal MI, stroke, or hospitalization for unstable angina over median follow-up of 550 days.

Purpose: A study of torcetrapib for prevention of MACE in high-risk patients.

Population: 15,067 patients with stable CVD or type 2 diabetes.

Treatment: Torcetrapib 60 mg daily, or placebo; all patients were on atorvastatin therapy to target LDL < 100 mg/dL.

Results: Patients taking torcetrapib had significantly higher HDL levels, by nearly 72.1%, and lower LDL levels (by 24.9%) at 12 months. However, there was a significantly higher rate of cardiovascular events (hazard ratio, 1.25, $p = 0.001$) and all-cause mortality (hazard ratio, 1.58, $p = 0.006$) in the *torcetrapib* group, compared with placebo (atorvastatin only). These were accompanied by significant decreases in serum potassium and increases in serum sodium, bicarbonate, and aldosterone.

Comment: Development of torcetrapib was subsequently abandoned.

77. Schwartz GG, et al.; for the dal-OUTCOMES Investigators. Effects of dalcetrapib in patients with a recent acute coronary syndrome. N Engl J Med 2012;367:2089–2099.

Design: Prospective, randomized, double-blind, placebo-controlled, multicenter trial. Primary end point was a composite of death from CHD, nonfatal MI, stroke, unstable angina, or resuscitated cardiac arrest.

Purpose: To evaluate the efficacy of dalcetrapib for the secondary prevention of cardiovascular events.

Population: 15,871 patients, age 45 or older, with ACS within the previous 6 months (mean: 61 days).

Treatment: Dalcetrapib 600 mg daily, or placebo; in addition to evidence-based post-ACS care (including statin in 97%).

Results: HDL cholesterol levels increased by 31% to 40% in the dalcetrapib group, compared to 4% to 11% in the placebo group. LDL levels were minimally affected by dalcetrapib, and SBPs were only 0.6 mm Hg higher in the dalcetrapib group compared to the usual-care group. However, dalcetrapib did not affect the risk of the primary end point (HR, 1.04; 95% CI, 0.93 to 1.16; $p = 0.52$) or any of its components.

Comment: The failure of the CETP inhibitors torcetrapib and dalcetrapib to produce meaningful improvements in clinical end points despite a favorable effect on lipid profiles remains poorly understood. Other CETP inhibitors, including anacetrapib and evacetrapib (see below), are in development.

78. Cannon CP, et al.; for the Determining Safety and Tolerability Investigators. Safety of anacetrapib in patients with or at high risk for coronary heart disease. N Engl J Med 2010;363:2406–2415.

Design: Prospective, randomized, double-blind, placebo-controlled, multicenter trial. Primary end points were the percent change from baseline in LDL at 24 weeks and the side effect and safety profile through 76 weeks.

Purpose: To evaluate the safety of anacetrapib, a novel CETP inhibitor, in primary and secondary prevention.

Population: 1,623 patients, 18 to 80 years old, with known stable CAD or 10-year Framingham Risk Score > 20%; all patients were taking a statin and had LDL between 50 and 100 mg/dL and HDL < 60 mg/dL.

Treatment: Anacetrapib, 100 mg daily, or placebo.

Results: At 24 weeks, LDL decreased from 81 to 45 mg/dL in the anacetrapib group and from 82 to 77 mg/dL in the control group ($p < 0.001$). Over the same time frame, HDL increased from 41 to 101 mg/dL in the anacetrapib group and from 40 to 46 mg/dL in the control group, a 138.1% increase in the anacetrapib group beyond that seen with placebo ($p < 0.001$). No changes in blood pressure or electrolytes were seen with anacetrapib compared with placebo. The trial was not powered to detect clinical end points.

79. Nicholls SJ, et al. Effects of the CETP inhibitor evacetrapib administered as monotherapy or in combination with statins on HDL and LDL cholesterol: a randomized controlled trial. *JAMA* 2011;306:2099–2109.

Design: Prospective, randomized, double-blind, placebo-controlled, multicenter trial. Coprimary end points were the percent change from baseline in LDL and HDL at 12 weeks of treatment.

Purpose: To evaluate the safety, tolerability, and effect on lipid profiles of evacetrapib, a novel CETP inhibitor.

Population: 398 patients with elevated LDL (based on NCEP ATP III goal) or low HDL (<45 mg/dL in men or <55 mg/dL in women).

Treatment: Evacetrapib at varying doses (30 mg, 100 mg, or 500 mg daily), evacetrapib 100 mg daily plus a statin (simvastatin 40, atorvastatin 30, or rosuvastatin 10 mg daily), statin alone, or placebo.

Results: Treatment with evacetrapib alone led to dose-dependent increases in HDL of 53.6% to 128.8%, compared to essentially no change with placebo ($p < 0.001$), and dose-dependent decreases in LDL of 13.6% to 35.9%, compared to an increase by 7.2 mg/dL with placebo ($p < 0.001$). When combined with a statin, evacetrapib 100 mg daily led to increases in HDL of 78.5% to 88.5% (variability was dependent on the statin used) and decreases in LDL of 11.2% to 13.9% ($p < 0.001$ compared to statin alone). The trial was not powered to detect clinical end points, but no adverse effects were noted.

Meta-analyses and General Studies

80. Briel M, et al. Association between change in high density lipoprotein cholesterol and cardiovascular disease morbidity and mortality: systematic review and meta-regression analysis. *BMJ* 2009;338:b92.

This meta-analysis of 108 trials of lipid therapy, measuring HDL and clinical outcomes, involved 299,310 patients at risk of CVD. After adjusting for LDL levels, they found little variability in outcomes with respect to HDL levels. While reducing LDL demonstrated a strong relationship with reduced clinical events, increasing HDL levels did not correlate with clinical improvements. Importantly, this analysis did not differentiate among the treatments used to increase HDL, and many different interventions were included in the group of studies.

81. Khera AV, et al. Cholesterol efflux capacity, high-density lipoprotein function, and atherosclerosis. *N Engl J Med* 2011;13:127–135.

The authors measured cholesterol efflux capacity, an indicator of HDL function, in 442 patients with angiographically confirmed CHD and 351 patients without CAD. They found that higher cholesterol efflux capacity was associated with a lower likelihood of CAD independent of HDL level. This study strengthened claims that HDL level is a less important determinant of atherosclerosis than HDL function, perhaps partly explaining the failure of HDL-raising therapies to meaningfully prevent adverse clinical outcomes.

NOVEL CLASSES OF LIPID-LOWERING AGENTS

82. Roth EM, et al. Atorvastatin with or without an antibody to PCSK9 in primary hypercholesterolemia. *N Engl J Med* 2012;367:1891.

Design: Placebo-controlled, double-blind, randomized, multicenter clinical trial. The primary outcome measure was percent change in LDL cholesterol.

Purpose: To assess safety and efficacy of a novel PCSK9 antibody in patients with hypercholesterolemia.

Population: 92 patients with primary hypercholesterolemia and LDL > 100 mg/dL despite atorvastatin treatment.

Treatment: Oral atorvastatin plus subcutaneous injection of SAR236553, a human monoclonal antibody to PCSK9, or atorvastatin plus placebo.

Results: After 8 weeks of treatment, LDL cholesterol was reduced by 73% in the atorvastatin plus SAR236553 group versus 17% in the atorvastatin plus placebo group. All of the patients who received atorvastatin plus SAR236553 reached an LDL level < 100 mg/dL, compared to 52% of patients who received atorvastatin plus placebo.

Comment: Renamed alirocumab, SAR236553 was further tested in the Long-term Safety and Tolerability of Alirocumab in High Cardiovascular Risk Patients with Hypercholesterolemia Not Adequately Controlled with Their Lipid Modifying Therapy (ODYSSEY LONG TERM) study, and demonstrated significant lipid-lowering effect with the suggestion of reduced clinical events (see *N Engl J Med.* 2015 Apr 16;372(16):1489–1499).

83. Giugliano RP, et al.; for the LAPLACE-TIMI 57 Investigators. Efficacy, safety, and tolerability of a monoclonal antibody to protein convertase subtilisin/kexin type 9 in combination with a statin in patients with hypercholesterolaemia (LAPLACE-TIMI 57): a randomised, placebo-controlled, dose-ranging, phase 2 study. *Lancet* 2012;380:2007–2017.

Design: Double-blind, placebo-controlled, international, multicenter randomized trial.

Purpose: To assess safety and efficacy of AMG145, a monoclonal antibody to PCSK9.

Population: 631 patients with LDL > 85 mg/dL on a stable dose of statin (with or without ezetimibe).

Treatment: Varying doses of AMG145 (70 mg, 105 mg, or 140 mg) administered subcutaneously every 2 or every 4 weeks, or to matching placebo.

Results: Mean LDL concentrations were decreased by AMG145 in a dose-dependent manner, with reductions ranging from 41.8% to 66.1% (50 to 78 mg/dL; $p < 0.0001$). Lipoprotein(a) concentrations were also reduced by AMG145 in a dose-dependent manner (see *Circulation* 2013;128:962–969). This larger study replicated the results of smaller studies in statin-intolerant patients (see *JAMA* 2012;308:2497–2506 and *Lancet* 2012;380:1995–2006).

Comment: AMG145, renamed evulocumab, was subsequently shown to reduce LDL over the long-term with potentially improved clinical outcomes in pooled analyses of the OSLER-1 and OSLER-2 trials (Open-Label Study of Long-Term Evaluation against LDL Cholesterol; see *N Engl J Med.* 2015 Apr 16;372(16):1500–1509).

84. Ladenson PW, et al. Use of the thyroid hormone analogue eprotirome in statin-treated dyslipidemia. *N Engl J Med* 2010;362(10):906–916.

Design: Randomized, placebo-controlled, double-blind multicenter trial.

Purpose: To assess the safety and efficacy of KB2115, a thyroid hormone analogue eprotirome.

Population: 189 patients with hyperlipidemia (LDL $\geq$ 116 mg/dL) despite statin treatment.

Treatment: Thyromimetic drug eprotirome at varying doses (25 μg, 50 μg, or 100 μg daily) or matching placebo for a 12-week treatment course.

Results: At the end of follow-up, patients treated with placebo, 25 μg eprotirome daily, 50 μg eprotirome daily, and 100 μg eprotirome daily had reductions in LDL by 7%, 22%, 28%, and 32% respectively. The trial was not powered to detect clinical outcomes, but no adverse effects were noted on the thyroid, heart, or bone.

85. Stein EA, et al. Apolipoprotein B synthesis inhibition with mipomersen in heterozygous familial hypercholesterolemia: results of a randomized, double-blind, placebo-controlled trial to assess efficacy and safety as add-on therapy in patients with coronary artery disease. *Circulation* 2012;126:2283–2292.

Design: Prospective, double-blind, placebo-controlled, multicenter randomized study. Patients were treated for 26 weeks, and the primary end point was change in LDL cholesterol at week 28.

Purpose: Assessment of safety and efficacy of mipomersen.

Population: 124 patients with heterozygous familial hyperlipidemia and LDL ≥ 100 mg/dL despite maximally tolerated statin for at least 12 weeks.

Treatment: 200 mg mipomersen, an inhibitor of apolipoprotein B synthesis injected subcutaneously each week, or matching placebo.

Results: LDL decreased by 28% with mipomersen compared to a 5% increase with placebo ($p < 0.001$). Mipomersen also effectively decreased Lp(a). It was, however, associated with elevations in ALT, increased hepatic fat, and influenza-like symptoms at the time of injection. The study was not powered to detect clinical end points. Separate placebo-controlled trials in 33 statin-intolerant patients (see *Eur Heart J* 2012;33:1142–1149) and 76 patients on stable statin therapy (see *J Am Coll Cardiol* 2010;55:1611–1618) demonstrated similar results.

86. Ballantyne, CM, et al. Efficacy and safety of a novel dual modulator of adenosine triphosphate-citrate lyase and adenosine monophosphate-activated protein kinase in patients with hypercholesterolemia: results of a multicenter, randomized, double-blind, placebo-controlled parallel-group trial. *J Am Coll Cardiol* 2013;62:1154–1162.

Design: Randomized, placebo-controlled, double-blind trial.

Purpose: To assess the safety and efficacy of ETC-1002, a small molecule modifier or lipid metabolism, in patients with hyperlipidemia.

Population: 177 patients with hyperlipidemia (LDL, 130 to 220 mg/dL).

Treatment: The novel small molecule ETC-1002 at varying doses or matching placebo for a 12-week treatment course.

Results: At the end of follow-up, patients treated with placebo, ETC-1002 40 mg, ETC-1002 80 mg, and ETC-1002 120 mg had reductions in LDL by 2.2%, 17.9%, 25%, and 26.6%, respectively ($p < 0.0001$ for all doses of ETC-1002 compared to placebo). ETC-1002 did not substantially change HDL or TGs. The trial was not powered to detect clinical end points, but adverse event rates were similar in all groups.

Antioxidants, Vitamins, Fish Oil, Chelation, and Hormones

OBSERVATIONAL STUDIES

87. Tomson J, et al. Vitamin D and risk of death from vascular and non-vascular causes in the Whitehall study and meta-analyses of 12,000 deaths. *Eur Heart J* 2013;34:1365–1374.

In this prospective survey of 5,409 elderly British men (mean baseline age 77 years) followed for 13 years, levels of 25-hydroxyvitamin D at baseline were inversely correlated with vascular and nonvascular mortality. After adjustment for confounders, a doubling in baseline 25-hydroxyvitamin D levels was associated with a relative risk of 0.80 (95% CI, 0.70 to 0.91) for 13-year vascular mortality and a relative risk of 0.77 (95% CI, 0.69 to 0.86) for 13-year nonvascular mortality in this elderly population.

88. Stampfer MJ, et al. Postmenopausal estrogen therapy and cardiovascular disease. *N Engl J Med* 1991;325:756–762.

This prospective cohort study was composed of 48,470 postmenopausal women without prior CVD or cancer. After adjustment for risk factors, at an average follow-up of 7 years, estrogen patients had a significant 11% lower total mortality, 28% lower cardiovascular mortality, and 44% RRR in the incidence of major coronary disease. No significant difference was found in stroke rates.

89. Grodstein F, et al. Postmenopausal estrogen and progestin use and the risk of cardiovascular disease. N Engl J Med 1996;335:453–461.

This prospective cohort analysis focused on 59,337 NHS participants who were aged 30 to 55 years and free of known CVD at baseline. At an average follow-up of 11.2 years, combined estrogen and progestin users had a lower incidence of major CHD (MI, death) compared with nonhormone and estrogen-only users (adjusted RRs, 0.39 and 0.60).

90. Lidegaard Ø, et al. Thrombotic stroke and myocardial infarction with hormonal contraception. N Engl J Med 2012;366:2257.

This cohort study examined 15 years of historical data regarding the rates of stroke and MI in nonpregnant Danish women without CVD, aged 15 to 49 years, both on and off hormonal contraception. Though the study found that the absolute rates of MI (10.1 per 100,000 person-years) and thrombotic stroke (21.4 per 100,000 years) were low, these rates were increased by a factor of 0.9 to 1.7 with low-dose ethinyl estrogen (20 μg daily) and by a factor of 1.3 to 2.3 with high-dose ethinyl estrogen (30 to 40 μg daily). The clinical significance of this increase is not clear.

CLINICAL TRIALS

91. Cambridge Heart Antioxidant Study (CHAOS). Randomised controlled trial of vitamin E in patients with coronary artery disease: CHAOS. Lancet 1996;347:781–786.

Design: Prospective, randomized, double-blind, placebo-controlled, single-center study. Primary end points were nonfatal MI and cardiovascular death plus nonfatal MI. The median follow-up period was 510 days.

Purpose: To evaluate whether high-dose α-tocopherol would reduce subsequent risk of MI and cardiovascular death in patients with known CAD.

Population: 2,002 patients with angiographically proven coronary atherosclerosis.

Exclusion Criteria: Prior use of vitamin supplements containing vitamin E.

Treatment: Vitamin E, 400 IU/day or 800 IU/day, or placebo.

Results: The treatment group had significant reduction in cardiovascular death and nonfatal MI (RR, 0.53; 95% CI, 0.34 to 0.083; $p = 0.005$). The beneficial effects on this composite end point were due to the 66% fewer nonfatal MIs (14 vs. 41 patients; $p = 0.005$); no difference in cardiovascular deaths was detected (27 vs. 23 patients; $p = 0.61$).

92. The Heart Outcome Prevention Evaluation (HOPE) Study Investigators. Vitamin E supplementation and cardiovascular events in high risk patients. N Engl J Med 2000;342:154–160.

This prospective, randomized, 2 × 2 factorial study of 9,541 high-risk patients aged 55 years or older with CAD, stroke, PVD, or diabetes plus one other cardiac risk factor included a randomization to vitamin E (400 IU daily) or placebo. Vitamin E supplementation use was not beneficial; the incidence of cardiovascular death, MI, and stroke was 16.0% in vitamin E–treated subjects versus 15.4% in placebo-treated subjects (see Ref. 228 for expanded summary and ramipril results).

93. Lee I-M, et al. Vitamin E in the primary prevention of cardiovascular disease and cancer: the Women's Health Study: a randomized controlled trial. JAMA 2005;294:56–65.

Design: Prospective, randomized, double-blind, multicenter study, with 2 × 2 factorial design evaluating vitamin E and aspirin, both compared with placebo. Primary end point was a composite of nonfatal MI, stroke, or cardiovascular death and total invasive cancer. Average follow-up was 10.1 years.

Purpose: To evaluate the efficacy of vitamin E supplementation for the prevention of CVD or cancer in women (the results of the aspirin arm were reported separately).

Population: 39,876 healthy women at least 45 years of age.

Treatment: Vitamin E 600 IU every other day versus placebo.

Results: There were no significant differences in outcomes between the two groups for incidence of MI (RR 1.01, $p = 0.96$), stroke (RR 0.98, $p = 0.82$), cancer (RR 1.01, $p = 0.87$), or all-cause mortality (RR 1.04, $p = 0.53$). There was significantly lower cardiovascular mortality in the vitamin E group (RR 0.76, $p = 0.03$).

Comments: While cardiovascular mortality was lower in those taking vitamin E, this was not consistent with the other end points, and vitamin E was not recommended for cardiovascular or cancer prevention for women.

94. Gaziano JM, et al. Multivitamins in the prevention of cardiovascular disease in men: the Physicians' Health Study II randomized clinical trial. JAMA 2012;308:1751–1760.

Design: Prospective, randomized, double-blind, placebo-controlled trial. Primary end point was a composite end point of nonfatal MI, nonfatal stroke, and cardiovascular death over a median follow-up of 11.2 years.

Purpose: To determine if long-term multivitamin supplements decrease the risk of CVD in men.

Population: 14,641 male physicians age 50 years or older at study entry; 754 men had CVD at randomization.

Treatment: Daily multivitamin or placebo continued through the end of the trial.

Results: At the end of the follow-up period, subjects randomized to placebo had no reduction in their incidence of the primary end point (11.0 events vs. 10.8 events per 1,000 person-years for subjects treated with multivitamin and placebo, respectively; HR, 1.01; 95% CI, 0.91 to 1.10; $p = 0.91$) nor in any of the components of the primary end point.

95. Hulley S, et al. Heart and Estrogen/Progestin Replacement Study (HERS). Randomized trial of estrogen and progestin for secondary prevention of coronary heart disease in postmenopausal women. JAMA 1998;280:605–613.

Design: Prospective, randomized, blinded, placebo-controlled, multicenter study. Primary outcome was a composite of nonfatal MI plus cardiovascular death. Average follow-up was 4.1 years.

Purpose: To determine whether estrogen plus progestin alters the risk for CHD events in postmenopausal women with known coronary disease.

Population: 2,763 women younger than 80 years (mean age, 66.7 years).

Exclusion Criteria: CHD event in previous 6 months, sexual hormone use in previous 3 months, history of pulmonary embolism (PE), deep venous thrombosis (DVT), breast cancer, and endometrial cancer.

Treatment: Conjugated equine estrogens (0.625 mg once daily) and medroxyprogesterone (2.5 mg once daily) or placebo.

Results: Compliance rates were 82% at 1 year and 75% at 3 years. No difference in the incidence of the primary outcome [relative hazard (RH), 0.99] was observed. Lack of effect was observed despite the hormone group having 11% lower LDL and 10% higher HDL (each $p < 0.001$). The hormone group had more events in year 1 and fewer in years 4 and 5. The hormone group had more venous thromboembolism (RH, 2.89; 95% CI, 1.50 to 5.58) and gallbladder disease (RH, 1.38; 95% CI, 1.00 to 1.92).

96. Writing Group for the Women's Health Initiative Investigators. Risks and benefits of estrogen plus progestin in healthy postmenopausal women: principal results from the Women's Health Initiative randomized controlled trial. JAMA 2002;288:321–333 (editorial, 366–368).

Design: Prospective, randomized, controlled, multicenter, primary prevention trial. Primary end point was CHD death and nonfatal MI. Primary adverse outcome was invasive breast cancer. A global index included the two primary outcomes plus stroke, PE, endometrial cancer, colorectal cancer, hip fracture, and death due to other causes.

Purpose: To assess the major health benefits and risks of the most commonly used combined hormone preparation in the United States.

Population: 16,608 postmenopausal women, aged 50 to 79 years, with an intact uterus.

Exclusion Criteria: Prior breast cancer, other prior cancer in previous 10 years, and low hematocrit or platelet counts.

Treatment: Equine estrogens, 0.625 mg/day, plus medroxyprogesterone acetate, 2.5 mg/day, in one tablet, or placebo.

Results: The estrogen/progestin arm of the trial was terminated early (at 5.2 years' follow-up rather than the planned 8.5 years) because of excessive risk of the global index in the hormone group compared with placebo (HR, 1.15; 95% CI, 1.03 to 1.28). The hormone group also had a significantly higher incidence of CHD (HR, 1.29; 95% CI, 1.02 to 1.63), breast cancer (HR, 1.26; 95% CI, 1.00 to 1.59), stroke (HR, 1.41; 95% CI, 1.07 to 1.85), and PE (HR, 2.13; 95% CI, 1.39 to 3.25). All-cause mortality rates were similar (HR, 0.98; 95% CI, 0.82 to 1.18).

Comments: Although mortality rates were similar, the overall risk–benefit profile in this trial is not consistent with the requirements for a clearly safe and efficacious intervention for primary prevention of chronic diseases.

97. Barrett-Connor E, et al.; for the MORE Investigators (Multiple Outcomes of Raloxifene Evaluation). Raloxifene and cardiovascular events in osteoporotic postmenopausal women: four-year results from the MORE (Multiple Outcomes of Raloxifene Evaluation) randomized trial. JAMA 2002;287:847–857.

Design: Prospective, randomized, double-blind, placebo-controlled, multicenter trial. Primary end point was MI, unstable angina, coronary ischemia, and stroke or TIA.

Purpose: To determine the effect of raloxifene on cardiovascular events in osteoporotic postmenopausal women.

Population: 7,705 osteoporotic postmenopausal women (mean age, 67 years); osteoporosis was documented by prior vertebral fracture or bone mineral density score (T score) < -2.5.

Exclusion Criteria: Stroke or venous thromboembolic disease in prior 10 years.

Treatment: Raloxifene, 60 mg/day; raloxifene, 120 mg/day; or placebo, for 4 years.

Results: No significant differences were noted between the three treatment groups in coronary and cerebrovascular events (raloxifene, 60 mg/day: 3.2%; raloxifene, 120 mg/day: 3.7%; placebo, 3.7%). Among the 1,035 women with increased cardiovascular risk at baseline, those assigned to raloxifene (either dose) had a significantly lower risk of cardiovascular events compared with placebo (RR, 0.60; 95% CI, 0.38 to 0.95). The number of cardiovascular events during the first year was not significantly different in the overall cohort, or among women at increased cardiovascular risk ($p = 0.86$) or with evidence of established CHD ($p = 0.60$).

98. Barret-Connor E, et al.; for the Raloxifene Use for The Heart (RUTH) Trial Investigators. Effects of raloxifene on cardiovascular events and breast cancer in postmenopausal women. N Engl J Med 2006;355:125–137.

Design: International, multicenter, randomized, double-blind, placebo-controlled trial. The two primary end points were coronary events (coronary death, MI, hospitalization for ACS) and invasive breast cancer. Median follow-up was 5.6 years.

Purpose: To evaluate the effects of raloxifene, an estrogen receptor modulator, on CHD and breast cancer.

Population: 10,101 postmenopausal women (average age 67.5 years) with CHD or multiple risk factors.

Treatment: Raloxifene, 60 mg daily, or placebo.

Results: There were a similar number of coronary events in each arm (HR 0.95, 95% CI, 0.84 to 1.07) over the follow-up period. Invasive breast cancer occurred in significantly fewer women in the raloxifene arm (40 vs. 70 events, respectively, HR 0.56, 95% CI, 0.38 to 0.83). This finding was mainly driven by a reduction in estrogen receptor–positive invasive cancers. Overall mortality was similar between the two groups; however, there were significantly increased rates of venous thromboembolism (HR, 1.44) and stroke (HR, 1.49) in the raloxifene arm.

Comment: While raloxifene did not contribute to coronary events and improved breast cancer outcomes, these benefits should be weighed against the risk for thromboembolic and cerebrovascular events.

99. Basaria S, et al. Adverse events associated with testosterone supplementation. N Engl J Med 2010;363:109.

In this prospective, randomized, double-blind, placebo-controlled, multicenter clinical trial, investigators assigned 291 elderly men, 65 years of age and older, with low testosterone (between 100 and 350 ng/dL) and impaired mobility to testosterone gel or placebo gel. The primary outcome was improvement in leg press strength. However, the trial was stopped prematurely when it was demonstrated that the group randomized to testosterone supplementation had a higher rate of cardiovascular adverse events.

100. GISSI-Prevenzione Investigators. Dietary supplementation with n-3 polyunsaturated fatty acids and vitamin E after myocardial infarction: results of the GISSI-Prevenzione trial. Lancet 1999;354:447–455.

Design: Prospective, randomized, open-label, multicenter study. Primary end point was death, nonfatal MI, and stroke. Average follow-up was 3.5 years.

Purpose: To evaluate the independent and combined effects of n-3 PUFAs and vitamin E on morbidity and mortality after MI.

Population: 11,324 patients with an MI in the previous 3 months.

Treatment: n-3 PUFA (1 g daily), vitamin E (300 mg/day), both, or none.

Results: The n-3 PUFA group had a significant reduction in death, MI, and stroke (12.3% vs. 14.6% in the control group; $p = 0.023$). All-cause mortality was 20% lower in the n-3 PUFA group (8.3% vs. 10.4%). The vitamin E group had a nonsignificant reduction in death, MI, and stroke (13.1% vs. 14.4%). Vitamin E use was associated with a significant 20% reduction in cardiovascular deaths.

Comment: At the start of the trial, statins were not in widespread use. Only 4.7% of participants were on cholesterol-lowering medications at the start of the study; 45.5% were taking cholesterol-lowering medications by 42-month follow-up.

101. Kromhout D, et al.; for the Alpha Omega Trial Group. n-3 fatty acids and cardiovascular events after myocardial infarction. N Engl J Med 2010;363:2015.

In this prospective, randomized, double-blind, placebo-controlled, multicenter study, investigators randomized 4,837 elderly (age 60 to 80 years) patients with prior MI and currently on evidence-based therapy for CAD (including lipid-modifying therapy) to receive one of three different margarines supplemented with low doses of n-3 fatty acids or a placebo margarine. None of the margarines was more effective at preventing a composite end point of fatal MI, nonfatal MI, or revascularization, though there was a trend toward benefit in the patients treated with margarine supplemented with the plant-derived alpha linolenic acid (HR, 0.91; 95% CI, 0.78 to 1.05; $p = 0.20$).

102. The ORIGIN trial investigators. n-3 fatty acids and cardiovascular outcomes in patients with dysglycemia. N Engl J Med 2012;367:309–318.

Design: Prospective, randomized, double-blind, placebo-controlled, multicenter study. The primary end point was death from cardiovascular causes. This substudy was part of a larger trial with a 2 × 2 factorial design that randomized the same patients to insulin glargine or standard care. Median follow-up was 6.2 years.

Purpose: To assess the efficacy of n-3 fatty acids in the prevention of adverse cardiac outcomes in patients with high cardiovascular risk and type 2 diabetes, impaired glucose tolerance, or impaired fasting glucose.

Population: 12,537 people with cardiovascular risk factors or known CVD in addition to impaired glucose tolerance, impaired fasting glucose, or type 2 diabetes mellitus.

Treatment: 1-g capsule containing at least 900 mg of ethyl esters of n-3 fatty acids daily, or placebo.

Results: Despite a decrease in TG by 14.5 mg/dL in patients receiving n-3 fatty acids, n-3 fatty acid supplementation did not reduce the incidence of cardiovascular death in these patients at high cardiovascular risk (HR, 0.98; 95% CI, 0.87 to 1.10; $p = 0.72$).

103. Risk and Prevention Study Collaborative Group. n-3 fatty acids in patients with multiple cardiac risk factors. *N Engl J Med* 2013;368:1800–1808.

Design: Prospective, randomized, double-blind, placebo-controlled, multicenter study. The primary end point was cardiovascular death or cardiac hospital admission. Median follow-up was 5 years.

Purpose: To assess the efficacy of n-3 fatty acids in the prevention of adverse cardiac outcomes in patients with high cardiovascular risk or known CVD.

Population: 12,513 patients with multiple cardiac risk factors (diabetes plus 1 of the following, or no diabetes plus ≥ 4 of the following: age ≥ 65, male sex, HTN, hyperlipidemia, current smoking, BMI ≥ 30 kg/m^2, or family history of early CAD) or known CVD (but without prior history of MI).

Treatment: 1 g/day n-3 fatty acids, or olive oil.

Results: There was no difference in the incidence of the primary end point between the two groups (11.7% in the n-3 PUFAs group vs. 11.9% of the olive oil group; HR 0.97; 95% CI, 0.88 to 1.08; $p = 0.58$). Secondary analyses did reveal a beneficial effect in women (HR, 0.82; 95% CI, 0.67 to 0.99; $p = 0.04$) and a reduction in heart failure hospitalizations ($p = 0.002$).

Comment: It has been hypothesized that the beneficial effect of n-3 fatty acids seen in some studies is due to n-3 fatty acids' protective effects against ventricular arrhythmias, which occurred at a high rate in the heart failure and post-MI patients enrolled in those trials. A recent meta-analysis of 9 trials enrolling 32,919 patients (see *Heart Lung* 2013;42: 251–256) reported a nonsignificant 18% reduction in SCD or ventricular arrhythmias in patients treated with n-3 fatty acids (OR, 0.82; 95% CI, 0.60 to 1.21; $p = 0.21$).

104. Lamas GA, et al.; for the TACT Investigators. Effect of disodium EDTA chelation regimen on cardiovascular events in patients with previous myocardial infarction: the TACT randomized trial. *JAMA* 2013;309:1241–1250.

Design: Prospective, randomized, double-blind, placebo-controlled multicenter study. The primary end point was a composite of overall mortality, recurrent MI, coronary artery revascularization, or hospitalization for angina. The overall study was part of a larger 2 × 2 factorial design that randomized the same patients to oral high-dose multivitamins or placebo.

Purpose: To assess the efficacy of chelation therapy with sodium EDTA, a treatment used for over 50 years without proof of efficacy, in preventing cardiovascular events.

Population: 1,708 patients 50 or older who had an MI at least 6 weeks prior to enrollment (median time from qualifying MI to enrollment was 4.6 years).

Exclusion Criteria: Creatinine > 2.0 mg/dL, platelet count < 100,000/μL, abnormal LFTs, BP > 160/100 mm Hg, chelation therapy within 5 years, cigarette smoking within 3 months, and heart failure hospitalization in the prior 6 months.

Treatment: A 10-component chelation solution, designed to closely match the solution used by chelation practitioners, consisting of 3-g disodium EDTA, 7-g ascorbic acid, 2-g magnesium chloride, 100-mg procaine hydrochloride, 2,500 units of unfractionated heparin, 2 mEq of potassium chloride, 840-mg sodium bicarbonate, 250-mg pantothenic acid, 100-mg thiamine, 100-mg pyridoxine, and sterile water to a total volume of 500 mL solution, or a placebo consisting of 500-mL normal saline and 2.5-g dextrose. The solutions were infused intravenously over 3 hours each week for 30 weeks, followed by 10 additional infusions 2 to 8 weeks apart. All participants received a daily low-dose vitamin intended to prevent depletion from the chelation regimen.

Results: At median 55 weeks' follow-up, 26% of patients randomized to chelation had met the primary end point, compared to 30% of patients randomized to placebo (HR, 0.82; 95% CI, 0.69 to 0.99; $p = 0.035$). None of the individual components of the primary end point, including overall mortality, were significantly reduced by the chelation regimen, but the point estimate of the magnitude of the treatment's effect was similar on all components of the primary end point (HRs, 0.72 to 0.81) except for overall mortality (HR, 0.93; 95% CI, 0.70 to 1.25). A majority of the 483 events that contributed to the primary end point were "soft outcomes"—revascularization procedures or hospitalizations for angina (67%).

Comment: Concerns were raised immediately about the reliability of this controversial trial (see JAMA 2013;309:1293–1294): 60% of enrolling sites were complementary and alternative medicine centers, 18% of randomized patients were lost to follow-up due to withdrawal of consent (largely from the placebo group), and the trial sponsors (NHLBI and NCCAM) performed 11 interim analyses with unblinded data. The authors themselves note that the lack of a well-established hypothesis for the mechanism of benefit makes interpretation of this trial difficult and forces consideration that the results could be a chance finding. These controversial findings will likely need to be replicated before they are widely accepted into clinical practice.

META-ANALYSES

105. Miller ER, et al. Meta-analysis: high-dosage vitamin E supplementation may increase all-cause mortality. *Ann Intern Med* 2005;142:37–46.

This is a review of 135,967 patients in 19 clinical trials of vitamin E supplementation, including both high-dose (≥ 400 IU daily) and standard-dose interventions. They found a pooled excess risk of all-cause mortality in the high-dose supplementation groups, at an overall rate of 39 per 10,000 persons ($p = 0.035$). There was a nonsignificant trend toward lower mortality in pooled analysis of low-dose trials, a reduction of 16 deals per 10,000 persons ($p > 0.2$). They identified a cutoff of 150 IU per day, over which an excess in mortality would be expected. Of note, this analysis did not include the WHS.

106. Hooper L, et al. Risks and benefits of omega 3 fats for mortality, cardiovascular disease, and cancer: systematic review. *BMJ* 2006;332:752–760.

The authors reviewed both randomized controlled trials (48 in total) and cohort studies (41 in total) that involved at least 6 months of omega-3 fat supplements. Treatment with omega-3 fat supplements did not produce a statistically significant reduction in total mortality (RR, 0.87; 95% CI, 0.73 to 1.03), and the results of individual studies were inconsistent. The authors could not conclude that there was any benefit to omega-3 supplementation, either for all-cause mortality or cardiovascular outcomes. However, based on their analyses, they could not detect a signal of harm for patients taking omega-3 fat supplements.

107. Rizos EC, et al. Association between omega-3 fatty acid supplementation and risk of major cardiovascular disease events: a systematic review and meta-analysis. *JAMA* 2012;308:1024–1033.

The authors reviewed 20 randomized controlled trials involving 68,680 patients treated with omega-3 fatty acids or placebo for 1 year or more. Using a threshold of $p < 0.0063$ to account for multiple comparisons, they found no statistically significant reduction in all-cause mortality (RR 0.96; 95% CI, 0.91 to 1.02), cardiovascular death (RR, 0.91; 95% CI, 0.85 to 0.98), SCD (RR, 0.87; 95% CI, 0.75 to 1.01), MI (RR, 0.89; 95% CI, 0.76 to 1.04), or stroke (RR, 1.05; 95% CI, 0.93 to 1.18). In their review, the authors note that the first randomized controlled trial comparing omega-3 fatty acid supplementation to placebo showed a strong effect on all cardiovascular outcomes, but with subsequent studies, the effect became weaker and lost statistical significance. The overall effect of omega-3 fatty acids on cardiovascular outcomes in clinical trials has remained small, despite multiple randomized clinical trials enrolling thousands of subjects. Additional meta-analyses including only secondary prevention trials also failed to find any clinical benefit (see *Arch Intern Med* 2012;172:686–694).

108. Myung SK, et al. Efficacy of vitamin and antioxidant supplements in prevention of cardiovascular disease: systematic review and meta-analysis of randomised controlled trials. *BMJ* 2013;346:f10.

In this meta-analysis of 50 randomized controlled trials involving 294,478 participants taking vitamin or antioxidant supplements, the authors found that supplementation did not reduce cardiovascular events (RR 1.00; 95% CI, 0.98 to 1.02). Subset analyses of vitamin B_6, vitamin B_{12}, folic acid, vitamin C, vitamin D, vitamin E, β-carotene, and selenium also failed to identify a statistically significant reduction in cardiovascular events with supplementation.

Diet

109. Kris-Etherton PM, et al.; for the AHA Nutrition Committee. Fish consumption, fish oil, omega-3 fatty acids, and cardiovascular disease. *Circulation* 2002;106:2747–2757.

The AHA recommends that patients with documented CHD should consume about 1 g of omega-3 fatty acids per day. In those unable to eat sufficient amounts of fish to meet this requirement, it recommends daily supplementation with 1-g fish oil capsules that contain 180 mg of eicosapentaenoic acid and 120 mg of docosahexaenoic acid. In individuals with high TG levels, higher amounts (2 to 4 g/day) can be taken. See "Lifestyle" for additional guidelines.

110. Mente A, et al. A systematic review of the evidence supporting a causal link between dietary factors and coronary heart disease. *Arch Intern Med* 2009;169:659–669.

The authors compiled prospective cohort or randomized studies of dietary interventions and CHD outcomes using Bradford Hill criteria to assess causation. Overall, 507 cohort studies and 94 randomized trials were included, yielding strong evidence to support the associations of protective dietary factors (vegetables, nuts, "Mediterranean" patterns) and harmful dietary factors (*trans*-fatty acids, high-glycemic-index foods). There was moderate evidence to suggest fish (omega-3 fatty acids), folate, whole grains, dietary vitamins E and C, β-carotene, alcohol, fruit, and fiber may be protective. When restricted to randomized trials, the Mediterranean dietary pattern was found to be protective. Overall, the review provides strong evidence for the role of diet in modulating the incidence of coronary disease.

OBSERVATIONAL STUDIES

111. Pietinen P, et al. Intake of dietary fiber and risk of coronary heart disease in a cohort of Finnish men. *Circulation* 1996;94:2720–2727.

This analysis focused on 21,930 ATBC patients (all male smokers aged 50 to 69 years). At follow-up (average, 6.1 years), MI and CHD deaths were found to be inversely associated with fiber intake. The highest quintile (34.8 g/day) versus lowest quintile (16.1 g/day) showed an RR of coronary death of 0.69 ($p < 0.001$ for trend). The same effect was evident after adjustment for cardiac risk factors and intake of β-carotene and vitamins C and E. The strongest association was seen with water-soluble and cereal (vs. vegetable or fruit) fibers. Again, the observational nature of this study limits conclusions.

112. Bernstein AM, et al. Major dietary protein sources and risk of coronary heart disease in women. *Circulation* 2010;122:876–883.

In a prospective analysis of 84,136 NHS participants free of CVD at baseline, researchers collected information on diet via a validated survey every 4 years. At 26 years' follow-up, higher intake of red meat and high-fat dairy were associated with higher rates of MI and cardiovascular death. Conversely, higher intake of fish, poultry, and nuts was associated with lower risk.

113. Dehghan M, et al.; for the ONTARGET/TRANSCEND Investigators. Relationship between healthy diet and risk of CVD among patients on drug therapies for secondary prevention: a prospective cohort study of 31.546 high-risk individuals from 40 countries. *Circulation* 2012;126:2705–2712.

In this prospective study, 31,546 patients with CAD or type 2 diabetes enrolled in two large clinical trials completed a validated qualitative food frequency questionnaire at the time of trial enrollment. The questionnaire recorded the subjects' recollections of the types of foods that comprised their diets over the prior 12 months; it did not record portion sizes. The diets were scored using two dietary indices. Subjects consuming a diet in the healthiest quintile had a hazard ratio of 0.78 (95% CI, 0.71 to 0.87) for a composite outcome of cardiovascular death, MI, stroke, or heart failure compared to diets in the least healthy quintile.

CLINICAL TRIALS

114. de Lorgeril M, et al.; Lyon Diet Heart Study. A Mediterranean diet reduced mortality after MI. *Lancet* 1994;343:1454–1459.

This prospective, randomized, secondary prevention study enrolled 605 patients with a first MI (91% men). The diet group underwent a 1-hour educational session. At 8 weeks and annually, a diet survey and counseling were administered. At follow-up (average, 27 months), the Mediterranean diet group had a 73% lower relative incidence of death and nonfatal MI compared with the prudent Western-type diet group (2.7% vs. 11%; $p = 0.001$). A subsequent report with a mean follow-up of 46 months showed persistent benefits.

115. Appel LJ, et al.; for the OmniHeart Collaborative Research Group. Effects of protein, monounsaturated fat, and carbohydrate intake on blood pressure and serum lipids: results of the OmniHeart randomized trial. *JAMA* 2005;294:2455–2464.

Design: Prospective, randomized, crossover, multicenter study. Primary end points were measures of BP and LDL at baseline, following each diet, and at the end of the study period.

Purpose: To evaluate the effects on cardiac risk factors of various diets, substituting alternative macronutrients for saturated fats.

Population: 164 adults with prehypertension or stage 1 HTN.

Treatment: A diet rich in carbohydrates, a diet rich in protein (about half from plant sources), and a diet rich in unsaturated fat (predominantly monounsaturated); each participant was exposed to each diet in a 6-week crossover feeding period.

Results: Overall, the protein and unsaturated fat diets both led to similar and lower 10-year CHD risk. There were significant reductions in BP, LDL, and TGs and increases in HDL for adults on the protein diet compared with the carbohydrate diet. For those on the unsaturated fat diet, there were significant reductions in BP and TGs, with increases in HDL. There was no effect on LDL when comparing the carbohydrate and unsaturated fat diets.

Comment: The study represents strong evidence that dietary modification, over a period as short as 6 weeks, can modify long-term cardiovascular risk (if maintained).

116. Dansinger ML, et al. Comparison of the Atkins, Ornish, Weight Watchers, and Zone diets for weight loss and heart disease risk reduction: a randomized trial. JAMA 2005;293:43–53.

Design: Prospective, randomized, single-center study. Primary end points were changes in weight, measures of cardiac risk (cholesterol, BP, glucose), and self-selected dietary adherence at 1 year.

Purpose: To evaluate the comparative efficacy of four different fad diets in producing and maintaining meaningful changes in weight and/or cardiovascular risk.

Population: 160 adults, aged 22 to 72 years, with mean BMI 35 kg/m^2 and known HTN, dyslipidemia, or fasting hyperglycemia.

Treatment: Randomization to four different popular diet groups, including the Atkins (carbohydrate restriction), Zone (macronutrient balance), Weight Watchers (calorie restriction), or Ornish (fat restriction) diets.

Results: Overall, each diet produced significant, yet modest, weight loss; adherence at 1 year was poor overall, yet reported better in patients with greater weight loss. There were significant improvements in LDL/HDL ratio from baseline for all diets (all $p < 0.05$), but not in BP or glucose at 1 year.

117. Estruch R, et al.; for the PREDIMED Study Investigators. Primary prevention of cardiovascular disease with a Mediterranean diet. N Engl J Med 2013;368:1279–1290.

Design: Prospective, randomized, controlled, multicenter study in Spain. Primary end point was major adverse cardiac events (cardiovascular death, stroke, or MI). The trial was stopped on the basis of an interim analysis, after participants were followed for 4.8 years.

Purpose: To evaluate the effectiveness of the Mediterranean diet compared to a control diet in the primary prevention of cardiovascular events.

Population: 7,447 adults aged 55 to 80 years with either type 2 diabetes mellitus or 3 of 6 major cardiovascular risk factors (smoking, HTN, elevated LDL, low HDL, overweight or obesity, or family history of CVD).

Treatment: Randomization to one of three different groups: a Mediterranean diet supplemented with extra-virgin olive oil, a Mediterranean diet supplemented with nuts, or a control low-fat diet. Both Mediterranean diets emphasized consumption of significant amounts of olive oil, tree nuts, fruits, vegetables, fish, legumes, wine, and sofrito (a sauce made with tomato and onion) and discouraged the consumption of soft drinks, baked goods, spread fats, and red meats.

Results: Adherence to all three dietary interventions was high. Major adverse cardiac events were reduced by 30% in the groups that received a Mediterranean diet compared to the control group (3.8% for Mediterranean diet supplemented with extra-virgin olive oil vs. 3.4% for the Mediterranean diet supplemented with nuts vs. 4.8% in the control group; $p = 0.015$). The reduction in the primary end point was mainly driven by a reduction in stroke in the Mediterranean diet groups, but there was a non-significant trend of a 20% reduction in MI. There was no effect on all-cause mortality.

Comment: This was the first trial to demonstrate the efficacy of a specific diet in primary prevention, but some have questioned whether it was truly a test of the Mediterranean diet or a test of supplementation with mixed nuts or extra-virgin olive oil, since the diets actually consumed by all groups were fairly similar once the supplementary foods were excluded (see N Engl J Med 2013;368:1353–1354).

Alcohol

118. de Lorgeril M, et al. Wine drinking and risks of cardiovascular complications after recent acute myocardial infarction. *Circulation* 2002;106:1465–1469.

This analysis examined 437 survivors of a recent MI who had at least two reliable assessments of drinking (and dietary) habits. In these patients, average ethanol intake was 7.6% of the total energy intake, of which wine ethanol represented 92%. At 4-year follow-up, 104 cardiovascular complications (23.8%) had occurred. In comparison with abstainers, the adjusted risk of complications was reduced by 59% in patients whose average ethanol intake was 7.7% of the total energy intake (about 2 drinks per day) and by 52% in those whose average ethanol intake was 16% of energy (about 4 drinks per day).

119. Mukamal KJ, et al. Roles of drinking pattern and type of alcohol consumed in coronary heart disease in men. *N Engl J Med* 2003;348:109–118.

This study assessed alcohol intake by questionnaire in 38,077 male health professionals free of CVD and cancer at baseline. At 12 years of follow-up, men who consumed alcohol 3 to 4 or 5 to 7 days per week had decreased risks of MI compared with those who had less than one drink per week [multivariate RR, 0.68 for 3 to 4 days per week (95% CI, 0.55 to 0.84) and 0.63 for 5 to 7 days per week (95% CI, 0.54 to 0.74)]. No single type of beverage conferred additional benefit. A 12.5-g increase in daily alcohol consumption over a 4-year follow-up period was associated with 22% reduction in the relative risk of MI compared to abstinence.

120. Maraldi C, et al. Impact of inflammation on the relationship among alcohol consumption, mortality, and cardiac events: the health, aging, and body composition study. *Arch Intern Med* 2006;166:1490–1497.

This analysis of 2,487 septuagenarians without baseline CHD or HF assessed alcohol consumption and serum inflammatory makers (IL-6 and CRP) at mean follow-up of 5.6 years. Light to moderate alcohol intake did not affect inflammatory markers, but was associated with significantly less cardiac morbidity and mortality.

Lifestyle

GUIDELINES AND GENERAL ARTICLES

121. Lichtenstein AH, et al. Diet and lifestyle recommendations revision 2006: a scientific statement from the American Heart Association Nutrition Committee. *Circulation* 2006;114:82–96.

The committee reviewed the most recent data on diet and lifestyle as they relate to CVD. Highlights of their recommendations include a balanced diet limiting intake of saturated fat, trans fat, and cholesterol. They stop short of recommending alcohol intake but stress its use in moderation.

122. Lloyd-Jones DM, et al. Defining and setting national goals for cardiovascular health promotion and disease reduction: the American Heart Association's strategic impact goal through 2020 and beyond. *Circulation* 2010;121:586–613.

As part of its overarching goal to "improve the cardiovascular health of all Americans by 20%" by the year 2020, the American Heart Association refocused on primordial prevention, avoiding the development of risk factors. In doing so, it defined ideal cardiovascular health as the presence of seven evidence-based metrics: abstinence from smoking, BMI < 25 kg/m^2, physical activity at goal, consumption of a heart healthy diet, untreated TC < 200 mg/dL, untreated BP < 120/80, and absence of diabetes mellitus. With some adjustments, the measures were also applied to a pediatric population (**Table 1.2**). The committee continues on to review the large body of evidence for the seven components of ideal cardiovascular health (individually and collectively), and a primordial prevention strategy in general, for the prevention of CVD.

| Table 1.2 | Guideline Comparisons of Goal BP and Initial Drug Therapy for Adults with Hypertension |

Guideline	Population	Goal BP, mm Hg	Initial Drug Treatment Options
2014 hypertension guideline	General ≥60 y	<150/90	Nonblack: thiazide-type diuretic, ACEI, ARB, or CCG; black: thiazide-type diuretic or CCB
	General <60 y	<140/90	
	Diabetes	<140/90	Thiazide-type diuretic, ACEI, ARB, or CCB
	CKD	<140/90	ACEI or ARB
ESH/ ESC 2013	General nonelderly	<140/90	Diuretic, β-blocker, CCB, ACEI, or ARB
	General elderly <80 y	<150/90	
	General ≥80 y	<150/90	
	Diabetes	<140/85	ACEI or ARB
	CKD nonproteinuria	<140/90	ACEI or ARB
	CKD + proteinuria	<130/90	
CHEP 2013	General <80 y	<140/90	Thiazide, β-blocker (age <60 y), ACEI (nonblack) or ARB
	General ≥80 y	<150/90	
	Diabetes	<130/80	ACEI or ARB with additional CVD risk ACEI, ARB, thiazide, or DHPCCB without additional CVD risk
	CKD	<140/90	ACEI or ARB
ADA 2013	Diabetes	<140/80	ACEI or ARB
KDIGO 2012	CKD no proteinuria	≤140/90	ACEI or ARB
	CKD + proteinuria	≤130/80	
NICE 2011	General <80 y	<140/90	<55 y: ACEI or ARB
	General ≥80 y	<150/90	≥55 y or black: CCB
ISHIB 2010	Black, lower risk	<135/85	Diuretic or CCB
	Target organ damage or CVD risk	<130/80	

Data from James PA, et al. 2014 evidence-based guideline for the management of high blood pressure in adults: report from the panel members appointed to the Eighth Joint National Committee (JNC 8). JAMA 2014;311(5):507–520.

123. Eckel, RH, et al. 2013 AHA/ACC guideline on lifestyle management to reduce cardiovascular risk: a report of the American College of Cardiology/American Heart Association Task Force on Practice Guidelines. *Circulation* 2014;129:S76–S99. doi: 10.1161/01.cir.0000437740.48606.d1.

Using a new approach to synthesizing the evidence and identifying relevant questions, as well as knowledge gaps, the task force updates their recommendations on lifestyle management for the prevention of CVD.

124. Jensen, MD, et al. 2013 AHA/ACC/TOS guideline for the management of overweight and obesity in adults: a report of the American College of Cardiology/American Heart Association Task Force on Practice Guidelines and The Obesity Society. *Circulation* 2014;129:S102–S138. doi 10.1161/01.cir.0000437739.71477.ee

These revised guidelines included measurements of waist circumference in overweight and obese adults and emphasized the use of calorie restriction for weight loss, in the setting of comprehensive lifestyle program. Methods for weight loss *maintenance* as well as considerations for bariatric surgery are also discussed.

125. Stampfer MJ, et al. Primary prevention of coronary heart disease in women through diet and lifestyle. N *Engl J Med* 2000;343:16–22.

This analysis examined the 84,129 NHS participants who were free of diagnosed CVD, cancer, and diabetes at baseline. During 14 years of follow-up, 296 CHD deaths and 832 nonfatal MIs occurred. Low-risk subjects (only 3% of cohort) were defined as follows: nonsmokers, BMI < 25 kg/m^2, alcohol consumption at least half a drink per day, moderate-to-vigorous physical activity for average of approximately 30 minutes per day, scored in highest 40% of cohort for consumption of a diet high in cereal fiber, marine n-3 fatty acids, and folate, with a high ratio of polyunsaturated to saturated fat and low in trans fat and glycemic load. After adjustment for age, family history, presence or absence of diagnosed HTN or diagnosed high cholesterol level, and menopausal status, all factors independently and significantly predicted risk. Low-risk women had an 83% RRR in CHD death or nonfatal MI compared with all the other women.

126. Chow CK, et al. Association of diet, exercise, and smoking modification with risk of early cardiovascular events after acute coronary syndromes. *Circulation* 2010;121:750–758.

In this prospective secondary analysis of a multicenter randomized clinical trial, 18,809 patients treated for UA/NSTEMI with fondaparinux or enoxaparin in the OASIS 5 clinical trial reported adherence to recommendations regarding diet, exercise, and smoking cessation 30 days after their index event. Though adherence to secondary prevention drugs was high, 35% of patients smoking at the time of their coronary event persisted in smoking, 41% of patients did not adhere to dietary recommendations, and 57% of patients did not exercise for > 30 minutes 3 times per week. At 6 months' follow-up, those patients who quit smoking had a decreased risk of recurrent MI compared to persistent smokers (OR, 0.57; 95% CI, 0.36 to 0.89), and those patients adherent to diet and exercise had a decreased risk of recurrent MI compared to nonadherents (OR, 0.52; 95% CI, 0.4 to 0.69). Overall, in patients who continued to smoke and did not adjust diet or exercise patterns, risk of recurrent MI was 3.8-fold higher than in those who adhered to all behavioral recommendations. Though this study is limited by its observational nature, the benefits of behavioral modification were substantial; the authors argue that advocating for behavioral modification should be as high a priority in the post-ACS period as prescribing appropriate secondary prevention medications.

127. Folsom AR, et al. Community prevalence of ideal cardiovascular health, by the American Heart Association definition, and relationship with cardiovascular disease incidence. J *Am Coll Cardiol* 2011;57:1690–1696.

Researchers retrospectively applied the American Heart Association's 2010 concept of ideal cardiovascular health to a population from the Atherosclerosis Risk in Communities

(ARIC) Study cohort free of CVD in 1987 to 1989 and measured the incidence of cardiovascular events until 2007. Subjects with ideal cardiovascular health across all 5 to 7 metrics in 1987 to 1989 were 5 times less likely to have cardiovascular events than those that met 0 metrics (7 per 1,000 person-years vs. 32.1 per 1,000 person-years).

128. Dong C, et al. Ideal cardiovascular health predicts lower risk of myocardial infarction, stroke, and vascular death across white, blacks, and Hispanics: the northern Manhattan study. *Circulation* 2012;125:2975.

In this prospective cohort study, 2,981 subjects free of vascular disease at baseline were followed for 11 years for the development of MI, stroke, and vascular death. The number of ideal cardiovascular health elements present at baseline was strongly predictive of incident CVD. Compared to a reference group with 0 or 1 ideal cardiovascular health metrics, adjusted hazard ratios were 0.73, 0.61, 0.49, and 0.41 for subjects with 2, 3, 4, and 5 or 6 metrics. These relationships were consistent across age and race. This association has been replicated across diverse populations (see also *Circulation* 2012;125:987–995).

129. Russ TC, et al. Association between psychological distress and mortality: individual participant pooled analysis of 10 prospective cohort studies. *BMJ* 2012;345:e4933.

In this analysis, authors included data from 10 prospective cohort studies involving 68,222 participants free of CVD at baseline, at which time each participant had baseline psychological distress measured by the General Health Questionnaire. At a mean 8.2 years' follow-up, there was a dose–response relationship between baseline psychological distress and subsequent cardiovascular and all-cause mortality.

130. Gullicksson M, et al. Randomized controlled trial of cognitive behavioral therapy vs standard treatment to prevent recurrent cardiovascular events in patients with coronary heart disease: Secondary Prevention in Uppsala Primary Health Care project (SUPRIM). *Arch Intern Med* 2011;171:134–140.

This single-center randomized controlled trial allocated 362 patients discharged from the hospital after MI, PCI, or CABG to either traditional care or traditional care plus a cognitive–behavioral therapy (CBT) program focused on stress management. After a mean 94 months' follow-up, the CBT group had a hazard ratio of 0.59 for recurrent cardiovascular events (95% CI, 0.42 to 0.83; $p = 0.002$) and 0.55 for recurrent acute MI (95% CI, 95% CI, 0.36 to 0.85; $p = 0.007$). There was a nonsignificant trend toward reduced overall mortality in the CBT group (HR 0.72; 95% CI, 0.40 to 1.30; $p = 0.28$).

OBESITY AND WEIGHT LOSS

131. Willett WC, et al. Weight, weight change and coronary heart disease in women: risk within the normal weight range. *JAMA* 1995;273:461–465.

This prospective cohort study was composed of 115,818 nurses aged 30 to 55 years with no history of CAD. Even modest weight gains after 18 years were associated with increased risk of death due to CVD and nonfatal MI: RR, 1.25 for 5- to 7.9-kg gain; RR, 1.64 for 8- to 10.9-kg gain; and 2.65 for 11- to 19-kg gain.

132. Wilson PW, et al. Overweight and obesity as determinants of cardiovascular risk: the Framingham experience. *Arch Intern Med* 2002;162:1867–1872.

This study examined Framingham Heart Study participants aged 35 to 75 years, who were monitored for up to 44 years. The primary outcome was new CVD, which included angina pectoris, MI, cerebrovascular disease, or stroke. Analyses compared overweight (BMI, 25.0 to 29.9 kg/m^2) and obese persons (BMI, 30 kg/m^2 or more) with a reference group of normal weight persons (BMI, 18.5 to 24.9 kg/m^2). Overweight status was associated with significantly increased risks of HTN (age-adjusted RR: men, 1.46; women, 1.75). New-onset hypercholesterolemia and diabetes mellitus were less highly associated with excess adiposity. The age-adjusted RR (CI) for CVD was increased among those who were overweight [men, 1.21 (95% CI, 1.05 to 1.40); women, 1.20 (95% CI, 1.03 to 1.41)] and obese [men, 1.46 (95% CI, 1.20 to 1.77); women, 1.64 (95% CI, 1.37 to 1.98)].

133. Flegal KM, et al. Prevalence and trends in obesity among U.S. adults, 1999–2000. JAMA 2002;288:1723–1727.

Information was obtained from 4,115 adult men and women who participated in the NHANES. The age-adjusted prevalence of obesity was 30.5% in 1999 to 2000 compared with 22.9% in NHANES III (1988 to 1994; $p < 0.001$). The prevalence of overweight also increased during this period from 55.9% to 64.5% ($p < 0.001$). Extreme obesity (BMI $\geq$ 40 kg/m^2) also increased significantly in the population, from 2.9% to 4.7% ($p = 0.002$).

134. Fontaine KR, et al. Years of life lost due to obesity. JAMA 2003;289:187–193.

This study examined data from U.S. Life Tables (1999), the Third National Health and Nutrition Examination Survey (NHANES III; 1988 to 1994), First National Health and Nutrition Epidemiologic Follow-up Study (NHANES I and II; 1971 to 1992), and NHANES II Mortality Study (1976 to 1992). Among whites, a U-shaped association was found between overweight or obesity and years of life lost (YLL). The optimal BMI (associated with the least YLL or greatest longevity) is 23 to 25 kg/m^2 for whites and 23 to 30 kg/m^2 for blacks. For any degree of overweight, younger adults typically had greater YLL than did older adults. White men between 20 and 30 years old with BMI > 45 kg/m^2 lost 13 years of life due to obesity; women in that age group with BMI > 45 kg/m^2 lost 8 years due to obesity. Among blacks older than 60 years, overweight and moderate obesity were not associated with an increased YLL; only severe obesity resulted in YLL. However, younger blacks with severe levels of obesity had a maximum YLL of 20 for men and 5 for women.

135. Bibbins-Domingo K, et al. Adolescent overweight and future adult coronary heart disease. N Engl J Med 2007;357:2371–2379.

On the basis of obesity rates in adolescents in 2000, the investigators estimated the prevalence of obese 35-year-olds in 2020 and the subsequent incidence of CHD based on models. Allowing for the expected shortcomings of such a study, the authors conclude there could be as many as 100,000 excess cases of CHD in 2035, attributable to the current epidemic of adolescent obesity.

136. Tirosh A, et al. Adolescent BMI trajectory and risk of diabetes versus coronary disease. N Engl J Med 2011;364:1315–1325.

In this prospective cohort study, the investigators examined the association between adolescent and adult BMI with incident CHD and diabetes over a mean 17.4 years of follow-up in 36,764 young male career Israeli Army personnel. After adjustment for other factors, adolescent BMI in the highest decile compared to the lowest decile was associated with a 2.76-fold increased risk of diabetes (95% CI, 2.11 to 3.58) and a 5.43-fold increased risk of angiographically confirmed CAD (95% CI, 2.77 to 10.62). Even after adjustment for adult BMI, the association between elevated adolescent BMI and incident CAD remained strong and significant. This study, along with many other similar cohort studies, has added weight to estimations of excess coronary disease due to pediatric overweight and obesity and led to an increased focus on primordial prevention of CAD through risk factor modification in children and adolescents.

137. James WP, et al.; for the SCOUT Investigators. Effect of sibutramine on cardiovascular outcomes in overweight and obese patients. N Engl J Med 2010;363:901–917.

In this prospective, double-blind, placebo-controlled, multicenter study, investigators randomized 10,744 overweight or obese patients with known CVD, type 2 diabetes, or both to sibutramine or placebo (after a 6-week single-blind run-in period where all patients received sibutramine) for a mean treatment duration of 3.4 years. The primary outcome measure was a composite of nonfatal MI, nonfatal stroke, resuscitated cardiac arrest, or cardiovascular death. Though patients in the sibutramine group maintained an excess 1.7-kg weight loss compared to the placebo group, the risk of reaching the primary end point was higher in the sibutramine group than the placebo group (11.4% vs. 10.0%; HR, 1.16; $p = 0.02$). This outcome was driven by nonfatal MI and stroke; the risks of cardiovascular and all-cause death were not different between the two groups.

138. Sjöström L, et al. Bariatric surgery and long-term cardiovascular events. JAMA 2012;307:56–65.

Design: Prospective, nonrandomized controlled multicenter study in Sweden. Primary end point was overall mortality; MI and stroke were secondary end points. Mean follow-up was 14.7 years.

Purpose: To examine the interaction between bariatric surgery, weight loss, and cardiovascular events.

Population: 2010 obese (BMI $\geq$ 34 kg/m^2 in men, $\geq$ 38 kg/m^2 in women) patients undergoing bariatric surgery between 1987 and 2001 and 2037 matched controls who did not undergo surgery.

Treatment: Most bariatric surgery patients underwent vertical banded gastroplasty (68.1%); the remainder underwent gastric bypass or gastric banding.

Results: Bariatric surgery was associated with a reduction in cardiovascular death (HR, 0.47; 95% CI, 0.29 to 0.76; $p = 0.002$) and cardiac events (HR, 0.67; 95% CI, 0.54 to 0.83; $p < 0.001$).

Comment: The primary analysis of this study (see N Engl J Med 2007;357:751–752) had already shown a statistically significant decrease in weight in subjects treated with bariatric surgery compared to controls and a reduction in overall mortality.

139. Ikramuddin S, et al. Roux-en-Y gastric bypass vs intensive medical management for the control of type 2 diabetes, hypertension, and hyperlipidemia: the Diabetes Surgery Study randomized clinical trial. JAMA 2013;309:2240–2249.

In this randomized controlled trial comparing Roux-en-Y gastric bypass to intensive medical management, investigators allocated 60 patients to intensive medical management plus Roux-en-Y gastric bypass and 60 to intensive medical management alone and followed them for the development of a primary composite end point comprising hemoglobin A1c < 7%, LDL < 100 mg/dL, and SBP < 130 mm Hg. After 12 months, 49% of patients in the gastric bypass group had reached the primary end point, compared to 19% in the medical management group (OR 4.8; 95% CI, 1.9 to 11.7). There were 22 serious adverse events in the gastric bypass group, compared to 15 in the medical management group.

140. Vest AR, et al. Surgical management of obesity and the relationship of cardiovascular disease. Circulation 2013;127:945–959.

The authors review existing data on the effectiveness of bariatric surgery in causing weight loss and improving metabolic and cardiovascular risk parameters. Though they point out that randomized, controlled trials with cardiovascular end points have been limited in sample size, they do note that observational studies have shown improved mortality in patients undergoing bariatric surgery compared to matched contemporary or historical controls. They conclude that the limited available data suggest that bariatric surgery is safe and effective, but that further studies are needed to ascertain long-term cardiovascular outcomes for patients undergoing bariatric surgery.

141. Steven R, et al.; the Behavioral Modification and Lorcaserin for Overweight and Obesity Management (BLOOM) Study Group. Multicenter, placebo-controlled trial of lorcaserin for weight management. N Engl J Med 2010;363:245–256.

Design: Prospective, randomized, placebo-controlled, double-blind trial. The coprimary end points were weight loss at 1 year and maintenance of weight loss at 2 years.

Purpose: To assess the efficacy and safety of lorcaserin, a selective serotonin 2C receptor agonist, for weight loss.

Population: 3,182 patients with BMI $\geq$30 kg/m^2 (or $\geq$27 kg/m^2 with at least one comorbidity).

Treatment: Lorcaserin 10 mg twice daily or placebo.

Results: A greater proportion of patients receiving lorcaserin lost 5% or more of body weight, compared to those receiving placebo (47.5% vs. 20.3%, $p < 0.001$). However, only 55.4% and 45.1% of patients, respectively, remained in the study at 1 year. Among those who lost at least 5% of body weight at year 1, those who continued to receive lorcaserin were more likely to maintain the weight loss, compared to those receiving placebo (67.9% vs. 50.3%, $p < 0.001$) (see also *Obesity* (Silver Spring) 2012;20(7):1426–1436).

142. Gadde KM, et al. Effects of low-dose, controlled-release, phentermine plus topiramate combination on weight and associated comorbidities in overweight and obese adults (CONQUER): a randomised, placebo-controlled, phase 3 trial. *Lancet* 2011;377(9774):1341–1352.

Design: Prospective, randomized, double-blind, placebo-controlled trial. The coprimary end points were the proportion of patients with 5% or more of weight loss and percentage change in body weight at 56 weeks' follow-up.

Purpose: To assess the safety and efficacy of combination therapy with phentermine and topiramate for weight loss.

Population: 2,487 patients with BMI 27 to 45 kg/m^2 and 2 or more comorbidities (HTN, dyslipidemia, diabetes, prediabetes, or abdominal obesity).

Treatment: Phentermine 7.5 mg plus topiramate 46.0 mg once daily, phentermine 15.0 mg plus topiramate 92.0 mg once daily, or placebo.

Results: Change in body weight was -1.4 kg for those on placebo, -8.1 kg for those on lower-dose phentermine/topiramate (-7.8%; $p < 0.0001$), and -10.2 kg (-9.8%; $p < 0.0001$) for those on higher-dose phentermine/topiramate. Loss of at least 5% of body weight occurred in 21%, 62% ($p < 0.0001$), and 70% ($p < 0.0001$), respectively.

143. Apovian CM, et al.; COR-II Study Group. A randomized, phase 3 trial of naltrexone SR/bupropion SR on weight and obesity-related risk factors (COR-II). *Obesity (Silver Spring)* 2013;21(5):935–943.

Design: Prospective, randomized, placebo-controlled, double-blind trial. The coprimary end points were change in weight and proportion with at least 5% weight loss at 28 weeks.

Purpose: To assess the safety and efficacy of combination therapy with naltrexone and bupropion for weight loss.

Population: 1,496 patients with BMI 30 to 45 kg/m^2 (or 27 to 45 kg/m^2 with HTN and/or dyslipidemia).

Treatment: Naltrexone sustained release (32 mg/day) plus bupropion SR (360 mg/day) or placebo.

Results: Patients assigned to naltrexone/bupropion had greater percentage weight loss at 28 weeks (6.5% vs. 1.9%, $p < 0.001$) and at 56 weeks (6.4% vs. 1.2%, $p < 0.0001$). More patients receiving naltrexone/bupropion had weight loss of at least 5% of body weight at 28 weeks (55.6% vs. 17.5%).

EXERCISE

144. Leon AS, et al. Physical activity and 10.5 year mortality in the Multiple Risk Factor Intervention Trial (MRFIT). *Int J Epidemiol* 1991;20:690–697.

This analysis focused on 12,138 male MRFIT subjects who had leisure time physical activity (LTPA) assessed by the Minnesota questionnaire. The level of LTPA was inversely related to all-cause mortality, CHD mortality, and cardiovascular mortality; those in the lowest LTPA tertile had excess mortality rates of 15%, 27%, and 22%, respectively, compared with men in the middle tertile. No significant further attenuation of risk was seen with additional LTPA.

145. Mittleman MA, et al. Triggering of acute MI by heavy physical exertion. N *Engl J Med* 1993;329:1677–1683.

This analysis focused on interviews with 1,228 patients an average of 4 days after MI. Heavy exertion (≥6 metabolic equivalents) within 1 hour had occurred in 4.4%. The RR of acute MI in the 1 hour after exertion was 5.9; however, risk correlated with the frequency of exercise (less than once per week: RR, 107; 1 to 2 times: RR, 19.4; 3 to 4 times: RR, 8.6; at least 5 times: RR, 2.4).

146. Willich SN, et al. Physical exertion as a trigger of AMI. N *Engl J Med* 1993;329:1684–1690.

This analysis focused on interviews with 1,194 patients at 13 ± 6 days after MI. An increased risk of MI was associated with strenuous activity (≥6 metabolic equivalents; 7.1% of patients) at onset of acute MI (RR, 2.1). The RR also was 2.1 for activity within 1 hour; infrequent exercise (less than four times per week) was associated with an RR of 6.9 (vs. 1.3).

147. Rognmo Ø, et al. Cardiovascular risk of high- versus moderate-intensity aerobic exercise in coronary heart disease patients. *Circulation* 2012;126:1436–1440.

In this prospective cohort study of 4,846 patients with CAD undergoing supervised high- and moderate-intensity exercise for a total of 175,820 exercise training hours at 3 Norwegian cardiac rehabilitation centers, the investigators found 1 fatal cardiac arrest that occurred during moderate-intensity training and 2 nonfatal cardiac arrests during high-intensity training. No patients had an MI during exercise training. The authors conclude that the absolute risk of acute adverse cardiac events during supervised exercise training is low and that the inclusion of high-intensity exercise in cardiac rehabilitation should be considered.

148. Kushi LH, et al. Physical activity and mortality in postmenopausal women. *JAMA* 1997;277:1287–1292.

This prospective cohort study of 40,417 postmenopausal Iowa women, aged 55 to 69 years at baseline (1986), assessed physical activity with a mailed questionnaire. After adjustment for confounders and excluding women with heart disease and those who died in the first 3 years of follow-up, women with regular physical activity had a lower risk of death during mean 7 years' follow-up than women who did not (RR, 0.77; 95% CI, 0.66 to 0.90). Increasing frequency of moderate activity was associated with reduced risk of death, and a similar pattern was seen for vigorous physical activity. Women with moderate activity but no vigorous activity also benefited; even moderate activity only once per week was associated with lower mortality (RR, 0.78; 95% CI, 0.64 to 0.96).

149. Manson JE, et al. A prospective study of walking as compared with vigorous exercise in the prevention of coronary heart disease in women. N *Engl J Med* 1999;341:650–658.

This prospective cohort study of 72,488 NHS participants found that brisk walking, as assessed by a self-administered questionnaire, was associated with fewer coronary events. In multivariate analyses, women in the highest quintile group (≥3 hours/week at a brisk pace) had an RR of 0.65 (95% CI, 0.47 to 0.91) compared with those who walked infrequently. Regular vigorous exercise (≥6 METs) was associated with similar risk reductions (30% to 40%).

150. Tanasescu M, et al. Exercise type and intensity in relation to coronary heart disease in men. *JAMA* 2002;288:1994–2000.

This cohort analysis examined the 44,452 US men enrolled in the Health Professionals' Follow-up Study. At follow-up (average, 10.7 years), 1,700 new cases of CHD were found. Total physical activity, running, weight training, and rowing were each inversely associated with risk of CHD. The adjusted RRs of nonfatal MI or fatal CHD corresponding to quintiles of METs for total physical activity were 1.0, 0.90 (95% CI, 0.78 to 1.04), 0.87 (0.75 to 1.00), 0.83 (0.71 to 0.96), and 0.70 (0.59 to 0.82; $p < 0.001$ for trend). Men who ran for an hour or more per week had a 42% risk reduction (RR, 0.58; 95% CI, 0.44 to 0.77) compared with men who did not run ($p < 0.001$ for trend). Weight training for 30 minutes or more per week was associated with a 23% risk reduction (RR, 0.77; 95% CI, 0.61 to 0.98; $p = 0.03$ for trend), whereas rowing for 1 hour or more per week was associated with an 18% risk reduction (RR, 0.82; 05% CI, 0.68 to 0.99). Average exercise intensity was associated with reduced CHD risk, independent of the total volume of physical activity: moderate (4 to 6 METs) and high (6 to 12 METs) activity intensities were associated with 6% and 17% RRRs compared with low activity intensity (<4 METs; $p = 0.02$ for trend).

151. Sattelmair J, et al. Dose response between physical activity and risk of coronary heart disease: a meta-analysis. *Circulation* 2011;124:789–795.

In this meta-analysis of nine studies that included quantitative estimates of LTPA, the authors found a 14% relative risk reduction in the incidence of CAD with 150 minutes/week of moderate exercise (RR, 0.86; 95% CI, 0.77 to 0.96) and a 20% relative risk reduction with 300 minutes/week of moderate exercise (RR, 0.80; 95% CI, 0.74 to 0.88). The weekly exercise durations were chosen based on US guidelines suggesting a minimum of 150 minutes of exercise per week and suggesting that additional benefits would be accrued in those participating in 300 minutes of exercise per week.

152. Carnethon MR, et al. Cardiorespiratory fitness in young adulthood and the development of cardiovascular disease risk factors. *JAMA* 2003;290:3092–3100.

As part of the Coronary Artery Risk Development in Young Adults (**CARDIA**) study, participants aged 18 to 30 years who had completed the treadmill examination in 1985 to 1986 were followed up in 2000 to 2001. Investigators measured the incidence of type 2 diabetes, HTN, metabolic syndrome, and hypercholesterolemia, stratified by cardiorespiratory fitness. After first adjusting for age, race, sex, smoking, and family history of risk factors (diabetes, HTN, premature MI), participants in the lowest quintile of fitness were significantly more likely to develop diabetes, HTN, and metabolic syndrome when compared with those in the top three quintiles ($p < 0.001$). Statistically, BMI partially accounted for such an effect. Interval increase in fitness did improve a participant's risk of developing such cardiovascular risk factors; however, this effect was mitigated when controlling for change in weight over the same period.

SMOKING

Epidemiology

153. Willett WC, et al. Relative and excess risks of coronary heart disease among women who smoke cigarettes. *N Engl J Med* 1987;317:1303–1309.

This analysis focused on 119,404 NHS participants with 6 years of follow-up; 30% were smokers. They found that number of cigarettes smoked per day correlated positively with risk of fatal and nonfatal CHD. Compared to a nonsmoker, smoking 1 to 4 cigarettes/day was associated with a 2.4-fold increased risk; 5 to 14 cigarettes/day, a 2.1-fold increased risk; 15 to 24 cigarettes/day, a 4.2-fold increased risk; 25 to 34 cigarettes/day, a 5.4-fold increased risk; 35 to 44 cigarettes/day, a 7.1-fold increased risk; and ≥ 45 cigarettes/day, a 10.8-fold increased risk. Overall, smoking was responsible for approximately 50% of events. The greatest absolute risks were seen with smoking in combination with other risk factors: smoking and HTN, RR, 22.2; smoking and hypercholesterolemia, RR, 18.9; and smoking and diabetes, RR, 22.3.

154. Kawachi I, et al. Smoking cessation and time course of decreased risks of coronary heart disease in middle-aged women. *Arch Intern Med* 1994;154:169–175.

This prospective cohort study was composed of 117,006 nurses free of CHD in 1976. The average follow-up period was 11.7 years. In a multivariate analysis, among current smokers versus never smokers, the RR was 4.23 (95% CI, 3.60 to 4.96); among those who started smoking before age 15 years, RR, 9.25; and among former smokers, RR, 1.48 (95% CI, 1.22 to 1.79). After quitting, one-third of the excess risk was gone at 3 years, and normal risk was attained after 10 to 14 years.

155. Colivicchi F, et al. Effect of smoking relapse on outcome after acute coronary syndromes. *Am J Cardiol* 2011;108:804–808.

In this prospective cohort study, investigators followed 1,294 active smokers who had stopped smoking after an admission for ACS for 1 year after hospital discharge to determine the number of patients that resumed smoking and the likelihood of cardiovascular events in abstainers and relapsers. On multivariate analysis, the resumption of smoking was associated with a 3.1-fold increased risk of 1-year mortality (95% CI, 1.3 to 5.7; $p = 0.004$).

156. Steenland K, et al. Environmental tobacco smoke and coronary heart disease in the ACS CPS-II cohort. *Circulation* 1996;94:622–628 (editorial, 596–599).

This prospective study included 353,180 female and 126,500 male nonsmokers. A 22% higher CHD mortality rate (95% CI, 7% to 40%) was observed among men married to current smokers compared to men married to never smokers; the corresponding RR for women married to current smokers was 1.1 (95% CI, 0.96 to 1.22). Living with a former smoker conferred no excess risk. The editorial provides an analysis of data from 14 studies that shows an approximate 20% increased risk of CHD death in nonsmokers married to smokers.

157. He J, et al. Passive smoking and the risk of coronary heart disease: a meta-analysis of epidemiologic studies. *N Engl J Med* 1999;340:920–926.

This analysis of 10 cohort and 8 case–control studies showed that nonsmokers exposed to environmental smoke had 25% increased risk of CHD (95% CI, 17% to 32%) compared with that of nonsmokers with no such exposure. This association was significant in both men and women and present in those exposed at home or in the workplace. A significant dose–response relation was demonstrated: the RR of CHD was 1.23 in those exposed to the smoke of 1 to 19 cigarettes/day compared to a RR of 1.31 in those exposed to $\geq$ 20 cigarettes/day ($p = 0.006$ for linear trend).

158. Hamer M, et al. Objectively measured secondhand smoke exposure and risk of cardiovascular disease: What is the mediating role of inflammatory and hemostatic factors? *J Am Coll Cardiol* 2010;56:18–23.

In this prospective study of 13,443 nonsmokers, researchers measured salivary cotinine (a marker of secondhand smoke exposure) and serum CRP and fibrinogen at baseline; participants were subsequently followed for a mean of 8 years for the development of cardiovascular death. At follow-up, high baseline salivary cotinine was significantly associated with all-cause mortality (HR, 1.25; 95% CI, 1.02 to 1.53) and CVD (HR, 2.44; 95% CI, 1.75 to 3.40). Secondhand smoke exposure was associated with elevated levels of CRP, which statistically explained 40% of the excess all-cause mortality associated with secondhand smoke exposure.

159. Centers for Disease Control and Prevention. Reduced hospitalizations for acute myocardial infarction after implementation of a smoke-free ordinance—City of Pueblo, Colorado, 2002–2006. *MMWR Morb Mortal Wkly Rep* 2009;57:1373–1377.

In this Colorado town, the authors identify significant declines in rates of acute MI after a city-wide smoking ban was implemented in July 1, 2003. They detected such a decline within only 18 months after the ban went into effect.

160. Tan CE, et al. Association between smoke-free legislation and hospitalization for cardiac, cerebrovascular, and respiratory diseases: a meta-analysis. *Circulation* 2012;126:2177–2183.

The authors combine 45 studies from 33 smoke-free laws to assess the impact of such ordinances on cardiovascular health. Risk of hospital admission or death dropped by 15% for coronary events, 39% for other heart disease, and 16% for cerebrovascular accidents. More comprehensive laws reduced risk more than less comprehensive laws.

Smoking Cessation

161. The Varenicline Phase 3 Study Group. See JAMA 2006;296:56–63, JAMA 2006;296:47–55, and JAMA 2006;296:64–71.

These three reports from the Varenicline Phase 3 Study Group compared varenicline, a partial nicotine receptor agonist, to placebo and sustained-release bupropion for effectiveness at achieving smoking cessation. In several thousand adult smokers, these series of reports demonstrated that patients taking varenicline were significantly more likely to abstain from cigarette smoking over follow-up periods up to 1 year. Abstinence was proven by carbon monoxide testing. Further monitoring has revealed a risk of significant psychiatric side effects with varenicline treatment, leading to FDA warnings for patients at high risk of such adverse events.

162. Rigotti NA, et al. Efficacy and safety of varenicline for smoking cessation in patients with cardiovascular disease: a randomized trial. *Circulation* 2010;121:221–229.

The investigators randomized 714 smokers with stable CVD to varenicline or placebo, with counseling for smoking cessation, over 12 weeks. Smoking abstinence was higher for those on varenicline, and there was no difference in adverse cardiovascular events over 52 weeks of follow-up.

Metabolic Syndrome and Diabetes

EPIDEMIOLOGY

163. Haffner SM, et al. Mortality from coronary heart disease in subjects with type 2 diabetes and in nondiabetic subjects with and without prior MI. *N Engl J Med* 1998;339:229–234.

This Finnish-based population study found that diabetic subjects ($n = 1,059$) without a prior MI had a similar risk of subsequent MI compared with nondiabetic subjects ($n = 1,373$) with a prior MI. The 7-year incidence rates of MI among diabetics with and without a prior MI were 45.0% and 22%, compared with 18.8% and 3.5% in nondiabetics. The risk factor–adjusted HR for death from CHD for diabetics without prior MI as compared with nondiabetics with a prior MI was 1.2 (95% CI, 0.6 to 2.4). This was one of the first population-based studies to establish diabetes as a CAD risk equivalent.

164. Gu K, et al. Diabetes and decline in heart disease mortality in U.S. adults. *JAMA* 1999;281:1291–1297.

This analysis of data from the First National Health and Nutrition Examination Survey (NHANES I; 1971 to 1975) and NHANES I Epidemiologic Follow-up Survey (1982 to 1984) showed that the declines in heart disease mortality seen in the general population have not occurred in diabetics. The two cohorts were followed up for mortality at an average of 8 to 9 years. Comparing the 1982 to 1984 period with the 1971 to 1975 period, nondiabetic men had a 36.4% decline in age-adjusted heart disease mortality compared with only a 13% decline for men with diabetes. Among women, nondiabetics had a 27% decline, whereas a 23% increase occurred in diabetics. A similar pattern was found for all-cause mortality.

165. Lotufo PA, et al. Diabetes and all-cause and coronary heart disease mortality among U.S. male physicians. *Arch Intern Med* 2001;161:242–247.

This prospective cohort study found that the increased overall mortality risk conferred by diabetes is similar to that conferred by a history of CHD, whereas for CHD mortality, a history of CHD is a more potent predictor than is diabetes. The total cohort of 91,285 US male physicians (aged 40 to 84 years) consisted of four groups: (a) reference group of 82,247 free of both diabetes and CHD (previous MI and/or angina) at baseline; (b) 2,317 with history of diabetes but not CHD; (c) 5,906 with history of CHD but not diabetes; and (d) 815 with a history of both diabetes and CHD. At follow-up (average 5.5 years), compared to the reference group of men without diabetes and CHD, the age-adjusted RR of mortality was 2.3 (95% CI, 2.0 to 2.6) among men with diabetes and without CHD, 2.2 (95% CI, 2.0 to 2.4) among men with CHD and without diabetes, and 4.7 (95% CI, 4.0 to 5.4) among men with both diabetes and CHD. The corresponding RRs of CHD death were 3.3, 5.6, and 12.0. Multivariate adjustment for BMI, smoking status, alcohol intake, and activity did not significantly alter these associations.

166. Wannamethee SG, et al. Impact of diabetes on cardiovascular risk and all-cause mortality in older men: influence of age at onset, diabetes duration, and established and novel risk factors. *Arch Intern Med* 2011;171:404–410.

In this prospective cohort study of 4045 60- to 79-year-old men with either diabetes or CAD followed for a mean of 9 years, investigators attempted to determine the risk of cardiovascular events conferred by early- or late-onset diabetes mellitus, as compared to CAD. Patients with both early-onset (diagnosed prior to age 60) and late-onset diabetes mellitus were at higher risk for cardiovascular events, compared to control patients without either diabetes or coronary disease (RR, 1.54 for late-onset diabetes and RR, 2.39 for early-onset diabetes), but only patients with early-onset diabetes mellitus had risk similar to those patients with prior MI (RR, 2.51). The authors conclude that only early-onset diabetes should be considered a true CAD risk equivalent.

167. Selvin E, et al. Glycated hemoglobin, diabetes, and cardiovascular risk in nondiabetic adults. *N Engl J Med* 2010;362:800–811.

In this prospective analysis of 11,092 middle-aged adults without diabetes or CVD at baseline enrolled in the ARIC study cohort, investigators measured glycated hemoglobin at baseline (1990 to 1992) and followed subjects for 15 years for the development of diabetes or CHD. Compared to a reference group of subjects with glycated hemoglobin 5% to 5.5% at baseline, subjects with glycated hemoglobin 5.5% to 6%, 6% to 6.5%, and >6.5% at baseline had hazard ratios for the 15-year development of CAD of 1.23 (95% CI, 1.07 to 1.41), 1.78 (95% CI, 1.48 to 2.15), and 1.95 (95% CI, 1.53 to 2.48), respectively. Elevated glycated hemoglobin at baseline was even more strongly associated with incident diabetes at 15-year follow-up.

168. Ford ES, et al. Prevalence of the metabolic syndrome among U.S. adults: findings from the third National Health and Nutrition Examination Survey. *JAMA* 2002;287:356–359.

This analysis examined data on 8,814 participants in the Third National Health and Nutrition Examination Survey (1988 to 1994). The ATP III definition of the metabolic syndrome was used (three or more of the following: waist circumference, >102 cm in men and >88 cm in women; TGs ≥ 150 mg/dL; HDL < 40 mg/dL in men or < 50 mg/dL in women; BP > 130/85 mm Hg; and glucose level ≥ 110 mg/dL). The unadjusted prevalence of metabolic syndrome was 21.8%. Prevalence increased from 6.7% in those aged 20 through 29 years to 43.5% and 42.0% for those aged 60 to 69 years and 70 years or older, respectively. Age-adjusted prevalences were similar in men (24.0%) and women (23.4%); however, among African Americans, women had a 57% higher prevalence than men, and among Mexican Americans, women had about a 26% higher prevalence than men.

169. Lakka HM, et al. The metabolic syndrome and total and cardiovascular disease mortality in middle-aged men. *JAMA* 2002;288:2709–2716.

This study analyzed data on 1,209 participants in a population-based, prospective cohort study of Finnish men who were initially free of CVD, cancer, or diabetes. At 11.4 years of follow-up, a total of 109 deaths had occurred, and the prevalence of the metabolic syndrome ranged from 8.8% to 14.3%, depending on the definition. After adjustment for conventional risk factors, the metabolic syndrome was associated with a significant 2.9- to 4.2-fold increased risk of CHD death (by both NCEP and WHO definitions). With the WHO definition, all-cause mortality was 1.9 times higher in those with the metabolic syndrome. The NCEP definition less consistently predicted CVD and all-cause mortality.

170. Peterson JL, et al. Metabolic syndrome is not associated with increased mortality or cardiovascular risk in nondiabetic patients with a new diagnosis of coronary artery disease. *Circ Cardiovasc Qual Outcomes* 2010;3:165–172.

In an observational analysis of patients with angiographically proven obstructive CAD, researchers assessed the prevalence of diabetes and the metabolic syndrome and assessed rates of the primary outcome of death, MI, or stroke at 6 months, 1 year, and then annually to a median of 5 years. For these patients with newly diagnosed CAD, diabetes, but *not* the metabolic syndrome, was significantly predictive of worse outcome, by all measures.

171. Arnlöv J, et al. Impact of body mass index and the metabolic syndrome on the risk of cardiovascular disease and death in middle-aged men. *Circulation* 2010;121:230–236.

In this cohort analysis, 1,758 subjects without CVD in 1970 to 1973 when enrolled in the Uppsala Longitudinal Study of Adult Men (USLAM) were retrospectively categorized by weight (normal, overweight, obese) and by the presence of the metabolic syndrome. At 30 years' follow-up, normal weight patients with the metabolic syndrome, overweight and obese patients with the metabolic syndrome, and overweight and obese patients without the metabolic syndrome all had increased risk of CVD as compared to normal weight patients without metabolic syndrome. These findings are contrary to other studies suggesting that overweight and obesity without the metabolic syndrome do not convey excess risk.

172. Motillo S, et al. Metabolic syndrome and cardiovascular risk: a systematic review and meta-analysis. *J Am Coll Cardiol* 2010;56:1113–1132.

This meta-analysis pooled the results of 87 studies including 951,083 patients to determine the cardiovascular risk associated with the metabolic syndrome, as defined by the NCEP definition. The metabolic syndrome was associated with an increased risk of CVD (RR, 2.35; 95% CI, 2.02 to 2.73), cardiovascular mortality (RR, 2.40; 95% CI, 1.87 to 3.08), all-cause mortality (RR, 1.58; 95% CI, 1.39 to 1.78), MI (RR, 1.99; 95% CI, 1.61 to 2.46), and stroke (RR, 2.27; 95% CI, 1.80 to 2.85). It was not clear whether the risk of the metabolic syndrome exceeded that of its component metabolic derangements.

TREATMENT

173. Gaede P, et al. STENO-2. Multifactorial intervention and cardiovascular disease in patients with type 2 diabetes. *N Engl J Med* 2003;348:383–393.

This prospective, open, parallel-group trial randomized 160 type 2 diabetics with microalbuminuria to conventional treatment, in accordance with national guidelines, or intensive treatment, with a step-wise implementation of behavior modification and drug therapy that targeted hyperglycemia, HTN, dyslipidemia, and microalbuminuria as well as secondary prevention of CVD with ASA. At follow-up (mean, 7.8 years), the intensive therapy group had a significantly lower risk of CVD (HR, 0.47; 95% CI, 0.24 to 0.73), nephropathy (HR, 0.39; 95% CI, 0.17 to 0.87), and retinopathy (HR, 0.42; 95% CI, 0.21 to 0.86).

174. The Look AHEAD Research Group. Cardiovascular effects of intensive lifestyle intervention in type 2 diabetes. *N Engl J Med* 2013;369:145–154.

In this trial involving 5,145 overweight or obese patients with type 2 diabetes, the researchers randomized half to an intensive lifestyle intervention (vs. usual care) in an effort to assess cardiovascular effects of weight loss. Subjects were assessed at 1 year for surrogate end points (see *Diabetes Care* 2007;30:1374–1383) and were followed for a median of 9.6 years for the incidence of a composite primary end point that incorporated cardiovascular death, nonfatal MI, nonfatal stroke, or hospitalization related to angina. Those in the intervention group lost significantly more weight than controls (8.6% body weight lost vs. 0.7%, $p < 0.001$ at 1 year; 6.0% vs. 3.5% at study end) and additionally had significant improvements in cardiac risk factors, such as hemoglobin A1c, BP, TGs, and HDL, at 1 year and at study end, though LDL cholesterol did not significantly differ between groups. However, at study end, the incidence of the primary outcome did not differ significantly between the intensive intervention and usual-care groups (HR, 0.95; 95% CI, 0.83 to 1.09; $p = 0.51$).

175. The Action to Control Cardiovascular Risk in Diabetes Study (ACCORD) Group. Effects of intensive glucose lowering in type 2 diabetes. N Engl J Med 2008;358:2545–2559.

Design: Prospective, randomized, multicenter study. The primary end point was a composite outcome of nonfatal MI, stroke, or death from cardiovascular causes. Mean follow-up was 3.5 years prior to study discontinuation.

Purpose: To test the hypothesis that more intensive glucose control would reduce cardiovascular events in patients with type 2 diabetes.

Population: 10,251 patients with type 2 diabetes and HbA1c $\geq$ 7.5%, who were either aged 40 to 79 years with CVD or aged 55 to 79 with anatomical evidence of significant diabetic end-organ damage or atherosclerosis risk factors.

Treatment: Intensive therapy targeting an HbA1c < 6.0% versus standard therapy targeting an HbA1c of 7.0% to 7.9%. Counseling and lifestyle modification were employed in both groups, and there were no particular restrictions on the type of pharmacotherapy implemented.

Results: The difference in mean HbA1c achieved was significant at 1 year (6.4% in the intensive therapy vs. 7.5% in the standard therapy). After a mean follow-up period of 3.5 years, the study was discontinued due to the finding of higher mortality in the intensive therapy group (257 deaths in the intensive arm vs. 203 in the standard group, $p = 0.04$). At the premature stopping point, a primary end point event had occurred in 352 patients in the intensive therapy group versus 371 in the standard therapy group (HR, 0.90; 95% CI, 0.78 to 1.04; $p = 0.16$). There were significantly more episodes of hypoglycemia requiring assistance in the intensive therapy group ($p < 0.001$).

Comment: The results of this study came as a surprise, and the underlying mechanism(s) explaining such an outcome are not clear. The intensive therapy arm may have had too aggressive of a goal, or perhaps, the *type* of hypoglycemic therapy is important, as well. Following the termination of this clinical trial, the approaches originally applied to patients in the standard group were applied to patients in the intensive therapy group. After 17 months of additional follow-up, the difference in overall mortality between the groups remained the same, despite similar incidences of severe hypoglycemia following the termination of the intensive therapy arm (see *N Engl J Med* 2011;364:818–828), strengthening claims that hypoglycemia was not the mediator of increased mortality in the intensive therapy group.

176. The Action in Diabetes and Vascular Disease: Preterax and Diamicron Modified Release Controlled Evaluation (ADVANCE) Collaborative Group. Intensive blood glucose control and vascular outcomes in patients with type 2 diabetes. N Engl J Med 2008;358:2560–2572.

Design: Prospective, randomized, multicenter study. The primary end point was a composite outcome of major macrovascular events (cardiovascular death, MI, stroke) and major microvascular events (nephropathy or retinopathy), both jointly and separately, after a median of 5 years of follow-up.

Purpose: To test the hypothesis that more intensive glucose control would reduce macro- and microvascular events in patients with type 2 diabetes.

Population: 11,140 patients with type 2 diabetes, diagnosed at age 30 years or older, who were 55 years or older at study entry and had a history of major macro- or microvascular disease, or at least one additional risk factor for vascular disease. Baseline HbA1c levels were not included in the inclusion or exclusion criteria.

Treatment: Intensive therapy targeting HbA1c ≤ 6.5% using glipizide plus other drugs as needed versus standard glucose control.

Results: At the conclusion of the study, mean HbA1c level was lower in the intensive therapy group (6.5%) than in the standard therapy arm (7.3%). Combined major macro- and microvascular events were lower in the intensive therapy group (18.1% vs. 20.0%; $p = 0.01$), which was primarily driven by a reduction in major microvascular events (9.4% vs. 10.9%; $p = 0.01$), specifically nephropathy. There were no differences in outcomes with regard to retinopathy or major macrovascular events between the two groups.

Comment: The composite end point of this contemporary trial summarizes the combined outcomes of several previous trials—aggressive glucose control in type 2 diabetes can have significant effects on *micro*vascular disease (retinopathy, nephropathy); however, it is difficult to improve on *macro*vascular events (MI, stroke). A subsequent analysis of the trial data demonstrated that a significantly higher number of patients in the intensive therapy group had an episode of severe hypoglycemia (defined as transient CNS impairment leaving patients unable to treat themselves) compared to the group assigned to standard control (2.7% vs. 1.2%). Patients with severe hypoglycemia were more likely to have major cardiac events (HR, 2.88), major microvascular events (HR, 1.81), cardiovascular death (HR, 2.68), and all-cause death (HR, 2.69) (see *N Engl J Med* 2010;363:1410–1418). Though the authors caution that hypoglycemia is as likely to be a marker of vulnerability to adverse events as it is to be a contributor to them, the results of ACCORD and ADVANCE together suggest that attempts at intensive glucose control will be limited by the substantial risks of hypoglycemia. It is unclear if different therapies (specifically, metformin) could have changed the outcome of this trial.

177. Hemmingsen B, et al. Intensive glycaemic control for patients with type 2 diabetes: systematic review with meta-analysis and trial sequential analysis of randomized controlled trials. *BMJ* 2011;343:d6898.

In this meta-analysis of 14 randomized controlled trials enrolling 28,614 patients with type 2 diabetes allocated to intensive or conventional glycemic control, investigators found no effect of tight glycemic control on all-cause mortality (RR, 1.02; 95% CI, 0.91 to 1.13) or cardiovascular mortality (RR, 1.11; 95% CI, 0.92 to 1.13). Intensive glycemic control was shown to reduce the risk of nonfatal MI (RR, 0.85; 95% CI, 0.76 to 0.95), microvascular adverse outcomes (RR, 0.88; 95% CI, 0.79 to 0.97), and retinopathy (RR, 0.80; 95% CI, 0.67 to 0.94), with no significant effect on nephropathy. The risk of hypoglycemia was significantly increased by intensive glycemic control (RR, 2.39; 95% CI, 1.71 to 3.34). This meta-analysis essentially synthesizes the findings of ACCORD and ADVANCE, trials that together contributed 75% of the total number of patients included in the meta-analysis.

178. Yakubovich N, et al. Serious cardiovascular outcomes in diabetes: the role of hypoglycemia. *Circulation* 2011;123:342–438.

In this review, the authors summarize clinical trial and epidemiologic data to determine whether interventions that increase the risk of hypoglycemia also increase the risk of adverse cardiac outcomes, whether hypoglycemic episodes are a risk factor for adverse cardiac events, and whether hypoglycemic episodes can precipitate cardiovascular events. They conclude that the data are mixed on whether interventions that cause hypoglycemia increase the risk of cardiac events, citing the different cardiovascular outcomes of ACCORD and ADVANCE (see above), as well as neutral data from trials in lower-risk patients and those using the thiazolidinediones pioglitazone and rosiglitazone.

179. The ORIGIN trial investigators. Basal insulin and cardiovascular and other outcomes in dysglycemia. *N Engl J Med* 2013;367:319–328.

Design: Prospective, randomized, multicenter study. The coprimary end points were (a) a composite of death from cardiovascular causes, nonfatal MI, and nonfatal stroke and (b) these events plus hospitalization for heart failure and revascularization. This substudy was part of a larger trial with a 2 × 2 factorial design that randomized the same patients to n-3 fatty acid supplementation or placebo. Median follow-up was 6.2 years.

Purpose: To assess the efficacy of insulin provision compared to standard care in the prevention of adverse cardiac outcomes in patients with cardiovascular risk factors and type 2 diabetes or impaired fasting glucose.

Population: 12,537 people with cardiovascular risk factors or known CVD in addition to impaired glucose tolerance, impaired fasting glucose, or type 2 diabetes mellitus not already on insulin therapy.

Treatment: Subcutaneous injection of insulin glargine (with a target fasting blood glucose ≤ 95 mg/dL) or standard care.

Results: Insulin provision was successful in reducing fasting glucose to ≤ 94 mg/dL in 50% of participants. Nevertheless, the incidence of both coprimary outcomes was similar between the insulin glargine and standard care groups (HR, 1.02, for the first coprimary outcome; HR, 1.04, for the second coprimary outcome). Rates of severe hypoglycemia were significantly higher in the insulin glargine group.

180. Home PD, et al.; for the RECORD Study Team. Rosiglitazone evaluated for cardiovascular outcomes in oral agent combination therapy for type 2 diabetes (RECORD): a multicentre, randomised, open-label trial. *Lancet* 2009;373:2125–2135.

Design: Open-label, multicenter randomized, active-controlled clinical trial. Primary outcome was a composite of cardiovascular death or hospitalization due to cardiovascular causes. Mean follow-up was 5.5 years.

Purpose: To determine the noninferiority of rosiglitazone, an insulin sensitizer, plus metformin and a sulfonylurea to a standard-of-care regimen including metformin and a sulfonylurea in the prevention of cardiovascular events. The prespecified noninferiority margin was HR ≤ 1.2.

Population: 4,447 patients, aged 40 to 75, with type 2 diabetes and mean HbA1c 7.9% on maximum tolerated doses of either metformin or sulfonylurea. Patients with known heart failure were excluded.

Treatment: Rosiglitazone 4 mg/day, titrated up to 8 mg/day targeting an HbA1c of ≤ 7%, plus metformin or a sulfonylurea, with the addition of a third agent for HbA1c ≥ 8.5%, or metformin plus sulfonylurea targeting an HbA1c of ≤ 7%.

Results: At 5 years' follow-up, the rosiglitazone group did have a lower mean HbA1c. Treatment with rosiglitazone plus either metformin or a sulfonylurea was noninferior to combination therapy with metformin plus a sulfonylurea in the prevention of the primary outcome (HR, 0.99; 95% CI, 0.85 to 1.16). The HRs for cardiovascular death, MI, and stroke were 0.84, 1.14, and 0.72, respectively; the upper limit of the 95% CI was greater than the noninferiority margin only for MI. However, patients treated with rosiglitazone did have a twofold increase in heart failure hospitalizations or death (risk difference, 2.6 deaths or hospitalizations per 1,000 person-years; HR 2.1; 95% CI, 1.35 to 3.27).

181. Scirica BM, et al.; for the SAVOR-TIMI 53 Steering Committee and Investigators. Saxagliptin and cardiovascular outcomes in patients with type 2 diabetes mellitus. *N Engl J Med* 2013;369(14):1317–1326.

Design: Multicenter, randomized, placebo-controlled multicenter study. Primary outcome was a composite of cardiovascular death, nonfatal MI, or nonfatal ischemic stroke. Median follow-up was 2.1 years.

Purpose: To assess the cardiovascular safety and efficacy of saxagliptin, a novel dipeptidyl peptidase 4 (DPP-4) inhibitor.

Patients: 16,492 patients with type 2 diabetes mellitus, HbA1c between 6.5% and 12%, and either ≥ 40 years old with established CVD or ≥ 55 years old (in men) or 60 years old (in women) with either hyperlipidemia, HTN, or active smoking. Nearly 80% of patients had established CVD.

Treatment: Saxagliptin 2.5 or 5 mg/day (adjusted for renal function), or matching placebo.

Results: At the end of the follow-up period, hemoglobin A1c levels were lower in the saxagliptin group than the placebo group (7.7% vs. 7.9%; $p < 0.001$), and these patients were less likely to require the initiation of a new oral hypoglycemic medication or insulin ($p < 0.001$ for both). A primary end point event occurred in 7.3% of patients in the saxagliptin group, compared to 7.2% of patients in the placebo group (HR, 1.00; 95% CI, 0.89 to 1.12). A prespecified noninferiority analysis demonstrated the noninferiority of saxagliptin compared to placebo with respect to the primary outcome (p for noninferiority < 0.001). Saxagliptin was noninferior to placebo in an on-treatment analysis, as well as in most secondary outcomes, though patients treated with saxagliptin were more likely to be hospitalized for heart failure (3.5% vs. 2.8%; HR, 1.27; 95% CI, 1.07 to 1.51; $p = 0.007$).

182. White WB, et al.; for the EXAMINE Investigators. Alogliptin after acute coronary syndrome in patients with type 2 diabetes. *N Engl J Med* 2013;369(14):1327–1335.

Design: Multicenter, randomized, placebo-controlled multicenter study. Primary outcome was a composite of cardiovascular death, nonfatal MI, or nonfatal ischemic stroke. Median follow-up was 18 months.

Purpose: To assess the noninferiority of the addition of alogliptin, a novel DPP-4 inhibitor, to usual care in patients with recent ACS. The prespecified noninferiority margin was HR ≤ 1.3.

Patients: 5,380 patients with type 2 diabetes mellitus, HbA1c between 6.5% and 11%, and recent ACS.

Treatment: Alogliptin 6.25 to 25 mg/day, or matching placebo.

Results: At the end of the follow-up period, absolute HbA1c levels had decreased by 0.33% in the alogliptin group and had increased by 0.03% in the placebo group ($p < 0.001$). A primary end point event occurred in 11.3% of patients in the alogliptin group, compared to 11.8% of patients in the placebo group (HR, 0.96; upper bound of a one-sided 95% CI, 1.16; p for noninferiority < 0.001). Analyses of various secondary end points and subgroups failed to show a difference between the groups.

Hypertension

183. Chobanian AV, et al.; JNC 7. The seventh report of the Joint National Committee on prevention, detection, evaluation, and treatment of high blood pressure: the JNC 7 report. *JAMA* 2003;289:2560–2571.

JNC 7 defines hypertension as SBP > 140 mm Hg or DBP > 90 mm Hg, or taking hypertensive medication(s). JNC 7 introduced a new BP category, prehypertension, that includes those with SBP 120 to 139 mm Hg or DBP 80 to 89 mm Hg. Blood pressure target is < 140/90 mm Hg in most patients, but < 130/80 in patients with diabetes and chronic kidney disease. When pharmacologic intervention is indicated, JNC 7 advocates the use of diuretics and β-blockers as first-line agents in most patients. As was the case with JNC VI, other therapies (e.g., ACE inhibitors) also are recommended for individuals with specific characteristics (see text for details, pages 19–21). If BP is > 20/10 mm Hg above target, initial therapy should be with two agents.

184. James, PA, et al. 2014 evidence-based guideline for the management of high blood pressure in adults: report from the panel members appointed to the Eighth Joint National Committee (JNC 8). JAMA 2014;311(5):507–520.

These most recent JNC guidelines dramatically changed the approach. There was a much more targeted and rigorous analysis of the evidence (or lack thereof), and where absolute cutoffs were not proven superior, recommendations were not made. Definitions of hypertension categories were no longer addressed, and targets became more consistent across populations, except where there was specific evidence for a different target. Medication selection *and* dose was guided by the outcomes trials (**Table 1.3** and **Fig. 1.2**).

Table 1.3	Definition of Ideal Cardiovascular Health
Goal/Metric	**Ideal Cardiovascular Health Definition**
Current smoking	
Adults >20 y of age	Never or quit >12 mo ago
Children 12–19 y of age	Never tried; never smoked whole cigarette
Body mass index	
Adults >20 y of age	$<25 \text{ kg/m}^2$
Children 2–19 y of age	<85th percentile
Physical activity	
Adults >20 y of age	≥150 min/wk moderate intensity or ≥75 min/wk vigorous intensity or combination
Children 12–19 y of age	≥60 min of moderate- or vigorous-intensity activity every day
Healthy diet score[a]	
Adults >20 y of age	4–5 components[a]
Children 5–19 y of age	4–5 components[a]
Total cholesterol	
Adults >20 y of age	$<200 \text{ mg/dL}^b$
Children 6–19 y of age	$<170 \text{ mg/dL}^b$
Blood pressure	
Adults >20 y of age	$<120/<80 \text{ mm Hg}^b$
Children 8–19 y of age	<90th percentile[b]
Fasting plasma glucose	
Adults >20 y of age	$<100 \text{ mg/dL}^b$
Children 8–19 y of age	$<100 \text{ mg/dL}^b$

[a]The committee selected 5 aspects of diet to define a healthy dietary score. The score is not intended to be comprehensive. Rather, it is a practical approach that provides individuals with a set of potential concrete actions.

[b]Untreated values.

Data from Lloyd-Jones DM, et al. Defining and setting national goals for cardiovascular health promotion and disease reduction: the American Heart Association's strategic impact goal through 2020 and beyond. *Circulation* 2010;121:586–613.

EPIDEMIOLOGY AND RISK FACTORS

185. O'Donnell CJ, et al. Hypertension and borderline isolated systolic hypertension increase risks of cardiovascular disease and mortality in male physicians. *Circulation* 1997;95:1132–1137.

This prospective cohort analysis focused on 18,682 PHS participants, with a mean follow-up of 11.7 years. Isolated elevated SBP (140 to 159 mm Hg) was associated with higher rates of stroke (RR, 1.42) and cardiovascular death (RR, 1.56) as well as a 22% higher all-cause mortality rate.

186. Kumbhani DJ, et al.; for the REACH Registry Investigators. Resistant hypertension: a frequent and ominous finding among hypertensive patients with atherothrombosis. *Eur Heart J* 2013;34:1204–1214.

This analysis of the prospective, international REACH registry examined the effect of resistant hypertension (BP above goal despite ≥ 3 antihypertensive medications, including a diuretic) on a primary outcome including MI, stroke, or cardiovascular death at 4 years' follow-up. Among 53,530 patients with hypertension, 12.7% had resistant hypertension, and resistant hypertension was associated by multivariate modeling with a 1.11-fold increased risk of the primary outcome (95% CI, 1.02 to 1.20; $p = 0.017$), with much of this increased risk due to fatal and nonfatal stroke.

187. Mosterd' A, et al. Trends in the prevalence of hypertension, antihypertensive therapy, and left ventricular hypertrophy from 1950 to 1989. *N Engl J Med* 1999;340:1221–1227.

This analysis focused on 10,333 Framingham Heart Study participants. From 1950 to 1989, the age-adjusted prevalence of SBP > 160 mm Hg, or DBP > 100 mm Hg, declined from 18.5% to 9.2% among men and from 28.0% to 7.7% among women. A decline was noted in ECG evidence of LV hypertrophy (LVH): 4.5% to 2.5% and 3.6% to 1.1%.

188. Vasan RS, et al. Residual lifetime risk for developing hypertension in middle-aged women and men: the Framingham Heart Study. *JAMA* 2002;287:1003–1010.

In this prospective cohort analysis of 1,298 Framingham Heart Study participants who were aged 55 to 65 years and free of hypertension at baseline (1976 to 1998), the residual lifetime risk for developing hypertension was determined to be 90% in both 55- and 65-year-old participants. The lifetime probability of receiving antihypertensive medication was 60%. The risk for hypertension remained unchanged for women, but it was approximately 60% higher for men in the 1976 to 1998 period compared with the 1952 to 1975 period. In contrast, the residual lifetime risk for stage 2 hypertension (≥160/100 mm Hg regardless of treatment) was lower in both sexes in the recent period, likely owing to a marked increase in pharmacologic treatment of individuals with substantially elevated BP.

STUDIES OF TREATMENT

Nonpharmacologic Therapies

189. Appel LJ, et al.; for the Dietary Approaches to Stop Hypertension (DASH) Research Group. A clinical trial of the effects of dietary patterns on blood pressure. *N Engl J Med* 1997;336:1117–1124.

This prospective, randomized study was composed of 459 adults with SBP < 160 mm Hg and DBP 80 to 95 mm Hg. For 3 weeks, all participants were fed a control diet that was low in fruits, vegetables, and dairy products. They were then randomized to the control diet or a diet rich in fruits and vegetables or a combination diet rich in fruits, vegetables, and low-fat dairy products and with reduced saturated fat and total fat. Body weight and sodium intake were not modified. The combination diet resulted in significant reductions in SBP and DBP compared with the control diet (11.4 and 5.5 mm Hg, respectively; both $p < 0.001$).

190. Sacks FM, et al.; for the DASH Sodium Collaborative Research Group. Effects on blood pressure of reduced dietary sodium and the dietary approaches to stop hypertension (DASH) diet. N Engl J Med 2001;344:3–10.

This prospective trial randomized 412 participants to a control diet typical of intake in the United States or the DASH diet (rich in vegetables, fruits, and low-fat dairy products). Within the assigned diet, participants ate foods with high, intermediate, and low levels of sodium for 30 consecutive days each, in random order. Decreasing sodium intake from the high to intermediate level reduced SBP by 2.1 mm Hg ($p < 0.001$) in subjects consuming the control diet and by 1.3 mm Hg ($p = 0.03$) in those consuming the DASH diet. Decreasing intake from the intermediate to low level resulted in further reductions of 4.6 mm Hg with the control diet ($p < 0.001$) and 1.7 mm Hg with the DASH diet ($p < 0.01$). The effects of sodium were seen in those with and without hypertension, blacks, and women and men. The benefits of the DASH diet and low sodium intake were additive, with the largest SBP difference seen between those on the control diet with high sodium intake and those on the DASH diet with low sodium (DASH diet with low sodium, 7.1 mm Hg lower in those without hypertension, 11.5 mm Hg lower in hypertensives). In summary, the reduction of sodium intake to levels below the current recommendation of 100 mmol/d and the DASH diet both reduce BP substantially, with greater effects in combination.

191. Marin JM, et al. Association between treated and untreated obstructive sleep apnea and risk of hypertension. JAMA 2012;307:2169–2176.

In this prospective cohort study, 1,889 patients free of hypertension who were referred by their physicians for polysomnography were followed for a median of 12.2 years after their sleep study and assessed for the development of hypertension. Ultimately, 310 patients were not diagnosed with obstructive sleep apnea (OSA) and served as controls. Over the follow-up period, patients with OSA not treated with CPAP (due to ineligibility, intolerance, or nonadherence) were more likely to develop hypertension than controls, whereas those patients with OSA treated with CPAP were actually less likely to develop hypertension than controls.

192. Barbé F, et al.; for the Spanish Sleep and Breathing Network. Effect of continuous positive airway pressure on the incidence of hypertension and cardiovascular events in nonsleepy patients with obstructive sleep apnea: a randomized controlled trial. JAMA 2012;307:2161–2168.

In this prospective, randomized, controlled, nonblinded clinical trial, investigators randomized 725 nonsleepy subjects with OSA based on polysomnography but no CVD to CPAP treatment or no intervention and followed them for a median of 4 years for the development of hypertension or a cardiovascular event. In an intention-to-treat analysis, CPAP did not significantly reduce the incidence of a composite end point of new-onset hypertension or cardiovascular event [incidence density ratio (IDR), 0.83; 95% CI, 0.63 to 1.1; $p = 0.20$]. However, in an exploratory secondary analysis, those patients who used their CPAP ≥ 4 hours/night did have a statistically significant reduction in the incidence of the composite end point (IDR, 0.72; 95% CI, 0.52 to 0.98; $p = 0.04$).

193. Durán-Cantolla J, et al.; for the Spanish Sleep and Breathing Group. Continuous positive airway pressure as treatment for systemic hypertension in people with obstructive sleep apnea: randomised controlled trial. BMJ 2010;341:c5991.

This prospective, randomized, sham-controlled, multicenter trial allocated 340 patients with OSA and recently diagnosed hypertension to either CPAP or sham CPAP for 3 months. The main outcome was change in 24-hour ambulatory BP at the end of the 3-month period. Compared with sham CPAP, optimal CPAP reduced mean ambulatory SBP by 2.1 mm Hg (95% CI, 0.4 to 3.7 mm Hg) and mean ambulatory DBP by 1.3 mm Hg (95% CI, 0.2 to 2.3 mm Hg). The investigators note that the clinical significance of this decrease in BP is uncertain.

Medical Therapy

194. Hansson L, et al. Randomised trial of effects of calcium antagonists compared with diuretics and beta-blockers on cardiovascular morbidity and mortality in hypertension: the Nordic Diltiazem (NORDIL) study. *Lancet* 2000;356:359–365.

Design: Prospective, randomized, open, blinded end point, multicenter trial. Primary end point was fatal and nonfatal stroke, MI, and other cardiovascular death. Mean follow-up was 4.5 years.

Purpose: To compare the effects of calcium antagonists with those of diuretics and β-blockers on major outcomes in middle-aged hypertensive individuals.

Population: 10,881 patients aged 50 to 74 years with DBP $\geq$ 100 mm Hg.

Treatment: Diltiazem (180 to 360 mg/day) versus diuretics, β-blockers, or both. Additional antihypertensives could be added to achieve DBP < 90 mm Hg.

Results: SBP and DBP were lowered effectively in both groups (reduction, 20.3/18.7 mm Hg with diltiazem vs. 23.3/18.7 mm Hg with diuretics/β-blockers; difference in systolic reduction, p < 0.001). No difference was found between the two groups in the incidence of the primary composite end point [16.6 (diltiazem) vs. 16.2 (diuretic/β-blocker) events per 1,000 patient-years]. The diltiazem group had a lower incidence of fatal and nonfatal stroke compared with the diuretic and β-blocker group [6.4 vs. 7.9 events per 1,000 patient-years; RR, 0.80 (95% CI, 0.65 to 0.99); p = 0.04], whereas the rates of fatal and nonfatal MI were not significantly different [7.4 vs. 6.3 events per 1,000 patient-years; RR, 1.16; 95% CI, 0.94 to 1.44; p = 0.17].

195. Pepine CJ, et al. A calcium antagonist vs. a non-calcium antagonist hypertension treatment strategy for patients with coronary artery disease. The International Verapamil-Trandolapril Study (INVEST): a randomized controlled trial. *JAMA* 2003;290: 2805–2816.

Design: Prospective, randomized, open-label, multicenter study with blinded end points. Primary end point was the first occurrence of death, nonfatal MI, or nonfatal stroke at 24 months.

Purpose: To compare clinical outcomes with calcium antagonists versus noncalcium antagonists in patients with CAD and hypertension.

Population: 22,576 patients, ages 50 years or older, with CAD and hypertension, at 862 sites in 14 countries.

Treatment: Calcium antagonist (verapamil sustained release, with trandolapril if needed) or noncalcium antagonist (atenolol with hydrochlorothiazide if needed).

Results: At follow-up (mean 2.7 years), there was no difference between the arms (RR 0.98) in the incidence of death, nonfatal stroke, or nonfatal MI. Achievement of guideline-recommended BP (systolic and/or diastolic) was roughly equivalent between the two strategies. The verapamil group did have a lower incidence of new-onset diabetes (6.2% vs. 7.3%).

196. Dahlöf B, et al.; for the ASCOT Investigators. Prevention of cardiovascular events with an antihypertensive regimen of amlodipine adding perindopril as required versus atenolol adding bendroflumethiazide as required, in the Anglo-Scandinavian Cardiac Outcomes Trial-Blood Pressure Lowering Arm (ASCOT-BPLA): a multicentre randomized controlled trial. *Lancet* 2005;366:895–906.

Design: Multicenter, prospective, randomized trial. Primary end point was fatal CHD or MI. Median follow-up was 5.5 years.

Purpose: To compare two regimens of BP control—a calcium channel blocker with ACEI addition versus β-blocker with diuretic addition.

Population: 19,257 patients, ages 40 to 79, with hypertension and at least three other CVD risk factors.

Treatment: Amlodipine, 5 to 10 mg/day, with perindopril, 4 to 8 mg/day, as needed versus atenolol, 50 to 100 mg/day, with bendroflumethiazide, 1.25 to 2.5 mg/day, as needed.

Results: Based on significantly higher mortality in the atenolol group, the trial was halted early, at median 5.5 years of follow-up. At this time, there was a nonsignificant trend in the primary end point, favoring the amlodipine group (unadjusted HR 0.90, $p = 0.11$). Additionally, stroke (0.77, $p = 0.003$) and all-cause mortality (0.89, $p = 0.025$) were both significantly lower in the amlodipine group.

197. Jamerson K, et al.; for the ACCOMPLISH trial investigators. Benazepril plus amlodipine or hydrochlorothiazide for hypertension in high-risk patients. N Engl J Med 2008;359:2417–2428.

Design: Prospective, randomized, double-blind trial. Primary end point was the composite of cardiovascular death, nonfatal MI, nonfatal stroke, hospitalization for angina, resuscitation from sudden cardiac arrest, or coronary revascularization.

Purpose: To compare hydrochlorothiazide in addition to benazepril, with amlodipine, also in addition to benazepril.

Population: 11,506 patients with hypertension at high risk for cardiovascular events (previous events, prior revascularization, impaired renal function, peripheral arterial disease, LVH, or diabetes mellitus).

Treatment: Hydrochlorothiazide plus benazepril, or amlodipine plus benazepril.

Results: After a mean follow-up of 36 months, the trial was halted early when the primary outcome significantly favored the benazepril–amlodipine arm (9.6% vs. 11.8%, $p < 0.001$), with a relative risk reduction of 19.6%. The narrower secondary end point, a composite of death, nonfatal MI, or nonfatal stroke, also significantly favored the amlodipine arm (HR, 0.79, $p = 0.002$). In the subset of patients with pre-existing CAD, the benefits of benazepril plus amlodipine persisted (see *Am J Cardiol* 2013;122:255–259).

198. Hansson L, et al. Effect of angiotensin-converting-enzyme inhibition compared with conventional therapy on cardiovascular morbidity and mortality in hypertension: the Captopril Prevention Project (CAPPP) randomised trial. **Lancet 1999;353:611–616.**

Design: Prospective, randomized, multicenter, open study. Primary composite end points were fatal and nonfatal MI, stroke, and other CV deaths. Mean follow-up period was 6.1 years.

Purpose: To compare the effectiveness of captopril with a conventional antihypertensive regimen of diuretics or β-blockers on cardiovascular morbidity and mortality.

Population: 10,985 patients aged 25 to 66 years with DBP ≥ 100 mm Hg on two occasions.

Exclusion Criteria: Secondary hypertension or serum creatinine >150 μmol/L (1.7 mg/dL).

Treatment: Captopril, 50 mg once or twice daily, versus β-blockers (most common: metoprolol and atenolol) or diuretics (most common, HCTZ and bendrofluazide).

Results: The two groups had a similar incidence of the composite end point (11.1 and 10.2 events per 1,000 patient-years in captopril and conventional therapy groups); the captopril group had a trend toward lower cardiovascular mortality (RR, 0.77; $p = 0.092$) but a higher incidence of fatal and nonfatal stroke (RR, 1.15; $p = 0.044$); MI rates were similar.

Comments: Lower stroke risk in conventional group may have been due to lower baseline BP (–2 mm Hg).

199. The Heart Outcome Prevention Evaluation (HOPE) Study Investigators. Effects of an ACE inhibitor, ramipril, on cardiovascular events in high risk patients. N Engl J Med 2000;342:145–153.

Design: Prospective, randomized, double-blind, 2 × 2 factorial, multicenter study. Primary end point was cardiovascular death, MI, or stroke. Mean follow-up was 4.5 years.

Purpose: To assess the role of an ACE inhibitor, ramipril, in patients at high risk for cardiovascular events but without LV dysfunction or HF.

Population: 9,297 high-risk patients aged 55 years or older with CAD, stroke, peripheral arterial disease, or diabetes plus one other cardiovascular risk factor (hypertension, elevated TC, low HDL, smoking, documented microalbuminuria).

Exclusion Criteria: HF, EF < 40%, uncontrolled hypertension, MI or stroke in previous 4 weeks, and overt nephropathy.

Treatment: Ramipril (10 mg/day), vitamin E (400 IU/day), both, or neither (2 placebos).

Results: The ramipril group had a 22% relative reduction in cardiovascular death, MI, or stroke compared with the placebo group (14.0% vs. 17.8%; $p < 0.001$). Ramipril was associated with significantly lower rates of cardiovascular death (6.1% vs. 8.1%; RR, 0.74; $p < 0.001$), MI (9.9% vs. 12.3%; RR, 0.80; $p < 0.001$), stroke (3.4% vs. 4.9%; RR, 0.68; $p < 0.001$), all-cause mortality (10.4% vs. 12.2%; RR, 0.84; $p = 0.005$), revascularization procedures (16.3% vs. 18.8%; RR, 0.85; $p < 0.001$), cardiac arrest [0.8% vs. 1.3%; RR, 0.62; $p = 0.02$ (corrected)], HF (9.1% vs. 11.6%; RR, 0.77; $p < 0.001$), and diabetes-related complications (6.4% vs. 7.6%; RR, 0.84; $p = 0.03$). In the MICRO-HOPE substudy of 3,577 diabetics (see *Lancet* 2000;355:253), ramipril reduced primary events by 25%, MI by 22%, stroke by 33%, CV death by 37%, total mortality by 24%, and overt nephropathy by 24% ($p = 0.027$). After adjustment for the anticipated effect on cardiovascular outcomes of ramipril's effect on SBP (−2.4 mm Hg) and DBP (−1.0 mm Hg), ramipril still reduced the risk of the combined primary outcome by 25%.

200. PROGRESS (Perindopril pROtection aGainst REcurrent Stroke Study) Collaborative Group. Randomised trial of a perindopril-based blood-pressure-lowering regimen among 6,105 individuals with previous stroke or transient ischaemic attack. *Lancet* 2001;358:1033–1041 (editorial, 1026–1027).

Design: Prospective, randomized, double-blind, placebo-controlled, multicenter trial. Primary end point was total stroke (fatal or nonfatal). Mean follow-up was 3.9 years.

Purpose: To determine the effects of a BP-lowering regimen in hypertensive and nonhypertensive patients with a history of stroke or TIA.

Population: 6,105 individuals with a stroke (hemorrhagic or ischemic) or TIA in the previous 5 years and no major disability.

Treatment: Perindopril, 4 mg daily, with addition of the diuretic indapamide, 2.5 mg daily, at physicians' discretion, versus placebo.

Results: At follow-up, active treatment reduced BP by 9/4 mm Hg. In the active treatment group, 60% received both drugs, and 40% received perindopril alone. The active treatment group had a significantly lower incidence of stroke compared with the placebo group (10% vs. 14%; RRR, 28%; $p < 0.0001$). Active treatment also reduced total major vascular events by 26%. Hypertensive and nonhypertensive subgroups had similar reductions in stroke (all values $p < 0.01$). Combination therapy with perindopril plus indapamide reduced BP by 12/5 mm Hg and stroke risk by 43%, whereas single-drug therapy reduced BP by 5/3 mm Hg and resulted in no significant reduction in stroke incidence.

Comments: Editorialists dispute study's conclusion that treatment with both agents be considered routinely for patients with a history of stroke or TIA, irrespective of BP, and advocate starting treatment with a diuretic, not with combination therapy. They also point out that the 5 mm Hg reduction in SBP seen in the perindopril group should translate into an approximate 20% reduction in stroke risk, as seen in many prior studies using diuretics and β-blockers.

201. Dahlof B, et al.; for the LIFE (Losartan Intervention For End point reduction in hypertension) Study Group. Cardiovascular morbidity and mortality in the losartan intervention for end point reduction in hypertension study (LIFE): a randomised trial against atenolol. *Lancet* 2002;359:995–1003.

Design: Prospective, randomized, placebo-controlled, blinded, parallel-group, multicenter trial. Primary end point was death, MI, or stroke. Mean follow-up was 4.8 years.

Purpose: To evaluate the use of losartan compared with atenolol in patients with hypertension and LVH in reducing adverse clinical outcomes.

Population: 9,193 patients aged 55 to 80 years with previously treated or untreated hypertension (SBP between 160 to 200 mm Hg and/or DBP between 95 to 115 mm Hg) and ECG signs of LVH.

Exclusion Criteria: Secondary hypertension; MI or stroke in previous 6 months; angina requiring β-blockers or calcium antagonists; HF or LVEF $\leq$ 40%; and compelling indication for treatment with any ARB, any β-blocker, any ACE inhibitor, or HCTZ.

Treatment: Losartan-based or atenolol-based regimen after 1 to 2 weeks of placebo washout. Drugs were dosed to reach a target BP < 140/90 mm Hg per titration schedule.

Results: BP was reduced by 30.2/16.6 mm Hg in the losartan group and 29.1/16.8 mm Hg in the atenolol group (treatment difference, $p = 0.017$ for SBP and $p = 0.37$ for DBP). The losartan group had a significantly lower incidence of death, MI, or stroke compared with the atenolol group (11% vs. 13%; HR, 0.87; $p = 0.021$), primarily driven by fewer strokes (5% vs. 7%; HR, 0.75; $p = 0.001$). Cardiovascular mortality rates were not significantly different (4% vs. 5%; HR, 0.89; $p = 0.21$). Losartan also was associated with a lower incidence of new-onset diabetes (6% vs. 8%; HR, 0.75; $p = 0.001$). A major LIFE substudy examined cardiovascular outcomes in 1,195 patients with diabetes, hypertension, and ECG signs of LVH (*Lancet* 2002;359:1004). At a mean follow-up of 4.7 years, mean BP decreased to similar levels (losartan, 146/79 mm Hg; atenolol, 148/79 mm Hg). However, the losartan group had a significant 24% RRR in death, MI, or stroke. The losartan group also had significant reductions in cardiovascular mortality (37% RRR; $p = 0.028$) and all-cause mortality (39% RRR; $p = 0.002$). These substudy results suggest that losartan has benefits beyond BP reduction. In the subgroup of patients with isolated systolic hypertension (DBP < 90 mm Hg) and LVH (by ECG), treatment with losartan was associated with 25% fewer primary events compared with atenolol (see *JAMA* 2002;288:1491).

Comments: These results are in contrast to those of the CAPPP, NORDIL, and STOP-HTN2 trials, which compared ACE inhibitors or calcium channel blockers with β-blockers and diuretics for treatment of hypertension and found no difference in efficacy. Because this trial examined the efficacy of losartan in *high-risk* hypertensive patients with signs of LVH, one cannot extrapolate these results to lower-risk patients.

202. Teo KK, et al.; for the ACE Inhibitors Collaborative Group. Effects of long-term treatment with angiotensin-converting-enzyme inhibitors in the presence or absence of aspirin: a systematic review. *Lancet* 2002;360:1037–1043.

This overview examined data on 22,060 patients from six long-term randomized trials evaluating ACE inhibitor therapy. Results from analyses of all trials, except SOLVD, found no significant differences between the risk reductions with ACE inhibitor therapy in the presence or absence of ASA in the composite of death, MI, stroke, HF hospitalization, or revascularization or in any of its individual components, except MI (interaction $p = 0.01$). Overall, ACE inhibitor therapy significantly reduced the risk of major clinical outcomes by 22% ($p < 0.0001$), with clear reductions in risk both among those receiving ASA at baseline (OR, 0.80; 99% CI, 0.73 to 0.88) and those who were not (OR, 0.71; 99% CI, 0.62 to 0.81; interaction $p = 0.07$).

203. van Vark LC, et al. Angiotensin-converting enzyme inhibitors reduce mortality in hypertension: a meta-analysis of randomized clinical trials of renin-angiotensin-aldosterone system inhibitors involving 158,998 patients. *Eur Heart J* 2012;33:2088–2097.

This meta-analysis included data from 20 large randomized controlled trials published between 2000 and 2011 allocating a total of 158,998 patients with hypertension to ACE inhibitor or ARB versus placebo or an active control. Of the 20 trials, 7 involved ACE inhibitor therapy and 13 involved ARB therapy; 7 were placebo controlled, and the rest had active controls. At a mean follow-up of 7 years, patients assigned to ACE inhibitor or ARB therapy had a 5% RRR in all-cause mortality (HR, 0.95; 95% CI, 0.91 to 1.00; $p = 0.032$) and a 7% RRR in cardiovascular mortality (HR, 0.93; 95% CI, 0.88 to 0.99; $p = 0.018$). In a stratified analysis according to the type of renin–angiotensin–aldosterone system inhibitor (ACE inhibitor vs. ARB), ACE inhibitor therapy was associated with a 10% RRR in all-cause mortality (HR, 0.90; 95% CI, 0.84 to 0.97; $p = 0.004$), but ARB therapy was not associated with a reduced incidence of all-cause mortality (HR, 0.99; 95% CI, 0.94 to 1.04, $p = 0.683$), despite the inclusion of similar numbers of patients allocated to each drug class.

204. McAlister FA, et al.; for the Renin Angiotensin System Modulator Meta-Analysis Investigators. Angiotensin-converting enzyme inhibitors or angiotensin receptor blockers are beneficial in normotensive atherosclerotic patients: a collaborative meta-analysis of randomized trials. *Eur Heart J* 2012;33:505–514.

In this meta-analysis, investigators included data from 13 randomized controlled trials involving 80,594 patients with CHD treated with ACE inhibitor or ARB versus placebo. Data from the trials were stratified by SBP at the time of trial entry; 23,922 patients enrolled in the 13 trials had SBP < 130 mm Hg at the time of trial entry. In these patients, the HR for a composite outcome including cardiovascular death, nonfatal stroke, or nonfatal MI with ACE inhibitor or ARB compared to placebo was 0.84 (95% CI, 0.77 to 0.90; $p < 0.00001$). This effect persisted in *post hoc* analyses of atherosclerotic patients without diabetes mellitus or congestive heart failure and in those with SBP < 120 mm Hg.

205. Wing LM, et al.; ANBP-2 (Second Australian National Blood Pressure Study). A comparison of outcomes with angiotensin-converting enzyme inhibitors and diuretics for hypertension in the elderly. *N Engl J Med* 2003;348:583–592.

Design: Prospective, randomized, open, multicenter study. Primary end point was death or any cardiovascular event. Median follow-up was 4.1 years.

Purpose: To compare outcomes in older hypertensive subjects receiving ACE inhibitors with those treated with diuretics.

Population: 6,083 subjects aged 65 to 84 years with hypertension.

Treatment: ACE inhibitor, or diuretic (enalapril and hydrochlorothiazide recommended, but not mandated).

Results: The ACE inhibitor group had a significant reduction in primary events compared to diuretic group (hazard ratio, 0.89, 95% CI, 0.71 to 1.00, $p = 0.05$). Among men, the HR was 0.83 (95% CI, 0.71 to 0.97, $p = 0.02$), while it was 1.00 for women.

Comments: Criticisms of this trial include the open-label design, no restrictions on drugs used, and inclusion of "soft" end points. Also of note, the study enrolled few or no black patients (% not reported).

206. The ONTARGET Investigators. Telmisartan, ramipril, or both in patients at high risk for vascular events. *N Engl J Med* 2008;358:1547–1559.

Design: Multicenter, randomized, double-blind, controlled trial. Primary end point was cardiovascular death, MI, stroke, or CHF hospitalization at median follow-up of 56 months.

Purpose: To compare ACE inhibitor, ARB, and their combination in prevention of cardiovascular events.

Population: 25,620 patients with CAD, peripheral arterial disease, cerebrovascular disease, or diabetes.

Exclusion Criteria: Those who could not tolerate ACEI were randomized in a separate trial to ARB or placebo.

Treatment: Ramipril, telmisartan, or both.

Results: Primary end point events occurred in 16.5% of patients in the ramipril group versus 16.7% in the telmisartan group and 16.3% in the combination therapy group (pair-wise comparisons not significant). There was more BP lowering and higher incidence of adverse events (hypotensive symptoms, syncope, and renal dysfunction) in the combination group, compared with the ramipril group.

207. Makani H, et al. Efficacy and safety of dual blockade of the renin-angiotensin system: meta-analysis of randomised trials. *BMJ* 2013;346:f360.

This meta-analysis of 33 randomized controlled trials apportioning 68,405 patients to either dual blockade of the renin–angiotensin system or monotherapy (including ONTARGET, described above) essentially recapitulated the results of ONTARGET. Dual blockade of the renin–angiotensin system did not reduce all-cause mortality (RR 0.97; 95% CI, 0.89 to 1.06) or cardiovascular mortality (RR 0.96; 95% CI, 0.88 to 1.05) compared to monotherapy. However, dual therapy did cause statistically significant increases in hyperkalemia (RR 1.55; 95% CI, 1.32 to 1.82), hypotension (RR 1.66; 95% CI, 1.38 to 1.98), and renal failure (RR 1.41; 95% CI, 1.09 to 1.84).

208. Parving HH, et al.; for the AVOID Study Investigators. Aliskiren combined with losartan in type 2 diabetes and nephropathy. *N Engl J Med* 2008;358:2433–2446.

Aliskiren, a novel direct renin inhibitor, was added to the ARB losartan in half of the 599 patients enrolled in this prospective, international, double-blind, randomized trial. The population included patients with hypertension and type 2 diabetes with nephropathy, and the primary end point was reduction in albumin-to-creatinine ratio at 6 months. Patients receiving aliskiren did have lower albumin-to-creatinine ratios, and it may provide a renoprotective effect. There was a mild, nonsignificant trend to lower SBP in the aliskiren group, and the adverse events were similar. The trial was not powered to detect clinical end points.

209. Nicholls SJ, et al. Effect of aliskiren on progression of coronary disease in patients with prehypertension: the AQUARIUS randomized clinical trial. *JAMA* 2013;310:1135–1144.

In this double-blind, randomized, placebo-controlled, multicenter clinical trial, investigators assigned 613 patients who had undergone coronary IVUS with CAD, prehypertension (SBP between 125 and 139 mm Hg), and 2 additional cardiac risk factors to either aliskiren or placebo. Participants were followed up with repeat IVUS after at least 72 weeks of treatment. The primary outcome measured, change in percent atheroma volume from baseline, did not differ significantly between groups, though there was a trend toward benefit with aliskiren (−0.33% with aliskiren vs. 0.11% with placebo; $p = 0.08$). Other angiographic variables also did not demonstrate a benefit from aliskiren.

210. Hansson L, et al.; for the Hypertension Optimal Treatment (HOT) study. Effects of intensive blood pressure lowering and low dose aspirin in patients with hypertension: principal results of the Hypertension Optimal Treatment (HOT) randomized trial. *Lancet* 1998;351:1755–1762.

Design: Prospective, randomized, partially open, partially blinded (ASA arm), multicenter study. Primary outcome was cardiovascular events. Mean follow-up period was 3.8 years.

Purpose: To (a) assess the association between major cardiovascular events and three different target BPs as well as the actual DBP achieved during treatment and (b) evaluate whether the addition of low-dose ASA to antihypertensive treatment reduces major cardiovascular events.

Population: 18,790 patients aged 50 to 80 years (mean, 61.5 years) with DBP between 100 and 115 mm Hg.

Treatment: Three different DBPs were targeted ($\leq$90 mm Hg, $\leq$ 85 mm Hg, and $\leq$ 80 mm Hg) using a five-step approach: step 1, felodipine, 5 mg/day; step 2, addition of low-dose ACE inhibitor or β-blocker; step 3, felodipine increased to 10 mg/day; step 4, dose of ACE inhibitor or β-blocker increased; and step 5, addition of low-dose alternative agent or HCTZ. All patients were randomized in double-blind fashion to ASA, 75 mg/day, or placebo.

Results: At 2 years, target DBP was achieved in 85%, 67%, and 75% of the patients in the $\leq$ 90 mm Hg, $\leq$ 85 mm Hg, and $\leq$ 80 mm Hg groups, respectively. Despite a goal of 5 mm Hg difference in DBPs, mean DBPs were closely grouped: 85.2, 83.2, and 81.1 mm Hg in the $\leq$ 90 mm Hg, $\leq$ 85 mm Hg, and $\leq$ 80 mm Hg groups, respectively. The incidence of cardiovascular events did not significantly differ between the three groups, but significantly fewer cardiovascular events and cardiovascular deaths were noted among diabetic patients assigned to a target DBP of $\leq$ 80 mm Hg compared with $\leq$ 90 mm Hg ($p = 0.005$ for events; $p = 0.016$ for deaths). No differences were found in BP between ASA- and placebo-treated patients, but ASA use was associated with 15% fewer major events ($p = 0.03$), a 36% reduction in fatal or nonfatal MI ($p = 0.002$), and similar rates of hemorrhagic and ischemic stroke.

Comments: The study was underpowered for two reasons: (a) actual mean DBPs were approximately 2 mm Hg apart instead of the planned 5 mm Hg and (b) only 724 major CV events occurred over a 3.8-year period versus projected 1,100 over a 2.5-year period.

211. The ALLHAT (Antihypertensive and Lipid-Lowering Treatment to Prevent Heart Attack Trial) Officers and Coordinators for the ALLHAT Collaborative Research Group. Major outcomes in high-risk hypertensive patients randomized to angiotensin-converting enzyme inhibitor or calcium channel blocker versus diuretic. JAMA 2002;288:2981–2997 (editorials, 3039–3044).

Design: Prospective, randomized, active-controlled, multicenter trial. Primary end point was fatal CHD or nonfatal MI. Secondary outcomes were all-cause mortality, stroke, combined CHD (primary outcome, plus coronary revascularization or hospitalization for angina), and combined CVD (CHD, stroke, treated angina without hospitalization, HF, and peripheral arterial disease). Mean follow-up was 4.9 years.

Purpose: To determine whether treatment with a calcium channel blocker or an ACE inhibitor lowers the incidence of CHD or other CVD events versus treatment with a diuretic.

Population: 33,357 participants, aged 55 years or older, with hypertension and at least one other CHD risk factor.

Exclusion Criteria: History of symptomatic HF and/or known EF < 35%.

Treatment: Chlorthalidone, 12.5 to 25 mg/day ($n = 15,255$); amlodipine, 2.5 to 10 mg/day ($n = 9,048$); or lisinopril, 10 to 40 mg/day ($n = 9,054$).

Results: No significant differences were found between the treatment groups in the incidence of fatal CHD or nonfatal MI (overall rate, 8.9%). Compared with chlorthalidone, the RRs of the primary end point with amlodipine and lisinopril were 0.98 (95% CI, 0.90 to 1.07) and 0.99 (95% CI, 0.91 to 1.08), respectively. All-cause mortality rates were also similar. SBP at 5 years was significantly lower in chlorthalidone-treated subjects compared to amlodipine-treated (–0.8 mm Hg; $p < 0.001$)

and lisinopril-treated subjects (−2 mm Hg; $p < 0.001$), whereas DBP was significantly higher with chlorthalidone compared with amlodipine (0.8 mm Hg; $p < 0.001$). For amlodipine versus chlorthalidone, secondary outcomes were similar except for a higher 6-year rate of HF with amlodipine (10.2% vs. 7.7%; RR, 1.38; 95% CI, 1.25 to 1.52). For lisinopril versus chlorthalidone, lisinopril had higher 6-year rates of combined CVD (33.3% vs. 30.9%; RR, 1.10; 95% CI, 1.05 to 1.16); stroke (6.3% vs. 5.6%; RR, 1.15; 95% CI, 1.02 to 1.30); and HF (8.7% vs. 7.7%; RR, 1.19; 95% CI, 1.07 to 1.31). The fourth arm of the trial testing the α-blocker doxazosin was discontinued in January 2000 because of increased cardiovascular events and HF hospitalizations for this agent compared with chlorthalidone (see JAMA 2000;283:1967).

Comments: The results from this very large trial suggest that in patients in which cardiovascular events are the greatest risk, a thiazide-type diuretic is clearly the preferred first agent; however, in patients with kidney disease or with major risk for renal events, ACE inhibitors should be considered. The study results contradict those observed in HOPE, especially the observation that ACE inhibitors conferred protection against stroke independent of BP. Major criticisms of the ALLHAT study include the following: (a) results have limited relevance because most patients require combination therapy for adequate BP control; (b) results appear driven by poor BP response to ACE inhibitors observed in black patients; and (c) add-on therapy to ACE inhibitor should have been a diuretic or calcium channel blocker, not a β-blocker.

212. Wright JT, et al.; for the ALLHAT Collaborative Research Group. ALLHAT Findings revisited in the context of subsequent analyses, other trials, and meta-analyses. *Arch Intern Med* 2009;169:832–842.

The ALLHAT investigators subsequently re-evaluated their results in the context of contemporary trials and meta-analyses. Overall, they find that the original trial's conclusions persist—that neither α-blockers, calcium channel antagonists, nor ACE inhibitors are superior to thiazide-type diuretics for the initial management of hypertension. They add that the new-onset diabetes associated with the diuretics did not lead to worse outcomes in the time frame studied.

213. Beckett NS, et al. Treatment of hypertension in patients 80 years of age or older. *N Engl J Med* 2008;358:1887–1898.

Design: Prospective, randomized, double-blind trial. Primary end point was fatal or nonfatal stroke.

Purpose: To determine if the treatment of very elderly hypertensive patients with antihypertensive agents is beneficial.

Population: 3,845 patients, aged 80 or older, with SBP between 160 mm Hg and 199 mm Hg off treatment.

Treatment: Indapamide, 1.5 mg/day, or matching placebo; if blood pressure remained above goal (150/90), perindopril, or matching placebo, could be added at escalating doses.

Results: After a mean follow-up of 1.8 years, 48% of patients randomized to the active treatment arm had an SBP < 150 mm Hg compared to 19% in the placebo arm ($p < 0.001$). The relative risk reduction for stroke in the active treatment arm was 30% (95% CI, −1% to 51%; $p = 0.06$); in secondary analyses, there was a 21% reduction in all-cause mortality in the treatment arm (95% CI, 4% to 35%; $p = 0.02$) and a 39% reduction in fatal stroke (95% CI, 1% to 62%; $p = 0.05$).

Comment: This trial demonstrated that treatment of hypertension in the very elderly does reduce the rate of fatal stroke and all-cause mortality. It should be noted that the blood pressure goals in this trial were much more liberal than JNC 7 guidelines; the benefit of tight blood pressure control in the very elderly is less well established, as reflected in the JNC 8 recommendations.

214. Hermida RC, et al. Influence of circadian time of hypertension treatment of cardiovascular risk: results of the MAPEC study. *Chronobiol Int* 2010;27:1629–1651.

Design: Prospective, unblinded, single-center study. Primary end point was total cardiovascular morbidity and mortality—a composite end point encompassing all-cause death, MI, angina, coronary revascularization, acute peripheral arterial occlusion, retinal artery thrombosis, hemorrhagic and ischemic stroke, and TIA. Median follow-up was 5.6 years.

Purpose: To determine if dosing one or more blood pressure medication at night reduced cardiovascular events compared to a traditional schedule with all medications dosed in the morning.

Population: 2,156 patients with either untreated or resistant hypertension confirmed by ambulatory blood pressure monitoring (awake mean BP ≥ 135/85, or asleep mean BP ≥ 120/70).

Treatment: All blood pressure medications upon awakening, or ≥ 1 blood pressure medication at bedtime. Class of antihypertensive was not specified by the trial protocol, but randomization was stratified by antihypertensive class.

Results: While mean awake blood pressure was similar between the two groups, asleep blood pressure was lower in the group taking ≥ 1 blood pressure medication at bedtime. In the group taking at least one blood pressure medication at bedtime, the relative risk of the primary end point was 0.39 (95% CI, 0.29 to 0.51; $p < 0.001$); this magnitude of this effect was consistent among a number of secondary outcomes, including total mortality, cardiovascular mortality, stroke, and MI.

Diabetes and Hypertension

215. UKPDS 38. Tight blood pressure control and risk of macrovascular and microvascular complications in type 2 diabetes: UK Prospective Diabetes Study Group. *BMJ* 1998;317:703–713.

This prospective, randomized, controlled, multicenter trial enrolled 1,148 type 2 diabetics with hypertension (mean entry BP 160/94 mm Hg). Patients were assigned to tight BP control (goal ≤ 150/85 mm Hg) using captopril or atenolol as the main treatment or less tight control (goal ≤ 180/105 mm Hg). At follow-up (median, 8.4 years), mean BP was significantly reduced in the group assigned tight BP control (144/82 mm Hg in the tight control group vs. 154/87 mm Hg in the looser control group; $p < 0.0001$). The tight-control group had significant relative reductions of 24% in diabetes-related end points, 32% in deaths related to diabetes, 44% in strokes, and 37% in microvascular end points. A nonsignificant reduction was found in all-cause mortality. The tight-control group also had a 34% risk reduction in the proportion of patients with deterioration of retinopathy by two steps and a 47% reduced risk of deterioration in visual acuity by three lines of the diabetic retinopathy study chart. In a predefined substudy of the tight-control patients (UKPDS 39; see *BMJ* 1998;317:713–720), captopril and atenolol were equally effective in reducing BP, risk of macrovascular end points, and deterioration in retinopathy.

216. Brenner BM, et al.; for the RENAAL (Reduction of End points in NIDDM with Angiotensin II Antagonist Losartan) Study Investigators. Effects of losartan on renal and cardiovascular outcomes in patients with type 2 diabetes and nephropathy. *N Engl J Med* 2001;345:861–869.

This prospective, randomized, double-blind, placebo-controlled, multicenter trial enrolled 1,513 type 2 diabetics with nephropathy (urinary albumin-to-creatinine ratio ≥ 300 and serum creatinine between 1.3 and 3.0 mg/dL). Patients received losartan, 50 to 100 mg once daily, or placebo. Both were taken in addition to conventional antihypertensive agents. At a mean follow-up of 3.4 years, the losartan group had a 16% RRR in primary events [doubling of baseline serum creatinine, end-stage renal disease (ESRD), or death] compared with the placebo group (43.5% vs. 47.1%; $p = 0.02$). Losartan reduced serum creatinine doubling by 25% ($p = 0.006$) and ESRD by 28% ($p = 0.002$) but had no significant effect on all-cause mortality. The benefits exceeded those attributable to changes in BP. Losartan also was associated with a lower rate of first hospitalization for HF (RRR, 32%; $p = 0.005$) and a 35% decline in proteinuria ($p < 0.001$ in comparison with placebo).

217. Lewis EJ, et al.; IDNT (Irbesartan Diabetic Nephropathy Trial). Renoprotective effect of the angiotensin-receptor antagonist irbesartan in patients with nephropathy due to type 2 diabetes. *N Engl J Med* 2001;345:851–860.

This prospective, randomized, double-blind, placebo-controlled, multicenter, primary trial enrolled 1,715 hypertensive patients with nephropathy due to type 2 diabetes. Patients received irbesartan (300 mg daily), amlodipine (10 mg daily), or placebo. Target BP was 135/85 mm Hg or less. At mean follow-up of 2.6 years, the irbesartan group had 20% and 23% fewer primary events (doubling of baseline serum creatinine, ESRD, or death) than did the placebo and amlodipine groups [32.6% vs. 39% ($p = 0.02$) and 41.1%; $p = 0.006$]. Irbesartan was associated with 33% and 37% lower rates of serum creatinine doubling [16.9% vs. 23.7% ($p = 0.003$) and 25.4% ($p < 0.001$)] and 23% lower RR of ESRD than both other groups (14.2% vs. 17.8% and 18.3%; $p = 0.07$ for both comparisons). These differences were not explained by the achieved BP differences. No significant differences were noted between the groups in all-cause mortality or the cardiovascular composite end point.

218. Parving HH, et al.; for the IRMA II (Irbesartan in patients with Type 2 Diabetes and Microalbuminuria) Study Group. The effect of irbesartan on the development of diabetic nephropathy in patients with type 2 diabetes. *N Engl J Med* 2001;345:870–878.

This prospective, randomized, double-blind, placebo-controlled, multicenter trial enrolled 590 hypertensive patients with type 2 diabetes and microalbuminuria. The primary end point was time to onset of diabetic nephropathy (defined as urinary albumin excretion rate > 200 μg/min and $\geq$ 30% higher than baseline level). Patients received irbesartan, 150 mg or 300 mg daily, or placebo. At 2-year follow-up, both irbesartan groups had a lower incidence of the primary end point compared with the placebo group [5.2% (300 mg) and 9.7% (150 mg) vs. 14.9% (placebo); HRs, 0.30 ($p < 0.001$) and 0.61 ($p = 0.081$)]. Average BPs were 141/83 mm Hg in the 300-mg group, 143/83 mm Hg in the 150-mg group, and 144/83 mm Hg in the placebo group ($p = 0.004$ for the comparison between SBP with placebo compared to SBP with either dose of irbesartan). Serious adverse events were less frequent among the patients treated with irbesartan ($p = 0.02$).

219. NAVIGATOR Study Group. Effect of valsartan on the incidence of diabetes and cardiovascular events. *N Engl J Med* 2010;362:1477–1490

In this prospective, randomized, double-blind, placebo-controlled clinical trial, investigators treated 9,306 patients with impaired glucose tolerance and either CVD or cardiovascular risk factors to valsartan (up to 160 mg daily) or placebo. The patients were followed for a median of 5 years for the development of one of three coprimary outcomes: a composite of cardiovascular death, nonfatal MI, UA, nonfatal stroke, HF hospitalization, or arterial revascularization; a composite of cardiovascular death, nonfatal MI, nonfatal stroke, or heart failure hospitalization; and new-onset diabetes. Valsartan did not significantly reduce the rate of either cardiovascular end point, but did reduce the rate of new-onset diabetes (33.1% in the valsartan group vs. 36.8% in the placebo group; HR, 0.86; 95% CI, 0.80 to 0.92; $p < 0.001$).

220. The ACCORD Study Group. Effects of intensive blood-pressure control in type 2 diabetes mellitus. *N Engl J Med* 2010;362:1575–1585.

The trial tested the hypothesis (and guideline recommendations) that reducing SBP below 140 mm Hg in patients with diabetes is beneficial to cardiovascular health. They randomized 4,733 patients with type 2 diabetes mellitus to intensive BP therapy targeted to reduce SBP to >120 mm Hg or conventional therapy with a goal of >140 mm Hg. At mean follow-up of 4.7 years, there was no statistically significant different in the rate of the primary end point of cardiovascular death, MI, or stroke (1.87% annually for intensive vs. 2.09% annually for standard, $p = 0.20$). There was, however, a surfeit of adverse events related to antihypertensive therapy in the intensive group (3.3% vs. 1.3%, $p < 0.001$).

221. McBrien K, et al. Intensive and standard blood pressure targets in patients with type 2 diabetes mellitus: systematic review and meta-analysis. *Arch Intern Med* 2012;172:1296–1303.

This meta-analysis of 5 randomized trials of intensive (<130/80) versus standard blood pressure control included 7,312 patients with diabetes mellitus. The investigators found a nonsignificant trend toward decreased mortality (RR, 0.76; 95% CI, 0.55 to 1.05) and MI (RR, 0.93; 95% CI, 0.80 to 1.08) in the group targeting BP < 130/80,and a significant decrease in stroke in this group (RR 0.65; 95% CI, 0.48 to 0.86). Absolute risk differences with tight blood pressure control were clinically and statistically insignificant.

Invasive Therapies

222. van Jaarsveld BC, et al.; for DRASTIC (Dutch Renal Artery Stenosis Intervention Cooperative) Study Group. The effect of balloon angioplasty on hypertension in atherosclerotic renal-artery stenosis. *N Engl J Med* 2000;342:1007–1014.

This prospective, randomized study enrolled 106 hypertensive patients (DBP > 95 mm Hg on ≥ 2 antihypertensive drugs) with atherosclerotic renal artery stenosis (50% or more stenosis) and a serum creatinine 2.3 mg/dL or less. Patients underwent percutaneous transluminal renal angioplasty (PTRA) or received drug therapy. BP, doses of antihypertensive drugs, and renal function were assessed at 3 and 12 months, and patency of the renal artery was assessed at 12 months. At 3 months, BPs were similar: 169/99 mm Hg in the PTRA group and 176/101 mm Hg in the control group. However, PTRA patients were taking fewer daily doses of medication compared with the drug therapy group (2.1 vs. 3.2; $p < 0.001$). In the drug group, 22 patients underwent PTRA after 3 months because of worsening renal function or persistent hypertension despite treatment with ≥ 3 antihypertensive drugs. At 1 year, no significant differences were found between the groups in SBP and DBP, daily drug doses, or renal function.

223. The ASTRAL Investigators. Revascularization versus medical therapy for renal-artery stenosis. *N Engl J Med* 2009;361:1953–1962.

To evaluate the utility of percutaneous renal artery stenting versus medical therapy in patients with significant renal artery stenosis, the investigators randomized 806 patients to stenting versus medical therapy alone. The primary outcome was renal function; secondary outcomes were BP, cardiovascular renal function, or any clinical outcomes between the two groups; moreover, revascularization was associated with a 9% risk of periprocedural complications.

224. Cooper CJ, et al.; CORAL Investigators. Stenting and medical therapy for atherosclerotic renal-artery stenosis. *N Engl J Med* 2014;370(1):13–22.

The investigators randomly assigned 947 patients with renal artery stenosis and either significant hypertension (treated with ≥2 drugs) or chronic kidney disease to either renal artery stenting (with medical therapy) or medical therapy alone. The primary end point was a composite of cardiovascular or renal death, MI stroke, heart failure hospitalization, progressive kidney disease, or need for dialysis, assessed at a median follow-up of 43 months. There was no significant difference in the rate of the primary end point (35.1% vs. 35.8%; hazard ratio for stenting, 0.94; 95% CI, 0.76 to 1.17; $p = 0.58$), and its components were also balanced. There was a modest effect on SBP (−2.3 mm Hg benefit of stenting; 95% CI, −4.4 to −0.2; $p = 0.03$).

225. Bisognano JD, et al. Baroreflex activation therapy lowers blood pressure in patients with resistant hypertension: results from the double-blind, randomized, placebo-controlled Rheos Pivotal Trial. *J Am Coll Cardiol* 2011;58:765–773.

To evaluate the safety and efficacy of an implanted baroreceptor activation device, investigators implanted the device into 265 subjects with resistant hypertension. Subjects were randomized to immediate baroreceptor activation therapy or delayed initiation of device therapy for 6 months. After 6 months, 42% of the group receiving active baroreceptor activation therapy had SBP ≤ 140 mm Hg, compared to 24% of the group with device implantation but no active therapy ($p = 0.005$).

226. Bhatt DL, et al.; The Symplicity-3 Investigators. A controlled trial of renal denervation for resistant hypertension. N Engl J Med 2014;370(15):1393–1401.

Design: Prospective, randomized, single-blinded, sham-controlled, multicenter trial. Primary end point was change in seated office-based measurement of SBP at 6 months.

Purpose: To ascertain the efficacy of renal sympathetic denervation in lowering BP in patients with treatment-resistant hypertension.

Population: 535 patients with treatment-resistant hypertension, defined as SBP ≥ 160 mm Hg despite treatment with 3 or more antihypertensive agents.

Results: SBP was reduced by 14.1 mm Hg in the denervation group versus 11.7 mm Hg in the sham-procedure group ($p < 0.001$ for each compared to baseline), with a between-group difference of −2.39 (95% CI, −6.89 to 2.12; $p = 0.26$ for superiority).

Comment: This was the first trial of denervation to include a sham-procedure arm, with single blinding. The lack of superiority of renal denervation raised serious questions about its future role in the treatment of hypertension.

META-ANALYSES

227. Johnson AG, et al. Do non-steroidal anti-inflammatory drugs affect blood pressure? A meta-analysis. Ann Intern Med 1994;121:289–300.

This analysis was performed on data from 38 randomized, placebo-controlled trials and 12 randomized but not placebo-controlled trials (comparing two NSAIDs). NSAID use was associated with a 5.0 mm Hg higher supine mean BP. NSAIDs also antagonized the antihypertensive effect of β-blockers (BP elevation, 6.2 mm Hg). Sulindac and ASA were found to have the least hypertensive effect.

228. Aburto NJ, et al. Effect of lower sodium intake on health: systemic review and meta-analysis. BMJ 2013;346:f1326.

This meta-analysis of 42 randomized controlled trials examined the effect of dietary sodium reduction on a number of clinical variables, including BP, serum lipid profile, and renal function. A reduction in sodium intake reduced SBP by 3.39 mm Hg (95% CI, 2.46 to 4.31) and DBP by 1.54 mm Hg (95% CI, 0.98 to 2.11) with no effect on lipid profile or renal function. The authors also undertook a separate analysis of 14 prospective cohort studies that reported clinical outcomes, including all-cause mortality. In this analysis, reduced sodium intake did not have an appreciable effect on all-cause mortality, cardiovascular mortality, or incident CVD, but *increased* sodium intake significantly increased the risk of stroke, death from stroke, and death from CVD.

229. He FJ, et al. Effect of longer term modest salt reduction on blood pressure: Cochrane systematic review and meta-analysis of randomised trials. BMJ 2013;346:f1325

In this meta-analysis of 34 randomized controlled trials involving patients that modestly reduced sodium intake (by 2.3 to 7.0 g salt per day, or 920 to 2,800 mg sodium per day) for at least 4 weeks, investigators report the effect of sodium restriction on a number of hemodynamic and hormonal variables. Similar to the above meta-analysis (137a), they demonstrate a reduction in SBP by 4.18 mm Hg (95% CI, 3.18 to 5.18) and DBP by 2.06 mm Hg (95% CI, 1.45 to 2.67). Meta-regression demonstrated that reduction in BP correlated with decrease in 24-hour urine sodium, suggesting causality. In an analysis restricted to patients with pre-existing hypertension, the reductions in blood pressure were even more significant; SBP fell by 5.39 mm Hg (95% CI, 4.15 to 6.62) with sodium restriction, and DBP declined by 2.82 mm Hg (95% CI, 2.11 to 3.54). Even normotensive individuals had a smaller but statistically significant decrease in BP with reduced sodium intake. Small physiologic increases in plasma renin, aldosterone, and norepinephrine were noted, but there was no significant change in serum lipid profile; this contradicted earlier meta-analyses that included trials with shorter duration and suggested a deleterious effect of sodium restriction on hormones and lipids.

230. Aburto NJ, et al. Effect of increased potassium intake on cardiovascular risk factors and disease: systematic review and meta-analyses. BMJ 2013;346:f1378.

This meta-analysis of 22 randomized controlled trials (involving 1,606 patients) and 11 prospective cohort studies (involving 127,038) investigated the association between potassium intake and BP, lipid parameters, and cardiovascular outcomes. Importantly, studies targeting those patients with impaired renal potassium handling were excluded from all analyses. In an analysis including both randomized controlled trials and cohort studies, increased potassium intake was demonstrated to reduce SBP by 3.49 mm Hg (95% CI, 1.82 to 5.15) and DBP by 1.96 mm Hg (95% CI, 0.86 to 3.06); this effect was seen only in patients with hypertension, not in those without hypertension. No association between potassium intake and lipid parameters, renal function, or neurohormones was noted. In an analysis including only prospective cohort studies, increased potassium intake was associated with a decreased risk of stroke (RR 0.76, 95% CI, 0.66 to 0.89); there was no statistically significant association between potassium intake and CVD, though there was a trend toward reduced mortality with increased potassium consumption (RR 0.88, 95% CI, 0.70 to 1.10).

231. Law MR, et al. Use of blood pressure lowering drugs in the prevention of cardiovascular disease: meta-analysis of 147 randomised trials in the context of expectations from prospective epidemiological studies. BMJ 2009;338:b1665.

The authors compile data from 147 randomized trials, including 464,000 patients to quantify the effect on BP of each class of antihypertensive medication. Overall, they found that the five different classes of medications (thiazide diuretics, β-blockers, ACE inhibitors, ARBs, and calcium channel blockers) all had similar BP lowering effects. However, β-blockers had the additional benefit of lowering risk of recurrent CHD events in those patients with a previous history of CAD. Similarly, calcium channel blockers had a small advantage in lowering risk of stroke. However, in the general population, the authors could not identify meaningful clinical outcome differences among the classes.

232. Thompson AM, et al. Antihypertensive treatment and secondary prevention of cardiovascular disease among persons without hypertension: a meta-analysis. JAMA 2011;305:913–922.

This meta-analysis of 25 randomized controlled trials of antihypertensive medications for the secondary prevention of CVD in patients without hypertension (blood pressure < 140/90 mm Hg) included 64,162 patients. The investigators found that treatment with antihypertensive drugs reduced the risk of stroke (RR, 0.77; 95% CI, 0.61 to 0.98), MI (RR, 0.80; 95% CI, 0.69 to 0.93), congestive heart failure (RR, 0.71; 95% CI, 0.65 to 0.77), composite cardiovascular events (RR 0.85; 95% CI, 0.69 to 0.99), and all-cause mortality (RR 0.87; 95% CI, 0.80 to 0.95). Studies included in the meta-analysis tested beta blockers, ACE inhibitors, calcium channel blockers, and diuretics, but the investigators did not report risk ratios by antihypertensive class.

233. Shen L, et al. Meta-analysis of cohort studies of baseline prehypertension and risk of coronary artery disease. Am J Cardiol 2013;112:266–271.

This meta-analysis of 18 cohort studies enrolling 934,106 participants with prehypertension (SBP, 120 to 139 mm Hg; DBP, 80 to 89 mm Hg) found that prehypertension is associated with a 36% increased risk of CHD (95% CI, 22% to 53%). When participants were stratified into low-range prehypertension (BP 120/80 to 129/84 mm Hg) and high-range prehypertension (BP 130/85 to 139/90 mm Hg), the risk of CHD was significantly increased in the high-range prehypertension subgroup (RR, 1.53; 95% CI, 1.19 to 1.97), but there was only a trend toward increased CHD risk in the low-range prehypertension group (RR 1.16; 95% CI, 0.96 to 1.42).

Nonmodifiable Risk Factors

AGE AND GENETICS

234. Wei JY. Age and the cardiovascular system. N Engl J Med 1992;327:1735–1739.

This review discusses the impact of age on the myocardium, vasculature, cardiac output, diastolic function, BP regulation, and effects of exercise training.

235. Andresdottir MB, et al. Fifteen percent of myocardial infarctions and coronary revascularizations explained by family history unrelated to conventional risk factors: the Reykjavik Cohort Study. Eur Heart J 2002;23:1655–1663.

This prospective cohort study examined 9,328 men and 10,062 women aged 33 to 81 years in the Reykjavik area, from 1967 to 1996. During follow-up (18 to 19 years), in 2,700 men and 1,070 women, CHD developed. After adjustment for other cardiac risk factors, the HR of family history of CHD was highly significant—1.66 (95% CI, 1.51 to 1.82) and 1.64 (95% CI, 1.43 to 1.89) for men and women, respectively. Family history of MI was calculated to be responsible for 15.1% of all cases of CHD in men and 16.6% in women, independent of other known risk factors.

236. Marenberg ME, et al. Genetic susceptibility to death from coronary heart disease in a study of twins. N Engl J Med 1994;330:1041–1046.

This analysis focused on 21,004 Swedish twins, with 26-year follow-up data. The RR of death due to CHD if one twin died of CHD at younger than 55 years was 8.1 in monozygous twins and 3.8 in dizygous twins. For women, the RRs were 15.0 and 2.6. Overall, the RRs decreased with increasing age at the time of the twin's death from CHD.

237. Palomaki GE, et al. Association between 9p21 genomic markers and heart disease: a meta-analysis. JAMA 2010;303:648–656.

The authors compiled data from 22 articles, on 47 different data sets, including 35,872 cases and 95,837 controls. The 9p21 allele proved significantly related to cardiovascular risk, the magnitude of which varied by the age of the individual. Overall, the effect was small, particularly in the context of more traditional risk factors.

238. Paynter NP, et al. Association between a literature-based genetic risk score and cardiovascular events in women. JAMA 2010;303:631–637.

In 19,313 participants in the Women's Genome Health Study, the authors constructed genetic risk scores based on the National Human Genome Research Institute's catalog of genome-wide association results. In all, 101 single nucleotide polymorphisms had been found to be significantly associated with CVD. While the collective genetic score did modestly but significantly predict CVD risk after controlling for age (HR, 1.02, $p = 0.006$), the effect was no longer significant after controlling for other traditional risk factors (HR 1.00).

239. O'Donnell CJ, et al. Genomics of CVD. N Engl J Med 2011;365:2098–2109.

In this review article, published 10 years after the publication of the human genome sequence, the authors provide an overview of advances made in cardiovascular genetics and genomics over the past decade. They briefly discuss Mendelian cardiovascular risk genes, such as those involving the LDL receptor, before moving on to the genome-wide association studies that have uncovered many of the common gene variants contributing to the risk of CAD. These genome-wide association studies have identified about 30 loci associated with MI and CAD and 10 loci associated with early-onset MI. While many of these loci contained genes that participated in pathways known to be involved in the development of CVD, others contained noncoding regions or genes involved in novel pathways. These genome-wide association studies have generated a number of hypotheses that have enabled a better understanding of the pathogenesis of CVD, but the authors caution that evidence has thus far been insufficient to warrant the creation or use of a genetic risk score.

240. Ashley EA, et al.; for the American Heart Association Advocacy Coordinating Committee. Genetics and cardiovascular disease: a policy statement from the American Heart Association. *Circulation* 2012;126:142–157.

In this wide-ranging review, the authors cover the implications of recent genetic and genomic developments that have made it possible for genetic evaluation to influence clinical medicine. In addition to making policy recommendations on issues such as the legal status of genes, nondiscrimination toward patients on the basis of genetic testing, and standards for laboratories conducting genetic testing for use in the clinical arena, the authors note that, despite robust evidence from genome-wide association studies linking multiple common genetic variants to CHD, there is no evidence suggesting a clinical benefit to informing patients of their genetic risk or clinical consensus on how to incorporate genetic risk into a clinical workup.

Inflammation

C-REACTIVE PROTEIN

241. Ridker PM, et al. Inflammation, aspirin, and the risk of cardiovascular disease in apparently healthy men. *N Engl J Med* 1997;336:973–979.

Case–control study of 543 PHS participants who had an MI, stroke, or venous thrombosis and 543 participants who did not have a vascular event at a long-term follow-up (>8 years). Baseline CRP concentrations were significantly higher in men who subsequently had an MI (1.51 vs. 1.13 mg/L; $p < 0.001$) or ischemic stroke (1.38 vs. 1.13 mg/L; $p = 0.02$), but not venous thrombosis (1.26 vs. 1.13 mg/L; $p = 0.34$), than among men without vascular events. Men in the highest quartile of CRP values had, as compared with those in the lowest quartile, an approximately threefold and twofold higher risk of MI and stroke, respectively (RR for MI, 2.9; $p < 0.001$; RR for stroke, 1.9; $p = 0.02$). The use of ASA was associated with a substantial (55.7%) reduction ($p = 0.02$) in MI among men in the highest CRP quartile, but only a nonsignificant (13.9%) reduction among those in the lowest quartile.

242. Ridker PM, et al.; for the Air Force/Texas Coronary Atherosclerosis Prevention Study Investigators. Measurement of C-reactive protein for the targeting of statin therapy in the primary prevention of acute coronary events. *N Engl J Med* 2001;344:1959–1965.

CRP was measured at baseline and 1 year in 5,742 AFCAPS/TexCAPS participants. At 5 years, higher baseline CRP levels were associated with higher coronary event rates. Lovastatin therapy reduced CRP levels by 14.8% ($p < 0.001$), an effect not explained by lovastatin-induced changes in the lipid profile. In particular, lovastatin was effective in those with TC/HDL ratio lower than the median and a CRP higher than the median ($p = 0.02$). In contrast, lovastatin was ineffective in those with TC/HDL ratio and a CRP level that were both lower than the median.

243. Heart Protection Study Collaborative Group. C-reactive protein concentration and the vascular benefits of statin therapy: an analysis of 20,536 patients in the Heart Protection Study. *Lancet* 2011;377:469–476.

In this secondary analysis of the Heart Protection Study (see Ref. 44), investigators studied whether baseline levels of CRP modified the relative risk reduction achieved with simvastatin therapy compared to placebo. They found that the relative risk reduction for major vascular events, major coronary events, stroke, and need for revascularization achieved with simvastatin therapy was not modified by baseline CRP level, with pretreatment CRP levels ranging from < 1.25 mg/dL to > 8 mg/dL. The relative reduction in major vascular events in the group treated with simvastatin persisted even in the subset of patients with LDL cholesterol and CRP below the median. Though the findings from this study contradict those from AFCAPS/TexCAPS (182), they have been replicated with rosuvastatin and pravastatin in the JUPITER (see *Am J Cardiol* 2010;106:204–209) and PROSPER (see *Circulation* 2007;115:981–989) trial populations, respectively.

244. Pradhan AD, et al. Inflammatory biomarkers, hormone replacement therapy, and incident coronary heart disease: prospective analysis from the Women's Health Initiative observational study. JAMA 2002;288:980–987.

This prospective, nested case–control study of postmenopausal women examined the 304 cases in which CHD developed during the Women's Health Initiative; 304 controls were matched by age, smoking status, ethnicity, and follow-up time (median, 2.9 years). Cases had significantly higher median baseline levels of CRP and IL-6 compared with controls (0.33 vs. 0.25 mg/dL CRP; $p < 0.001$; 1.81 vs. 1.47 pg/mL IL-6; $p < 0.001$). In matched analyses, the OR for incident CHD in the highest versus lowest quartile was 2.3 for CRP (95% CI, 1.4 to 3.7; p for trend = 0.002) and 3.3 for IL-6 (95% CI, 2.0 to 5.5; p for trend < 0.001). After additional adjustment for lipid and nonlipid risk factors, both inflammatory markers were associated with significant twofold increases in risk of CHD events. Current use of HRT was associated with elevated median CRP levels, but showed no association with IL-6. In analyses comparing individuals with similar baseline levels of either CRP or IL-6, those taking or not taking HRT had similar CHD ORs. Thus, use or nonuse of HRT had less importance as a predictor of cardiovascular risk than did baseline levels of either CRP or IL-6.

245. Ridker PM, et al. Comparison of C-reactive protein and low-density lipoprotein cholesterol levels in the prediction of first cardiovascular events. N Engl J Med 2002;347:1557–1565.

This study measured baseline LDL and CRP in 27,939 WHS participants. At a mean follow-up of 8 years, both measures had a strong linear relation with the incidence of cardiovascular events, although the two were minimally correlated ($r = 0.08$). After adjustment for age, smoking status, diabetes, BP, use or nonuse of HRT, the RRs of first cardiovascular event (MI, ischemic stroke, coronary revascularization, or cardiovascular death) according to increasing quintiles of CRP, as compared with the women in the lowest quintile, were 1.4, 1.6, 2.0, and 2.3 ($p < 0.001$). Corresponding RRs in increasing quintiles of LDL, as compared with the lowest, were 0.9, 1.1, 1.3, and 1.5 ($p < 0.001$). Similar effects were observed in separate analyses of each component of the composite end point. Overall, 46% of major events occurred among those with LDL < 130 mg/dL. Importantly, because CRP and LDL measurements tended to identify different high-risk groups, screening for both biologic markers provided better prognostic information than did screening for either alone.

246. Mueller C, et al. Inflammation and long-term mortality after non–ST elevation acute coronary syndrome treated with a very early invasive strategy in 1042 consecutive patients. Circulation 2002;105:1412–1415.

In this prospective cohort study of 1,042 patients with NSTEMI undergoing coronary angiography and subsequent culprit artery stenting within 24 hours, CRP levels were determined on admission. In-hospital mortality was significantly higher in patients with a CRP > 10 mg/L (3.7% vs. 1.2% with CRP < 3 mg/L and 0.8% with CRP of 3 to 10 mg/L; RR, 4.2 for CRP > 10 mg/L vs. CRP ≤ 10 mg/L; $p = 0.004$). At follow-up (mean, 20 months), mortality was 3.4% with CRP < 3 mg/L, 4.4% with CRP between 3 and 10 mg/L, and 12.7% with CRP > 10 mg/L (RR, 3.8 for CRP > 10 mg/L vs. CRP ≤ 10 mg/L). In multivariate analysis, CRP remained an independent predictor of long-term mortality.

247. Ray KK, et al.; for the PROVE IT-TIMI 22 Investigators. Relationship between uncontrolled risk factors and C-reactive protein levels in patients receiving standard or intensive statin therapy for acute coronary syndromes in the PROVE IT-TIMI 22 trial. *J Am Coll Cardiol* 2005;46:1417–1424.

This additional analysis of the PROVE IT-TIMI 22 trial demonstrated that intensive statin therapy led to lower CRP levels, independent of other risk factors. Furthermore, CRP level correlated significantly with a number of other clinical risk factors such as age, gender, BMI, smoking, LDL, glucose, HDL, and TGs. This suggests that, in addition to pharmacotherapy, other means of reducing CRP, such as lifestyle intervention, may be appropriate in the secondary prevention of CHD.

248. Zacho J, et al. Genetically elevated C-reactive protein and ischemic vascular disease. *N Engl J Med* 2008;359:1897–1908.

In subgroups of two observational cohorts, the authors compared the DNA polymorphisms of 2,238 patients with IHD with 4,474 controls and 612 patients with ischemic cerebrovascular disease with 1,224 controls. They identified four polymorphisms that were significantly linked with elevated CRP levels. However, while elevated CRP in the general population was predictive of ischemic events, patients with such polymorphisms were not at significantly increased risk of events. The authors conclude that these data demonstrate that CRP does not play a *causal* role in ischemic atherosclerotic disease.

249. The Emerging Risk Factors Collaboration. C-reactive protein concentration and risk of coronary heart disease, stroke, and mortality: an individual participant meta-analysis. *Lancet* 2010;375:132–140.

In a meta-analysis of 54 prospective studies with 160,309 participants free of vascular disease at baseline, the investigators measured CRP and assessed risk for cardiovascular events. After controlling for variation in risk factors among participants, CRP proved significantly predictive of CAD, ischemic stroke, cardiovascular mortality, and death, as well as lung disease and several cancers. The predictive effect of CRP for CVD was significantly attenuated by incorporation of conventional risk factors. These data support the idea of CRP as a marker of underlying inflammation of unclear pathophysiology, representing elevated risk for such disease processes.

HOMOCYSTEINE AND B VITAMINS

Observational Studies

250. Homocysteine Studies Collaboration. Homocysteine and risk of ischemic heart disease and stroke: a meta-analysis. *JAMA* 2002;288:2015–2022.

This meta-analysis included data from 30 prospective or retrospective studies involving a total of 5,073 IHD events and 1,113 stroke events. Allowances were made for differences between studies, for confounding by known cardiac risk factors, and for regression dilution bias. Stronger associations were observed in retrospective studies of homocysteine measured in blood collected after the onset of disease than in prospective studies among individuals who had no history of CVD when blood was collected. After adjustment for cardiac risk factors in the prospective studies, a 25% lower than usual homocysteine level [about 3 mmol/L (0.41 mg/L)] was associated with an 11% lower IHD risk (OR, 0.89; 95% CI, 0.83 to 0.96) and 19% lower stroke risk (OR, 0.81; 95% CI, 0.69 to 0.95).

251. Morrison HI, et al. Serum folate and the risk of fatal coronary heart disease. *JAMA* 1996;275:1893–1896.

This retrospective study of 5,056 patients showed that 15-year CHD mortality was correlated with serum folate levels; < 3 ng/mL conferred a 69% excess risk of CHD mortality compared with > 6 ng/mL.

252. Jacques PF, et al. The effect of folic acid fortification on plasma folate and total homocysteine concentrations. N Engl J Med 1999;340:1449–1454.

This study analyzed blood samples of Framingham Offspring Study participants taken from January 1991 to December 1994 and compared them with subsequent samples obtained before fortification of enriched grain with folic acid (January 1995 to September 1996; control group) and after fortification was implemented (September 1997 to March 1998; study group). Among study-group subjects who did not use vitamin supplements, mean folate concentrations more than doubled from the baseline to follow-up visit (4.6 to 10.0 ng/mL; $p < 0.001$), and the prevalence of low folate levels (<3 ng/mL) markedly decreased from 22.0% to 1.7% ($p < 0.001$). The mean total homocysteine concentration decreased from 10.1 to 9.4 μmol/L, and the prevalence of high homocysteine levels (more than 13 μmol/L) decreased from 18.7% to 9.8% ($p < 0.001$). No significant changes were noted in folate or homocysteine concentrations in control group subjects.

253. Bostom AG, et al. Nonfasting plasma total homocysteine levels and all-cause and cardiovascular disease mortality in elderly Framingham men and women. Arch Intern Med 1999;159:1077–1080.

Nonfasting plasma homocysteine levels were obtained in 1933 Framingham Study participants between 1979 and 1982; mean age was 70 years. At follow-up (median, 10.0 years), proportional hazard modeling showed that homocysteine levels in the upper quartile ($\geq$14.26 μmol/L) compared with levels in the lower three quartiles were associated with RRs of all-cause and cardiovascular mortality of 2.18 and 2.17, respectively (95% CIs, 1.86 to 2.56, and 1.68 to 2.82). These RR estimates were attenuated but remained significant [1.54 (95% CI, 1.31 to 1.82), 1.52 (1.16 to 1.98)] after adjustment for age, sex, SBP, diabetes, smoking, TC, and HDL.

254. Nurk E, et al. Plasma total homocysteine and hospitalizations for cardiovascular disease: the Hordaland Homocysteine Study. Arch Intern Med 2002;162:1374–1381.

This prospective cohort study of 17,361 individuals aged 40 to 42 or 65 to 67 years was conducted from April 1992 to May 1998 (mean follow-up, 5.3 years) in western Norway. At baseline, those with pre-existing CVD had higher mean total plasma homocysteine values than did individuals without CVD. Risk of CVD hospitalizations increased significantly with increasing baseline plasma homocysteine only in the older age group. In this group, multiple risk factor–adjusted hospitalization rate ratios in 5 plasma homocysteine categories (<9, 9 to 11.9, 12 to 14.9, 15 to 19.9, and $\geq$ 20 μmol/L) were as follows: 1.00 (reference level), 1.00, 1.34, 1.67, and 1.94, respectively (p for trend < 0.001). The relation between plasma homocysteine level and CVD hospitalizations was significantly stronger among individuals with pre-existing CVD than in those without (hospitalization rate ratio per 5 μmol/L increment, 1.29 vs. 1.10; p for interaction = 0.02).

255. Ridker PM, et al.; for Air Force/Texas Coronary Atherosclerosis Prevention Study (AFCAPS/TexCAPS) Investigators. Plasma homocysteine concentration, statin therapy, and the risk of first acute coronary events. Circulation 2002;105:1776–1779.

A total of 5,569 AFCAPS/TexCAPS participants had homocysteine measured at baseline and 1 year. Median baseline homocysteine levels were significantly higher in those with subsequent ACS (12.1 vs. 10.9 μmol/L; $p < 0.001$). The RRs of future events from lowest to highest quartile of homocysteine were 1.0, 1.6, 1.6, and 2.2 ($p < 0.001$). This increased risk was only modestly attenuated after adjustment for other traditional risk factors. The subgroup of participants with elevated LDL and elevated homocysteine levels were at high risk and benefited significantly from lovastatin therapy (RR, 0.46; 95% CI, 0.29 to 0.75). However, in contrast to findings in this trial for CRP, homocysteine levels did not help to define low LDL subgroups with different responses to lovastatin therapy.

Trials and Meta-analyses

256. Bønaa KH.; for the NORVIT Trial Investigators. Homocysteine lowering and cardiovascular events after acute myocardial infarction. *N Engl J Med* 2006;354:1578–1588.

In 3,749 patients with recent acute MI, treatment with a variety of B vitamins (or placebo) lowered homocysteine levels, but had no effect on recurrent events (MI, stroke, or sudden CAD death).

257. The Heart Outcomes Prevention Evaluation (HOPE) 2 Investigators. Homocysteine lowering with folic acid and B vitamins in vascular disease. *N Engl J Med* 2006;354:1567–1577.

5,522 patients with CVD or diabetes were randomized to combination folate, vitamin B_6, vitamin B_{12}, or placebo. Over an average follow-up of 5 years, there was no significant effect of supplementation on the primary end point of cardiovascular death, MI, or stroke.

258. Jamison RL, et al. Effect of homocysteine lowering on mortality and vascular disease in advanced chronic kidney disease and end-stage renal disease a randomized controlled trial. *JAMA* 2007;298:1163–1170.

In this double-blind, randomized controlled trial, 2,056 veterans with advanced chronic kidney disease and elevated homocysteine levels (>15 μmol/L) were assigned to either a multivitamin with folate, vitamin B_6, and vitamin B_{12} or matching placebo. Despite decreased homocysteine in the multivitamin group compared to the placebo group, there was no difference in all-cause mortality at 3 years, or any of the additional secondary end points.

259. Bostom AG, et al. Homocysteine-lowering and cardiovascular disease outcomes in kidney transplant recipients: primary results from the Folic Acid for Vascular Outcome Reduction in Transplantation trial. *Circulation* 2011;123:1763–1770.

In this double-blind, placebo-controlled trial, researchers randomized 4,100 kidney transplant patients to a high-dose folic acid, B_6, and B_{12} multivitamin, or matching placebo. After a median 4 years' follow-up, the multivitamin-treated patients had lower homocysteine than control patients, but there was no difference in the rate of cardiovascular events, dialysis-dependent renal failure, or all-cause mortality.

260. Ebbing M, et al.; for the WENBIT Trial. Mortality and cardiovascular events in patients treated with homocysteine-lowering B vitamins after coronary angiography: a randomized controlled trial. *JAMA* 2008;300:795–804.

In patients undergoing coronary angiography (acutely or electively), 3,096 were randomized to combinations of folate, B_{12}, B_6, or placebo (in a factorial design) for the prevention of death, MI, UA, or stroke. No combination of the above vitamins or folate provided reduction in the primary end point.

261. Study of the Effectiveness of Additional Reductions in Cholesterol and Homocysteine (SEARCH) Collaborative Group. Effects of homocysteine-lowering with folic acid plus vitamin B_{12} on mortality and major morbidity in myocardial infarction survivors: a randomized trial. *JAMA* 2010;303:2486–2494.

This international trial randomized 12,064 men and women aged 18 to 80 years with a previous MI to either simvastatin, 80 mg or 20 mg daily, and homocysteine-lowering therapy with folic acid and vitamin B_{12}, in a 2 × 2 factorial design. Patients were followed for a mean of 6.7 years for the development of a composite primary end point of major coronary events (nonfatal MI, coronary revascularization, or CHD death), any stroke, or revascularization (including coronary and noncoronary surgery, angioplasty, or amputation). In the folate/B_{12} group, homocysteine was reduced by an average of 3.8 μmol/L, yet there was no difference in incidence of primary outcome events (25.5% in the treatment group vs. 24.8% in the placebo control).

262. Clarke R, et al.; for the B-Vitamin Treatment Trialists' Collaboration. Effects of lowering homocysteine levels with B vitamins on cardiovascular disease, cancer, and cause-specific mortality: Meta-analysis of 8 randomized trials involving 37,485 individuals. *Arch Intern Med* 2010;170:1622–1631.

In this meta-analysis, authors found that supplementation with folic acid produced an average 25% reduction in plasma homocysteine levels, but that at a median 5 years' follow-up, there was no significant effect on vascular outcomes, including major vascular events (RR, 1.01; 95% CI, 0.97 to 1.05), major coronary events (RR, 1.03; 95% CI, 0.97 to 1.10), or stroke (RR, 0.96; 95% CI, 0.87 to 1.06).

LIPOPROTEIN-ASSOCIATED PHOSPHOLIPASE A_2 (LP-PLA_2)

263. O'Donoghue M, et al. Lipoprotein-associated phospholipase A2 and its association with cardiovascular outcomes in patients with acute coronary syndromes in the PROVE IT-TIMI 22 (PRavastatin Or atorVastatin Evaluation and Infection Therapy—Thrombolysis In Myocardial Infarction) trial. *Circulation* 2006;113: 1745–1752.

The investigators measured levels of Lp-PLA$_2$ in patients in the PROVE IT-TIMI 22 trial immediately following ACS and again at 30 days. While levels in the setting of ACS were not useful in predicting clinical outcomes, elevation of Lp-PLA2 at 30 days following ACS was found to be associated with a higher risk of clinical cardiovascular events, independent of LDL or CRP.

264. Lp-PLA(2) Studies Collaboration, et al. Lipoprotein-associated phospholipase A(2) and risk of coronary disease, stroke, and mortality: collaborative analysis of 32 prospective studies. *Lancet* 2010;375:1536–1544.

In this meta-analysis involving 79,036 participants from 32 prospective studies, a 1 standard deviation increase in Lp-PLA2 activity or mass was associated with small but significant increases in the risk of CAD (RR, 1.10 for Lp-PLA2 activity, and 1.11 for Lp-PLA2 mass), vascular death, and nonvascular death.

265. Mohler ER, et al.; for the Darapladib Investigators. The effect of darapladib on plasma lipoprotein-associated phospholipase A2 activity and cardiovascular biomarkers in patients with stable coronary heart disease or coronary heart disease risk equivalent: the results of a multicenter, randomized, double-blind, placebo-controlled study. *J Am Coll Cardiol* 2008;51:1632–1641.

Darapladib is a selective inhibitor of Lp-PLA$_2$; the investigators sought to measure its effect on other biomarkers of cardiovascular risk in 959 patients with CVD or its risk equivalents. All patients were already receiving atorvastatin. Darapladib at doses of 40, 80, and 160 mg daily inhibited Lp-PLA$_2$ activity in a dose–response fashion ($p < 0.001$); at the highest dose of 160 mg, darapladib significantly decreased IL-6 and hsCRP at 12 weeks. No clinical adverse effects or detrimental platelet function effects were detected during the brief study—this suggests that therapy with darapladib as an inhibitor of Lp-PLA$_2$ may be beneficial in reducing the inflammation associated with CVD. Studies powered to detect differences in clinical events, as well as rare adverse effects, are needed.

266. Rosenson RS, et al.; for the PLASMA II Investigators. Randomized trial of an inhibitor of secretory phospholipase A2 on atherogenic lipoprotein subclasses in statin-treated patients with coronary heart disease. *Eur Heart J* 2011;32:999–1005.

In this randomized, placebo-controlled trial, investigators studied the effect of varespladib, an oral inhibitor of secretory PLA$_2$, on lipid profile in 135 patients with stable CAD. Compared with placebo, varespladib reduced LDL and non-HDL cholesterol by 15% ($p < 0.001$) over 8-week follow-up.

INFECTIONS AND CARDIOVASCULAR DISEASE

Antibiotic Trials

267. O'Connor CM, et al.; Azithromycin for the secondary prevention of coronary heart disease events: the Investigators in the WIZARD (Weekly Intervention with Zithromax for Atherosclerosis and its Related Disorders) Study. JAMA 2003;290:1459–1466.

This prospective, randomized, placebo-controlled multicenter trial enrolled 7,747 post-MI patients with elevated C. pneumoniae titers. Patients received azithromycin (600 mg daily for the first 3 days and then 600 mg/week for 11 weeks), or placebo. At 2-year follow-up, no significant difference was found between the two groups in the primary composite end point of all-cause mortality, recurrent MI, revascularization, and hospitalization for angina (7% reduction in azithromycin group; HR, 0.93; $p = 0.23$).

268. Cannon CP, et al.; for the Pravastatin or Atorvastatin Evaluation and Infection Therapy—Thrombolysis in Myocardial Infarction 22 Investigators. Antibiotic treatment of Chlamydia pneumoniae after acute coronary syndrome. N Engl J Med 2005;352:1646–1654.

In the antibiotic arm of the PROVE IT-TIMI 22 trial, the 4,162 patients enrolled during hospitalization for ACS were randomized to treatment with gatifloxacin (a bactericidal antibiotic with known efficacy against C. pneumoniae), or placebo, in a randomized, double-blind fashion. Subjects received therapy for an initial 2-week course beginning 2 weeks after randomization and then a 10-day course every month over the duration of the trial (a mean of 2 years). The primary end point was a composite of all-cause mortality, MI, hospitalization for UA, revascularization, or stroke. There were no significant differences between the groups in this primary end point, or several secondary end points, over the follow-up period. This provided the most convincing data to date that, despite evidence suggesting a causal link, antibiotic therapy against C. pneumoniae is not an effective strategy to reduce cardiovascular events.

269. Grayston JT, et al.; ACES Investigators. Azithromycin for the secondary prevention of coronary events. N Engl J Med 2005;352:1637–1645.

Investigators randomized 4,012 patients with stable CAD to 600-mg azithromycin weekly or placebo for 1 year. Over follow-up period of a mean of 3.9 years, there was no significant difference in the composite rate of cardiovascular death, MI, coronary revascularization, or hospitalization for UA between the azithromycin (446 events) and placebo groups (449 events).

HIV-Related Cardiovascular Risk

270. Freiberg MS, et al. HIV infection and the risk of acute myocardial infarction. JAMA Intern Med 2013;173:614–622.

In this prospective cohort study lasting from 2003 to 2009, investigators measured the 6-year rate of MI in 27,350 HIV-infected veterans and 55,109 controls matched demographically and behaviorally. After controlling for substance use, comorbidities, and Framingham risk factors, HIV-infected veterans had an increased risk of MI compared to controls (HR, 1.48; 95% CI, 1.27 to 1.72). This increased risk persisted among veterans with good virologic control (HIV RNA level < 500 copies/mL).

271. Boccara F, et al. HIV and coronary heart disease: time for a better understanding. J Am Coll Cardiol 2013;61:511–523.

In this review, the authors discuss the scope of CHD in the HIV-infected population. They note that cardiovascular causes account for 15% of deaths in HIV-infected patients and that HIV-infected patients suffer MI at a younger mean age (48) than the general population. This excess risk is explained by a combination of the higher prevalence of traditional risk factors in patients with HIV (including smoking, hypertension, hyperlipidemia, and diabetes mellitus), dysmetabolic effects of antiretroviral drugs (especially protease inhibitors), and the inflammatory effect of chronic infection.

272. Friis-Møller N, et al.; for The Data Collection on Adverse Events of Anti-HIV Drugs (DAD) Study Group. Combination antiretroviral therapy and the risk of myocardial infarction. *N Engl J Med* 2003;349:1993–2003.

This prospective cohort study enrolled 23,468 patients with HIV and followed them for a 2.5 years for the development of MI. Per year of exposure to antiretroviral therapy, the relative risk of MI was increased by 26% (95% CI, 21% to 41%; $p < 0.001$), though the absolute risk of MI was just 3.5 events per 1,000 person-years in this cohort with median age of 39 years.

273. DAD Study Group. Class of antiretroviral drugs and the risk of myocardial infarction. *N Engl J Med* 2007;356:1723–1735.

This prospective observational study of 23,437 patients with HIV investigated the association between exposure to protease inhibitors and development of MI. Though the overall risk of MI was low (3.65 events per 1,000 person-years), exposure to protease inhibitors increased the relative risk of MI by 16% per year (95% CI, 10% to 23%) after adjustment for cardiovascular risk factors. Based on these findings, researchers created a risk model for the prediction of CVD in HIV-infected patients that incorporates traditional risk factors as well as protease inhibitor exposure (see *Eur J Cardiovasc Prev Rehabil* 2010;17:491–501). This risk model outperformed the Framingham risk model in predicting incident cardiovascular events in HIV-infected patients.

MISCELLANEOUS

274. Tang WH, et al. Intestinal microbial metabolism of phosphatidylcholine and cardiovascular risk. *N Engl J Med* 2013;368:1575–1584.

In this prospective cohort analysis, the investigators quantified plasma and urine levels of trimethylamine-N-oxide (TMAO), a proatherosclerotic metabolite produced by gut microbiota, before and after antibiotic challenge in 4,007 patients who underwent elective coronary angiography. Levels of TMAO were suppressed by antibiotics and then rose again when antibiotics were withdrawn. At 3 years' follow-up, those patients in the highest quartile for baseline TMAO levels were more likely to have major adverse cardiac events (stroke, MI, or death) than those in the lowest quartile (HR, 2.54; 95% CI, 1.96 to 3.28) even after adjustment for traditional risk factors.

275. März W, et al. Homoarginine, cardiovascular risk, and mortality. *Circulation* 2010;122:967–975.

In this cohort analysis of 3,305 patients in the LUdwigshafen RIsk and Cardiovascular Health (LURIC) study undergoing angiography, researchers measured serum homoarginine levels at the time of angiography and monitored the patients for cardiovascular death over a median of 7.7 years. At follow-up, those subjects with serum homoarginine levels in the lowest quartile had 4.1-fold increased risk of death (95% CI, 3.0 to 5.7) compared to patients in the highest quartile. The investigators confirmed the association between low serum homoarginine and cardiovascular mortality in a second, higher-risk population of patients with diabetes and dialysis-dependent renal failure from the 4D (Die Deutsche Diabetes Dialyse) study.

276. Tonelli M, et al. Risk of coronary events in people with chronic kidney disease compared with those with diabetes: a population-level cohort study. *Lancet* 2012;380:807–814.

This prospective cohort study in Alberta, Canada, followed 1,268,029 participants for a median of 4 years. Participants with chronic kidney disease (GFR 15 to 59 mL/min per 1.73 m^2) had a higher risk of MI than patients with diabetes (6.9 per 1,000 person-years vs. 5.4 per 1,000 person-years; $p < 0.001$), though their risk of MI was not as high as participants with prior MI. The authors suggest on the basis of these data that patients with chronic kidney disease, like those with diabetes, should be considered at the highest risk of future cardiovascular events.

Antiplatelet Drugs for Primary and Secondary Prevention

PRIMARY PREVENTION

277. Physicians' Health Study, Steering Committee of the Physicians Health Study Research Group. Final report on aspirin component of the ongoing Physicians' Health Study. N Engl J Med 1989;321:129–135.

Design: Prospective, randomized, double-blind, placebo-controlled study. Primary end point was the incidence of cardiovascular mortality. Average follow-up was 5 years.

Purpose: To determine whether low-dose aspirin (ASA) decreases cardiovascular mortality.

Population: 22,071 male physicians aged 40 to 84 years.

Treatment: ASA, 325 mg every other day, or placebo.

Results: The ASA group had a 44% reduction in the risk of MI (0.255%/year vs. 0.44%/year; $p < 0.00001$). This benefit was restricted to those older than 50 years. The ASA group also had a nonsignificant reduction in cardiovascular mortality (RR, 0.96) as well as a nonsignificant increase in stroke rate (RR, 2.1; $p = 0.06$). Among 333 patients with chronic stable angina, the risk of MI was reduced by 87%.

Comments: This study was stopped early because of the highly significant reduction in nonfatal MIs. However, as a result, the evidence regarding stroke and total cardiovascular deaths is inconclusive because of the very low event rates.

278. de Gaetano G; for the Collaborative Group of the Primary Prevention Project. Low-dose aspirin and vitamin E in people at cardiovascular risk: a randomised trial. Lancet 2001;357:89–95.

Design: Prospective, randomized, open-label, 2 × 2 factorial, multicenter trial. Primary end point was cardiovascular death, nonfatal MI, and nonfatal stroke.

Purpose: To determine the benefit of ASA and vitamin E for primary prevention of cardiovascular events in a clinical practice setting.

Population: 4,495 patients, aged 50 years or older, with one or more cardiac risk factors, including HTN, hypercholesterolemia, diabetes, obesity, family history of premature MI, or age 65 years or older; approximately 70% had two or more risk factors.

Treatment: Low-dose ASA (100 mg/day) and vitamin E (300 mg/day), either, or neither.

Results: Study was terminated prematurely at a mean follow-up of 3.6 years because the benefit of ASA was demonstrated in similar trials. ASA use was associated with a significantly lower incidence of cardiovascular death (0.8% vs. 1.4%; RR, 0.56) and a composite outcome comprising cardiovascular death, MI, or stroke (6.3% vs. 8.2%; RR, 0.77). Bleeding occurred more frequently in the ASA group (1.1% vs. 0.3%). Vitamin E showed no effect on any end points.

Comments: The evidence in support of ASA for primary prevention of cardiovascular events has mounted and appears to be independent of dose (75 to 325 mg), age, gender, and cardiovascular risk status; however, in low-risk patients, large relative risk reductions for cardiovascular events may correspond to minimal absolute risk reductions, which may be outweighed by the increased bleeding risk with ASA.

279. Ridker PM, et al. A randomized trial of low-dose aspirin in the primary prevention of cardiovascular disease in women. N Engl J Med 2005;352:1293–1304.

Design: Prospective, randomized, double-blind, placebo-controlled study. Average follow-up period was 10 years. Primary end point was a composite of nonfatal MI, nonfatal stroke, or cardiovascular death.

Purpose: To assess the efficacy of aspirin for primary prevention of CVD in apparently healthy women.

Population: 39,876 healthy women, aged 45 years or older.

Treatment: ASA, 100 mg every other day, or placebo.

Results: There was a nonsignificant reduction in the primary end point, favoring the aspirin group (relative risk, 0.91; $p = 0.13$). However, there was a significant 24% reduction in ischemic stroke, favoring the aspirin group ($p = 0.009$), at the expense of a nonsignificant increase in hemorrhagic stroke (RR 1.24, $p = 0.31$). There were no significant differences in the risk of MI or cardiovascular death between the two groups. The risk of GI bleeding was significantly higher in the aspirin group (RR 1.40; $p = 0.02$).

SECONDARY PREVENTION

280. Gent M, et al. Clopidogrel versus aspirin in patients at risk of ischaemic events (CAPRIE). A randomised, blinded trial of clopidogrel versus aspirin in patients at risk of ischaemic events (CAPRIE). *Lancet* 1996;348:1329–1339.

Design: Prospective, randomized, multicenter study. Primary end point was ischemic stroke, MI, and vascular death. Mean follow-up period was 1.9 years.

Purpose: To compare the effectiveness of clopidogrel with ASA in preventing major vascular events.

Population: 19,185 patients with a history of recent ischemic stroke (1 week to 6 months earlier), MI (≥35 days earlier), or symptomatic peripheral arterial disease.

Treatment: Clopidogrel, 75 mg once daily, or ASA, 325 mg/day.

Exclusion Criteria: Carotid endarterectomy or severe deficit after stroke, uncontrolled HTN, and scheduled major surgery.

Results: Clopidogrel group had a significant 8.7% relative reduction in the primary composite end point (5.32 vs. 5.83%/year; $p = 0.043$). The subgroup of patients with peripheral arterial disease had a significant 23.8% reduction in the primary end point ($p = 0.003$), whereas the stroke patients had a nonsignificant 7.3% reduction ($p = 0.26$), and MI patients had a nonsignificant 3.7% *increase*. A subsequent analysis of all 8,446 patients with any history of MI showed that clopidogrel was associated with a statistically insignificant 7.4% decrease in the combined end point. No difference was found in incidence of side effects, including neutropenia (clopidogrel, 0.1%; ASA, 0.17%).

281. Mangano DT, et al.; for the Multicenter Study of Perioperative Ischemia Research Group. Aspirin and mortality from coronary bypass surgery. *N Engl J Med* 2002;347:1309–1317.

This prospective, multicenter study of 5,065 patients undergoing CABG found that early use of ASA is associated with a reduced risk of mortality and ischemic complications. During hospitalization, overall mortality was 3.2%, whereas the incidence of nonfatal cardiac, cerebral, renal, or GI ischemic complications was 16.0%. Among patients who received ASA (up to 650 mg) within 48 hours, mortality was nearly 70% lower (1.3% vs. 4.0% with no ASA; $p < 0.001$). ASA therapy also was associated with a 48% lower incidence of MI (2.8% vs. 5.4%; $p < 0.001$), a 50% lower incidence of stroke (1.3% vs. 2.6%; $p = 0.01$), lower incidence of renal failure (0.9% vs. 3.4%; $p < 0.001$), and a 62% lower rate of bowel infarction (0.3% vs. 0.8%; $p = 0.01$). Multivariate analysis showed that no other factor or medication was independently associated with reduced rates of these outcomes. Furthermore, the risk of hemorrhage, gastritis, infection, or impaired wound healing was not increased with ASA use (OR, 0.63; 95% CI, 0.54 to 0.74).

282. Bhatt DL, et al.; for the CHARISMA Investigators. Clopidogrel and aspirin versus aspirin alone for the prevention of atherothrombotic events. *N Engl J Med* 2006;354:1706–1717.

Design: Prospective, randomized, multicenter study. Primary end point was a composite of MI, stroke, or cardiovascular death.

Purpose: To compare the effectiveness of dual antiplatelet therapy with clopidogrel with ASA versus ASA alone in preventing major vascular events in a population of both primary and secondary prevention.

Population: 15,603 patients with either known CVD (secondary prevention group) or multiple risk factors (primary prevention group); randomization was not stratified by group.

Treatment: Clopidogrel, 75 mg daily, or placebo; both groups received low-dose aspirin (75 to 162 mg daily).

Results: A primary end point event occurred in 6.8% of patients in the clopidogrel plus aspirin group versus 7.3% in the aspirin only group ($p = 0.22$). Rates of severe bleeding were higher in the clopidogrel plus aspirin group (1.7% vs. 1.3%, $p = 0.09$). In the subgroup without known disease but with multiple risk factors, those in the clopidogrel plus aspirin group had a similar number of primary end point events to the aspirin only group, but a significantly higher risk of cardiovascular death (3.9% vs. 2.2%, $p = 0.01$). In the subgroup with known disease, the addition of clopidogrel to aspirin yielded a 12% lower risk of cardiovascular events ($p = 0.046$).

Comment: While the overall primary end point of this trial was negative, it is important to note that results from the secondary prevention group (the "CAPRIE-like" cohort) were consistent with previous trials. However, it does not appear that dual antiplatelet therapy is appropriate for patients with multiple risk factors but no known CVD.

283. Morrow DA, et al.; for the TRA 2P-TIMI 50 Steering Committee and Investigators. Vorapaxar in the secondary prevention of atherothrombotic events. *N Engl J Med* 2012;366:1404–1413.

Design: Prospective, randomized, double-blind, placebo-controlled multicenter study. Primary end point was a composite of stroke, MI, or death from cardiovascular causes. Patients were followed for a median of 30 months.

Purpose: To evaluate the efficacy of vorapaxar, a novel protease-activated receptor-1 (PAR-1) inhibitor, in the secondary prevention of cardiovascular events.

Population: 26,449 patients with known stable atherosclerotic vascular disease (history of peripheral arterial disease, stroke, or MI); 2 years into the 3-year-long study, the safety monitoring board recommended discontinuation of vorapaxar in patients with a history of stroke, due to an excess of intracranial hemorrhages in these patients.

Treatment: Vorapaxar 2.5 mg daily, or matching placebo.

Results: The primary end point occurred in 9.3% of patients in the vorapaxar group versus 10.5% of patients in the placebo group (HR, 0.87; 95% CI, 0.80 to 0.94; $p < 0.001$). However, moderate or severe bleeding was also more common in the vorapaxar group (HR, 1.66; $p < 0.001$), as was intracranial hemorrhage (1% in the vorapaxar group vs. 0.5% in the placebo group; $p < 0.001$).

GENERAL REVIEW ARTICLES AND META-ANALYSES

284. Weisman SM, et al. Evaluation of the benefits and risks of low-dose aspirin in the secondary prevention of cardiovascular and cerebrovascular events. *Arch Intern Med* 2002;162:2197–2202.

This meta-analysis analyzed data from six trials (6,300 patients) that used low-dose ASA (<325 mg/day) in approved secondary prevention indications. ASA reduced the incidence of all-cause mortality by 18%, stroke by 20%, MI by 30%, and other "vascular events" by 30%. GI tract bleeding was 2.5 times more common in those taking ASA compared with placebo. Overall, the NNT for ASA to prevent one death from any cause was 67, whereas the NNT was 100 for detection of one nonfatal GI bleeding event. In summary, ASA use for the secondary prevention of thromboembolic events has a favorable risk–benefit profile and should be encouraged in those at high risk.

285. Antithrombotic Trialists' Collaboration. Collaborative meta-analysis of randomised trials of antiplatelet therapy for prevention of death, myocardial infarction, and stroke in high risk patients. *BMJ* 2002;324:71–86.

This analysis examined 287 randomized studies involving 135,000 patients in comparisons of antiplatelet therapy versus control and 77,000 in comparisons of different antiplatelet regimens. Among high-risk patients (e.g., acute MI, acute stroke, previous stroke or TIA, peripheral arterial disease, atrial fibrillation), antiplatelet therapy reduced the incidence of serious vascular events (nonfatal MI or stroke, vascular death) by approximately 25%, nonfatal MI by approximately 33%, nonfatal stroke by approximately 25%, and vascular mortality by approximately 17% (all p-values < 0.00001). No adverse effects were noted on other deaths. In each of the high-risk categories, the absolute benefits outweighed the absolute risks of major extracranial bleeding. Clopidogrel reduced serious vascular events by 10% compared with ASA. Among patients at high risk of immediate coronary occlusion, short-term addition of an intravenous GP IIb/IIIa antagonist to ASA prevented a further 20 vascular events per 1,000 ($p < 0.0001$) but caused 23 major (but rarely fatal) extracranial bleeds per 1,000.

286. Berger JS, et al. Aspirin for the primary prevention of cardiovascular events in women and men: a sex-specific meta-analysis of randomized controlled trials. *JAMA* 2006;295:306–313.

In this meta-analysis of 51,342 women and 44,114 men without CVD enrolled in six trials comparing aspirin therapy to placebo, investigators found that, in women, aspirin reduced the risk of cardiovascular events by 12% compared to placebo (95% CI, 1% to 21%; $p = 0.03$), driven by a 17% reduction in stroke (95% CI, 3% to 30%; $p = 0.02$) without any significant reduction in MI or cardiovascular death. By contrast, in men, aspirin reduced cardiovascular events by 14% (95% CI, 6% to 22%; $p = 0.01$) and MI by 32% (95% CI, 14% to 46%; $p = 0.001$) with no significant reduction in stroke or cardiovascular mortality. Bleeding risk was increased in both men and women.

287. Antithrombotic Trialists' (ATT) Collaboration. Aspirin in the primary and secondary prevention of vascular disease: collaborative meta-analysis of individual participant data from randomised trials. *Lancet* 2009;373:1849–1860.

Using individual patient-level data from the various trials included in the original meta-analysis (above), the ATT investigators reviewed the benefit in vascular events prevented versus the risks of bleeding events caused, when using aspirin for primary prevention. They found aspirin accountable for a 12% relative reduction in serious vascular events (MI, stroke, vascular death, $p = 0.0001$), largely due to a dramatic reduction in nonfatal MI (absolute reduction of 5%). The net effect on stroke incidence was not significant, given a nonsignificant increase in hemorrhagic strokes on aspirin. These effects appeared similar between men and women. However, aspirin increased all bleeding, GI and extracranial (0.10% vs. 0.07%, $p < 0.0001$). Thus, the authors conclude that for primary prevention, in patients without known vascular disease, the benefits of aspirin must be heavily weighed against a nonsignificant risk of adverse bleeding events.

288. Seshasai SR, et al. Effect of aspirin on vascular and nonvascular outcomes: Meta-analysis of randomized controlled trials. *Arch Intern Med* 2012;172:209–216.

This meta-analysis of nine randomized controlled trials comparing low-dose aspirin to placebo for primary prevention in over 100,000 participants demonstrated a significant reduction in the risk of total cardiovascular events (OR, 0.90; 95% CI, 0.85 to 0.96) driven largely by a reduction in the rate of nonfatal MI with low-dose aspirin; there was no significant reduction in the risk of cardiovascular or cancer death. By contrast, aspirin therapy was associated with a significantly increased risk of bleeding (OR 1.31; 95% CI, 1.14 to 1.50). The authors report a NNT to prevent one cardiovascular event of 120 and an NNT to cause one clinically significant bleeding event of 73. Based on these results, the authors caution against the routine use of aspirin for primary prevention and advocate for its use only on a case-by-case basis.

chapter 2

Coronary Revascularization and Percutaneous Procedures

Christopher P. Cannon, Benjamin A. Steinberg, and Justin M. Dunn

This chapter focuses on the evidence for coronary angiography, revascularization, and other common percutaneous vascular procedures. While there are many exciting developments for procedural-based therapies in cardiovascular disease, we focus on the most common, evidence-based interventions currently approved and widely adopted.

CORONARY ANGIOGRAPHY

Indications

1. Positive stress test result (e.g., exercise, echo, nuclear)
2. Unstable angina and non–ST elevation myocardial infarction (NSTEMI; see Chapter 3) or STEMI (see Chapter 4)
3. Incapacitating angina pectoris despite medical therapy
4. Complicated myocardial infarction [MI; e.g., recurrent ischemia, heart failure or hypotension, ventricular septal defect, mitral regurgitation, ventricular tachycardia (VT), failed thrombolysis]
5. Preoperative assessment (valve repair/replacement, other high-risk surgery)
6. Recurrent angina after percutaneous coronary intervention (PCI) or after coronary artery bypass graft (CABG) surgery
7. Miscellaneous: aortic dissection, unexplained ventricular failure, suspected congenital heart disease, postcardiac transplantation, pericardial tamponade or constriction, persistent precordial chest pain of unclear etiology

Flow Grade

The Thrombolysis in Myocardial Infarction (TIMI) flow grade system is the most commonly used classification system to assess flow:

- Grade 0, no anterograde flow beyond the point of occlusion.
- Grade 1, contrast goes beyond occlusion but fails to opacify the entire distal bed.

- Grade 2, entire vessel opacified, but the rate of entry to and clearance from the distal bed of the contrast is slower than normal.
- Grade 3, normal flow.

The TIMI corrected frame count is a more precise method and allows quantitative assessment of flow as a continuous variable (6). The TIMI myocardial perfusion grade system (grades 0 through 3) provides additional prognostic information to epicardial flow assessment (TIMI grade flow) in acute MI patients receiving thrombolytic therapy (see Chapter 4).

Stenosis Morphology

The American College of Cardiology (ACC)/American Heart Association (AHA) Classification (7) is enumerated as follows:

Type A: discrete, concentric, readily accessible, nonangulated segment, smooth contour, little or no calcification, nonostial, no major side branch involved, no thrombus present, <10 mm in length

Type B: tubular, eccentric, moderate tortuosity, moderately angulated segment (45 to 90 degrees), irregular contour, moderate to heavy calcification, total occlusion for ≤3 months, ostial location, bifurcation lesion, thrombus present, longer than 10 mm

Type B1: one B characteristic

Type B2: two B characteristics

Type C: diffuse, excessive tortuosity, extremely angulated segment (>90 degrees), total occlusion for more than 3 months, inability to protect major side branch, degenerated vein graft lesion

Procedural success rates are typically lower and restenosis rates higher for type B and especially type C lesions.

PERCUTANEOUS CORONARY INTERVENTION

Uses and Indications

1. Stable angina/coronary artery disease (CAD) with significant ischemia in medically optimized patients
2. Unstable angina/non–ST elevation MI (see Chapter 3)
3. Acute ST elevation MI (see Chapter 4)

Although stenting is almost always preferable to balloon angioplasty alone for these indications (see later section), stenting is especially effective (or required) for the following:

1. Dissection or abrupt vessel closure.
2. High-risk lesions (e.g., left main CAD).

3. Saphenous vein grafts (SVGs). Lower restenosis rates have been reported in two retrospective analyses [17% vs. 50% with percutaneous transluminal coronary angioplasty (PTCA)] (135,136), whereas the randomized Saphenous Vein De Novo (SAVED) trial found a nonsignificant reduction in restenosis (37% vs. 46%) (149).

4. Diabetic patients. One study found that stenting was associated with a 56% relative reduction in restenosis at 6 months compared with PTCA alone (27% vs. 62%; $p < 0.0001$); furthermore, the stent group had lower incidence of cardiac death and nonfatal MI at 4 years (14.8% vs. 26.0%; $p = 0.02$).

The superiority of stenting compared with balloon angioplasty alone is related mostly to a lower incidence of abrupt closure (<1% vs. 5%) and lower restenosis rates (15% to 20% for most lesions). Two disadvantages of stenting are difficulty in treating restenosis when it occurs and stent thrombosis [however, the incidence is now <1% with contemporary antiplatelet regimens (see page below)].

As compared with bare-metal stents (BMS), stents coated with antiproliferative agents or drug-eluting stents (DES) have markedly reduced the risk of restenosis in numerous trials (see "Restenosis" section later). However, the risk of stent thrombosis, especially after 1 year, is higher in DES versus BMS. Differences have now been seen with improved outcomes with the next-generation DES (see below).

Operator and Hospital Volume

Substantial data accumulated in the early and mid-1990s showed better outcomes in patients undergoing PCI performed by high-volume operators and high-volume hospitals (8–11). The best outcomes were achieved by high-volume operators at high-volume facilities (more than 400 cases per year). The recent widespread use of newer stent technology has reduced overall major adverse event rates but has not attenuated the significant difference between high- and low-volume operators and hospitals (12). Current recommendations of the ACC/AHA Joint Committee and Society for Cardiac Angiography and Intervention (SCAI) suggest a minimum of 75 cases per year per operator, at a center performing more than 400 procedures yearly (200 minimum) to maintain proficiency (1). In the treatment of acute MI with primary PCI, outcomes also are better in high-volume centers (recommended level is 36 or more cases per year); some of this benefit is likely related to the shorter door-to-balloon times obtained at such centers (see Chapter 4). Some observational data have demonstrated increased mortality in patients undergoing PCI at centers without on-site cardiac surgery backup (15), but the most recent ACC/AHA Guidelines state it may be reasonable to perform primary or elective PCI without on-site surgical backup as long as certain criteria are met such as an established transfer plan and the ability to provide hemodynamic support during transport.

Procedural Details

ACCESS

The right femoral artery is the most common arterial access site, though radial access is increasingly being used for both elective and primary PCI (see below). A 6-French (F) catheter is now most commonly used for diagnostic catheterization. In one study, the use of 6-F catheters showed less bleeding and similar procedural success compared with 7-F and 8-F catheters (17). For femoral access, some observational studies have suggested a benefit of vascular closure devices (instead of manual compression for hemostasis) in achieving earlier hemostasis, but these devices have not been shown to decrease vascular complications or bleeding and they remain a Class III indication (no benefit) in ACC/AHA Guidelines.

More contemporary data suggest that the use of radial access for angiography and PCI may reduce rates of bleeding complications, especially in primary PCI (18,19). Data on the use of radial artery vascular access approaches have demonstrated impressive safety and efficacy with this approach. The largest trial comparing radial to femoral access in PCI is the RadIal Vs. femorAL access for coronary intervention (RIVAL) trial, which randomized 7.021 ACS patients to radial versus femoral access during coronary angiography (20). There was no significant difference between the groups in the primary end point, a composite of death/MI/stroke/major bleeding at 30 days. However, radial access did result in a 63% decrease in vascular access complications. The Radial versus Femoral Randomized Investigation in ST Elevation Acute Coronary Syndrome (RIFLE STEACS) trial focused on STEMI patients and randomized 1,001 STEMI patients to radial versus femoral access for primary PCI. The primary end point was a composite of bleeding and MACCE at 30 days and occurred significantly less frequently in the radial arm (13.6% radial, 21% femoral, $p = 0.003$) (21). The patients in the radial arm also had significantly less Bleeding Academic Research Consortium (BARC) type ≥ 2 bleeding (12.2% vs. 7.8%; $p = 0.026$) and 30-day cardiac mortality (9.2% vs. 5.2%; $p = 0.020$). These findings were confirmed in the ST-segment elevation MI treated by radial or femoral approach in a multicenter randomized clinical trial (STEMI-RADIAL) (22).

CONTRAST AGENT

Some observational and nonrandomized studies have found low-osmolar ionic contrast agents to result in fewer recurrent ischemic events than did nonionic agents, whereas others found no significant reductions in major events with nonionic agents. Randomized trials also produced conflicting results (23–27); however, the data are consistent in regard to a significant reduction in hypersensitivity and allergic reactions with nonionic agents compared with ionic agents.

LESION EVALUATION

The severity of stenoses is typically first assessed by angiography. Subjective visual assessment and quantitative coronary angiography (QCA) are used to grade stenoses from 0% to 100%; the latter is used in clinical trials and usually performed by an independent core laboratory.

Intravascular ultrasound (IVUS) provides three-dimensional imaging, which can better estimate the severity of complex and eccentric lesions; it is more sensitive than are fluoroscopy and angiography in detecting coronary calcification. IVUS can assess atheroma within the vessel walls, which often goes undetected by angiography because vascular "remodeling" due to outward displacement of the vessel wall allows early atheroma accumulation without impairing lumen diameter. IVUS also is used after stent deployment and can reveal suboptimal results due to edge dissections [if deep or long (longer than 5 mm), additional stenting is indicated] and malexpansion or malapposition (treated with balloon angioplasty with larger and/or higher-pressure balloons).

In the REStenosis after IVUS-guided Stenting (RESIST) study, 155 patients who had successful stenting were randomized to no further balloon dilatation or additional balloon dilatation(s) until IVUS criterion was achieved for adequate stent expansion. At 6 months, the lumen cross-sectional area was 20% larger in the IVUS-guided group, but no significant differences were found between the groups in mean luminal diameter or restenosis (4.47 vs. 5.36 mm²; $p = 0.03$). In the Can Routine Ultrasound Influence Stent Expansion (CRUISE) study (29), 522 patients from the Stent Antithrombotic Regimen Study (STARS) were enrolled in an IVUS substudy to determine whether IVUS-assisted stenting results in better outcomes when compared with angiography-assisted stenting. At 9 months, the IVUS-guided group had a larger minimal luminal diameter (MLD), a lower residual diameter stenosis, and a significantly lower target vessel revascularization (TVR) rate (8.5% vs. 15.3%; $p < 0.05$), but no significant differences occurred in death or MI rates. In the OPTimization with ICUS to reduce stent restenosis (OPTICUS) study (34), a less selected group of 550 patients with a symptomatic coronary lesion or silent ischemia were assigned to either IVUS-guided or angiography-guided implantation of two or more stents. At 6-month angiography, no significant differences appeared between the two groups in MLD or restenosis rate, and at 1 year, similar incidences were found of major adverse cardiac events (MACEs) and repeated PCI. Current guidelines state it is reasonable to use IVUS in angiographically indeterminate left main disease, 4 to 6 weeks and 1 year after cardiac transplant to assess for cardiac allograft vasculopathy and to determine the mechanism of in-stent restenosis (ISR).

Measurement of fractional flow reserve (FFR) provides quantitative assessment of the hemodynamic significance of a lesion and is an effective method to evaluate stenoses of moderate severity. It can be performed immediately before a potential intervention and requires the use of a pressure wire and administration of adenosine. FFR is defined as the maximal blood flow to the myocardium in a stenotic segment divided by the theoretic normal maximal flow in the same distribution. The normal value is 1.0, whereas an FFR of 0.75 or less is associated with inducible myocardial ischemia. In one study (28), all patients with an FFR < 0.75 had reversible myocardial ischemia evident on at least one noninvasive test (bicycle exercise testing, thallium scintigraphy, dobutamine stress echocardiography). After revascularization was performed (PTCA or CABG surgery), all the positive test results reverted to normal. In contrast, 88% of patients with an FFR of 0.75 or more tested negative for reversible ischemia on all the noninvasive tests, and none underwent revascularization (more than 1 year follow-up). In a larger, randomized study of 325 patients (30), 144 patients with an FFR < 0.75 underwent routine PTCA (reference group), whereas those with an FFR 0.75 or more were randomized to optimal intervention (performance group) or medical therapy (deferral group). At 2 years, the event-free survival was significantly higher in the performance and deferral groups (83% and 89%) compared with the reference group (78%). Additional, larger, contemporary randomized data have confirmed these findings—that is, percutaneous revascularization guided by angiography *and* FFR yielded better clinical outcomes when compared with angiography alone guiding revascularization (32). Most recently, the Fractional Flow Reserve–Guided PCI versus Medical Therapy in Stable Coronary Disease (FAME 2) trial showed a significant benefit of using an FFR cutoff of ≤0.80 in patients with stable coronary disease (33). The benefit was driven by a decrease in urgent revascularization in the FFR group rather than by MI or mortality; however, it was significant enough that the trial was stopped early. Current ACC/AHA Guidelines give FFR a Class IIa (LOA: A) recommendation in patients with stable ischemic heart disease and an angiographic 50% to 70% lesion.

Another alternative for noninvasive lesion evaluation is coronary flow velocity reserve (CFVR). A DEBATE II substudy (35) of 379 patients found that a low CFVR (<2.5) at the end of PCI was an independent predictor of MACEs at 30 days [odds ratio (OR), 4.71; $p = 0.034$] and at 1 year (OR, 2.06; $p = 0.014$). In another study, a lower CFVR cutoff of <2.0 was a more accurate measure of major cardiac events than was single photon emission computed tomography (SPECT) imaging; also, a multivariate analysis found CFVR was the only significant predictor for cardiac events. Of note, discordant results between CFVR and FFR have been observed in 25% to 30% of intermediate lesions.

BALLOON ANGIOPLASTY

Success rates with balloon angioplasty of approximately 90% to 95% have been achieved in most institutions [vs. 64% success rate in the first major report (16)]. Failures occur when the lesion cannot be crossed, inadequate balloon dilatation is achieved, and abrupt closure occurs. Predictors of failure include chronic occlusion; stenoses that are long, angulated, eccentric, at an ostium or branch point, calcified, and/or associated with intraluminal thrombus; hospital with low volume; operator with low volume; SVGs (especially if older than 3 years); female gender; and advanced age.

One specific type of balloon deserves mention. The cutting balloon, which consists of several microblades attached to a balloon, permits effective dilatation at lower inflation pressures and thus, hypothetically, causes less vessel stretching and trauma. In the CUBA study, the cutting balloon was compared with conventional PTCA. Mean luminal diameter at 6 months was larger for the cutting balloon group, but there was no significant difference between groups in the incidence of death, MI, or any target lesion revascularization. In the randomized CAPAS trial (73), lesions in smaller vessels were examined [<3.0 mm (mean, 2.2 mm), compared with 2.5 to 4.0 mm in CUBA]. The cutting balloon group had a significantly lower 3-month restenosis rate than did the PTCA group (25% vs. 42%) and a better 1-year event-free survival rate (72.8% vs. 61.0%). A third, larger randomized trial (1,238 patients) found the cutting balloon associated with a slightly lower TVR rate (11.5% vs. 15.4%; $p = 0.04$) but no difference in the rates of binary restenosis or MACE (75). A more recent meta-analysis including several of the above-mentioned trials demonstrated a lack of clinical benefit to routinely sectioning atheromas during PCI (78). Current PCI guidelines give the cutting balloon a Class IIb indication for IST or ostial lesions in side branches to avoid slippage-induced trauma to the vessel, but a Class III recommendation (no benefit) is given for routine use during PCI.

STENTING

First-generation stents [Palmaz–Schatz (PS) and Gianturco–Roubin] became available in the early 1990s and resulted in lower restenosis rates compared with PTCA in major randomized trials. As a result, subsequent second-generation stents were compared with the earlier stents (vs. PTCA) in trials designed to show "equivalence." A number of these trials were performed [e.g., ASCENT (MULTI-LINK), BEST (BeStent), EXTRA (XT), GR-II (Gianturco–Roubin II), SCORES (Radius), SMART (Microstent II)] (42,43,47). The GR-II stent had inferior results compared with the PS stent (42), whereas the others were found to be equivalent but not superior to the PS. However, these trials excluded the most difficult lesion types (e.g., severe calcification and tortuosity), which compose the majority of stent targets. Because these difficult lesions were less amenable to PS stenting, the newer-generation stents were rapidly adopted. Randomized stent versus stent trials are similarly designed but have compared newer stents with second-generation stents [e.g., TENISS (Tenax coated vs. Nir), MULTI-LINK DUET (MULTI-LINK vs. MULTI-LINK DUET)]; numerous observational and registry studies also compared different stents.

The majority of currently available stents are balloon-expandable, slotted-tube stents, whereas there are fewer self-expanding stents; the latter are very flexible and can be delivered through tortuous vessels, but accurate sizing and placement are challenging. As the technology has advanced, lower profile and smaller stents have become available (2.5 mm, 2.25 mm, 2.0 mm). A post hoc analysis of 331 STRESS I–II patients found that stenting resulted in lower restenosis rates than did PTCA in vessels smaller than 3.0 mm (154). Data from several randomized trials, however, yielded conflicting results with small-vessel lesions, with three showing similar outcomes between stenting and PTCA (ISAR-SMART, SISA, and COAST studies) (155,157), whereas two found lower restenosis rates with stenting [BESMART (156)]. The more robust, significant benefits of stents compared with PTCA have been clearly demonstrated in larger vessels, total occlusions, and SVG lesions (see below).

Medications

ASPIRIN

Use of aspirin significantly reduces ischemic complications in PTCA (190); however, use in conjunction with a thienopyridine provides even better outcomes in stenting (see below). These recommendations are predominantly based on the dosing of aspirin used in clinical trials of stenting. Data from the CURRENT-OASIS 7 trial found no difference in CV death, MI, or stroke at 30 days between 75 and 325 mg of ASA in ACS patients managed invasively, including those who underwent PCI. Current guidelines recommend a 325-mg loading dose of aspirin prior to PCI followed by 81 mg daily indefinitely.

HEPARIN

Heparin, initial bolus 50 to 70 U/kg, is used in conjunction with a GP IIb/IIIa inhibitor; higher dosing typically is used when administered alone. The target activated clotting time (ACT) when used alone is 250 to 350 seconds; a low periprocedural ACT is associated with increased complications while higher ACTs (400 to 600 seconds) are associated with increased bleeding. One study found that even less heparin (2,500 U; mean ACT, 207) appears safe in elective cases (113). Unless PCI is complicated (e.g., residual thrombus), a prolonged heparin infusion is not necessary because it is does not decrease ischemic complications and results in more frequent bleeding (111).

LOW MOLECULAR WEIGHT HEPARIN

Several studies have compared unfractionated heparin (UFH) with LWMH during coronary interventions. Observations from the National Investigators Collaborating on Enoxaparin (NICE-1 and NICE-4) trials in which enoxaparin was used with and without GP IIb/IIIa inhibitors also show that the use of enoxaparin appeared safe and effective in the interventional setting. The Superior Yield of the New Strategy of Enoxaparin, Revascularization and Glycoprotein IIb/IIIa Inhibitors (SYNERGY) trial of over 10,000 patients with high-risk unstable angina or NSTEMI demonstrated noninferiority of enoxaparin in this setting, though the trial was open label (115). A substudy of the ExTRACT-TIMI 25 trial (see Chapter 4) demonstrated superiority of enoxaparin in patients with STEMI undergoing subsequent PCI following fibrinolysis therapy (116). The Safety and Efficacy of Intravenous Enoxaparin in Elective Percutaneous Coronary Intervention (STEEPLE) trial randomized 3,528 patients to enoxaparin 0.5 mg/kg, 0.75 mg/kg, or UFH. At 48 hours, there was significantly less bleeding in the enoxaparin groups than in the UFH groups (117). However, when necessary to monitor low molecular weight heparin (LMWH), this can be less convenient. Anti-Xa levels have been obtained in some studies but take longer to measure than does an ACT. Thus, despite significant clinical evidence of noninferiority and in certain situations superiority of enoxaparin over UFH, many operators continue to use UFH due to familiarity and ease of monitoring intraprocedure.

DIRECT THROMBIN INHIBITORS

Direct thrombin inhibitors (e.g., argatroban or bivalirudin) represent an alternative to heparins for anticoagulation during cardiac catheterization. The 6,010-patient REPLACE 2 trial compared heparin plus eptifibatide or abciximab versus bivalirudin alone (provisional GP IIb/IIIa inhibitor if needed) (143). Provisional IIb/IIIa inhibitor treatment was given to only 7.2% of the bivalirudin group. The bivalirudin group had a nonsignificant reduction in death, MI, urgent revascularization at 30 days, and major in-hospital bleeding (primary end point) compared with heparin plus GP IIb/IIIa inhibitor (9.2% vs. 10.0%). Bivalirudin was associated with a significantly lower incidence of bleeding (2.4% vs. 4.1%), whereas there was a nonsignificant excess of MI with bivalirudin (7.0% vs. 6.2%). Contemporary data of bivalirudin, as compared with UFH, in stable or low-risk unstable coronary disease patients undergoing PCI with clopidogrel pretreatment were provided by the ISAR-REACT 3 trial (144). While there was no net clinical benefit (the combination of ischemic and bleeding events) of bivalirudin over UFH, patients receiving bivalirudin had lower bleeding events. Currently, only bivalirudin and UFH carry a Class I ACC/AHA recommendation for anticoagulation during PCI. In the wake of the HEAT-PPCI trial (see Chapter 4), the advantage of bivalirudin over UFH in reducing bleeding during primary PCI is being questioned.

THIENOPYRIDINES/ADP RECEPTOR ANTAGONISTS

The first agent available was *ticlopidine* (250 mg twice daily for 2 to 4 weeks), which, when given in conjunction with aspirin and heparin, is more effective at preventing recurrent events than is an anticoagulant regimen (e.g., intravenous heparin followed by warfarin). In three randomized studies [Intracoronary Stenting and Antithrombotic Regimen (ISAR), Full Anticoagulation versus Aspirin and Ticlopidine (FANTASTIC), and Stent Anticoagulation Restenosis Study (STARS)] (118,119), 50% to 80% fewer cardiac end points were reached (**Fig. 2.1**).

Clopidogrel was developed as an alternative to ticlopidine. Clopidogrel 75 mg daily provides similar levels of platelet inhibition as ticlopidine, 250 mg twice daily. Results of the Clopidogrel Aspirin Stent International Cooperative Study (CLASSICS) showed clopidogrel (75 mg once daily for 4 weeks ± 300 mg loading dose) to be as effective as ticlopidine in preventing stent thrombosis and clinical events, but it is much better tolerated (121) (see **Fig. 2.1**). More important, as shown in the large Clopidogrel versus Aspirin in Patients at Risk of Ischaemic Events (CAPRIE) trial (see Chapter 1), the risk of neutropenia (a well-known limitation of ticlopidine) with clopidogrel is very low (0.1%) and similar to aspirin.

In the PCI-CURE study (122), pretreatment with clopidogrel before PCI was associated with a significantly lower incidence of cardiovascular death, MI, or urgent revascularization at 30 days compared with placebo [4.5% vs. 6.4%; relative risk (RR), 0.70; $p = 0.03$]. Long-term administration of clopidogrel also

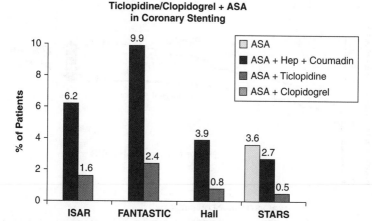

Figure 2.1 • These data from major coronary stent studies show the superiority of a regimen consisting of aspirin and/or ticlopidine or clopidogrel at reducing cardiovascular events. (Data from Refs. 119, 21, and 123.)

led to a 31% RR reduction in cardiovascular death or MI (8.8% vs. 12.6%; $p = 0.002$; see **Fig. 2.2**).

The Clopidogrel in Unstable Angina to Prevent Recurrent Events (CREDO) trial (126) found that a preprocedural loading dose followed by

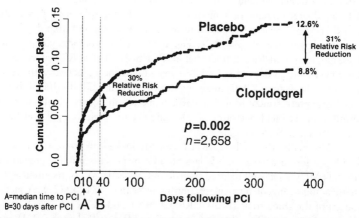

Figure 2.2 • The 2,658-patient Percutaneous Coronary Intervention-Clopidogrel in Unstable angina to prevent Recurrent ischemic Events (PCI-CURE) (122) study evaluated pretreatment and extended clopidogrel therapy and found it to be associated with a 31% relative reduction in cardiovascular death or nonfatal MI. (Data from PCI-CURE (Clopidogrel in Unstable angina to prevent Recurrent ischemic Events); Mehta SR, et al. Effects of pretreatment with clopidogrel and aspirin followed by long-term therapy in patients undergoing percutaneous coronary intervention: the PCI-CURE study. *Lancet* 2001;358:527–533.)

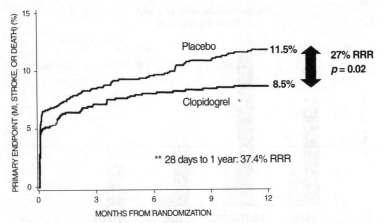

Figure 2.3 • The 2,116-patient CREDO (126) trial demonstrated a substantial 27% reduction in major events (death, MI, stroke) at 1 year. Continued clopidogrel therapy from 28 d to 1 y was associated with a further 37% relative reduction in events compared with placebo. (Data from **Steinhubl SR, et al.; for the Clopidogrel in Unstable angina to Prevent Recurrent Events CREDO Investigators.** Early and sustained dual oral antiplatelet therapy following percutaneous coronary intervention. *JAMA* 2002;288:2411–2420.)

long-term treatment (1 year) with clopidogrel after elective PCI was associated with a 26.9% relative reduction in death, MI, or stroke compared with post-PCI clopidogrel therapy for 1 month [8.5% vs. 11.5% (placebo); $p = 0.02$]. A further 37.4% relative reduction in major events occurred from day 29 to 1 year with clopidogrel ($p = 0.04$; **Fig. 2.3**). As for pretreatment, patients given clopidogrel at least 6 hours before PCI had a 38.6% RR reduction in major events at 28 days ($p = 0.05$) compared with no reduction with treatment <6 hours before PCI. Even among those receiving a GP IIb/IIIa inhibitor, clopidogrel pretreatment provided a 30% reduction in events. Finally, a trend toward a higher incidence of major bleeding occurred with clopidogrel (at 1 year, 8.8% vs. 6.7%; $p = 0.07$).

Additionally, the PCI-CLARITY analysis looked at pretreatment with clopidogrel for an average of 3.5 days pre-PCI in patients initially presenting with STEMI. Clopidogrel reduced the risk of CV death, MI, or recurrent ischemia leading to urgent revascularization by 46% ($p < 0.001$) (127). A meta-analysis of the three trials (PCI-CURE, CREDO, and PCI-CLARITY) found a highly significant 29% reduction in death or MI post-PCI ($p = 0.004$) and a significant 31% reduction in MI pre-PCI ($p = 0.005$) (127), supporting the routine and *early* use of clopidogrel in patients subsequently undergoing PCI. In summary, the results of these three trials support preprocedural loading and long-term therapy with clopidogrel in those scheduled for or expected to undergo PCI. The significant benefits do not appear attenuated by use of GP IIb/IIIa inhibitors.

On the other hand, if high-dose clopidogrel is used, one study found it may eliminate the need for GP IIb/IIIa inhibition during PCI. A total of 2,159 low-risk patients (excluded if MI within 14 days, ACS, or elevated troponin) undergoing elective PCI were all given 600 mg ≥2 hours before PCI and then randomized to abciximab or placebo (129). At 30 days, there was no difference in death, MI, or urgent TVR between the two groups (4% each in each group; $p = 0.82$). Observational data suggest that some patients may have reduced response to clopidogrel based on their cytochrome P450 genotypes; in these patients, more potent antiplatelet agents such as prasugrel or ticagrelor (see Chapters 3 and 4) may provide a substantial benefit; however, this remains to be validated in large, prospective, randomized trials (128). It should be noted that ticagrelor and prasugrel have not been rigorously studied in elective PCI, only in ACS patients (see Chapters 3 and 4).

GLYCOPROTEIN IIB/IIIA INHIBITORS

GP IIb/IIIa inhibitors have been used in patients with acute coronary syndromes and those undergoing PCI (**Fig. 2.4**). However, they were often not studied in patients at high risk of bleeding, and most of the studies of these agents were performed before the routine use of dual antiplatelet therapy. If used, lower heparin dosage is indicated, with a target ACT of approximately 250 seconds, as the use of a higher ACT target in early trials resulted in increased bleeding. The following agents are currently the most widely used:

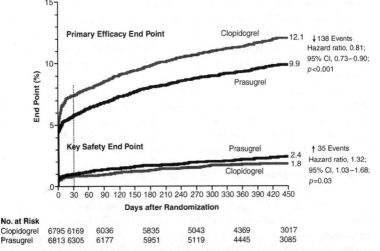

Figure 2.4 • Benefit of the more potent P2Y12 inhibitor prasugrel over clopidogrel in preventing CV death, MI, or stroke in patients undergoing high-risk PCI. Higher rates of bleeding were also seen with prasugrel. (From **Wiviott SD, et al.** Prasugrel versus clopidogrel in patients with acute coronary syndromes. *NEJM* 2007;357:2001–2015.)

Abciximab (ReoPro)

The monoclonal antibody fragment abciximab binds tightly to the GP IIb/IIIa receptor and has shown impressive results in certain patients undergoing PCI. In the Evaluation of 7E3 for the Prevention of Ischemic Complications (EPIC) trial (131), composed of 2,099 high-risk patients [acute MI, postinfarct angina with electrocardiographic (ECG) changes, high-risk clinical or angiographic features], the group receiving abciximab, 0.25 mg/kg intravenous bolus, and then 10 mg/min infusion for 12 hours, had 35% fewer end points compared with the placebo group. At 3-year follow-up, this benefit was still present. In the c7E3 Fab Antiplatelet Therapy in Unstable Refractory Angina (CAPTURE) trial (133), composed of 1,265 unstable angina patients, the abciximab group had a significant 29% reduction in primary composite end point at 30 days but not at 6 months. This loss of benefit is attributed to abciximab infusion being stopped 1 hour after PCI. In the Evaluation in PTCA to Improve Long-term Outcome with Abciximab Glycoprotein IIb/IIIa Blockade (EPILOG) trial (134), composed of 2,792 nonacute coronary syndrome patients, abciximab showed a >50% reduction in primary composite end point at 30 days, and the reduction remained significant at 6 months and 1 year.

In the Evaluation of Platelet IIb/IIIa Inhibitor for Stenting (EPISTENT) trial (136), composed of 2,399 CAD patients randomized to stent plus placebo, stent plus abciximab, or balloon angioplasty plus abciximab, the 2 abciximab groups had a significantly lower incidence of death, MI, and urgent revascularization at 30 days (5.3% and 6.9% vs. 10.8%). One-year mortality was also lower. A meta-analysis of all abciximab trials showed a nearly 30% lower mortality during 6-month to 3-year follow-up ($p = 0.003$; see *J Am Coll Cardiol* 2002;37:2059). Lastly, use of intracoronary administration of abciximab in unstable angina or acute MI patients resulted in 50% fewer major cardiac events at 30 days compared with IV administration (see *Circulation* 2003;107:1840); similar findings have been seen with another GP IIb/IIIa inhibitor (140).

Although an antibody response develops in 6% to 7% of patients receiving abciximab after first administration, the ReoPro Readministration Registry (R3) reported no significant differences in the incidence of adverse allergic or clinical events or thrombocytopenia in 500 patients receiving repeated abciximab compared with 23,000 patients treated for the first time.

Eptifibatide (Integrilin)

In the Novel Dosing Regimen of Eptifibatide in Planned Coronary Stent Implantation (ESPRIT) study (99), which randomized 2,064 patients undergoing stenting to *double-bolus* eptifibatide (two 180 μg/kg boluses 10 minutes apart and then 2 μg/kg/min for 18 to 24 hours) or placebo, eptifibatide had a significantly lower incidence of death, MI, urgent TVR, and thrombotic bailout GP IIb/IIIa inhibitor therapy within 48 hours (6.4% vs. 10.5%; $p = 0.0015$). This benefit was consistent across different components of the primary end point, including death/MI/TVR [RR, 0.65; 95% confidence interval (CI), 0.47

to 0.87], death/MI (RR, 0.60; CI, 0.44 to 0.82), and death (RR, 0.5; CI, 0.05 to 5.42). Kaplan–Meier survival curves appeared to separate over time, with most of the difference in mortality occurring between 30 days and 6 months (137). In the Platelet Glycoprotein IIb/IIIa in Unstable Angina Receptor Suppression Using Integrilin Therapy (PURSUIT) trial (see Chapter 3), a significant reduction in death or MI at 30 days of 31% was observed in patients undergoing PCI.

Tirofiban (Aggrastat)

The peptidomimetic tirofiban is currently approved by the U.S. FDA for use in acute coronary syndromes with or without PCI, but not in elective PCI. In the Randomized Efficacy Study of Tirofiban for Outcomes and Restenosis (RESTORE) (135), composed of 2,139 patients randomized to tirofiban, 10 μg/kg bolus and then 0.15 μg/kg/min for 36 hours, or placebo, the tirofiban group had significantly fewer events at 2 and 7 days but not at 30 days. In the Platelet Receptor Inhibition in Ischemic Syndrome Management in Patients Limited by Unstable Signs and Symptoms (PRISM-PLUS) trial (see Chapter 3), PCI patients showed a reduction in death or MI of approximately 35%. The TARGET trial (138) compared the safety and efficacy of tirofiban with abciximab, randomizing 5,308 patients scheduled for coronary stenting to tirofiban (10 μg/kg bolus, then 0.15 μg/kg/min for 18 to 24 hours) or abciximab. The tirofiban group had a significantly higher incidence of the primary composite end point of death, nonfatal MI, or urgent TVR at 30 days compared with the abciximab group (7.6% vs. 6.0%; $p = 0.038$). This significant difference did not persist at 6-month follow-up. Several investigators suggested that these results were due to underdosing of tirofiban, and subsequent data documented only 70% platelet inhibition over the first hour, which could explain the poorer outcomes (*Am J Cardiol* 2002;89:647; *Circulation* 2002;106:1470). Accordingly, some newer trials used a higher loading dose of 25 μg/kg bolus and found benefit (4,141).

A broad meta-analysis of 19 trials involving all available GP IIb/IIIa inhibitors (including those above) pooled 20,137 patients with death as the primary outcome. In these patients undergoing PCI (either urgently for acute MI or electively), use of a GP IIb/IIIA inhibitor significantly reduced overall mortality at 30 days (RR, 0.69; 95% CI, 0.53 to 0.90), as well as at 6 months (RR 0.79; 95% CI, 0.64 to 0.97). Additional composite clinical outcome was also reduced, and there was little heterogeneity across the spectra of trials (139). See Chapters 3 and 4 for more detailed discussion of the use of GP IIb/IIIa inhibitors in UA/NSTEMI and STEMI, respectively.

Applications of PCI

STABLE ANGINA

The Angioplasty Compared to Medicine (ACME) study (36) compared PTCA with medical therapy in patients with stable, single-vessel CAD. The PTCA group had increased exercise time and less use of antianginal medications but had a higher frequency of MI (4%) and emergency coronary artery bypass surgery (2%). The Veterans Administration Angioplasty Compared to Medicine (VA ACME) study (37) also showed that PTCA in patients with single-vessel CAD resulted in improved exercise time, less angina, and better quality-of-life score. The Randomized Intervention Treatment of Angina (RITA-2) trial (38) showed that angioplasty was associated with less angina and longer treadmill time but with an increased incidence of death or MI due to procedure-related MI events.

The Clinical Outcomes Utilizing Revascularization and Aggressive Drug Evaluation (COURAGE) trial enrolled more than 2,000 patients with objective CAD by noninvasive testing and compared aggressive medical therapy alone with aggressive medical therapy with added PCI in all but the highest-risk patients with CAD (39). At the follow-up median time of 4.6 years, patients in the PCI group had no better rates of death, MI, or other cardiovascular events than did those who were maximally medically managed (19% for PCI vs. 18.5% for medical management). The results of this trial underscored the pathophysiology of CAD—only medical management has the potential to reduce the burden of atherosclerotic disease, whereas PCI is the therapy of choice for *acute* or *severe* coronary obstructions.

UNSTABLE ANGINA/NON–ST ELEVATION MYOCARDIAL INFARCTION

Recent major trials have shown that an early invasive strategy is superior to a conservative approach, especially in high-risk patients (e.g., ST segment depression, positive cardiac troponin I; see Chapter 3).

ACUTE ST ELEVATION MYOCARDIAL INFARCTION

In experienced centers with short door-to-balloon times, primary PCI has been associated with lower mortality than has thrombolytic therapy (see Chapter 4). However, the availability and institutional volume and experience are limiting factors.

AFTER THROMBOLYTIC THERAPY

Studies performed in the 1980s found that routine immediate PTCA PCI was harmful (TAMI I, TIMI IIA, and ECSG trials; see Chapter 4), whereas delayed PTCA (at 18 to 48 hours) was associated with similar outcomes (SWIFT and TIMI IIB; see Chapter 4). PTCA PCI is indicated in patients with high-risk features, such as cardiogenic shock, persistent pain or ischemia, and VT or ventricular fibrillation (VF). The data suggest that it can now be performed routinely and safely early after thrombolysis (PACT, TIMI 14, ExTRACT-TIMI 25; see also *Am J Cardiol* 2001;88:831–836; see Chapter 4). For high-risk patients, with extensive anterior MI, early transfer (<6 hours) postfibrinolysis is now recommended on the basis of the TRANSFER-AMI and CARESS-AMI studies (see Chapter 4).

STENTING VERSUS PERCUTANEOUS TRANSLUMINAL CORONARY ANGIOPLASTY: MAJOR TRIALS

Consistently, major trials have shown a substantial reduction in restenosis rates with stenting compared with balloon angioplasty alone. Important results include the following:

1. In the Stent Restenosis Study (STRESS) (40), composed of 410 patients, stenting was associated with higher procedural success, less restenosis at 6 months (31% vs. 46%; $p = 0.046$), and a trend toward less revascularization ($p = 0.06$), but there was no significant reduction in clinical events.
2. In the EPISTENT study (133,134), composed of 2,399 patients, the rates of TVR at 6 months for stent and stent plus abciximab were significantly lower than those for PTCA and abciximab (10.6% and 8.7% vs. 15.4%; $p = 0.005$, $p < 0.001$).

Primary stenting versus PTCA with stenting *has become the standard of care for coronary lesions, and balloon angioplasty* is typically only performed when stenting is not feasible.

DIRECT STENTING VERSUS BALLOON PREDILATATION

Direct stenting potentially offers numerous advantages, including shorter procedure time, less radiation exposure and contrast use, and overall reduced costs. Possible disadvantages include increased risk of guide trauma and deployment failure. However, with the exclusion criteria used in several trials, such as excessive calcification, severe proximal tortuosity, and occlusion, crossover rates from direct stenting to predilatation have been low (3% to 6%). Most studies comparing direct stenting with predilatation followed by stenting have found no significant difference in major clinical outcomes (48,50); one study did find a lower TLR in a direct stenting group (18% vs. 28%; $p = 0.03$) (49). In summary, with careful lesion selection, direct stenting is typically successful, has at least similar clinical outcomes, and provides cost and procedural advantages compared with predilatation.

REPEATED INTERVENTION

PCI has a high initial success rate (95% to 100%) because restenosis is typically characterized by fibroproliferative tissue as opposed to atherosclerotic plaque. However, recurrent restenosis rates are high, exceeding 50% for diffuse ISR lesions. For treatment of restenosis after prior PTCA, stenting results in better outcomes compared with repeated PTCA; in the randomized REST study (182), the stent group had much lower restenosis and TVR rates compared with PTCA (18% vs. 32% and 10% vs. 27%, respectively).

For treatment of ISR, debulking techniques such as rotational atherectomy (RA) and directional atherectomy appear to be more effective than PTCA alone, but restenosis still occurs in about 30% of cases. Repeated stenting to treat ISR was examined in the RIBS (Restenosis Intrastent: Balloon vs. Stent) study (183). Results from this 450-patient study revealed that repeated stenting provided a larger MLD immediately after the procedure (2.77 mm vs. 2.25 mm; $p < 0.001$) and persisted to a lesser degree at 6-month follow-up (1.69 mm vs. 1.54 mm; $p = 0.046$). In a prespecified subgroup analysis, it was shown that patients whose target vessel was more than 3 mm in diameter had a lower restenosis rate and a better event-free survival with repeated stenting (27% vs. 49%, $p = 0.007$; 84% vs. 62%, $p = 0.002$).

Contemporary data from the ISAR-DESIRE trial of 300 patients with ISR demonstrated that DES were likely superior to balloon angioplasty in terms of recurrent restenosis at 6 months (185). The primary end point of angiographic restenosis based on "in-segment" analysis occurred in 44.6% in the balloon angioplasty group versus 14.3% in the sirolimus stent group, and 21.7% in the paclitaxel-stenting group ($p < 0.001$ for each stent compared with balloon angioplasty).

Complications

EARLY COMPLICATIONS

1. Death (<0.65%) in elective PCI, according to analysis of the NCDR from 2004 to 2007.
2. MI (<5%, varies depending on definition used). Causes include distal embolization, side-branch occlusion, and obstructive lesion complications such as thrombus, abrupt closure, or severe dissection. Retrospective analyses suggest that even small non–Q-wave MIs [often occurring in the absence of symptoms or ECG changes and detected by routine creatine kinase (CK) and CK-MB measurement] result in increased incidence of ischemic complications and subsequent recurrent MI, revascularization, and death (162).

   Post-PCI elevations of the more sensitive troponin assays occur even more frequently. In the TOPSTAR study (165), more than half of patients had an elevated troponin T level at 24 hours after PCI. Larger studies are needed to further investigate these findings, especially whether small troponin elevations with normal CK-MB levels are correlated with worse prognosis.

3. Severe dissection and abrupt closure (<1%). Closure results from extensive dissection, thrombosis, or vasospasm and is more likely to occur if ACT is low (164). Aspirin has been proven to decrease its incidence, whereas GP IIb/IIIa inhibitor use has resulted in a lower incidence of urgent revascularization. Treatment options include (a) conservative medical therapy (reasonable if collateralization is adequate or the amount of jeopardized myocardium is small), (b) stent placement [restores flow in more than 90% of patients, but infarcts occur in up to 20% and reocclusion (over days to weeks) occurs in about 10%], (c) repeated PTCA (50% success rate; perfusion catheter often is used, which allows balloon inflation for 10 to 30 minutes), or (d) emergency CABG (25% to 50% still have a Q-wave MI).

4. Perforation (<0.5%). Small perforations can be sealed with prolonged balloon inflations and/or covered stent(s). Large perforations typically result in pericardial tamponade. Delayed cardiac tamponade occurred in 45% of cases (mean time from PCI, 4.4 hours); thus, tamponade should be considered a cause of late hypotension after PCI.

5. Emergency CABG surgery is required in <0.5% according to recent data from the NCDR. As PCI technology improves, the need for emergency CABG is declining.

6. Other acute complications: (a) Allergic reactions, usually due to contrast agent. If severe, treat with epinephrine. If known, premedication is indicated with prednisone, diphenhydramine, and H_2 blocker. (b) Hypotension. Multiple causes include hypovolemia (inadequate hydration, blood loss), reduced cardiac output (ischemia, tamponade, arrhythmia), or severe arteriolar vasodilation (vasovagal reaction [especially with femoral sheath placement], excessive nitrates). (c) Arrhythmias: bradycardia (3%) is most often due to vasovagal reaction and conduction disturbances (bundle branch block or complete AV block); VT and VF (<0.5%) occur most commonly from intracoronary contrast injection (especially right coronary artery).

LATER COMPLICATIONS

Stent Thrombosis

Subacute stent thrombosis occurs in <1% of procedures [used to be more than 5% before high-pressure balloon inflation and antiplatelet regimens were introduced] and results in MI or death 20% to 45%. Subacute and *late* stent thrombosis is particularly a problem in the era of DES, as the same agents that inhibit neointimal hyperplasia also slow endothelialization over the stent (see later). For patients who receive DES, the number one predictor of stent thrombosis often is discontinuation of thienopyridine (clopidogrel) therapy (169,170). Additional data have shown that patients with STEMI secondary to stent thrombosis have worse outcomes than do those with STEMI from de novo coronary lesions (171).

Restenosis

Restenosis is typically a subacute to chronic phenomenon that occurs anywhere from 2 months to years following PCI and results from neointimal hyperplasia and vascular remodeling (less commonly progression of atherosclerosis). The incidence within the first year is approximately 30% to 40% for angioplasty alone (up to 50% to 60% for chronic occlusions), 15% to 20% bare metal for stenting, and as low as 5% for DES (based on the need for repeat revascularization). Risk factors can be categorized as clinical (diabetes, unstable angina, smoking, male gender, hypertension, end-stage renal disease, high cholesterol), anatomic [angiographically visible thrombus (181), aorto-ostial or proximal location, SVG, left anterior descending (LAD) artery, chronic occlusion, target vessel diameter, target lesion length], or procedural (residual stenosis more than 30%). Some studies have focused on the effect of stent strut thickness on restenosis rates. The ISAR-STEREO and ISAR-STEREO 2 trials (187,188) were randomized studies that found that thin-strut stents had lower rates of restenosis and TVR compared with thick-strut stents. Critics have asserted that potential confounders occur in these studies, such as stent-deployment pressure and other differences in design and mechanical properties of the tested stents. DES have been shown to reduce restenosis rates markedly (see later section).

Renal Dysfunction

The risk of contrast-induced acute kidney injury is increased with excessive contrast dye load (more than 3 mL/kg); other risk factors include diabetes, advanced age (over 75), periprocedural dehydration, heart failure, comorbid cirrhosis, nephrosis, hypertension, proteinuria, use of NSAIDs, and intra-arterial injection. If baseline creatinine is elevated, adequate prehydration and posthydration are clearly beneficial (172). The use of N-acetylcysteine (Mucomyst) does not appear to provide protection in those with baseline renal dysfunction and now has a Class III (no benefit) ACC/AHA recommendation after the publication of the acetylcysteine for prevention of renal outcomes in patients undergoing coronary and peripheral vascular angiography, main results from the randomized Acetylcysteine for Contrast-Induced Nephropathy Trial (ACT).

Fenoldopam, a selective agonist of the dopamine-1 receptor, showed no benefit in the randomized, 315-patient CONTRAST study (176). Early data suggested that hydration with sodium bicarbonate may be superior to normal saline (177); however, more recent clinical data have contradicted that finding (178). Finally, cholesterol embolization can cause a late increase in creatinine levels (weeks to months vs. 1 to 2 days with contrast nephropathy), and treatment is supportive, with frank renal failure developing in up to 50%.

OTHER POSTPROCEDURAL COMPLICATIONS

Thrombocytopenia can be caused by either heparin (heparin-induced thrombocytopenia [HIT]) or GP IIb/IIIa inhibitors (incidence approximately 1%); if there is a known history of HIT, direct thrombin inhibitors (e.g., bivalirudin) should be used preferentially.

Infection: there is a higher risk with brachial versus femoral approach; some centers administer prophylactic antibiotics when a delayed intervention after sheath exchange is performed.

Vascular complications include femoral or retroperitoneal hematoma, arteriovenous fistula, and pseudoaneurysm (18,180). They may vary from benign or requiring manual compression to severe bleeding or vascular compromise requiring urgent or emergent surgical intervention. Alternative access, such as the radial artery, appears to reduce this risk (see "Access" above).

Treatment and Prevention of Restenosis

DRUG STUDIES

Numerous therapies have shown no benefit in randomized trials, including aspirin (190), LWMH (191,196,207), subcutaneous (s.c.) UFH (194), abciximab (205), hirudin (193), 3-hydroxy 3-methyl-glutaryl coenzyme A (HMG-CoA) reductase inhibitors (statins, 192,197), angiotensin-converting enzyme (ACE) inhibitors, β-blockers (208), calcium channel blockers (199,206), n-3 fatty acids (204), nitric oxide donors, antibiotics (209), and antiallergic drugs [e.g., tranilast (210)].

Cilostazol, a platelet aggregation inhibitor (currently approved in the United States for treatment of claudication), has shown promise in several small studies (200). In patients with diabetes undergoing PCI, cilostazol (when added to aspirin and clopidogrel) did reduce target lesion revascularization at 9 months, when compared with only aspirin and clopidogrel (202). The DECLARE-LONG II trial evaluated the addition of cilostazol versus placebo to dual antiplatelet therapy in patients with lesions ≥25 mm in length stented with a zotarolimus-eluting stent (ZES) and found a significantly lower incidence of in-stent late loss in the cilostazol group (203). Current guidelines however do not recommend the addition of cilostazol to dual antiplatelet therapy in patients undergoing PCI.

RADIATION THERAPY

Intravascular radiation therapy (IVRT) yielded promising results in initial studies of ISR, with restenosis rates typically <20%. Gamma radiation sources were used in the Scripps Coronary Radiation to Inhibit Proliferation Poststenting (SCRIPPS) trials, Washington Radiation for In-Stent Restenosis Trial (WRIST), and GAMMA trials (86–88), whereas beta sources were used in the Beta Energy Restenosis Trial (BERT) and BETA-WRIST, INHIBIT, START, and BRITE II trials (95,96,98,99). The LONG WRIST study examined lesions 36 to 80 mm in length and found gamma radiation reduced major cardiac events by one-third at 1 year; additional benefit was seen with use of 18 Gy versus 15 Gy (22% vs. 42%; $p < 0.05$) (93). Data from SVG WRIST demonstrated that the ability of gamma radiation to reduce restenosis also extends to SVGs (92).

One issue noted early in the radiation experience was late (more than 1 month) stent thrombosis, which occurred in 6.6% of radiation-treated patients in one study (159). These late events likely occur because radiation delays the healing process. Subsequent studies, such as WRIST and WRIST 12 (89,91), used longer courses of thienopyridine therapy with lower stent thrombosis rates. Current recommendations are to avoid new stenting at the time of brachytherapy (if possible) and to continue dual antiplatelet therapy for at least 6 to 12 months following radiation.

DRUG-ELUTING STENTS

The most effective development for the prevention of ISR has been the implantation of DES. These stents slowly release drugs that inhibit smooth muscle cell proliferation, neointimal hyperplasia, and inflammation. Sirolimus (rapamycin) is a naturally occurring macrolide antibiotic that has immunosuppressive properties. It inhibits smooth muscle cell proliferation and migration by blocking certain aspects of cellular metabolism and thereby preventing mitosis.

The Sirolimus-Eluting Stent in Coronary Lesions (SIRIUS) trial (53) examined the use of this stent in longer lesions (15 to 30 mm) and in a more typical patient population (28% with diabetes, 72% with hyperlipidemia, 70% with hypertension, 37% with previous PCI or CABG surgery). In 8-month angiographic data on the first 400 patients, the sirolimus stent group had only a 2% incidence of ISR versus 31.1% of controls; total in-segment restenosis rates were 9.2% and 32.3%, respectively. Long-term data were compiled in a 2009 meta-analysis of the four major SES trials (54). In this comparison of the SES to BMS in 1,748 patients who underwent nonemergent PCI, rates of TVR continued to favor SES (15.2% vs. 30.1%; $p < 0.0001$), with no overall increase in death, MI, or stent thrombosis over 5 years.

Paclitaxel-eluting stents were the next DES to hit the market. Paclitaxel is a taxane derivative that blocks mitosis by interfering with microtubule function; it is cytotoxic at higher doses. The TAXUS IV trial enrolled 1,314 patients with de novo lesions and compared the paclitaxel stent with an uncoated stent with the primary end point of angiographic follow-up at 9 months (57). Composite clinical end points of cardiac death, MI, or stent thrombosis were equal in the two groups, whereas rates of angiographic restenosis (26.6% for BMS vs. 7.9% for PES; $p < 0.001$) and TLR (11.3% for BMS vs. 3.0% for PES; $p < 0.001$) were significantly reduced.

Thus, while initial trials may have hinted at improved MACE outcomes for DES, it has become increasingly clear that the major benefit of DES lies in prevention of repeat TVR, that is, ISR is reduced. The second-generation DES has not necessarily led to reductions in deaths or MIs (58).

Importantly, DES were predominantly tested and approved for use in stable CAD in straightforward patient populations who have simple, de novo, short lesions in relatively large vessels. One exception was the TAXUS V trial, which randomized 1,156 patients with complex lesions (longer and narrower than previously studied) to either BMS or PES, often requiring multiple stents (59). At 9 months, the primary end point of ischemia-driven TVR was significantly lower in the PES group (8.6% vs. 15.7%; $p < 0.001$). While additional data have yielded good results in alternative lesions and patient populations (e.g., those with diabetes, use in acute STEMI, use for ISR), these remain "off-label" uses of DES (60).

The latest DES on the market include a ZES (Endeavor, Resolute) and an everolimus-eluting stent [EES (Xience, Promus)]. The Endeavor stent demonstrated superiority to BMS in the Endeavor II trial (64); however, it was not superior to SES for angiographic outcomes at 8 months in the ENDEAVOR III trial (65) and was noninferior to PES for 9-month TVF in the ENDEAVOR IV trial (66). Advantages of the second-generation DES include refined pharmacokinetics of drug delivery from the polymer and a stent delivery system that many intervention lists prefer. The Resolute ZES was compared to the Xience V EES in the Resolute All-Comers trial (67) and the TWENTE trial (68). Both studies found similar safety and efficacy between the two stents.

Several trials of second-generation DES have demonstrated favorable results, particularly the Xience stent, when compared with its first-generation counterparts. In the SPIRIT III trial, use of the EES in 1,002 patients with stable CAD was compared with PES, for intervention in lesions <28 mm in length and with reference vessel diameter between 2.5 and 3.75 mm. Major cardiac events (including MI and TVR) were lower in the EES group at 9 months ($p = 0.03$) and 1 year ($p = 0.02$). At follow-up extended to 2 years, a signal of reduced stent thrombosis favoring EES was also detected. These data are supported by the SPIRIT IV trial (69).

In February 2012, the FDA approved the Resolute Integrity ZES, the first in the so-called third-generation DES, which differ from second-generation stents in the platform used rather than the drug eluted. The DUrable Polymer-based STent CHallenge of Promus Element Versus ReSolute Integrity in an All Comers Population (DUTCH PEERS) trial (also called the TWENTE II trial) compared two third-generation stents: the Resolute Integrity ZES and the Promus Element EES (70). This trial found no difference in safety or efficacy between the two stents.

These stents are now being compared with newer, biodegradable stents, which are resorbed by the body over time. Their advantages are that they provide the immediate scaffolding to maintain patency, can deliver drug to prevent ISR, and then dissolve over the long term to avoid late complications and imaging distraction. The latest is an EES build from a dissolvable polymer (71). Long-term results up to 2 years have demonstrated its safety and efficacy by multiple imaging techniques.

As previously mentioned, drugs released by the stents not only prevent restenosis, but also slow endothelialization of the stent, increasing the risk of stent thrombosis. These concerns led to multiple analyses of long-term data from DES trials. Pooled experience from the early nine trials of PES and SES demonstrated an increased risk of stent thrombosis at 1 year (63), when compared with their older, BMS counterparts (despite no difference in clinical outcomes at 4 years) (**Fig. 2.5**). However, other long-term analyses have failed to detect this signal at a statistically significant level (54). It is based on these data and concerns over *late* stent thrombosis that current recommendations are for at least 1 year of dual antiplatelet therapy (aspirin plus thienopyridine) following DES implantation, bleeding risks notwithstanding.

DIRECTIONAL ATHERECTOMY

Directional coronary atherectomy (DCA) is an effective debulking technique that uses a cutting device to excise atheromas. DCA requires an 8-F or 9-F sheath, results in frequent distal embolization, and is a difficult technique with a narrow therapeutic window. Eccentric, noncalcified, short lesions in nontortuous vessel segments are ideal lesions.

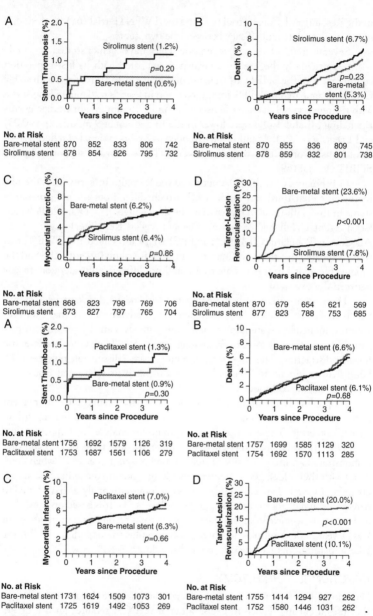

Figure 2.5 • Rates of stent thrombosis, death, MI, and TLR in patients receiving SES (panel A, graphs 1 to 4) or PES (panel B, graphs 1 to 4) versus BMS. (From Stone GW, et al. Safety and efficacy of sirolimus- and paclitaxel-eluting coronary stents. *N Engl J Med* 2007;356:998–1008.)

The Coronary Angioplasty versus Excisional Atherectomy Trial (CAVEAT) I and CAVEAT II (79) both showed that DCA achieved better initial success rates compared with balloon angioplasty within native-vessel and SVG lesions, respectively. However, the atherectomy groups did not have significantly lower restenosis rates, and the incidence of death and MI was higher. The Optimal Atherectomy Restenosis Study (OARS) and Balloon versus Optimal Atherectomy Trial (BOAT) (81,82) showed lower restenosis rates with atherectomy and similar major complication rates. In the BOAT, directional atherectomy was performed with adjunctive PTCA if indicated.

None of the trials mentioned earlier compared atherectomy with stenting. Given the advancement of newer stent technologies, directional atherectomy devices are no longer marketed for coronary use in the United States. There may be a role for these devices in the area of peripheral vascular disease of the lower extremities, however.

ROTATIONAL ATHERECTOMY

RA uses a diamond-coated burr that preferentially ablates atherosclerotic plaque while deflecting away from healthy elastic tissue ("differential cutting"). This technique can facilitate stent delivery and expansion by increasing arterial compliance and lumen diameter in complex, calcified, and diffusely atherosclerotic lesions.

RA was evaluated in the Excimer Laser, Rotational Atherectomy, and Balloon Angioplasty Comparison (ERBAC) trial in patients with type B or C lesions, and the atherectomy group was found to have a better procedural success rate than did the balloon angioplasty (PTCA) or excimer laser groups, but the 6-month restenosis rate was higher compared with that observed with PTCA (57% vs. 47%; $p < 0.05$).

After this trial was completed, substantial technical improvements were made, so additional studies were performed. The Study to Determine Rotablator and Transluminal Angioplasty Strategy (STRATAS) randomized 497 patients to aggressive rotablator therapy (70% to 90% burr-to-artery ratio) or standard rotablator (50% to 70% burr-to-artery ratio). At 6 months, no significant differences were observed between the two groups in mean luminal diameter, restenosis, or clinical events. Similar results were seen in the COBRA study (83).

The Rotational Atherectomy Does Not Reduce Recurrent In-Stent Restenosis (ARTIST) study (84) examined the use of RA for the treatment of ISR. The RA and balloon angioplasty (PTCA) group had a higher restenosis at 6 months compared with PTCA alone (65% vs. 51%; $p = 0.039$).

Prevention of Distal Embolization

THROMBECTOMY

The Possis AngioJet catheter uses high-speed saline jets to generate intense local suction by the Venturi effect, which pulls thrombus into the jets, where it is macerated and then driven down the catheter lumen for external collection. The Vein Graft AngioJet Study randomized 352 patients with angina or MI more than 24 hours before the procedure and thrombus on angiography with intracoronary or graft urokinase (more than 6-hour infusion) or thrombectomy by using the AngioJet system (100). At 30 days, significantly fewer AngioJet patients had experienced MACEs (death, MI, revascularization; 16% vs. 33%; $p < 0.001$). Bradycardia occurred in 24% of those treated with AngioJet and was managed successfully with atropine and temporary pacing.

Additional data on the AngioJet rheolytic device came from the JETSTENT trial. Five-hundred and one patients with STEMI and at least modest thrombus burden were randomized to either direct stenting or stenting following AngioJet rheolytic thrombectomy (101). Not only was the primary outcome (ST-segment resolution at 30 minutes) significantly improved in the AngioJet group, but so were clinical adverse cardiac events at 6 months.

Similar data from the TAPAS study support aspiration of thrombus during primary PCI (106). In 1,071 patients undergoing primary PCI, those randomly assigned to thrombus aspiration had more complete ST-segment resolution and improved myocardial blush and better clinical outcomes in those with better myocardial perfusion grades. In summary, this technique allows rapid thrombus removal and stenting during the same catheterization session and may be particularly beneficial in patients with acute MI who typically have a high thrombus burden. The Thrombus Aspiration during ST-Segment Elevation Myocardial Infarction (TASTE) trial, however, showed no mortality benefit at 30 days in 7,244 patients with STEMI randomly assigned to manual thrombus aspiration followed by PCI versus PCI only (2.8% vs. 3.0%, respectively; HR, 0.94; 95% CI, 0.72 to 1.22; $p = 0.63$).

DISTAL PROTECTION

Distal embolization of friable debris is common during SVG interventions, is a main cause of no reflow, and frequently results in CK release. The Saphenous vein graft Angioplasty Free of Emboli Randomized (SAFER) trial (103) randomized 801 patients with a history of angina, evidence of myocardial ischemia, and more than 50% stenosis in the mid-portion of an SVG with a diameter of 3 to 6 mm, to the GuardWire (Medtronic/PercuSurge) balloon occlusion device or a conventional angioplasty guide wire. The embolic protection group had an impressive 42% relative reduction in MACEs at 30 days (9.6% vs. 16.5%; $p = 0.004$). This reduction was due primarily to fewer MIs (8.6% vs. 14.7%; $p = 0.008$) and "no reflow" (3% vs. 9%; $p = 0.02$). The benefit of the distal protection device was evident both with and without the use of concomitant GP IIb/IIIa–receptor blockers.

Filter devices provide another method of distal protection that permits TIMI 3 flow during the intervention. In the FilterWire EX During Transluminal Intervention of Saphenous Vein Grafts (FIRE) trial, the FilterWire EX device was compared with the GuardWire; 30-day MACE rates were similar (9.9% vs. 11.6%) (104).

However, use of distal protection devices does not provide substantial benefit in urgent PCI, as demonstrated in the Enhanced Myocardial Efficacy and Recovery by Aspiration of Liberated Debris (EMERALD) trial (105). Two-hundred and fifty-two patients with STEMI undergoing primary PCI were randomized to routine PCI or balloon occlusion and aspiration distal microcirculatory protection system during PCI. Despite effectively retrieving embolic debris, the distal protection system did not affect microvascular flow, infarct dimensions, or clinical outcomes. Current recommendations are that distal embolic protection devices be used for SVG interventions, when technically possible.

CORONARY ARTERY BYPASS SURGERY

Risk factors for operative mortality include advanced age, female gender, smoking, left ventricular dysfunction, and the urgency of the operation, as well as anatomic variables.

Coronary Artery Bypass Surgery versus Medical Therapy

Three major clinical trials—the European Coronary Surgery Study (ECSS), CASS, and Veterans Administration (VA) study—helped to define the groups of patients that benefit from bypass surgery. These three studies were performed before the common use of the IMA for revascularization. The ECSS enrolled 768 men aged 65 years or younger and found that surgery resulted in improved survival compared with medical therapy. The majority of the benefit was seen in patients with proximal LAD artery stenoses (216). The CASS enrolled 780 patients aged 65 years or younger and found CABG to be associated with a trend toward lower mortality in patients with triple vessel disease and an ejection fraction of 50% or less (217). Long-term follow-up showed better survival with CABG in patients with left main equivalent disease (severe proximal LAD and left circumflex disease) and left ventricular dysfunction. The VA study found no significant mortality difference between groups at 11-year follow-up, but CABG was beneficial in certain patient subgroups: (a) triple vessel disease and left ventricular dysfunction, and (b) clinically high-risk patients (at least two of the following: resting ST depression, history of MI, or history of hypertension) (28).

An overview of 2,649 patients from these 3 trials and 4 smaller studies showed that CABG was associated with a significantly lower mortality rate at 5 years compared with initial medical management (OR, 0.61), 7 years (OR, 0.68), and 10 years (OR, 0.83) (212). The risk reduction was most marked in patients with left main disease and triple vessel disease (ORs, 0.32 and 0.58). High-risk patients (defined as those with two of the following: severe angina, history of hypertension, prior MI, and ST segment depression at rest) had a 29% mortality reduction with CABG at 10 years compared with a nonsignificant trend toward higher mortality in low-risk patients (no severe angina, hypertension, or prior MI). Overall, these results demonstrate that patients with more severe coronary disease, poor LV dysfunction, and high-risk clinical characteristics derive a significant benefit from bypass surgery versus medical therapy (243; see Chapter 5 for additional discussion of CABG in patients with heart failure).

Coronary Artery Bypass Surgery versus Percutaneous Coronary Intervention

The RITA-1, German Angioplasty Bypass Surgery Investigation (GABI), Emory Angioplasty versus Surgery Trial (EAST), Coronary Angioplasty versus Bypass Revascularization Investigation (CABRI), and Estudio Randomizado Argentino de Angioplastia versus Cirugia (ERACI) (219–222) all enrolled stable patients with single- to triple-vessel CAD. Overall, they showed no mortality difference between CABG and PTCA groups. CABG patients did have longer hospitalizations, fewer repeated interventions, and better quality of life (e.g., less angina and better functional status) at follow-up. The Bypass Angioplasty Revascularization Investigation (BARI) study enrolled 1,829 patients (41% with triple-vessel CAD); the CABG group had an 85% lower revascularization rate at 5 years, but there was no significant mortality reduction (223). Importantly, a 44% lower rate of mortality ($p = 0.003$) was found among diabetic patients who underwent bypass surgery versus PTCA.

A meta-analysis of eight trials with 3,371 patients published through 1996 (214) showed no significant mortality differences between CABG and PTCA. CABG patients had 90% fewer interventions at 1 year. Only a small proportion of patients screened for these trials (5% to 10%) were actually randomized; thus, these findings cannot be readily extrapolated to groups of patients with high-risk characteristics (e.g., left main disease, severe LV dysfunction, chronically occluded vessels). It also is important to note that these trials were completed before the frequent use of stenting.

The Arterial Revascularization Therapy Study (ARTS) (225), which compared stenting with bypass surgery in 1,200 patients with multivessel CAD, found similar rates of adverse outcomes at 30 days [6.8% (surgery) and 8.7% (stenting)] but a significantly lower incidence of repeated revascularization among bypass patients [0.8% vs. 3.7% (at 1 year, 3.5% vs. 16.8%)]. In the Stent or Surgery (SoS) trial, 988 patients with multivessel CAD were randomized to PCI (78% of lesions stented) or CABG. The CABG group had a lower 1-year revascularization rate (5.8% vs. 20.3%), whereas mortality rates were not significantly different (227). ERACI II was a similarly designed study, which enrolled 450 patients and also found a higher revascularization rate in the PCI group [at 18-month follow-up, 16.8% vs. 4.8% (CABG); $p < 0.002$]. However, the PCI group had a significantly lower 30-day and 18-month mortality (0.9% vs. 5.7%; $p < 0.013$; 3.1% vs. 7.5%; $p < 0.017$). A fourth study, the Angina with Extremely Serious Operative Mortality Evaluation (AWESOME), enrolled 554 high-risk VA patients (226). The PCI group had a slightly lower mortality at 30 days and 6 months, but the rates were similar at 3-year follow-up. Once again, the CABG group had a lower revascularization rate (4% vs. 11%). Subsequent

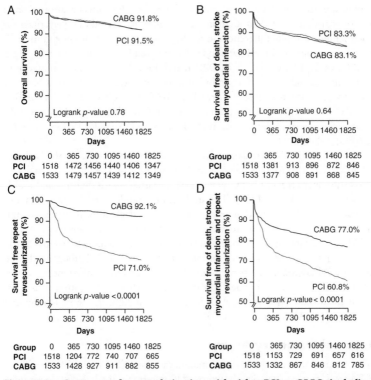

Figure 2.6 • Outcomes of revascularization with either PCI or CABG, including mortality (A); death, stroke, or MI (B); repeat revascularization (C); or the composite of death, stroke, MI, or repeat revascularization (D). (From Daemen J, et al. Long-term safety and efficacy of percutaneous coronary intervention with stenting and coronary artery bypass surgery for multivessel coronary artery disease: a meta-analysis with 5-year patient-level data from the ARTS, ERACI-II, MASS-II, and SoS trials. *Circulation* 2008;118:1146–1154.)

meta-analyses of several of the above trials have confirmed the overall comparable safety between surgical and percutaneous approaches, with revascularization rates heavily favoring surgery (229–231) (**Fig. 2.6**).

While it is reasonable to believe the use of DES will further narrow the gap between multivessel PCI and CABG surgery, this has not yet been observed in large randomized trials. Early data comparing CABG to DES are largely observational registries and continued to demonstrate revascularization rates heavily favoring CABG. Perhaps the most notable yet comparison of CABG versus DES has been the Synergy between PCI with Taxus and Cardiac Surgery (SYNTAX) trial (235). Investigators prospectively randomized 1,800 patients with left main or triple-vessel CAD to either PCI with DES or CABG, the primary end point being a composite of death, stroke, MI, or repeat revascularization at 12 months.

Notably, both an interventional cardiologist and cardiac surgeon were on hand to confirm that equivalent anatomic revascularization could be performed for each patient. Despite differences in medical management that favored the PCI group, outcomes of the primary end point favored CABG at 12 months (17.8 for PCI vs. 12.1 for CABG; $p = 0.0015$), and thus, PCI failed the noninferiority test. Clinical end points of death or MI were not statistically different between the groups, and stroke rates favored PCI (0.6% for PCI vs. 2.2% for CABG; $p = 0.003$). As expected, the primary end point was driven by a highly significant excess of revascularizations in the PCI group (13.7% for PCI vs. 5.9% for CABG; $p < 0.0001$).

The Future Revascularization Evaluation in Patients with Diabetes Mellitus: Optimal Management of Multivessel Disease (FREEDOM) trial suggests the superiority of CABG versus PCI in patients with diabetes and multivessel coronary disease (237). The investigators randomized 1,900 patients to CABG versus PCI (predominantly sirolimus- and paclitaxel-eluting stents). The primary outcome measure was a composite of death from any cause, nonfatal MI, or nonfatal stroke. The primary outcome occurred more frequently in the PCI group ($p = 0.005$), with 5-year rates of 26.6% in the PCI group and 18.7% in the CABG group. The benefit of CABG was driven by differences in rates of both MI ($p < 0.001$) and death from any cause ($p = 0.049$). Stroke was more frequent in the CABG group, with 5-year rates of 2.4% in the PCI group and 5.2% in the CABG group ($p = 0.03$).

Internal Mammary Artery

The patency rate for the internal mammary artery (IMA) is 85% to 95% at 10 years. Use is associated with improved long-term survival. A 27% lower mortality rate was observed in the Coronary Artery Surgery Study (CASS) registry analysis (238). In another analysis, IMA use was associated with a 40% lower 10-year mortality rate among triple vessel disease patients (227).

Saphenous Vein Grafts

From 8% to 12% of SVGs occlude in the early postoperative period (most because of technical factors), and 12% to 20% more occlude in the first year (typically because of intimal proliferation and thrombosis), and then 2% to 4% per year (overall 50% at 10 years). Results of the Post-CABG trial (see Chapter 1) showed a 30% to 40% slowing of graft atherosclerosis with very aggressive low-density lipoprotein (LDL)–lowering therapy (average achieved, LDL 90 mg/dL).

TRANSCATHETER AORTIC VALVE REPLACEMENT

The development and approval of transcatheter aortic valve replacement (TAVR) devices has created a paradigm shift in the management of aortic stenosis. Aortic valve surgery was previously the standard of care for the treatment of severe aortic stenosis in all patients, though a significant number of patients were deemed poor surgical candidates. With disappointing longevity of balloon aortic valvuloplasty (and no mortality benefit), percutaneous options were limited. In 1991, Dr. Henning Rud Andersen patented the TAVR technology, and Dr. Alain Cribier performed the first-in-man TAVR procedure in 2002. Since that time, several large randomized clinical trials have established the safety and efficacy of TAVR, and continued research is widening the patient population with proven benefit from TAVR.

Balloon-Expandable TAVR

The first major trial was the Transcatheter Aortic Valve Implantation for Aortic Stenosis in Patients Who Cannot Undergo Surgery [Placement of Aortic Transcatheter Valves (PARTNER) investigators, cohort B] multicenter trial comparing balloon-expandable transfemoral TAVR to standard medical care in 358 patients with severe aortic stenosis deemed inoperable (245). The primary end point was the rate of death from any cause, which occurred in 30.7% of patients with TAVR and 50.7% of patients with standard therapy including balloon aortic valvuloplasty (HR 0.55; 95% CI, 0.40 to 0.74; $p < 0.001$). The stroke rate at 30 days was higher in the TAVR group (6.7% vs. 1.7%).

Subsequently, the Transcatheter versus Surgical Aortic Valve Replacement in High-Risk Patients (PARTNER, cohort A) trial was published (246). This noninferiority trial was a parallel trial to the PARTNER cohort B trial and randomized 699 high-risk patients with severe AS to TAVR versus surgical aortic valve replacement (SAVR). The rates of death from any cause were 3.4% in the transcatheter group and 6.5% in the surgical group at 30 days ($p = 0.07$) and 24.2% and 26.8%, respectively, at 1 year ($p = 0.44$) (noninferiority $p = 0.001$). The rate of major stroke at 30 days was 3.8% in the TAVR group and 2.1% in the SAVR group. Vascular complications and paravalvular regurgitation were significantly more common in the TAVR group, but major bleeding and new-onset atrial fibrillation were significantly more common in the SAVR group.

Self-expanding TAVR

The PARTNER trials used a balloon-expandable bovine pericardial valve as this was the initial valve design. However, multiple new designs were and currently are being developed, most notably the self-expanding CoreValve. The Transcatheter Aortic Valve Replacement with a Self-Expanding Prosthesis (US CoreValve High Risk Study) trial randomized 795 high-risk patients with severe AS to TAVR with a self-expanding valve versus SAVR (247). The primary end point was the rate of death from any cause at 1 year and was significantly lower in the TAVR arm (14.2% vs. 19.1%; $p < 0.001$ for noninferiority; $p = 0.04$ for superiority).

The Comparison of Balloon-Expandable vs. Self-expandable Valves in Patients Undergoing Transcatheter Aortic Valve Replacement (CHOICE) trial was a large comparison trial between the two major types of valves studied in

TAVR. This trial randomized 240 high-risk patients with severe aortic stenosis to a balloon-expandable versus a self-expandable valve during TAVR. The primary end point was device success and occurred more frequently in the balloon-expandable arm (95.9% vs. 77.5%; RR, 1.24; 95% CI, 1.12 to 1.37; $p < 0.001$).

TAVR is quickly becoming the standard of care for patients with severe aortic stenosis deemed inoperable or very high-risk surgical candidates. In the 2014 ACC/AHA Guidelines for management of valvular heart disease, TAVR is a Class I recommendation in patients who meet an indication for AVR for AS who have a prohibitive surgical risk and a predicted post-TAVR survival >12 months. Two randomized trials are currently underway comparing TAVR to SAVR in intermediate risk patients: PARTNER II (balloon-expandable valve) and SURTAVI (self-expandable valve). Results of these and other trials and registries may continue to expand the indications and patient population for this exciting new technology.

REFERENCES

Guidelines and Classification

1. Levine GN, et al. 2011 ACCF/AHA/SCAI Guideline for Percutaneous Coronary Intervention: a Report of the American College of Cardiology Foundation/American Heart Association Task Force on Practice Guidelines and the Society for Cardiovascular Angiography and Interventions. *J Am Coll Cardiol* 2011;58(24):e44–e122.

These comprehensive guidelines discuss everything from the expected outcomes and standards for competency to the indications and medical management for patients undergoing angiography and PCI. They also address state-of-the-art percutaneous adjunctive technology.

2. Hillis L, et al. 2011 ACCF/AHA Guideline for Coronary Artery Bypass Graft Surgery: a Report of the American College of Cardiology Foundation/American Heart Association Task Force on Practice Guidelines Developed in Collaboration With the American Association for Thoracic Surgery, Society of Cardiovascular Anesthesiologists, and Society of Thoracic Surgeons. *J Am Coll Cardiol* 2011;58(24):e123–e210.

In collaboration with the American Association for Thoracic Surgery, Society of Cardiovascular Anesthesiologists, and the Society of Thoracic Surgeons (STS), the authors review outcomes and complications of surgery, comparisons with medical therapy and percutaneous revascularization, as well as perioperative and postoperative management of patients undergoing CABG. Special populations, such as the elderly, certain comorbidities, poor LV function, or transplant patients are also discussed.

3. Fihn SD, et al. 2012 ACCF/AHA/ACP/AATS/PCNA/SCAI/STS guideline for the diagnosis and management of patients with stable ischemic heart disease: a report of the American College of Cardiology Foundation/American Heart Association Task Force on Practice Guidelines, and the American College of Physicians, American Association for Thoracic Surgery, Preventive Cardiovascular Nurses Association, Society for Cardiovascular Angiography and Interventions, and Society of Thoracic Surgeons. *Circulation* 2012;126:e354–e471.

4. Fihn SD, et al. 2014 ACC/AHA/AATS/PCNA/SCAI/STS focused update of the guideline for the diagnosis and management of patients with stable ischemic heart disease: a report of the American College of Cardiology/American Heart Association Task Force on Practice Guidelines, and the American Association for Thoracic Surgery, Preventive Cardiovascular Nurses Association, Society for Cardiovascular Angiography and Interventions, and Society of Thoracic Surgeons. *Circulation* 2014;130 (online first).

This update to the 2012 full text regarding patients with stable ischemic heart disease adds a new section of recommendations addressing invasive testing for the diagnosis of CAD in patients with suspected stable ischemic heart disease.

5. Nishimura RA, et al. 2014 AHA/ACC guideline for the management of patients with valvular heart disease: a report of the American College of Cardiology/American Heart Association Task Force on Practice Guidelines. *J Am Coll Cardiol* 2014;63:e57–e185.

In collaboration with the American Association for Thoracic Surgery, American Society of Echocardiography, Society for Cardiovascular Angiography and Interventions, Society of Cardiovascular Anesthesiologists, and STS, the authors provide a comprehensive overview of the recommended diagnosis, medical management, and interventional treatment of all major forms of valvular disease including TAVR for aortic stenosis.

6. Gibson CM, et al. TIMI frame count. *Circulation* 1996;93:879–888.

This article describes a new method that quantifies coronary artery flow as a continuous variable [vs. assignment to one of four flow grades (i.e., TIMI grade 0, 1, 2, or 3)]. A total of 393 patients (315 TIMI 4 acute MI patients and 78 subjects without MI) were analyzed. The method was found to be reproducible (difference between two injections, 4.7 ± 3.9). Among normal patients, the LAD artery took 1.7 times longer to fill completely than did the right coronary artery and circumflex arteries (36.2 vs. 20.4, 22.2; both $p < 0.001$). After thrombolysis, mean corrected counts (LAD, divided by 1.7) were 39.2 at 90 minutes and 31.7 by 18 to 36 hours ($p < 0.001$); both were higher than were those in patients without acute MI.

7. Zaacks SM, et al. Value of the ACC/AHA stenosis morphology classification for coronary interventions in the late 1990s. *Am J Cardiol* 1998;82:43–49.

This prospective analysis was derived from 957 consecutive interventions in 1,404 lesions from June 1994 to October 1996. The overall procedural success rate was 91.9%. No significant differences in success rates were found between type A, B1, and B2 lesions (96.3%, 95.5%, 95.1%), but all were better than type C (88.2%; $p < 0.003$, $p < 0.004$, $p = 0.0001$, respectively). Multiple regression analysis showed that total occlusion and vessel tortuosity were predictive of procedural failure. Lesion type did not predict device use or complications. Actual predictors of complications were bifurcation lesions ($p = 0.0045$), presence of thrombus ($p = 0.0001$), inability to protect a major side branch ($p = 0.0468$), and degenerated vein graft lesions ($p = 0.0283$).

Operator and Hospital Characteristics

8. Jollis JG, et al. The relation between the volume of coronary angioplasty procedures at hospitals treating Medicare beneficiaries and short-term mortality. *N Engl J Med* 1994;331:1625–1629.

This analysis was conducted on 218,000 Medicare patients who underwent PTCA from 1987 to 1990. A significant mortality difference was found between the 10% treated at the highest- and lowest-volume (fewer than 50 procedures per year) centers (2.5% vs. 3.9%). A difference in the CABG surgery rate was found (2.8% vs. 5.3%).

9. Kimmel SE, et al. The relationship between coronary angioplasty procedure volume and major complications. *JAMA* 1995;274:1137–1142.

This cohort study showed an association between low hospital volume and increased complications. The cohort consisted of 19,594 non-MI patients undergoing a first PTCA.

Higher volume was associated with lower mortality ($p = 0.04$), emergency bypass surgery ($p < 0.001$), and major complications ($p < 0.001$). Multivariate analysis (adjusted for case mix) showed that the associations persisted, but the mortality difference was not significant. No difference was demonstrated in outcomes when comparing hospitals performing 200 versus more than 200 procedures. However, for hospitals performing 400 to 599 and 600 versus fewer than 200 procedures per year, the adjusted ORs for major complications were 0.66 and 0.54 ($p = 0.03$; $p = 0.001$).

10. Jollis JG, et al. Relationship between physician and hospital coronary angioplasty volume and outcome in elderly patients. *Circulation* 1997;95:2485–2491 (editorial, 2467–2470).

This analysis focused on 97,478 Medicare patients treated by 6,115 physicians at 984 hospitals in 1992. Median procedure volume was only 13 per operator; hospital median was 98. After risk factor adjustment, low-volume operators were associated with an increased rate of bypass surgery (fewer than 25, 3.8%; 25 to 50, 3.4%; more than 50, 2.6%; $p < 0.001$), and low-volume hospitals were associated with higher bypass surgery and mortality rates (fewer than 100, 3.9%/2.9%; 100 to 200, 3.5%/2.5%; more than 200, 3.0%/2.3%; $p < 0.001$). Improved outcomes were seen with up to 75 and 200 Medicare cases per year, respectively. The accompanying editorial points out that data were acquired in the early stent era and before the use of GP IIb/IIIa inhibition.

11. Ritchie JL, et al. Association between percutaneous transluminal coronary angioplasty volumes and outcomes in the Healthcare Cost and Utilization Project 1993–1994. *Am J Cardiol* 1999;83:493–497.

This analysis of 163,527 procedures from 214 centers demonstrated superior outcomes in high-volume institutions (more than 400 cases per year) compared with low-volume centers (fewer than 200 cases per year).

12. McGrath PD, et al. Relation between operator and hospital volume and outcomes following percutaneous coronary interventions in the era of the coronary stent. *JAMA* 2000;284:3139–3144.

Analysis of Medicare patients aged 65 to 99 years who underwent PCI in 1997. Low-volume operators were defined as those who performed fewer than 30 Medicare interventions per year, whereas high-volume operators performed more than 60 per year. Low-volume institutions were defined as those performing fewer than 80 Medicare interventions per year, whereas high volume was considered as more than 160 per year. The lowest incidence of 30-day mortality and CABG (4.6%) occurred at high-volume hospitals with a high-volume interventionalist, whereas the highest incidence (6.1%) was seen at low-volume hospitals with low-volume interventionalists.

13. Srinivas VS, et al. Effect of physician volume on the relationship between hospital volume and mortality during primary angioplasty. *J Am Coll Cardiol* 2009;53:574–579.

Data from 7,321 patients in the New York State PCI Registry for acute MI demonstrated significant variation of outcomes based on physician experience and hospital volumes. Within high-volume hospitals, risk-adjusted mortality was higher for low-volume physicians than for high-volume physicians (OR, 0.58; 95% CI, 0.39 to 0.86). While high-volume physicians in high-volume hospitals had a lower unadjusted mortality than low-volume physicians in low-volume hospitals (3.2% vs. 6.7%; $p = 0.03$), after risk adjustment, this difference was no longer statistically significant (3.8% vs. 8.4%; $p = 0.09$).

14. Nallamothu BK, et al. Relation between hospital specialization with primary percutaneous coronary intervention and clinical outcomes in ST-segment elevation myocardial infarction national registry of myocardial infarction-4 analysis. *Circulation* 2006;113:222–229.

The investigators stratified hospitals in NRMI by the proportion of STEMI patients who undergo primary PCI versus thrombolytics and assessed outcomes based on this stratification. Centers with the highest proportion of patients undergoing primary PCI (>88.5%) had lower in-hospital mortality (adjusted RR 0.64; $p = 0.006$ for highest vs. lowest quartiles). These differences did not extend to patients treated with fibrinolytic therapy. Additionally, door-to-balloon time was significantly shorter in the high-percentage PCI group (99.6 vs. 118.3 minutes; $p < 0.001$).

15. Pride YB, et al. Outcomes among patients with non–ST segment elevation myocardial infarction presenting to interventional hospitals with and without on-site cardiac surgery. *JACC Cardiovasc Interv* 2009;2(10):944–952.

In the 100,071 patients with NSTEMI in NRMI from 2004 to 2006, the authors assessed in-hospital mortality in patients treated at hospitals with on-site cardiac surgery versus those without on-site cardiac surgery. In the overall population, irrespective of PCI, in-hospital mortality was significantly lower at centers with surgery (5.0% vs. 8.8%; $p < 0.001$), and patients at these centers were more likely to receive aspirin, beta blockers, and statins ($p < 0.05$ for all). They were also more likely to undergo PCI at centers with on-site cardiac surgery (38.4% vs. 14.1%; $p < 0.001$); however, in propensity-adjusted analyses (including adjustment for medications and hospital characteristics), differences in mortality were nearly abolished (HR, 0.98; $p = 0.050$) and mortality for patients undergoing PCI was nearly identical (1.3% vs. 1.0%; $p = 0.51$).

Catheterization Technique

16. Gruntzig AR, et al. Nonoperative dilatation of coronary-artery stenosis: percutaneous transluminal coronary angioplasty. *N Engl J Med* 1979;301:61–68.

In this first major report of balloon angioplasty, 50 patients with angina (mean duration, 13 months) underwent angioplasty. All patients received aspirin, 1 g/day for 3 days (starting 1 day before), heparin and dextran during the procedure, and warfarin through follow-up (6 to 9 months). The procedural success rate was 64%. Five patients required CABG surgery, and three had an MI.

17. Metz D, et al. Comparison of 6F with 7F and 8F guiding catheters for elective coronary angioplasty: results of a prospective, multicenter randomized trial. *Am Heart J* 1997;134:131–137.

This study showed that bleeding and procedural complications decreased with the use of 6-F catheters. Four hundred and sixty patients with an ejection fraction of 30% and target lesions that could accommodate a 6-F catheter were enrolled. No differences were observed in procedural success rates (87%, 6F; 88%, 7F and 8F) or stenting rates (21%, 6F; 25%, 7F and 8F). The 6-F group had approximately 40% fewer femoral access site complications (13.8% vs. 23.5%; $p < 0.01$), had shorter procedure and fluoroscopy times, used less contrast, and had shorter post–sheath-removal femoral compression times (11.7 vs. 14.1 minutes; $p < 0.01$).

18. Sciahbasi A, et al. Arterial access-site-related outcomes of patients undergoing invasive coronary procedures for acute coronary syndromes (from the PRESTO-ACS vascular substudy). *Am J Cardiol* 2009;103:796–800.

The investigators examined access-related complications in a subset of patients in the PRESTO-ACS study undergoing PCI. All patients underwent PCI for NSTEMI ACS, and there was no difference in clinical events outcomes between those who had PCI via femoral site and those via radial approach (2.9% femoral vs. 2.6% radial; $p = 0.79$). Radial access was associated with less bleeding (2.4% vs. 0.7%; $p = 0.05$); at 1-year follow-up, patients who underwent radial approach had significantly lower rates of death or MI (8.3% vs. 4.9%; $p = 0.05$) and bleeding (2.7% vs. 0.7%; $p = 0.03$). It is important to highlight that this is a post hoc analysis of a trial that did *not* randomly assign patients to each access site.

19. Pristipino C, et al. Major improvement of percutaneous cardiovascular procedure outcomes with radial artery catheterization: results from the PREVAIL study. *Heart* 2009;95:476–482.

This real-world observational study looked at 1,052 consecutive patients undergoing PCI at nine centers: 509 via radial access and 543 via femoral. The primary end point was a composite of major and minor bleeding, periprocedural stroke, or access-site complication; a lower rate of such events occurred in the radial-access group (1.96% vs. 4.2%; $p = 0.03$). This result persisted in multivariable analysis (OR, 0.37 for radial access; 95% CI, 0.16 to 0.84).

20. Jolly SS, et al. Radial versus femoral access for coronary angiography and intervention in patients with acute coronary syndromes (RIVAL): a randomised, parallel group, multicentre trial. *Lancet* 2011;377:1409–1420.

This randomized study of 7,021 patients with ACS found no significant difference between radial and femoral access in the primary end point of death/MI/stroke/bleeding at 30 days (radial 3.7% vs. femoral 4.0%; $p = 0.50$). However, bleeding rates were low in both groups, and the study was underpowered to detect a difference in bleeding as defined in the study, and only 32% of the bleeding events were at the access site. Major vascular access site complications were significantly lower in the radial versus femoral group (1.4% vs. 3.7%; $p < 0.0001$), and a post hoc analysis showed no major access site bleeds in the radial group and 18 major bleeds in the femoral group.

21. Romagnoli E, et al. Radial versus femoral randomized investigation in ST-segment elevation acute coronary syndrome: the RIFLE-STEACS (Radial Versus Femoral Randomized Investigation in ST Elevation Acute Coronary Syndrome) study. *J Am Coll Cardiol* 2012;60(24):2481–2489.

This multicenter trial randomized 1,001 patients with STEMI to primary PCI with radial versus femoral approach at 4 high-volume centers. The primary end point of net adverse clinical events (NACE)—a composite of cardiac death, stroke, MI, target lesion revascularization, and bleeding—occurred less frequently in the radial (13.6%) versus the femoral arm (21%; $p = 0.003$). Radial access was also associated with significantly lower rates of cardiac mortality (5.2% vs. 9.2%; $p = 0.020$), bleeding (7.8% vs. 12.2%; $p = 0.026$), and shorter hospital stay (5 vs. 6 days; $p = 0.03$).

22. Bernat I, et al. ST-segment elevation myocardial infarction treated by radial or femoral approach in a multicenter randomized clinical trial: the STEMI-RADIAL trial. *J Am Coll Cardiol* 2014;63(10):964–972.

This trial randomized 707 patients with STEMI to radial versus femoral access at 4 high-volume radial centers. The primary end point of cumulative incidence of major bleeding and vascular access site complications at 30 days occurred in 1.4% of the radial group ($n = 348$) and 7.2% of the femoral group ($n = 359$; $p = 0.0001$). The radial approach also reduced ICU stays and contrast volume.

Contrast Agents

23. Grines CL, et al. A randomized trial of low-osmolar ionic versus nonionic contrast media in patients with MI or unstable angina undergoing percutaneous transluminal coronary angioplasty. *J Am Coll Cardiol* 1996;27:1381–1386 (editorial, 1387–1389).

This randomized study of 211 patients with acute MI or unstable angina showed that the use of ionic low-osmolar contrast media reduced the risk of ischemic complications.

Patients received nonionic or ionic low-osmolar contrast media during coronary angiography. The ionic media group had fewer recurrent ischemic events requiring repeated catheterization (3.0% vs. 11.4%; $p = 0.02$) and repeated angioplasty during initial hospitalization (1.0% vs. 5.8%; $p = 0.06$). At 1 month, the ionic contrast group had a reduced need for bypass surgery (none vs. 5.9%; $p = 0.04$) and reported fewer symptoms of any angina or angina at rest (8.5% vs. 20.0%, $p = 0.04$; none vs. 5.9%, $p = 0.04$).

24. Schrader R, et al. A randomized trial comparing the impact of nonionic (iomeprol) versus an ionic (ioxaglate) low-osmolar contrast medium on abrupt vessel closure and ischemic complications after coronary angioplasty. *J Am Coll Cardiol* 1999;33:395–402.

This prospective, randomized trial was composed of 2,000 patients undergoing PTCA. The frequency of reocclusions requiring repeated intervention was similar in both groups [in laboratory, 2.9% (iomeprol) and 3.0% (ioxaglate); out of laboratory, 3.1% and 4.1%]. Major ischemic complication rates also were similar (emergency CABG, 0.8% and 0.7%; MI, 1.8% and 2.0%; in-hospital cardiac death, 0.2% and 0.2%). The iomeprol group had higher rates of dissection and stenting (31.6% vs. 25.7%, $p = 0.004$; 31.6% vs. 25.7%, $p = 0.004$), whereas allergic reactions requiring treatment occurred only in the ioxaglate group (0.9%; $p = 0.002$).

25. Davidson CJ, et al. Randomized trial of contrast media utilization in high-risk PTCA: the COURT trial. *Circulation* 2000;101:2172–2177.

A total of 856 patients undergoing high-risk interventions were randomized to a nonionic iso-osmolar contrast agent (iodixanol) or an ionic low-osmolar contrast agent (ioxaglate). Angiographic success was significantly better in the nonionic contrast patients (92.2% vs. 85.9%; $p = 0.004$). The nonionic contrast group had a significantly lower incidence of the primary composite end point of in-hospital MI, abrupt closure, recatheterization, or emergency revascularization (5.4% vs. 9.5%; $p = 0.027$). The difference persisted in multivariable analyses ($p = 0.01$).

26. Bertrand ME, et al.; for the Visipaque in PTCA (VIP) Investigators. Influence of a nonionic, iso-osmolar contrast medium (iodixanol) versus an ionic, low-osmolar contrast medium (ioxaglate) on major adverse cardiac events in patients undergoing percutaneous transluminal coronary angioplasty: a multicenter, randomized, double-blind study. *Circulation* 2000;101:131–136.

This prospective, randomized, parallel-group, double-blind study enrolled 1,411 patients. Patients received either iodixanol (a nonionic, iso-osmolar contrast medium) or ioxaglate (an ionic, low-osmolar contrast medium) during PTCA. No significant differences were found between the groups in the incidence of the primary composite end point, consisting of death, stroke, MI, CABG surgery, and repeated PTCA at 2 days (iodixanol, 4.7%; ioxaglate, 3.9%; $p = 0.45$) and at 1 month. However, the iodixanol group had a lower incidence of hypersensitivity reactions ($p = 0.007$) and adverse drug reactions ($p = 0.002$) compared with the ioxaglate group.

27. Solomon RJ, et al. Cardiac angiography in renally impaired patients (CARE) study a randomized double-blind trial of contrast-induced nephropathy in patients with chronic kidney disease. *Circulation* 2007;115(25):3189–3196.

The investigators performed a multicenter, randomized, double-blind comparison of iopamidol (796 mOsm/kg) and iodixanol (290 mOsm/kg) for patients with chronic kidney disease undergoing coronary angiography. In the 414 patients included, 4.4% in the iopamidol group and 6.7% in the iodixanol group had increases in serum creatinine of ≥ 5 mg/dL ($p = 0.39$ for the primary outcome); however, in the subgroup of patients with diabetes, such an increase occurred in 5.1% with iopamidol and 13.0% with iodixanol ($p = 0.11$). Though numerically trending in favor of iopamidol, the authors conclude the differences between the two agents are small and unlikely to be clinically significant.

Lesion Evaluation (Fractional Flow Reserve, Intravascular Ultrasound)

28. Pijls NHJ, et al. Measurement of fractional flow reserve to assess the functional severity of coronary-artery stenoses. *N Engl J Med* 1996;334:1703–1708.

A total of 45 consecutive patients with chest pain and a moderate coronary stenosis of approximately 50% underwent bicycle testing, thallium scintigraphy, dobutamine stress echocardiography, and coronary arteriography. In all patients (21) with an FFR < 0.75, reversible ischemia was evident on at least one noninvasive test. After revascularization was performed (PTCA or CABG surgery), all positive test results reverted to normal. In contrast, 21 of 24 patients with an FFR of 0.75 or more tested negative for reversible ischemia on all the noninvasive tests. None of these patients underwent revascularization through 14 months of follow-up. The sensitivity of FFR in detecting reversible ischemia was 88%, specificity was 100%, positive predictive value was 100%, negative predictive value was 88%, and the accuracy was 93%.

29. Fitzgerald PJ, et al. Final results of the Can Routine Ultrasound Influence Stent Expansion (CRUISE) Study. *Circulation* 2000;102:523–530.

A total of 522 patients from 16 of 45 centers in the STARS were enrolled in this IVUS substudy to determine if IVUS-assisted stenting results in better outcomes when compared with angiography-assisted stenting. At 9 months, the IVUS-guided group had a larger MLD (2.9 mm vs. 2.7 mm; $p < 0.001$), a lower residual diameter stenosis (7.6% vs. 9.8%; $p < 0.001$), and higher final balloon size and inflation pressure (3.88 mm vs. 3.69 mm, and 18.0 atm vs. 16.6 atm; both $p < 0.001$). The IVUS group had a significantly lower TVR rate (8.5% vs. 15.3%; $p < 0.05$), whereas no differences were found in death or MI rates. Additional therapy based on IVUS information was used in 36% of patients (higher pressures in 59%, larger balloons in 33.7%, and an additional stent in 7%). In summary, IVUS-guided stent deployment results in improved stent expansion and a lower TVR compared with angiographic guidance alone.

30. Bech GJW, et al. Fractional flow reserve to determine the appropriateness of angioplasty in moderate coronary stenosis. *Circulation* 2001;103:2928–2934.

This study of 325 scheduled to undergo PTCA of a more than 50% native coronary artery stenosis in a larger than 2.5-mm vessel examined whether deferring PTCA, based on FFR of 0.75 or more, is safe and as least efficacious as performing PTCA. Patients were excluded if they had evidence of reversible ischemia in the previous 2 months. FFR was <0.75 for 144 patients, who underwent routine PTCA (reference group). Another 181 patients had an FFR of 0.75 or more and were randomized to optimal intervention (performance group) or medical therapy (deferral group) in a 1:1 fashion. Primary end point was absence of adverse cardiac events at 2 years, consisting of death, MI, PTCA, and any procedure-related complication requiring major intervention. At 2 years, event-free survival was significantly higher in the performance and deferral groups (83% and 89%) compared with the reference group (78%). The performance and deferral groups had similar rates of freedom from angina (50% vs. 49% at 1 year and 51% vs. 70% at 2 years), whereas the incidence was significantly higher in the reference group (67% at 1 year and 80% at 2 years).

31. Christou MA, et al. Meta-analysis of fractional flow reserve versus quantitative coronary angiography and noninvasive imaging for evaluation of myocardial ischemia. *Am J Cardiol* 2007;99(4):450–456.

A compilation of 31 studies comparing lesion assessment with FFR versus QCA and/or noninvasive imaging. The investigators assign sensitivity and specificity for each technique, as well as receiver–operator curves. The authors conclude that quantitative angiography does not predict functional stenosis, as predicted by FFR or dobutamine stress echocardiography.

32. Tonino PAL, et al.; for the FAME Study Investigators. Fractional flow reserve versus angiography for guiding percutaneous coronary intervention. *N Engl J Med* 2009; 360(3):213–224.

Investigators from 20 centers randomized 1,005 patients with multivessel CAD to undergo PCI with routine angiography guiding DES placement, versus that guided by FFR along with angiography. Lesions initially identified for stenting on angiography were only stented in the FFR group if the FFR was 0.80 or less and the primary end point was a composite of death, MI, or repeat revascularization at 1 year. This occurred in 18.3% of patients in the angiography group, versus 13.2% in the FFR group (p = 0.02); additionally, the number of stents used was lower in the FFR group (2.7 vs. 1.3; p < 0.001), though the number of lesions stented was similar (2.7 vs. 2.8; p = 0.34). In this contemporary trial involving patients with multivessel diseases receiving DES, using FFR to guide stent placement not only reduced the number of stents used but also improved clinical outcomes at 1 year.

33. De Bruyne B, et al. Fractional Flow Reserve-Guided PCI versus Medical Therapy in Stable Coronary Disease (FAME 2). *N Engl J Med* 2012;367:991–1001.

The FAME investigators randomized 888 patients with stable CAD and at least 1 functionally significant stenosis (FFR ≤0.80) to FFR-guided PCI plus the best available medical therapy versus the best available medical therapy alone. An additional 332 patients without a functionally significant lesion were enrolled in a registry with best available medical therapy. The trial recruitment was halted early because of a significant early difference in the primary end point, a composite of death from any cause/nonfatal MI/unplanned hospitalization leading to urgent revascularization during the first 2 years (4.3% FFR group, 12.7% medical group; HR, 0.32 [95% CI, 0.19 to 0.53]; p < 0.001). This difference was driven by a lower rate of urgent revascularization in the PCI group (1.6% vs. 11.1%; HR, 0.13 [95% CI, 0.06 to 0.30]; p < 0.001).

34. Mudra H, et al.; for the OPTICUS (OPTimization with ICUS to reduce stent restenosis) Study Investigators. Randomized comparison of coronary stent implantation under ultrasound or angiographic guidance to reduce stent restenosis (OPTICUS Study). *Circulation* 2001;104:1343–1349.

Prospective, randomized trial of 550 patients with a symptomatic coronary lesion or silent ischemia. Patients were assigned to either IVUS-guided or angiography-guided implantation of two or fewer stents. At 6-month angiography, no significant differences were seen between the two groups in MLD [1.95 mm (IVUS guided) vs. 1.91 mm] or restenosis rate (24.5% vs. 22.8%). At 1 year, the groups also had similar incidences of MACEs and repeated PCI.

35. Albertal M, et al.; for the Doppler Endpoints Balloon Angioplasty Trial Europe (DEBATE) II Study Group. Coronary flow velocity reserve after percutaneous interventions is predictive of periprocedural outcome. *Circulation* 2002;105:1573–1578.

A total of 379 DEBATE II study patients underwent Doppler flow–guided angioplasty. CFVR measured before PTCA and CFVR in the reference artery were independent predictors of an optimal CFVR (2.5 or more) after balloon angioplasty. A low CFVR (<2.5) at the end of the procedure was an independent predictor of MACEs at 30 days (OR, 4.71; p = 0.034) and at 1 year (OR, 2.06; p = 0.014). After excluding MACE at 30 days, no difference in MACE at 1 year was observed between the patients with and without a CFVR <2.5 at the end of the procedure.

Comparison of Revascularization with Medical Therapy

36. Parisi AF, et al. Angioplasty compared to medicine (ACME): a comparison of angioplasty with medical therapy in the treatment of single-vessel coronary artery disease. *N Engl J Med* 1992;326:10–16.

Design: Prospective, randomized, multicenter study. Primary end point was change in exercise tolerance, frequency of angina attacks, and nitroglycerin use.

Purpose: To compare medical therapy with balloon angioplasty in patients with one significant coronary artery stenosis.

Population: 212 patients with a single 70% to 99% stenosis.

Treatment: The drug therapy group included oral isosorbide dinitrate with sublingual glyceryl trinitrate and/or β-blockers and/or calcium antagonists. The balloon angioplasty group was given calcium antagonists before and for 1 month after the procedure and heparin and glyceryl trinitrate during and until 12 hours after the procedure. All patients received aspirin, 325 mg orally daily.

Results: Balloon angioplasty (PTCA) was successful in 80% and reduced stenoses from 76% to 36%. The PTCA group had less angina (64% vs. 46%; $p < 0.01$), better exercise performance [+2.1 minutes (6 months vs. baseline exercise test) vs. +0.5 minutes; $p < 0.0001$], and more improvement in quality-of-life score (+8.6 units vs. +2.4 units; $p = 0.03$). However, the PTCA group did have more complications [emergency bypass surgery in two patients, MIs in 5 (vs. 3), and repeated PTCA in 16].

37. Folland ED, et al. VA Angioplasty Compared to Medicine (VA ACME). Percutaneous transluminal coronary angioplasty vs medical therapy for stable angina pectoris. *J Am Coll Cardiol* 1997;29:1505–1511.

Design: Prospective, randomized, double-blind, multicenter study.

Purpose: To compare balloon angioplasty with medical therapy in patients with documented coronary disease and chronic stable angina.

Population: 328 patients with stable angina and positive exercise treadmill test; 101 patients had two-vessel disease ($\geq$70% stenosis in proximal two-thirds), and 227 had single-vessel disease.

Exclusion Criteria: Medically refractory unstable angina, prior coronary revascularization, ejection fraction $\leq$30%.

Treatment: Medical therapy or balloon angioplasty.

Results: Among two-vessel patients, no significant changes were found between treatment groups in exercise treadmill test duration (performed at 2 to 3 years) or freedom from angina and quality of life. However, fewer angioplasty patients had improved perfusion imaging results (59% vs. 75%) and higher average stenosis of worst lesions (74% vs. 56%). Among single-vessel disease patients, the angioplasty group had more improvement in exercise time (+2.1 vs. +0.6 minutes; $p < 0.001$) and quality-of-life score (+7.1 vs. +1.5; $p = 0.01$) and were more angina free (63% vs. 48%; $p = 0.02$).

38. Randomized Intervention Treatment of Angina (RITA-2) Trial participants. Coronary angioplasty vs. medical therapy for angina: the RITA-2 trial. *Lancet* 1997;350:461–468.

Design: Prospective, randomized, double-blind, multicenter study. Primary end point was death and nonfatal MI. Follow-up period was 2.7 years.

Purpose: To compare the effects of coronary angioplasty and conservative medical care in patients considered suitable for either treatment.

Population: 1,018 patients, 53% with grade 2 angina, 47% with prior MI, and only 7% with three-vessel disease.

Exclusion Criteria: Unstable angina in prior 7 days, left main CAD, and early revascularization necessary or planned.

Treatment: Medical therapy or balloon angioplasty (in the latter group, the procedure was performed in 93% at a median of 5 weeks).

Results: Angioplasty group had increased rates of death and MI (6.3% vs. 3.3%; $p = 0.02$). Benefit was attributable mostly to procedure-related events. However, the PTCA group had 7% less grade 2 angina at 2 years and longer exercise treadmill test time at 3 months (+35 seconds; $p < 0.001$).

39. Boden WE, et al.; for the COURAGE Trial Research Group. Optimal medical therapy with or without PCI for stable coronary disease. N Engl J Med 2007;356: 1503–1516.

Design: Prospective, randomized, multicenter trial. Primary outcome was a combined incidence of death or nonfatal MI at a median of 4.6 years of follow-up.

Purpose: To assess the advantage of stenting over optimal medical therapy to prevent clinical events in patients with stable CAD.

Population: A total of 2,287 patients with significant coronary disease (>70% stenosis of at least 1 epicardial vessel) and objective signs of ischemia (on ECG or by stress), without unstable disease.

Treatment: Patients were randomized to optimal medical therapy alone or in combination with revascularization by stenting. Optimal medical therapy included dual antiplatelet therapy in patients with stents, as well as long-acting metoprolol, amlodipine, isosorbide mononitrate, aggressive lipid lowering (to a goal LDL of 60 to 85 mg/dL), inhibitors of renin–angiotensin system, and additional HDL-raising therapy. In the group undergoing PCI, few received DES, as they were not approved until the final 6 months of the study.

Results: There was no statistical difference in the number of primary end points in the two groups (19.0% in the PCI group vs. 18.5% in the medical therapy group; $p = 0.62$). This was true when stroke was added to the end point, as well as for comparisons of rates of hospitalizations for ACS or MI. There was a significantly higher rate of revascularization (PCI or CABG) procedures in the medical therapy group (32.6% for the medical therapy group vs. 21.1% for the PCI group; $p < 0.001$).

Comments: This pivotal study attempted to address the goals of stenting in patients with stable, fixed coronary disease. Significant caveats are that (a) few patients received DES and (b) patients were only randomized *after* their angiogram was done and viewed by the enrolling investigators (a potential source of significant enrollment bias). However, the trial does lend support to the idea that it is not the tight lesions identified at angiography that are rupturing to cause acute MIs.

Stent Studies

EARLY STENT COMPARISONS

40. Fischman DL, et al.; Stent Restenosis Study (STRESS). A randomized comparison of coronary-stent placement and balloon angioplasty in the treatment of coronary artery disease. N Engl J Med 1994;331:496–501.

Design: Prospective, randomized, open-label, multicenter study. Primary end point was angiographic restenosis.

Purpose: To compare the results of elective balloon angioplasty with PS stent implantation on clinical outcomes and restenosis in patients with de novo coronary lesions.

Population: 410 patients with de novo 70% stenotic lesions ≤15 mm long and in vessels with a diameter of ≥3 mm

Exclusion Criteria: MI in previous 7 days, EF < 40%, diffuse coronary or left main artery disease, and angiographic evidence of thrombus.

Treatment: Balloon angioplasty or PS stent. All patients received aspirin, 325 mg daily. Stented patients received dextran (started 2 hours before the procedure); heparin,

10,000 to 15,000 U before the procedure and infusion for 4 to 6 hours after sheath removal; dipyridamole, 75 mg three times daily for 1 month; and warfarin for 1 month.

Results: Stent group had better procedural success (96.1% vs. 89.6%; $p = 0.011$), greater increase in lumen diameter (1.7 mm vs. 1.2 mm; $p < 0.001$; at 6 months, 1.56 mm vs. 1.24 mm; $p < 0.01$), and a lower rate of restenosis at 6 months (31% vs. 42%; $p = 0.046$). No significant difference in early clinical events (days 0 to 14) was observed between the two groups (19.5% vs. 23.8%). The stent group had a nonsignificant reduction in revascularization rate (10% vs. 15%; $p = 0.06$). At 1-year follow-up, 154 (75%) patients assigned to stent implantation and 141 (70%) to PTCA were free of all clinical events (death, MI, or any revascularization procedure).

Comments: The 1-year cost analysis showed the cost of stenting to be $800 more per patient despite lower costs during follow-up.

41. Benestent I, et al. A comparison of balloon-expandable stent implantation with balloon angioplasty in patients with coronary artery disease. N *Engl J Med* 1994;331:489–495.

Design: Prospective, randomized, multicenter study. Primary end point was death, stroke, MI, CABG, or need for repeated percutaneous intervention during hospitalization.

Purpose: To compare elective balloon angioplasty with PS stenting in patients with stable angina and de novo coronary lesions.

Population: 520 patients aged 30 to 75 years with stable angina and one de novo coronary lesion shorter than 15 mm and in vessel larger than 3 mm in diameter.

Treatment: Balloon angioplasty or PS stenting. All patients received aspirin, 250 to 500 mg/day, and dipyridamole, 75 mg three times daily (started 1 day before procedure and continued for more than 6 months); heparin, 10,000 U was given before the procedure. Stented patients received dextran, 1,000 mL over 6 to 8 hours, and then warfarin for 3 months (target international normalized ratio, 2.5 to 3.5).

Results: No differences were observed between groups in incidence of death, stroke, MI, or subsequent revascularization during index hospitalization, and no differences were observed in composite end point of in-hospital clinical events (6.2% and 6.9%). At 7 months, the stent group had a significant reduction in primary composite end point (20.1% vs. 29.6%; $p = 0.02$), with the majority of this difference attributed to fewer second angioplasties (10% vs. 20.6%; $p = 0.001$). The stent group had more vascular complications (13.5% vs. 3.1%; $p < 0.001$) and longer hospital stays (8.5 vs. 3.1 days; $p = 0.001$). The 1-year follow-up data showed similar rates of death, stroke, MI, and CABG, but the stent group had 26% fewer primary end points (23% vs. 31%; $p = 0.04$), primarily because of approximately 50% fewer repeated PTCAs (10% vs. 21%; $p = 0.001$). At 5-year follow-up, the stent group still had an approximate 10% absolute lower incidence of TVR (17.2% vs. 27.3%; $p = 0.008$; see *J Am Coll Cardiol* 2001;37:1598–1600).

Comments: Results suggest that stenting reduces repeated interventions but not major clinical events. Longer hospital stay with stenting was attributable to the aggressive antithrombotic regimen.

42. Lansky AJ, et al. Randomized comparison of GR-II stent and Palmaz–Schatz stent for elective treatment of coronary stenoses. *Circulation* 2000;102:1364–1368.

This prospective study randomized 755 patients to either Gianturco–Roubin (GR)-II or PS stent implantation. At 30 days, the composite MACE rate was significantly higher in the GR-II group compared with the PS group (4.2% vs. 1.3%; $p < 0.01$). This difference was mostly owing to more frequent subacute stent thrombosis in the GR-II group (3.9% vs. 0.3%; $p = 0.001$). At 1 year, the TLR rate (primary end point) also was significantly higher in the GR-II group (27.4% vs. 15.3%; $p < 0.001$).

43. Baim DS, et al.; for the ASCENT Investigators (ACS MultLink Stent Clinical Equivalence in De Novo Lesions Trial). Final results of a randomized trial comparing the MULTI-LINK stent with the Palmaz–Schatz stent for narrowings in native coronary arteries. *Am J Cardiol* 2001;87:157–162.

This prospective, randomized, multicenter trial enrolled 1,040 patients with single, de novo native-vessel lesions. Patients received ACS MULTI-LINK (ML) stent or PS stent. At 30 days, no significant differences were found between the groups in MACEs [5.0% (ML) vs. 6.5%]. The primary end point of target vessel failure at 9 months occurred in 15.1% of ML-treated patients compared with 16.7% of PS-treated patients, with the ML proving to be equal or superior to the PS stent ($p < 0.001$ by test for equivalency). Angiographic restudy in a prespecified subgroup showed a nonsignificant trend toward reduced restenosis with the ML stent (16.0% vs. 22.1%).

PROVISIONAL STENTING

44. Weaver WD, et al. Optimum percutaneous transluminal coronary angioplasty compared with routine stent strategy trial (OPUS-1): a randomised trial. *Lancet* 2000;355:2199–2203.

Design: Prospective, randomized, open, multicenter study. Primary end point was death, MI, and TVR at 6 months.

Purpose: Whether routine implantation of coronary stents is the best strategy to treat flow-limiting coronary stenoses is unclear. An alternative approach is to do balloon angioplasty and provisionally use stents only to treat suboptimal results. The multicenter trial compared the outcomes of patients treated with these strategies.

Population: 479 patients aged 21 to 81 years with stable or unstable angina or MI more than 24 hours earlier and 70% coronary artery stenosis (≤ 2 mm length, vessel diameter ≥ 3 mm).

Treatment: Systematic stenting or provisional stenting (undertaken if >20% residual stenosis, impending abrupt closure, ≥ 2 mm stenosis, or flow-limiting dissection). IVUS was used at the physician's discretion. Abciximab was used in fewer than 15% of patients. All patients received aspirin and ticlopidine.

Results: Stents were implanted in 98.7% of the routine stenting group, whereas 37% of patients assigned to initial PTCA had more than one stent placed because of suboptimal angioplasty results. At 6 months, the primary stenting group had a significantly lower incidence of death, MI, or TVR (6.1% vs. 14.9%; $p = 0.003$). The majority of this benefit was owing to a lower TVR rate (4% vs. 10%; $p = 0.007$). The provisional stent group had higher initial costs, but the overall costs at 6 months were similar in both groups.

45. Lafont A, et al. The French Randomized Optimal Stenting Trial (FROST): a prospective evaluation of provisional stenting guided by coronary velocity reserve and quantitative coronary angiography. *J Am Coll Cardiol* 2000;36:404–409.

Design: Prospective, randomized, open, multicenter study. Primary end point was the 6-month angiographic MLD.

Purpose: To compare systematic stenting with provisional stenting guided by Doppler measurements of coronary velocity reserve and QCA.

Population: 251 patients undergoing elective PTCA.

Treatment: Provisional stenting (stenting performed if post-PTCA coronary velocity reserve was <2.2 and/or residual stenosis 35% or more or as bailout) or to systematic stenting.

Results: Stenting was performed in 48.4% of the provisional stenting group and all systematic stenting patients. At 6 months, no significant differences were found between the groups in MLD [1.90 mm (provisional) vs. 1.99 mm; $p = 0.39$] or binary restenosis rate (27.1% vs. 21.4%; $p = 0.37$). The rates of TLR and MACEs (death, acute MI, and TLR) were similar in both groups (15.1% vs. 14.4%; 15.1% vs. 16.0%).

46. Serruys PW; on behalf of Doppler Endpoints Balloon Angioplasty Trial Europe (DEBATE) II Study Group. Randomized comparison of primary stenting and provisional balloon angioplasty guided by flow velocity measurement. *Circulation* 2000;102:2930–2937.

Design: Prospective, randomized, double-blind, multicenter study. Primary end point was death, nonfatal MI, and TLR.

Purpose: To determine if provisional stenting is as effective as and less expensive than primary stenting.

Population: 620 patients scheduled to undergo angioplasty for stable or unstable angina pectoris and with documented myocardial ischemia due to a single de novo lesion shorter than 25 mm.

Exclusion Criteria: MI in prior week, total occlusion, ostial or bifurcation lesions, vessel with target lesion previously bypassed, and vessel tortuous or containing thrombus.

Treatment: Primary stenting or balloon angioplasty guided by Doppler flow velocity and angiography. Patients in the latter group were further randomized after optimization to either additional stenting or termination of the procedure. Optimal result defined as flow reserve >2.5 and diameter stenosis 35% or greater.

Results: Bailout stenting occurred in 25% of patients in the balloon angioplasty group. No differences were found between the two groups in event-free survival at 1 year (primary stenting, 86.6%; provisional angioplasty, 85.6%). Costs at 1 year were higher in the provisional angioplasty group (EUR 6573 vs. EUR 5885; $p = 0.014$), primarily because of longer hospitalizations and higher rate of surgical revascularization. After the second randomization, stenting was associated with better 1-year event-free survival after both optimal balloon angioplasty (93.5% vs. 84.1%; $p = 0.066$) and suboptimal balloon angioplasty (89.3% vs. 73.3%; $p = 0.005$).

Comments: An unexpected observation was a further reduction in MACEs in patients stented after optimal balloon angioplasty.

47. Di Mario C, et al. Randomized comparison of elective stent implantation and coronary balloon angioplasty and intracoronary Doppler. *Circulation* 2000;102:2938–2944.

Design: Prospective, randomized, double-blind, multicenter study. Primary end point was a composite of death, MI, and TLR at 1 year.

Purpose: To compare the outcomes of balloon angioplasty with provisional stenting with primary stenting.

Population: 738 patients with lesions suitable for stent implantation.

Exclusion Criteria: Recent MI (24 hours or less), prior MI with akinesis or dyskinesis in target vessel territory, chronic total occlusion, graft and ostial stenoses, second restenosis after PTCA, stent restenosis, and planned rotational or directional atherectomy.

Treatment: Elective stent implantations (370 patients, 386 lesions) or PTCA guided by QCA and Doppler coronary flow reserve (CFR) analysis (368 patients, 384 lesions). Balloon angioplasty result was considered "optimal" if the final lesion diameter by QCA was <35%; no type C through F dissections were found, and CFR distal to the stenosis was >2.0.

Results: Optimal PTCA was achieved in 166 (43%) lesions. The main reasons for suboptimal PTCA were CFR 2.0 or less (62% cases) and significant residual stenosis (44% of cases). At 1 year, no significant difference was found in the primary composite end point of death, MI, and TLR (17.8% in elective stent group and 18.9% in guided PTCA group). When compared with provisional stenting, *optimal* PTCA was associated with a similar incidence of TLR (17.6% vs. 14.1% for provisional stenting; $p = $ NS) and death, MI, and TLR (20.1% and 18.0%, respectively; $p = $ NS).

Comments: Optimal PTCA achieved only in 43% of cases. Capacity to measure CFR is not available in every interventional laboratory, and it requires both operator and laboratory experience.

DIRECT STENTING

48. Brito FS Jr, et al.; for The DIRECT Study Investigators. Comparison of direct stenting versus stenting with predilatation for the treatment of selected coronary narrowings. *Am J Cardiol* 2002;89:115–120.

This prospective, multicenter trial randomized 411 patients to direct stenting or balloon predilatation followed by stent implantation. Lesions with severe calcification were excluded. Angiographic success rates were 100% with direct stenting (2.8% requiring balloon predilatation) and 98.6% with routine predilatation ($p = 0.12$). Direct stenting was associated with decreased use of balloons and a trend toward reduced procedure time (22.7 vs. 25.6 minutes; $p = 0.07$). Fluoroscopy time and contrast volume were not different between groups. At 6 months, mortality, MI, and TVR rates were similar in both groups. MACE-free survival rates were 87.5% for direct stenting and 85.5% for the predilatation group ($p = 0.0002$ for equivalence).

49. Brueck M, et al. Direct coronary stenting versus predilatation followed by stent placement. *Am J Cardiol* 2002;90:1187–1192.

This prospective, randomized study enrolled 335 symptomatic patients with single or multiple coronary lesions (severity, 60% to 95%; length, 30 mm or shorter; diameter, 2.5 to 4.0 mm). Lesion exclusion criteria were excessive calcification, severe proximal tortuosity, and occlusion. Patients were assigned to direct stenting or stenting after predilatation. In the direct stent group, there was a 5% crossover rate to predilatation. Direct stenting was associated with shorter procedural time (42.1 vs. 51.5 minutes; $p = 0.004$), less radiation exposure time (10.3 vs. 12.5 minutes; $p = 0.002$), less contrast dye used (163 vs. 197 mL; $p < 0.0001$), and lower procedural costs. In-hospital complication rates were similar. At 6 months, direct stenting was associated with a lower rate of angiographic binary restenosis (20% vs. 31%; $p = 0.048$) and target lesion revascularization (18% vs. 28%; $p = 0.03$).

50. Dawkins KD, et al. Effectiveness of "direct" stenting without balloon predilatation (from the Multilink Tetra Randomised European Direct Stent Study [TRENDS]). *Am J Cardiol* 2006;97(3):316–21.

This prospective, randomized, multicenter trial of 1000 patients showed that direct stenting and stenting with predilatation yield comparable angiographic and clinical results. Both treatment groups had similar characteristics, with eccentric and type B lesions predominating. Exclusion criteria included chronic occlusions and unprotected left main stenoses. Only 5.7% of patients in the direct stenting group crossed over to predilatation; this was because of failure to cross the target lesion in 25 of 31 cases. At 6-month angiography, no difference was found between the groups in MLD [2.91 mm (direct stenting) vs. 2.95 mm] or binary restenosis (12.3% vs. 11.4%). Resource use was less with the direct stent approach, including shorter procedure time (34.3 minutes vs. 37.5 minutes; $p = 0.01$) and less contrast use (175 mL vs. 186 mL; $p = 0.05$). No significant difference was found between the groups in death, MI, and TLR.

DRUG-ELUTING STENTS

51. Serruys PW, et al. Coronary-artery stents. *N Engl J Med* 2006;354:483–495.

The authors provide a review of coronary stenting, specifically the genesis of implanting vascular stents, through to the pathophysiologic basis for DES and the clinical data to support their use.

52. Morice M-C, et al.; for the RAVEL (Randomized BX VELocity) Study Group. Randomized comparison of a sirolimus-eluting stent with a standard stent for coronary revascularization. N Engl J Med 2002;346:1773–1780.

Design: Prospective, randomized, double-blind, multicenter study. Primary end points were mean lumen diameter and late lumen loss at 6 months.

Purpose: To determine whether implantation of a sirolimus-eluting stent in de novo lesions will result in decreased restenosis compared with a bare stent.

Population: 238 patients with stable or unstable angina pectoris or silent ischemia who needed treatment of a single de novo lesion in a native vessel (2.5 to 3.5 mm or larger) that could be covered by a single 18-mm stent.

Exclusion Criteria: Included evolving MI, left main stenosis, ostial lesion location, calcified lesion that could not be completely dilated before stenting, angiographically visible thrombus within target lesion, and ejection fraction <30%.

Treatment: Sirolimus-eluting stent or uncoated BX Velocity balloon-expandable stent. All received ticlopidine or clopidogrel for 2 months.

Results: Rapamycin group had a mean late loss of 0.01 mm compared with 0.80 mm in the control group ($p < 0.0001$). Restenosis occurred in none of the rapamycin patients versus 26% of controls ($p < 0.0001$). Freedom from MACE (death, MI, repeated PCI, and CABG) was 96.7% in the rapamycin group compared with 72.9% in the control group ($p < 0.0001$). No cases of subacute stent thromboses were found.

53. Moses JW, et al.; for the Sirolimus-Eluting Stent in Coronary Lesions (SIRIUS) Investigators. Sirolimus-eluting stents versus standard stents in patients with stenosis in a native coronary artery. N Engl J Med 2003;349:1315–1323.

Design: Prospective, randomized, double-blind, placebo-controlled, study. Primary end point was target vessel failure defined as cardiac death, MI, or TVR at 9 months.

Purpose: To establish the safety and efficacy of the sirolimus-eluting BX Velocity stent in decreasing target vessel failure in de novo native coronary artery lesions compared with the uncoated BX Velocity stent.

Population: 1,058 patients requiring single-vessel treatment of de novo higher-risk lesions (2.5 to 3.5 mm diameter and 15 to 30 mm long) in native vessels. Of note, 26% had diabetes, and 42% had multivessel disease. Most lesions were type B2 or C.

Exclusion Criteria: Included recent MI (<24 hours), unprotected left main disease, ostial location, total occlusion, angiographic evidence of thrombus, calcified lesion that could not be predilated, left ventricular ejection fraction (LVEF) < 25%, impaired renal function, pretreatment with devices other than balloon angioplasty, and prior or planned intervention within 30 days.

Treatment: Sirolimus-eluting stent or uncoated stent. Antiplatelet therapy given for 3 months.

Results: Target vessel failure (primary end point) was reduced by nearly 60% in the sirolimus group compared with the BMS group (from 21.0% to 8.6%; $p < 0.001$). The sirolimus stent group had a 91% reduction in ISR compared with BMS (3.2% vs. 35.4%; $p < 0.001$). ISR, which included the 5-mm segments proximal and distal to the stent, was reduced by 75% in the sirolimus group (8.9% vs. 36.3%; $p < 0.001$). Among diabetics, restenosis in the stent and in the segment was 8.3% and 17.6%, respectively, for sirolimus, compared with 48.5% and 50.5% for the bare stent. The distal margin had an equal treatment effect to that seen within the stent, whereas there was less intense effect but still significant effect in the proximal margin (late loss, 0.17 mm vs. 0.33 mm; $p < 0.001$). ISR increased by 13% for every additional 10 mm of implanted stent length in controls, compared with only 1.6% in the sirolimus group. Aneurysms occurred in two (0.6%) patients in the sirolimus group and in four (1.1%) patients in the control group. Stent thrombosis rates were also similar (0.6% and 1.1%). An IVUS study of 141 patients found an overall 90% reduction in neointimal volume in the coated-stent group; the lowest reduction was seen at the proximal margin in smaller vessels.

Comments: SIRIUS cohort had more patients with clinical characteristics associated with higher rates of restenosis as well as more complex lesions than the RAVEL cohort. However, several types of lesions were still excluded (see earlier), and ongoing studies are addressing these issues. The proximal margin findings suggest that balloon injury in this area is associated with pre-/postdilatation or stent delivery. However, the above findings in SIRIUS were confirmed Canadian cohorts in C-SIRIUS (see *J Am Coll Cardiol* 2004;43:1110–1115), as well as European cohorts in E-SIRIUS (see *Lancet* 2003;362:1093–1099). Results of cost-effectiveness analysis of the SIRIUS trial did not find DES implantation to be consistently cost-effective (see *Circulation* 2004;110:508–514).

54. Caixeta A, et al. 5-Year clinical outcomes after sirolimus-eluting stent implantation insights from a patient-level pooled analysis of 4 randomized trials comparing sirolimus-eluting stents with bare-metal stents. *J Am Coll Cardiol* 2009;54:894–902.

This combination of four trials of SES versus BMS (RAVEL, SIRIUS, E-SIRIUS, and C-SIRIUS) included 1,748 patients with follow-up to 5 years. While there was no difference in the rate of death or MI (15.15% for SES vs. 13.6% for BMS; $p = 0.36$), TVR was significantly reduced in the SES group (15.2% vs. 30.1%; $p < 0.0001$). Notably, rates of stent thrombosis, using a variety of definitions, were not different at 5 years (definite/probable stent thrombosis at 5 years, 2.1% vs. 2.0%; $p = 0.99$), using the Academic Research Consortium definition.

55. ASPECT (Asian Paclitaxel-Eluting Stent Clinical Trial); Park SJ, et al. A paclitaxel eluting stent for the prevention of coronary restenosis. *N Engl J Med* 2003;348:1537–1545.

This prospective, randomized, triple-blind, multicenter study enrolled 177 patients with discrete coronary lesions (<15 mm in length, 2.25 to 3.25 mm in diameter). Patients received a low-dose (1.3 μg/mm^2) or high-dose (3.1 μg/mm^2) paclitaxel mounted on a nonpolymerized stent or a BMS. At 4- to 6-month angiographic follow-up, the high-dose group had better results for the degree of stenosis (mean 14% vs. 39%; $p < 0.001$), late loss of luminal diameter (0.29 mm vs. 1.04 mm; $p < 0.001$), and binary restenosis (4% vs. 27%; $p < 0.001$).

56. Colomboa A, et al.; for the TAXUS II Study Group. Randomized study to assess the effectiveness of slow- and moderate-release polymer-based paclitaxel-eluting stents for coronary artery lesions. *Circulation* 2003;108:788–794.

This prospective, randomized, multicenter trial enrolled a total of 536 patients and compared a bare stent with two formulations of a paclitaxel-eluting stent [slow release (drug released over a 1-month period) or moderate release (most released in the first 2 days)]. Lesions were standard-risk de novo lesions (average length, approximately 10 mm; average reference vessel diameter, approximately 2.75 mm). Patients received aspirin and clopidogrel for 6 months. Both paclitaxel-eluting stents demonstrated substantial reductions in the primary end point, percentage of in-stent net volume obstruction (by IVUS), compared with the bare stent group (60% reduction with slow-release version and 62% with moderate-release version). At 12 months, MACE was significantly reduced with the DES [slow release, 10.9% vs. 22.0% (control); $p = 0.02$; moderate release, 9.9% vs. 21.4%; $p = 0.017$]. These reductions were driven by lower rates of TVR (slow release, 10.1% vs. 15.9%; $p = 0.20$; moderate release, 6.9% vs. 19.1%; $p = 0.005$) and TLR (slow release, 4.7% vs. 12.9%; $p = 0.03$; moderate release, 3.8% vs. 16.0%; $p = 0.002$). Importantly, no sign of edge effect was found, with nonsignificant *reductions* seen both in the proximal and in the distal segments of the segment with the DES versus controls.

57. Stone G, et al.; for the TAXUS IV Investigators. A polymer-based, paclitaxel-eluting stent in patients with coronary artery disease. N Engl J Med 2004;350:221–231.

This prospective randomized, multicenter trial enrolled 1,314 patients undergoing stenting for de novo lesions and assigned them to either a BMS or slow-release PES, in a double-blind fashion. Angiographic follow-up at 9 months was prespecified in 732 patients. At 9 months, incidence of ischemia-driven TVR was 12% for the BMS group and 4.7% for the PES group ($p < 0.001$). Rates of TLR (11.3% vs. 3.0%; $p < 0.001$) and binary angiographic restenosis (26.6% vs. 7.9%; $p < 0.001$) were also significantly reduced. However, rates of death or MI and stent thrombosis were similar.

58. Malenka DJ, et al. Outcomes following coronary stenting in the era of bare-metal vs the era of drug-eluting stents. JAMA 2008;299(24):2868–2876.

This observational study included 38,917 Medicare patients who received BMS prior to the release of DES and 28,068 who underwent stenting after DES came about (61.5% received DES, 38.5% BMS). After risk adjustment, rates of repeat revascularizations at 2 years were significantly lower for patients treated in the DES era (HR, 0.82; 95% CI, 0.79 to 0.85). Composite death or STEMI at 2 years was similar (HR, 0.96; 95% CI, 0.92 to 1.01).

59. Stone G, et al.; for the TAXUS V Investigators. Comparison of a polymer-based paclitaxel-eluting stent with a bare metal stent in patients with complex coronary artery disease: a randomized controlled trial. JAMA 2005;294:1215–1223.

Design: Prospective, randomized, double-blind, placebo-controlled, multicenter study. Primary end point was ischemia-driven TVR at 9 months.

Purpose: To establish the safety and efficacy of PES in more complex lesions, specifically those with narrower, longer stenoses and those requiring multiple stents.

Population: 1,156 patients with de novo lesions of a single coronary artery, without evidence of recent MI.

Treatment: Paclitaxel-eluting stent or uncoated stent. Antiplatelet therapy given for 6 months.

Results: Rates of the primary end point, TVR, were significantly reduced in the PES group (17.3% vs. 12.1%; $p = 0.02$), as were rates of TLR (15.7% vs. 8.6%; $p < 0.001$). Overall, 78% of lesions were B2/C, and patients received a mean of 1.38 stents with an average reference vessel diameter of 2.69 mm and a lesion length of 17.2 mm. Binary angiographic restenosis was reduced in the PES group (33.9% vs. 18.9%; $p < 0.001$), and this was a consistent effect for smaller vessels, larger vessels, as well as patients who received multiple stents. There were no differences in the rates of death or MI (5.5% vs. 5.7%) or stent thrombosis (0.7% for both).

60. Marroquin OC, et al. A comparison of bare-metal and drug-eluting stents for off-label indications. N Engl J Med 2008;358:342–352.

In this observational study of 6,551 patients in the National Heart, Lung, and Blood Institute Dynamic Registry, the investigators looked at 1-year outcomes in patients who received either BMS or DES, and whether their use was off-label. This included stenting for restenosis, bypass groups, left main disease, and ostial, bifurcated, or totally occluded lesions or stenting in vessels with reference diameter of <2.5 mm, more than 3.75, or longer than 30 mm. This off-label use occurred in 54.7% of patients who received BMS and 48.7% of those who got DES. Those who received stents for an off-label indication had higher unadjusted 1-year mortality (5.3% vs. 2.7%; $p < 0.001$) and rates of MI (5.3% vs. 3.8%; $p = 0.0002$). However, these were lower for the DES off-label group, compared with the BMS off-label group. Overall, after risk adjustment, rates of death or MI were no different for the DES group, compared with the BMS group. There were significantly lower rates of repeat PCI or revascularization in patients who received DES.

61. James SK, et al. Long-term safety and efficacy of drug-eluting versus bare-metal stents in Sweden. N Engl J Med 2009;360:1933–1945.

In a countrywide registry of patients undergoing PCI, the investigators examined 47,967 patients who received coronary stents, with mean follow-up of 2.7 years. In comparison between patients who received a single BMS (18,659) to those who received a single DES (10,294), there were no differences in the rates of death or MI, after risk adjustment. Rates of restenosis were significantly lower in the DES cohort (3.0 per 100 patient-years vs. 4.7; RR, 0.43; 95% CI, 0.36 to 0.52).

62. De Luca G, et al. Efficacy and safety of drug-eluting stents in ST-segment elevation myocardial infarction: a meta-analysis of randomized trials. Int J Cardiol 2009;133:213–22.

The authors combined 11 trials of DES versus BMS for primary PCI in STEMI, encompassing 3,605 patients. All trials had end points up to 12 months, and there were no differences in the combined rates of death (4.1% for DES vs. 4.4% for BMS; $p = 0.59$), recurrent MI (3.1% vs. 3.4%; $p = 0.38$), or stent thrombosis (1.6% vs. 2.2%; $p = 0.22$). Patients who got DES had significantly lower rates of TVR (5.0% vs. 12.6%; $p < 0.0001$). In a subset of four trials of 1,178, these outcomes were similar up to 18 to 24 months.

63. Stone GW, et al. Safety and efficacy of sirolimus- and paclitaxel-eluting coronary stents. N Engl J Med 2007;356:998–1008.

The investigators combined data from the early nine randomized trials of both SES (1,748 patients) and PES (3,513 patients) to assess clinical end points and, specifically, rates of late stent thrombosis in DES. At 4 years of follow-up, rates of death or MI were similar among the groups of SES, PES, and BMS; TLR rates were significantly lower in the DES groups, compared with the BMS groups. However, after 4 years, there were more stent thromboses in the SES group (1.2%) compared with the BMS group (0.9%; $p = 0.20$), as well as the PES group (1.3%; $p = 0.30$). Notably, of the five patients in the SES group who had stent thromboses within 1 year, only two were taking aspirin and clopidogrel, whereas two were taking only aspirin and one was taking no antiplatelet agent at all. Similarly, in the PES group of nine patients with late stent thromboses, three were only taking aspirin and five were taking no antiplatelet agents at all (the medication status of one patient was unknown). Subsequently, guidelines have been updated to recommend a minimum of 1 year of dual antiplatelet therapy (aspirin plus a thienopyridine) following any DES implant.

64. Fajadet J, et al.; for the ENDEAVOR II Investigators. Randomized, double-blind, multicenter study of the endeavor zotarolimus-eluting phosphorylcholine-encapsulated stent for treatment of native coronary artery lesions: clinical and angiographic results of the ENDEAVOR II trial. Circulation 2006;114:798–806.

This prospective, randomized, double-blind study assigned 1,197 patients with single, de novo coronary lesions to receive either a ZES or similar BMS. Mean reference vessel diameter was 2.75 mm and mean lesion length was 14.2 mm. At 9 months, the primary end point of target vessel failure was lower in the ZES group (7.9% vs. 15.1%; $p = 0.0001$), as were rates of TLR (4.6% vs. 11.8%; $p = 0.0001$). In a subset of 531 patients with follow-up angiography, restenosis was lower for the ZES group (13.2% vs. 35%; $p < 0.0001$).

65. Kandzari DE, et al.; for the ENDEAVOR III Investigators. Comparison of zotarolimus-eluting and sirolimus-eluting stents in patients with native coronary artery disease: a randomized controlled trial. J Am Coll Cardiol 2006;48:2440–2447.

The investigators randomized 436 patients undergoing PCI for stable de novo, native coronary lesions in a 3:1 fashion to receive either a new ZES or older SES. Primary end point was in-segment late lumen loss at 8-month angiography. This was significantly higher in the ZES group (0.34 mm vs. 0.13 mm; $p < 0.001$), as was binary in-segment restenosis (11.7% vs. 4.3%; $p = 0.04$). Rates of clinically driven TLR and target vessel failure were similar between the ZES and SES groups. However, in-hospital MACE rates were lower in the ZES group (0.6% vs. 3.5%; $p = 0.04$).

66. Leon MB, et al. A randomized comparison of the Endeavor zotarolimus-eluting stent versus the TAXUS paclitaxel-eluting stent in de novo native coronary lesions 12-month outcomes from the ENDEAVOR IV trial. *J Am Coll Cardiol* 2010;55(6):543–554.

Prospective, randomized, single-blind, multicenter controlled trial, which randomized 1,548 patients with single de novo coronary lesions to ZES versus paclitaxel-eluting stents. The primary end point was noninferiority of 9-month target vessel failure defined as cardiac death, MI, or TVR. ZES was noninferior to PES with rates of target vessel failure 6.6% versus 7.1%, respectively (noninferiority $p \leq 0.001$).

67. Serruys PW, et al. Comparison of Zotarolimus-Eluting and Everolimus-Eluting Coronary Stents (Resolute All-Comers trial). *N Engl J Med* 2010;363:136–146.

Design: Prospective, randomized, multicenter, noninferiority trial comparing Resolute ZES to Xience V EES. The primary end point was target lesion failure, defined as a composite of death from cardiac causes, any MI, or clinically indicated target lesion revascularization within 12 months.

Purpose: To compare two second-generation stents with two different drug coatings, ZES and EES, and evaluation noninferiority.

Population: 2,292 patients with stable ischemic heart disease or ACS with minimal exclusion criteria.

Major Exclusion Criteria: Known intolerance to a study drug/metal alloys/contrast media, planned surgery within 6 months, or participation in another trial prior to reaching the primary end point.

Results: The primary end point occurred in 8.2% of the ZES group and in 8.3% of the EES group ($p = 0.92$; noninferiority $p < 0.001$).

Comment: Rates of definite stent thrombosis occurred significantly more frequently in the ZES group (1.2% vs. 0.3%; $p = 0.01$), but the number of events was small and the study was not powered for this outcome.

68. von Biergelen C, et al. A Randomized Controlled Trial in Second-Generation Zotarolimus-Eluting Resolute Stents Versus Everolimus-Eluting Xience V Stents in Real-World Patients (The TWENTE Trial). *J Am Coll Cardiol* 2012;59:1350–1361.

The investigators randomized 1,391 patients with stable ischemic heart disease or UA/NSTEMI (STEMI was one of the few exclusion criteria) to Resolute ZES versus Xience V EES. The primary end point was target vessel failure, defined as a composite of cardiac death/MI/clinically indicated TVR, at 12 months. There was no significant difference between the groups (8.2% ZES vs. 8.1% EES, noninferiority $p = 0.001$). Between Resolute ZES and Xience V EES groups, there was also no difference in the components of the primary endpoint: cardiac death (1.0% vs. 1.4%; $p = 0.46$), target vessel–related MI (4.6% vs. 4.6%; $p = 0.99$), and clinically driven TVR at 12-month follow-up (3.3% vs. 2.7%; $p = 0.54$).

69. Stone G, et al.; for the SPIRIT III Investigators. Comparison of an everolimus-eluting stent and a paclitaxel-eluting stent in patients with coronary artery disease: a randomized trial. *JAMA* 2008;299:1903–1913.

Design: Prospective, randomized, single-blind study. Primary end point was in-segment late lumen loss on follow-up angiography at 8 months.

Purpose: To compare a contemporary EES to an older PES.

Population: 1,002 patients with stable CAD undergoing PCI for lesions <28 mm in length and with reference vessel diameter between 2.5 and 3.75 mm.

Results: Late lumen loss was significantly lower for patients in the EES group versus PES (0.14 mm vs. 0.28 mm, $p \leq 0.004$). At 9 months, target vessel failure was similar (7.2% vs. 9.0%, p for noninferiority < 0.001). Based on fewer MIs and a lower rate of TVR, MACE rates were lower in the EES group at 9 months (4.6% vs. 8.1%; $p = 0.03$) and 1 year (6.0% vs. 10.3%; $p = 0.02$).

Comment: At 2-year follow-up, clinical outcomes continued to favor the EES group, including rates of stent thrombosis (see *Circulation* 2009;119:680–686). Results of the upcoming SPIRIT IV trial similarly favored EES over PES with a significantly lower rate of target lesion failure 4.2% vs. 6.8% and relative risk 0.62 $p = 0.001$. Stone et al. *NEJM* 2010;362:1663–1674.

70. von Birgelen C, et al. Third-generation zotarolimus-eluting and everolimus-eluting stents in all-comer patients requiring a percutaneous coronary intervention (DUTCH PEERS): a randomised, single-blind, multicentre, non-inferiority trial. *Lancet* 2014;383(9915):413.

Prospective, randomized, multicenter, single-blinded trial comparing Resolute Integrity ZES versus Promus Element EES in 1811 all-comer patients. The primary end point was target vessel failure, a composite of safety (cardiac death or target vessel–related MI) and efficacy (TVR) at 12 months. The primary end point was not significantly different between the two groups (6% ZES vs. 5% EES; $p = 0.42$). Notably, the Promus Element stent was more susceptible to longitudinal stent deformation, prompting Boston Scientific to release the Promus Premier stent with strut reinforcement to help correct the problem.

71. Ormiston JA, et al. A bioabsorbable everolimus-eluting coronary stent system for patients with single de-novo coronary artery lesions (ABSORB): a prospective open-label trial. *Lancet* 2008;371:899–907.

In a prospective, open-label fashion, the investigators implanted a novel absorbable EES in 30 patients with stable, de novo coronary artery lesions. Previous studies had indicated 30% absorption (loss of stent mass) at 12 months and 60% at 18 months. Stent sizes were limited to either 3.0 × 12 mm or 3.0 × 18 mm. One-year event rates were low, with only one patient (3.3%) experiencing MI, and there were no TLRs or late stent thromboses. In-stent late loss was 0.44 mm on IVUS. Clinical events were confirmed in further analyses at 2 years, at which time the stent was bioabsorbed (see *Lancet* 2009;373:897–910).

72. Vavry AA, et al. Appropriate use of drug-eluting stents: balancing the reduction in restenosis with the concern of late thrombosis. *Lancet* 2008;371:2134–2143.

In light of significant data on late stent thromboses in patients who received DES without long-term dual-antiplatelet therapy, the authors review the indications for stenting as well as highlight patients who may be more appropriate for bare-metal stenting (e.g., those with poor access to medicines, at increased bleeding risk, or those likely to undergo invasive procedures in the near future). They emphasize the more-than-acceptable outcomes with BMS, specifically in patients at lower risk for ISR.

Additional Devices/Techniques

CUTTING BALLOON

73. Izumi M, et al. Final results of the CAPAS trial. *Am Heart J* 2001;142:782–789.

A total of 248 type B/C lesions in small vessels (smaller than 3 mm diameter) were randomly assigned to cutting balloon angioplasty (CBA) or conventional balloon angioplasty (PTCA). At follow-up angiography (3 months), restenosis was significantly lower in the CBA group compared with the PTCA group (25.2% vs. 41.5%; $p = 0.009$). At 1 year, the event-free survival rate was 72.8% in the cutting balloon group and 61.0% in the PTCA group ($p = 0.047$).

74. Adamian M, et al. Cutting balloon angioplasty for the treatment of in-stent restenosis: a matched comparison with rotational atherectomy, additional stent implantation and balloon angioplasty. *J Am Coll Cardiol* 2001;38:672–679.

A total of 648 lesions with ISR were divided into four groups according to treatment strategy: CBA, RA, additional stenting, and PTCA. After the matching process, 258 lesions were entered into the analysis. Acute lumen gain was significantly higher in the stent group (2.12 mm) compared with the CBA, RA, and PTCA groups (1.70 mm, 1.79 mm, and 1.56 mm, respectively). However, the lumen loss at follow-up was lower for the CBA versus RA and stent groups (0.63 mm vs. 1.30 mm and 1.36 mm, respectively; $p < 0.0001$), resulting in a lower recurrent restenosis rate in CBA group (20% vs. 35.9% and 41.4%, respectively; $p < 0.05$). By multivariate analysis, predictors of TLR were CBA (OR, 0.17; $p = 0.001$) and diffuse restenosis at baseline (OR, 2.07; $p = 0.02$).

75. Mauri L, et al. Cutting balloon angioplasty for the prevention of restenosis: results of the Cutting Balloon Global Randomized Trial. *Am J Cardiol* 2002;90:1079–1083.

This prospective, multicenter center randomized 1,238 patients to CB treatment or standard PTCA. At 6 months, binary angiographic restenosis rates (primary end point) were 31.4% for CB and 30.4% for PTCA. Freedom from TVR was slightly higher in the CB group (88.5% vs. 84.6%; log-rank $p = 0.04$). Coronary perforations occurred only in CB arm (0.8% vs. none; $p = 0.03$). At 270 days, the rates of MI, death, and total MACEs for CB and PTCA were 4.7% versus 2.4% ($p = 0.03$), 1.3% versus 0.3% ($p = 0.06$), and 13.6% versus 15.1% ($p = 0.34$), respectively.

76. Albiero R, et al. Cutting balloon versus conventional balloon angioplasty for the treatment of in-stent restenosis: results of the restenosis cutting balloon evaluation trial (RESCUT). *J Am Coll Cardiol* 2004;43(6):943–949.

This prospective, randomized trial was conducted at 23 European centers and enrolled 428 patients with ISR of all types, the majority of which were short (<20 mm) lesions. Patients were assigned to CB or standard balloon angioplasty (PTCA). Total number of balloons used was less in the CB group, and a single balloon was used more often in the CB group (82.3% for CB vs. 75% for PTCA; $p = 0.03$). Balloon slippage also occurred much less often with the CB (6.5% vs. 25.%; $p < 0.01$), and there was a trend toward less stenting in the CB group (3.9% vs. 8.0%; $p = 0.07$). However, at 7 months, no significant differences were found between the CB and PTCA groups in the rates of binary restenosis by QCA (29.8% vs. 31.4%; $p = 0.82$) or a clinical event composite of death, MI, or TLR (16.4% vs. 15.4%; $p = 0.79$).

77. REDUCE II (Restenosis Reduction by Cutting Balloon Evaluation). Preliminary results presented at Transcatheter Cardiovascular Therapeutics meeting, Washington, DC September 2002 [not subsequently published].

This prospective, randomized, multicenter trial enrolled 466 patients with ISR. Patients were treated with the CB or a standard balloon. Procedural results were similar with both balloons, with no significant differences in QCA parameters. The CB group had a lower incidence of in-hospital death, MI, or TLR (4.0% vs. 8.2% for the standard balloon; $p = 0.049$). However, at 6-month angiographic follow-up, no significant differences were found between the groups in the rates of binary restenosis, percentage stenosis, and MLD.

78. Bittl JA, et al. Meta-analysis of randomized trials of percutaneous transluminal coronary angioplasty versus atherectomy, cutting balloon atherotomy, or laser angioplasty. *J Am Coll Cardiol* 2004;43:936–942.

The authors review 16 trials of 9,222 patients to compare balloon angioplasty versus coronary atherectomy, laser angioplasty, or cutting balloon atherotomy. End points throughout the trials included both angiography improvement and clinical events. None of the adjunctive procedures improved 30-day mortality (OR, 0.94; 95% CI, 0.46 to 1.92), angiographic restenosis rates (OR, 1.06; 95% CI, 0.97 to 1.17), repeat revascularization

(OR, 1.04; 95% CI, 0.94 to 1.14), or cumulative adverse cardiac events at 1 year (OR, 1.09; 95% CI, 0.99 to 1.20). There was an early (30-day), significant increase in periprocedural MI (OR, 1.83; 95% CI, 1.43 to 2.34) and MACEs (OR, 1.54; 95% CI, 1.25 to 1.89) in the adjunctive procedures group.

ATHERECTOMY STUDIES

79. Topol EJ, et al.; Coronary Angioplasty versus Excisional Atherectomy Trial (CAVEAT). A comparison of directional atherectomy with coronary angioplasty in patients with coronary artery disease. N Engl J Med 1993;329:221–227.

Design: Prospective, randomized, controlled, multicenter study. Primary end point was angiographic restenosis at 6 months.

Purpose: To compare outcomes in patients undergoing balloon angioplasty (PTCA) with those having DCA.

Population: 1,012 patients with symptomatic CAD and no prior intracoronary interventions.

Treatment: PTCA or DCA.

Results: The atherectomy group had a higher initial success rate ($\leq$50% stenosis; 89% vs. 80%) but was associated with a higher rate of early complications (11% vs. 5%) and higher hospital costs. At 6-month angiography, the atherectomy group showed a trend toward lower restenosis (50% vs. 57%; $p = 0.06$) and a higher probability of death or MI (8.6% vs. 4.6%; $p = 0$).

80. Adelman AG, et al.; Canadian Coronary Atherectomy Trial (CCAT). A comparison of directional atherectomy with balloon angioplasty for lesions of the left anterior descending coronary artery. N Engl J Med 1993;329:228–233.

Design: Prospective, randomized, open-label, multicenter study. Primary end point was restenosis at follow-up angiography (median, 5.9 months).

Purpose: To compare restenosis rates for balloon angioplasty and directional atherectomy in lesions of the proximal LAD artery.

Population: 274 patients with de novo 60% stenosis of the LAD artery.

Treatment: Balloon angioplasty or directional atherectomy.

Results: Atherectomy group had a nonsignificantly higher success rate (94% vs. 88%; $p = 0.06$); no difference in complication rates was observed (5% vs. 6%). At follow-up angiography, restenosis rates and MLDs were similar [43% (angioplasty) vs. 46% (atherectomy); 1.61 vs. 1.55 mm].

81. Simonton CA, et al. Optimal directional atherectomy: final results of the Optimal Atherectomy Restenosis Study (OARS). Circulation 1998;97:332–339.

Design: Prospective, multicenter registry study. Primary end point was angiographic restenosis at 6 months.

Purpose: To determine if use of an optimal atherectomy technique would translate into a lower rate of late clinical and angiographic restenosis.

Population: 199 patients aged 18 to 80 years with angina or a positive functional study and after angiographic criteria: (a) target vessel reference diameter, 3.0 to 4.5 mm; (b) culprit lesion(s) with 60% stenosis; and (c) mild to moderate tortuosity and mild or no target lesion calcification. DCA and adjunctive angioplasty were performed if necessary to achieve <15% residual stenosis; 213 lesions met the criteria.

Treatment: DCA (7-F device).

Results: Frequent (87%) postatherectomy angioplasty was performed. The short-term procedural success rate was 97.5%. The mean rate of residual stenosis was only 7%.

The major complication rate was 2.5% (death, emergency bypass surgery, Q-wave MI). Non–Q-wave MI (CK-MB more than three times normal) occurred in 14%. At 1-year follow-up, the TLR rate was 17.8%. The 6-month restenosis rate was 28.9% (major predictor: smaller postprocedural lumen diameter).

Comments: A lower restenosis rate was observed than in prior directional atherectomy trials.

82. Baim DS, et al.; for the Balloon vs Optimal Atherectomy Trial (BOAT) Investigators. Final results of the Balloon vs. Optimal Atherectomy Trial (BOAT). Circulation 1998;97:322–331.

Design: Prospective, randomized, double-blind, multicenter study. Primary end point was restenosis rate at follow-up angiography (median, 6.9 months).

Purpose: To compare the optimal DCA technique with conventional balloon angioplasty on restenosis.

Population: 1,000 patients with single de novo, native-vessel lesions in vessels larger than 3 mm in diameter.

Treatment: DCA (large device used) with aggressive tissue removal and use of adjunctive PTCA if indicated or PTCA alone.

Results: DCA group had a higher procedural success rate (99% vs. 97%; $p = 0.02$) and a lower rate of residual stenosis (15% vs. 28%; $p < 0.0001$). Similar rates of major complication were observed (2.8% vs. 3.3%). However, DCA was associated with more frequent CK-MB elevations (more than three times normal; 16% vs. 6%; $p < 0.0001$). At follow-up angiography, the DCA group had a lower restenosis rate (primary end point): 31.4% versus 39.8% ($p = 0.016$). At 1-year follow-up, the DCA group had nonsignificant reductions in mortality (0.6% vs. 1.6%; $p = 0.14$), TVR (17.1% vs. 19.7%; $p = 0.33$), target site revascularization (15.3% vs. 18.3%; $p = 0.23$), and target vessel failure (death, Q-wave MI, or TVR; 21.1% vs. 24.8%; $p = 0.17$).

83. Dill T, et al. A randomized comparison of balloon angioplasty versus rotational atherectomy in complex coronary lesions (COBRA study). Eur Heart J 2000;21:1759–1766.

Design: Prospective, randomized, open-label, multicenter study. Primary end points were procedural success, 6-month restenosis rates in the treated segments, and major cardiac events during follow-up.

Purpose: To compare outcomes between RA and balloon angioplasty for the treatment of complex coronary artery lesions.

Population: 502 patients aged 20 to 80 years with angina and angiographic CAD with target lesion stenosis of 70% to 99% and mean lumen diameter of 1 mm or less for a length of 5 mm or more. Lesions were required to be complex (calcified, ostial or bifurcational, eccentric, diffuse, or within angulated segment).

Exclusion Criteria: Unstable angina, MI in previous 4 weeks, prior PCI of target vessel within 2 months, and LVEF < 30%.

Treatment: Rotablation (burr sizes, 1.25 to 2.5) or balloon angioplasty. All received ASA, nitroglycerin, nifedipine, and heparin (15 to 20 KU with target ACT, 350 seconds or more). Stenting allowed bailout for unsatisfactory outcomes.

Results: Procedural success was achieved more frequently with rotablation compared with angioplasty (85% vs. 78%; $p = 0.038$). No difference was found between PTCA and rotablation with respect to procedure-related complications such as Q-wave infarctions (both groups, 2.4%), emergency bypass surgery (1.2% vs. 2.4%), and death (1.6% vs. 0.4%). A higher incidence of stenting occurred after PTCA (14.9% vs. 6.4%; $p < 0.002$), mostly because of bailout or unsatisfactory results. If bailout stenting is included as an end point, procedural success rates were 84% for rotablation and were 73% for angioplasty ($p = 0.006$). At 6 months, the restenosis rates were similar in both groups (rotablation, 49%; PTCA, 51%).

84. vom Dahl J, et al. Rotational atherectomy does not reduce recurrent in-stent restenosis: results of the Angioplasty Versus Rotational Atherectomy for Treatment of Diffuse In-Stent Restenosis Trial (ARTIST). *Circulation* 2002;105:583–588.

Design: Prospective, randomized, multicenter (24 European sites). Primary end point was MLD assessed by QCA at 6 months.

Purpose: To determine the safety and efficacy of RA with balloon angioplasty (PTCA) compared with PTCA alone for the treatment of diffuse ISR.

Population: 298 patients with angina and/or objective evidence of target vessel–related ischemia and all of the following: documented ISR more than 70% within a stent ±5 mm of stent edges, stent diameter 2.5 mm or more, ISR as only lesion for treatment, length of ISR of 10 to 50 mm, and lesion accessible for rotablation.

Treatment: RA with PTCA or PTCA alone. Rotablation was performed by using a stepped-burr approach followed by adjunctive PTCA with low (6 atm) inflation pressure. Use of GP IIb/IIIa inhibitors was discouraged.

Results: Initial procedural success rates (residual stenosis <30%) were similar in both groups (89% PTCA, 88% RA). However, at 6-month angiography, the PTCA group had superior results with a mean net gain in MLD of 0.67 mm versus 0.45 mm for RA ($p = 0.0019$). The mean gain in diameter of stenosis was 25% and 17% ($p = 0.002$), resulting in binary restenosis rates of 51% (PTCA) and 65% (RA; $p = 0.039$). Six-month event-free survival also was significantly higher after PTCA (91.3%) compared with RA (79.6%; $p = 0.0052$).

85. Stankovic G, et al.; AMIGO Investigators. Comparison of directional coronary atherectomy and stenting versus stenting alone for the treatment of de novo and restenotic coronary artery narrowing. *J Am Coll Cardiol* 2004;93:9.

This prospective, multicenter (46 European sites) study randomized 753 patients to DCA plus stenting or stenting alone. The average lesion length was 14.6 mm in the DCA/stent group and 14.3 mm in the stent-only group. At 8 months, no significant overall difference was found in binary restenosis rates, in the subgroup (74%) with follow-up angiography available (26.7% in DCA/stent group vs. 22.1% in the stent-only group; $p = $ NS). Rates of mortality (1.3% vs. 0.8%; $p = 0.725$) and target vessel failure, the composite of death, MI, or TVR (23.9% vs. 21.5%; $p = 0.487$) were similar between the two groups at 12 months.

RADIATION THERAPY

86. Teirstein PS, et al.; Scripps Coronary Radiation to Inhibit Proliferation Post-Stenting (SCRIPPS). Catheter-based radiotherapy to inhibit restenosis after coronary stenting. *N Engl J Med* 1997;336:1697–1703 (editorial, 1748–1749).

Fifty-five patients with restenosis (in-stent, 62%) were randomized to [192]Ir (20- to 45-minute exposure; dose of 800 to 3,000 cGy) or placebo. The iridium group had less diabetes mellitus. Angiographic follow-up in 53 patients at 6.7 ± 2.2 months showed that the iridium group had a larger mean luminal diameter (2.43 vs. 1.85 mm; $p = 0.02$) and an impressive 69% lower restenosis rate (17% vs. 54%; $p = 0.01$). No apparent complications were seen with iridium use, although long-term follow-up is necessary. At 2-year follow-up, the incidence of death, MI, or TLR was 55% lower in the radiation group (23.1% vs. 51.7%; $p = 0.03$). Most of this benefit was owing to a 75% lower TLR rate (15.4% vs. 44.8%; $p < 0.001$).

87. Waksman R, et al.; Washington Radiation for In-Stent Restenosis Trial (WRIST). Intracoronary γ-radiation therapy after angioplasty inhibits recurrence in patients with in-stent restenosis. *Circulation* 2000;101:2165–2171.

Design: Prospective, randomized, blinded, placebo-controlled study. Primary clinical end point was cumulative composite of death, MI, and repeated TLR.

Purpose: To evaluate the effectiveness of gamma radiation as adjunctive therapy for patients with ISR.

Population: 130 patients with ISR in native coronary arteries ($n = 100$) and SVGs ($n = 30$) with reference diameter 3.0 to 5.0 mm and lesion length <47 mm.

Treatment: Catheter-delivered gamma radiation (^{192}Ir source; mean dwell time, 22 minutes) or placebo.

Results: At 6 months, the radiation therapy group had a significant reduction in the primary composite end point of death, MI, and TLR (29.2% vs. 67.6%; $p < 0.001$), primarily owing to a lower TLR rate (13.8% vs. 63.1%; $p < 0.001$). The death rates were 4.6% in the radiated group and 6.2% in the nonradiated groups; no patients had Q-wave infarcts. TLR also was lower in the radiation group (13.8%) versus the placebo group (63.1%), and the same pattern was seen at 12 months.

Comment: Most restenosis in the radiation group occurred at the edges of the stent.

88. Leon MB, et al.; GAMMA-1. Localized intracoronary gamma-radiation therapy to inhibit the recurrence of restenosis after stenting. N *Engl J Med* 2001;344: 250–256.

Design: Prospective, randomized, double-blind, multicenter study. Primary composite end point was death, MI, emergency CABG, or need for TLR at 9 months.

Purpose: To assess whether gamma radiation can prevent ISR.

Population: 252 patients with 60% restenosis of stented native vessels 2.75 to 4 mm in diameter and lesion length ≤45 mm.

Exclusion Criteria: Included MI in prior 72 hours, visible thrombus, ejection fraction <40%, and anticipated abciximab administration (actual use, <10%).

Treatment: Gamma radiation by using an ^{192}Ir ribbon or placebo. Lesions were irradiated with 800 to 3,000 cGy used (6, 10, or 14 seeds); delivery device dwell time was approximately 20 minutes. Most treated lesions (more than 70%) were complex (type B2 or C).

Results: Radiation group had a 58% lower stent restenosis rate ($p < 0.001$). At 9 months, the radiation group also had a significantly lower incidence of primary composite end point compared with the placebo group (28.2% vs. 43.8%; $p = 0.02$). Late thrombosis occurred in 5.3% (^{192}Ir) versus 0.8% (placebo; $p = 0.07$). A subsequent cost-effectiveness study found that initial costs were increased by nearly $4,100 per patient ($15,724 vs. $11,675; $p < 0.001$) and by $2,200 per patient at 1 year. However, if late thrombosis can be eliminated with extended antiplatelet therapy, long-term medical care costs will likely be lower with brachytherapy (see *Circulation* 2002;106:691–697).

89. Waksman R, et al.; WRIST PLUS. Prolonged antiplatelet therapy to prevent late thrombosis after intracoronary gamma-radiation in patients with in-stent restenosis. *Circulation* 2001;103:2332–2335.

A total of 120 consecutive patients with diffuse ISR in native coronary arteries and vein grafts with lesions smaller than 80 mm underwent PCI, including stenting in 28.3%. After PCI, gamma radiation was administered (^{192}Ir seeds; 14 Gy to 2 mm). All received clopidogrel for 6 months. Late occlusion and thrombosis rates were compared with the 125 gamma radiation–treated patients and 126 placebo patients from WRIST and LONG WRIST (only 1 month of antiplatelet therapy). At 6 months, prolonged antiplatelet therapy resulted in total occlusion in 5.8%, and late thrombosis, in 2.5%; these rates were lower than those in the active gamma radiation group and similar to those in the placebo historical control group.

90. Waksman R, et al.; WRIST 12. Twelve versus six months of clopidogrel to reduce major cardiac events in patients undergoing gamma-radiation therapy for in-stent restenosis. *Circulation* 2002;106:776–778.

A total of 120 consecutive patients with diffuse ISR underwent PCI, including additional stent placement in 33%, followed by gamma radiation (^{192}Ir; 14 Gy at 2 mm). All patients received clopidogrel for 12 months. Clinical event rates at 15 months were compared with those of WRIST PLUS patients who received clopidogrel for 6 months. Late thrombosis rates were not significantly different [3.3% (12 months vs. 4.2%); $p = 0.72$]; no cases in the 12-month group were seen between 12 and 15 months. The 12-month group did have a significantly lower incidence of MACE (21% vs. 36%; $p = 0.01$) and TLR (20% vs. 35%; $p = 0.009$).

91. Waksman R, et al.; SVG WRIST. Intravascular gamma radiation for in-stent restenosis in saphenous-vein bypass grafts. *N Engl J Med* 2002;346:1194–1199.

Design: Prospective, randomized, placebo-controlled, double-blind study. Primary end points were death from cardiac causes, Q-wave MI, TVR, and a composite of these events at 12 months.

Purpose: To examine the effects of i.v. gamma radiation in patients with ISR of saphenous vein bypass grafts.

Population: 120 patients with angina and evidence of ISR in SVGs who underwent successful PTCA with provisional stenting, laser, or atherectomy.

Treatment: Gamma radiation (^{192}Ir source; 14 to 15 Gy in 2.5- to 4.0-mm vessels and 18 Gy if diameter >4.0 mm) or placebo.

Results: At 6 months, the gamma-radiation group had more than a 50% relative reduction in restenosis compared with placebo (21% vs. 44%; $p = 0.005$). Restenosis rates were significantly lower in all segments (i.e., stented, injured, irradiated). No significant differences were found between the groups in the incidence of death or Q-wave MI, but the radiation group had much lower revascularization rates (1 year TVR, 17% vs. 57%; $p < 0.001$). Late thrombosis rates were similar (both 1.7%).

92. LONG WRIST; Waksman R, et al. Intracoronary radiation therapy improves the clinical and angiographic outcomes of diffuse in-stent restenotic lesions. *Circulation* 2003;107:1744–1749.

Design: Prospective, randomized, placebo-controlled; registry group: open label. Primary 1 year clinical end point: deaths, MI, and target lesion revascularization.

Purpose: To determine the safety and efficacy of vascular brachytherapy for the treatment of diffuse ISR.

Population: 120 patients with lesions 36 to 88 mm in length; additional 120 patients were treated with 18 Gy (registry patients).

Treatment: ^{192}Ir with 15 Gy at 2 mm or placebo; registry group: 18 Gy.

Results: At 6 months, binary restenosis rates were 73%, 45%, and 38% in placebo and 15 Gy and 18 Gy groups. One-year primary event rates were 63% in placebo group compared with 42% in 15 Gy group ($p < 0.05$) and only 22% with 18 Gy.

93. Limpijankit T, et al. Long-term follow-up of patients after gamma intracoronary brachytherapy failure (from GAMMA-I, GAMMA-II, and SCRIPPS-III). *J Am Coll Cardiol* 2003;92:315–318.

The investigators combine outcomes from the GAMMA-1, GAMMA-II, and SCRIPPS-III studies report outcomes in a subset of 225 patients who failed brachytherapy for ISR and subsequently survived to receive repeat PCI or CABG. They report worse total adverse events (including death, TVR, or MI) in the group that underwent PCI, as compared with CABG. It should be noted that these studies predate the use of DES for either de novo or in-stent lesions.

94. King SB III, et al.; Beta Energy Restenosis Trial (BERT). Endovascular beta-radiation to reduce restenosis after coronary balloon angioplasty. *Circulation* 1998;97:2025–2030.

This small study (23 patients) demonstrated the safety and feasibility of beta radiation after angioplasty. A ^{90}Sr/Y source was used to deliver 12, 14, or 16 Gy at 2 mm. Source delivery was successful in 21 (91%) of 23 patients. No in-hospital morbidity or mortality occurred, and follow-up angiography in 20 patients showed a late lumen loss of only 0.5 mm and restenosis in 15%. A larger, randomized, double-blind study is ongoing. Subsequent 6-month follow-up data on 64 patients showed an overall restenosis rate of 14% (20% in the 12-Gy group and 11% in the 14- and 16-Gy groups).

95. Waksman R, et al.; BETA-WRIST. Intracoronary β-radiation therapy inhibits recurrence of in-stent restenosis. *Circulation* 2000;101:1895–1898.

This small prospective study enrolled 50 patients with in-stent stenosis >50%; lesion length, <47 mm; and vessel diameter, 2.5 to 4.0 mm and who had successful primary treatment (<30% residual stenosis without complications). Exclusion criteria were recent acute MI (<72 hours), ejection fraction <20%, angiographic thrombus, and multiple lesions in the same vessel. Patients received beta radiation with yttrium 90 at a dose of 20.6 Gy at 1.0 mm. At 6 months, the binary angiographic restenosis rate was 22%, the TLR rate was 26%, and the TVR rate was 34%.

96. Serruys PW, et al. Safety and performance of 90-strontium for treatment of de novo and restenotic lesions: the BRIE Trial (Beta Radiation in Europe). *Circulation* 2000;102:II-750.

This prospective, randomized, multicenter study enrolled 150 patients with de novo lesions. Patients were treated with the Novoste Beta-Cath system (30-mm source) after angioplasty/stenting. At follow-up (6 months), angiographic restenosis had occurred in 33.6% and TVR in 15.4%. Geographic miss occurred in 41% of the patients and led to increased rates of restenosis (16.3% vs. 4.3%), especially at the edges of treated area (see *J Am Coll Cardiol* 2001;38:415–420). Geographic miss of stent-injured segments resulted in increased restenosis rates, whereas geographic miss of balloon-injured segments did not statistically increase restenosis.

97. Waksman R, et al. Use of localised intracoronary beta radiation in treatment of in-stent restenosis: the INHIBIT (Intimal Hyperplasia Inhibition with Beta In-stent Trial) randomised controlled trial. *Lancet* 2002;359:551–557.

Design: Prospective, randomized, blinded, multicenter study. Primary composite safety end point was death, Q-wave MI, and TLR at 9 months. Angiographic end point was binary restenosis.

Purpose: To evaluate whether beta-radiation brachytherapy with a P-32 source can reduce MACE and restenosis after treatment of ISR.

Population: 332 patients who underwent PTCA for single native-vessel ISR. Reference vessel diameter was 2.4 to 3.7 mm, and lesion length, <45 mm.

Exclusion Criteria: Acute MI in previous 72 hours, previous radiation treatment to chest, thrombus by angiogram, multiple lesions in target vessel.

Treatment: P-32 beta emitter versus placebo delivered through a centering catheter via an automatic afterloader.

Results: The P-32 beta-irradiation group had a 56% reduction compared with the control group in the composite end point of death, Q-wave MI, and TLR (15% vs. 31%; $p = 0.0006$) and a 50% reduction in the angiographic binary restenosis rate (26% vs. 52% control; $p < 0.0001$).

98. Popma JJ, et al.; for the Stents and Radiation Therapy (START) Investigators. Randomized trial of ^{90}Sr/^{90}Y β-radiation versus placebo control for treatment of in-stent restenosis. *Circulation* 2002;106:1090.

This prospective, randomized, placebo-controlled, multicenter study enrolled 476 patients with native coronary ISR in lesions shorter than 20 mm. After angioplasty, patients were assigned to either 16 or 20 Gy of beta radiation (depending on diameter of vessel) or placebo. Primary end points at 8 months were restenosis, TLR, TVR, and MACE. Beta radiation was associated with significantly lower restenosis rates compared with placebo (in-stent 14% vs. 41%, analysis segment 28.8% vs. 45.2%). Radiation group also had improved clinical outcomes (TLR, 13.6% vs. 24.4%; TVR, 17% vs. 26.8%; and MACE, 18.6% vs. 27.7%).

THROMBECTOMY

99. Kuntz RE, et al. A trial comparing rheolytic thrombectomy with intracoronary urokinase for coronary and vein graft thrombus [the Vein Graft AngioJet Study (VeGAS 2)]. *Am J Cardiol* 2002;89:326–330.

Design: Prospective, randomized, open, multicenter study. Primary end point was death, Q-wave MI, emergency coronary bypass surgery, TLR, stroke, or stent thrombosis at 30 days.

Purpose: To evaluate the safety and efficacy of rheolytic thrombectomy in CAD. Comparison of safety and efficacy of rheolytic thrombectomy (AngioJet) versus thrombolytic therapy (intracoronary urokinase).

Population: 352 patients with angina or MI more than 24 hours before the procedure and thrombus on angiography with discrete, mobile, intraluminal defect or a total occlusion with thrombus confirmed by multisidehole infusion catheter.

Exclusion Criteria: MI or thrombolytic therapy in previous 24 hours, more than two vessels requiring treatment, target vessel smaller than 2.0 mm diameter.

Treatment: Standard intracoronary or graft urokinase (more than 6-hour continuous infusion) or thrombectomy using the AngioJet system. Adjunctive thrombolytics and abciximab were discouraged, and crossover to AngioJet was prohibited. Short-term 30-day success was defined as more than 20% improvement in MLD, a final diameter stenosis of $\leq$50%, TIMI grade III flow, and freedom from major coronary events.

Results: Procedural success was significantly higher in the AngioJet group than in the urokinase group (86% vs. 72%; $p = 0.002$). Both treatments were equally effective with respect to the 30-day primary end point (AngioJet, 29%; urokinase, 30%). However, AngioJet patients had fewer MACEs (death, MI, revascularization; 16% vs. 33%; $p < 0.001$). Bradycardia occurred in 24% of those treated with AngioJet and was managed successfully with atropine and temporary pacing.

Comments: Trial was terminated early because of the growing safety difference between the two groups as well as reservations of investigators about using urokinase. Furthermore, mechanical thrombectomy allowed rapid thrombus removal and stenting during the same catheterization session.

100. Migliorini A, et al. Comparison of AngioJet rheolytic thrombectomy before direct infarct artery stenting with direct stenting alone in patients with acute myocardial infarction. The JETSTENT trial. *J Am Coll Cardiol* 2010;56(16):1298–306.

The investigators randomized 501 patients with STEMI and at least modest thrombus burden to either direct stenting or stenting following AngioJet rheolytic thrombectomy therapy. All patients received abciximab, and temporary pacing and balloon predilatation were discouraged. Primary outcome of ST-segment resolution at 30 minutes significantly favored the AngioJet group (86% vs. 79%; $p = 0.043$). Additionally, the AngioJet group had significantly more favorable clinical outcomes of lower major cardiac events at 6 months (11.2% vs. 19.4%; $p = 0.011$). Though the AngioJet group had longer procedure times, periprocedural complication rates, including bleeding, need for pacing, and perforation, were all similar in the two groups.

101. Sardella G, et al. **Thrombus aspiration during primary percutaneous coronary intervention improves myocardial reperfusion and reduces infarct size: the EXPIRA (thrombectomy with export catheter in infarct-related artery during primary percutaneous coronary intervention) prospective, randomized trial.** *J Am Coll Cardiol* 2009;53(4):309–315.

Design: Prospective, randomized, study. Primary end points were the occurrence of myocardial blush grade ≥ 2 and the rate of 90-min ST-segment resolution >70%.

Purpose: To evaluate the effect on infarct size and microvascular perfusion of mechanical thrombectomy during primary PCI for anterior STEMI.

Population: 175 patients with anterior STEMI were randomized to PCI or manual thrombectomy with PCI. Additionally, a subset underwent contrast-enhanced MRI at follow-up, to assess the resulting infarct.

Results: There was a lower rate of cardiac death in the thrombectomy group at 9 months (4.6% vs. 0%; $p = 0.02$). Additionally, patients in the thrombectomy group more frequently had myocardial blush grade ≥ 2 (88% vs. 60%; $p = 0.001$) and ST-segment resolution (64% vs. 39%; $p = 0.001$). At 3 months, infarct size was reduced in the thrombectomy group.

Comment: Subsequent 2-year data suggested such mechanical aspiration may reduce mortality (presented at the American Heart Association, 2009).

DISTAL PROTECTION

102. Baim DS, et al.; on behalf of Saphenous vein graft Angioplasty Free of Emboli Randomized (SAFER) Trial Investigators. Randomized trial of a distal embolic protection device during percutaneous intervention of saphenous vein aorto-coronary bypass grafts. *Circulation* 2002;105:1285–1290.

Design: Prospective, randomized, controlled, multicenter study. Primary end point was death, MI, emergency bypass surgery, or TVR (MACE) at 30 days.

Purpose: To compare clinical outcomes after SVG stenting plus GuardWire distal protection versus that performed over a conventional guide wire (control arm).

Population: 801 patients with a history of angina, evidence of myocardial ischemia, and >50% stenosis in the mid-portion of an SVG with a diameter of 3 to 6 mm. In the first 142 patients, the lesion could not occupy more than one-third of graft length.

Exclusion Criteria: Recent MI, ejection fraction <25%, creatinine >2.5 mg/dL (unless receiving long-term hemodialysis), and planned use of an atherectomy device.

Treatment: The 0.014-inch PercuSurge GuardWire balloon occlusion device or conventional 0.014-inch angioplasty guide wire. GP IIb/IIIa–receptor blocker could be used at the discretion of the operator.

Results: The embolic protection group had a 42% relative reduction in MACE at 30 days (9.6% vs. 16.5%; $p = 0.004$). This reduction was due primarily to fewer MIs (8.6% vs. 14.7%; $p = 0.008$) and "no reflow" (3% vs. 9%; $p = 0.02$). The benefit of the distal protection device was evident both with and without the use of concomitant GP IIb/IIIa–receptor blockers.

Comments: The use of distal embolization protection devices in other territories, such as native coronary, carotid, and renal arteries, has yet to be fully examined.

103. Stone GW, et al.; for the FilterWire EX Randomized Evaluation (FIRE) Investigators. Randomized comparison of distal protection with a filter-based catheter and a balloon occlusion and aspiration system during percutaneous intervention of diseased saphenous vein aorto-coronary bypass grafts. *Circulation* 2003;108:548–553.

This prospective, randomized, open, multicenter trial enrolled 651 patients with SVG lesion(s). Patients were treated using the GuardWire or FilterWire Ex devices. Device success was 95.5% for FilterWire EX and 97.2% for GuardWire ($p = 0.25$), with postprocedural epicardial patency also similar. At 30 days, MACE rates were similar [9.9% (FilterWire Ex) vs. 11.6%, p for superiority = 0.53, p for noninferiority = 0.0008].

104. Stone GW, et al.; for the Enhanced Myocardial Efficacy and Recovery by Aspiration of Liberated Debris (EMERALD) Investigators. Distal microcirculatory protection during percutaneous coronary intervention in acute ST-segment elevation myocardial infarction: a randomized controlled trial. JAMA 2005;293:1063–1072.

Design: Prospective, multicenter, randomized, controlled trial. The primary end points were ST-segment resolution at 30 minutes after PCI and infarct size as measured by sestamibi imaging at 5 to 14 days post-PCI.

Purpose: To assess effects on infarct size and reperfusion of distal embolic protection during primary PCI.

Population: 501 patients with acute STEMI undergoing primary PCI or rescue intervention after failed thrombolysis.

Treatment: Routine PCI or PCI with a balloon occlusion and aspiration of distal microcirculatory protection system.

Results: Of the 252 patients who received distal protection, visible debris was aspirated in 73% of the cases. There was no difference in ST-segment resolution or infarct size between the two groups. MACEs at 6 months were also similar (10.0% for distal protection vs. 11.0% for routine PCI; $p = 0.66$).

105. Svilaas T, et al. Thrombus aspiration during primary percutaneous coronary intervention (TAPAS). N Engl J Med 2008;358(6):557–567.

Design: Prospective, single-center, randomized, controlled trial. The primary end point was myocardial blush grade of 0 or 1 (poor myocardial perfusion grades). Secondarily, outcomes of ST-segment resolution and clinical events were also recorded.

Purpose: To assess effects on microvascular perfection of thrombus aspiration during primary PCI for acute STEMI.

Population: 1,071 patients with acute STEMI undergoing primary PCI.

Treatment: Routine PCI or PCI with adjunctive thrombus aspiration (confirmed by histopathologic evidence of atherothrombotic material).

Results: Patients in the thrombus-aspiration group had a lower rate of myocardial blush grade of 0 or 1 (17.1% vs. 26.3%; $p < 0.001$) and improved resolution of ST segments (56.6% vs. 442.%; $p < 0.001$). Independent of randomization category, rates of death, and adverse events at 30 days were inversely related to myocardial blush grades—the lower the blush grade, the poorer the clinical outcomes ($p < 0.01$ for both death and adverse clinical events by blush grade).

106. Fröbert O, et al. Thrombus Aspiration during ST-Segment Elevation Myocardial Infarction (TASTE). N Engl J Med 2013;369:1587–1597.

Design: Multicenter, prospective, randomized, controlled, open-label trial, with enrollment of patients from the national comprehensive Swedish Coronary Angiography and Angioplasty Registry (SCAAR). The primary end point was all-cause mortality at 30 days.

Purpose: To evaluate whether thrombus aspiration reduced mortality in STEMI patients undergoing primary PCI.

Population: 7,244 patients with STEMI undergoing primary PCI.

Treatment: Manual thrombus aspiration followed by PCI versus PCI only. The type of stent and P2Y12 inhibitor were left up to physician discretion.

Results: There was no significant difference in the primary end point between the two groups (2.8% in the aspiration group vs. 3.0% in the PCI only group, HR 0.94; 95% CI, 0.72 to 1.22; $p = 0.63$). This was consistent throughout all prespecified subgroups, including those patients with TIMI 0 or 1 flow and high thrombus burden. There was a trend toward decreased rehospitalization for reinfarction in the aspiration group, but this did not reach statistical significance ($p = 0.09$).

107. Haeck JDE, et al. Randomized comparison of primary percutaneous coronary intervention with combined proximal embolic protection and thrombus aspiration versus primary percutaneous coronary intervention alone in ST-segment elevation myocardial infarction: the PREPARE (PRoximal Embolic Protection in Acute myocardial infarction and Resolution of ST Elevation) study. *J Am Coll Cardiol Interv* 2009;2:934–943.

The investigators randomized 284 patients with STEMI undergoing primary PCI to the Proxis system of combined proximal embolic protection with thrombus aspiration or routine PCI. There was no significant difference in the primary end point of ST-segment resolution at 60 minutes (80% vs. 72%; $p = 0.14$). However, there were significant improvements in immediate complete ST resolution (66% vs. 50%; $p = 0.009$) and lower ST-segment curve area; however, clinical cardiac and cerebral end points were similar at 30 days (albeit with a low number of events).

108. Srinivasan M, et al. Adjunctive thrombectomy and distal protection in primary percutaneous coronary intervention impact on microvascular perfusion and outcomes. *Circulation* 2009;119:1311–1319.

In light of the recent Thrombus Aspiration During Percutaneous Coronary Intervention in Acute Myocardial Infarction Study (see above), the authors review the prior evidence for and current role of mechanical thrombectomy and distal embolic protection in primary PCI.

Adjunctive Pharmacologic Therapy

ASPIRIN

109. Schwartz L, et al. Aspirin and dipyridamole in the prevention of restenosis after percutaneous transluminal coronary angioplasty. *N Engl J Med* 1988;318:1714–1719.

This prospective, randomized, double-blind, placebo-controlled study enrolled 376 patients undergoing planned PTCA. Patients received an aspirin–dipyridamole combination (330 to 75 mg t.i.d.), beginning 24 hours before PTCA and until follow-up angiography, or placebo. At follow-up angiography (249 patients), no differences were observed between the two groups in binary restenosis rates [37.7% vs. 38.6% (placebo)]. However, the aspirin–dipyridamole group had significantly fewer periprocedural Q-wave MIs compared with the placebo group (6.9% vs. 1.6%; $p = 0.0113$).

For additional aspirin and antiplatelet studies, see Chapters 1, 3, and 4.

HEPARIN

110. Garachemani AR, et al. Prolonged heparin after uncomplicated coronary interventions: a prospective, randomized trial. *Am Heart J* 1998;136:352–356 (editorial, 183–185).

This prospective randomized trial was composed of 191 consecutive patients who underwent successful coronary angioplasty. Patients received prolonged intravenous heparin

(12 to 20 hours) or no postprocedural heparin. Stents were used in 33% and 36% of patients. MIs occurred in 3% and 4%, whereas vascular complications were seen in 3% and 1%. Accompanying editorial contains results from a meta-analysis of six studies comprising 2,186 patients. Postprocedural heparin was associated with a nonsignificant OR of 0.91 (0.45 to 1.84) for ischemic complications and an OR of 2.54 (1.44 to 4.47) for bleeding complications (27 additional episodes/1,000 patients treated).

111. Lincoff AM, et al.; Precursor to EPILOG (PROLOG) Investigators. Standard versus low-dose, weight-adjusted heparin in patients treated with the platelet glycoprotein IIb/IIIa receptor antibody fragment abciximab (c7E3 Fab) during percutaneous coronary revascularization. *Am J Cardiol* 1997;79:286–291.

This randomized 2 × 2 factorial pilot study was composed of a total of 103 patients undergoing PCI with concomitant abciximab (0.25 mg/kg intravenous bolus and then 10 μg/min for 12 hours) who were randomized to standard or high-dose heparin (100 U/kg bolus before PCI and then hourly boluses to keep ACT 300 to 350 seconds or continuous infusion at 10 U/kg/h without further ACT measurements) or low-dose heparin (70 U/kg and then 30 U/kg boluses during the procedure or continuous infusion at 7 U/kg/h without further ACT measurements). There was a separate randomization to early or late sheath removal. The early sheath-removal group had heparin discontinued immediately after PCI and sheaths removed at 6 hours, whereas the late group had heparin continued for 12 hours and sheaths removed 4 to 6 hours later. No difference was found between the groups in the incidence of ischemic events at 7 days. The early sheath-removal group had a smaller decrease in mean hemoglobin from baseline ($p = 0.03$), and nonsignificant trends occurred toward less minor non-CABG bleeding with low-dose heparin and early sheath removal.

112. Kaluski E, et al. Minimal heparinization in coronary angioplasty: how much heparin is really warranted? *Am J Cardiol* 2000;85:953–956.

Prospective, randomized, open study of 341 consecutive patients undergoing nonemergency PTCA. Patients received 2,500 U of UFH before PTCA with the intention of no additional boluses. Mean ACT at 5 minutes was 185 seconds. Two in-hospital deaths and one Q-wave MI occurred. Six (2%) patients had abrupt coronary occlusion within 14 days after PTCA, requiring repeated TVR. Six-month clinical follow-up in 184 patients revealed three cardiac deaths (one arrhythmic, two after cardiac surgery), one Q-wave MI, and 9.7% repeated TVR. These results warrant larger, randomized, double-blind heparin dose-optimization studies.

LOW MOLECULAR WEIGHT HEPARIN

113. Kereiakes DJ, et al. Enoxaparin and abciximab adjunctive pharmacotherapy during percutaneous coronary intervention (NICE 1 and NICE 4 Investigators. National Investigators Collaborating on Enoxaparin). *J Invasive Cardiol* 2001;13(4):272–278.

The NICE studies evaluated enoxaparin with (NICE-4) and without (NICE-1) abciximab in patients undergoing elective or urgent PCI. The NICE-1 trial assessed enoxaparin 1.0 mg/kg IV in 828 patients prior to PCI. All patients received aspirin and clopidogrel was left to the discretion of the interventionalist. In the NICE-4 trial, the enoxaparin dose was 0.75 mg/kg IV with standard dosing of abciximab. The primary end point was in-hospital and 30-day major hemorrhage. Bleeding events were low in both studies and appeared to establish the potential safety of LMWH during PCI, leading to further study.

114. The SYNERGY Trial Investigators. Enoxaparin vs unfractionated heparin in high-risk patients with non–ST segment elevation acute coronary syndromes managed with an intended early invasive strategy primary results of the SYNERGY randomized trial. *JAMA* 2004;292:45–54.

Design: Prospective, randomized, open, multicenter study. Primary end point was a composite of death or MI within 30 days. Safety outcomes of major bleeding or stroke were also assessed.

Purpose: To assess outcomes of patients with NSTEMI, undergoing an early invasive strategy with either UFH or enoxaparin.

Population: 10,027 patients with NSTEMI being treated with an intended early invasive strategy.

Treatment: s.c. enoxaparin versus intravenous UFH, both started at the time of enrollment and continued for a duration at the discretion of the treating physician.

Results: There was no difference in occurrence of the primary outcome for enoxaparin (14.0%) versus UFH (14.5%) or any other clinical ischemic outcomes. There were, however, increased rates of TIMI major bleeding in the enoxaparin group (9.1% vs. 7.6%; $p = 0.008$). The trial met the noninferiority margin for enoxaparin compared with UFH.

115. Gibson CM, et al. Percutaneous coronary intervention in patients receiving enoxaparin or unfractionated heparin after fibrinolytic therapy for ST-segment elevation myocardial infarction in the ExTRACT-TIMI 25 trial. *J Am Coll Cardiol* 2007;49:2238–2246.

The investigators performed a subgroup analysis of the 20,479 patients enrolled in the ExTRACT-TIMI 25 trial. The broader trial randomized patients with STEMI undergoing fibrinolytic therapy to either UFH or enoxaparin; however, a subgroup of 4,676 patients subsequently underwent PCI and were included in this analysis. It should first be noted that treatment remained blinded for the duration of hospitalization, and fewer patients initially randomized to enoxaparin actually underwent subsequent PCI. Of the group that did get PCI, those who received enoxaparin had a lower rate of death or MI at 30 days (10.7% vs. 13.8% for UFH; $p < 0.001$), the primary end point. Within this PCI subgroup, there were no differences in major bleeding rates (1.4% for enoxaparin vs. 1.6% for UFH; $p = NS$). For additional details on the full ExTRACT-TIMI 25 study, see Chapter 4.

116. Montalescot G, et al.; STEEPLE Investigators. Enoxaparin versus unfractionated heparin in elective percutaneous coronary intervention. *N Engl J Med* 2006;355(10):1006–1017.

Design: Prospective, randomized, open-label, multicenter trial. The primary end point was major or minor (non-CABG) bleeding; achievement of target anticoagulation was a secondary end point.

Purpose: To assess the safety of enoxaparin, compared with UFH, for elective PCI.

Population: 3,528 patients undergoing elective PCI, stratified by use of GP IIb/IIIa inhibitor.

Major Exclusion Criteria: Recent thrombolysis, high risk of bleeding, and use of any parenteral antithrombotic agent before PCI.

Treatment: Intravenous enoxaparin (0.5 or 0.75 mg/kg) or UFH adjusted for ACT.

Results: Lower-dose enoxaparin (0.5 mg/kg) was associated with significantly less bleeding (5.9% vs. 8.5%; $p = 0.01$); however, the higher dose (0.75 mg/kg) was not (6.5% vs. 8.5%; $p = 0.051$). The trial was not powered to assess efficacy end points.

THIENOPYRIDINES

117. Schomig A, et al.; Intracoronary stenting and antithrombotic regimen (ISAR). A randomized comparison of antiplatelet and anticoagulant therapy after the placement of coronary artery stents. *N Engl J Med* 1996;334:1084–1089.

Design: Prospective, randomized, open, multicenter study. Primary cardiac end points were cardiovascular death, MI, bypass surgery, and repeated target vessel intervention. Additional noncardiac end point was death from noncardiac causes, cerebrovascular accidents, severe hemorrhage, and peripheral vascular events.

Purpose: To compare the early outcome of patients given a combined antiplatelet regimen or conventional anticoagulation after coronary stent placement.

Population: 517 patients who underwent successful stenting.

Exclusion Criteria: Cardiogenic shock and stenting intended as a bridge to CABG surgery.

Treatment: Intravenous heparin for 12 hours; ticlopidine, 250 mg twice daily and aspirin; or intravenous heparin for 5 to 10 days, phenprocoumon, and aspirin.

Results: At 30 days, the antiplatelet group had 75% fewer cardiac end points (1.6% vs. 6.2%), including a significant reduction in MI (0.8% vs. 4.2%; $p = 0.02$). The antiplatelet group had a 90% reduction in the primary noncardiac end point (1.2% vs. 12.3%; $p < 0.001$), including an 87% reduction in peripheral vascular events (0.8% vs. 6.2%; $p = 0.001$) and no bleeding complications (vs. 6.5%; $p < 0.001$). Antiplatelet therapy also was associated with 86% fewer stent reocclusions (0.8% vs. 5.4%; $p = 0.004$).

118. Bertrand ME, et al.; Full Anticoagulation versus Aspirin and Ticlopidine (FANTASTIC). Randomized multicenter comparison of conventional anticoagulation versus antiplatelet therapy in unplanned and elective coronary stenting. *Circulation* 1998;98:1597–1603.

Design: Prospective, randomized, multicenter study. Primary end point was bleeding and peripheral vascular complications. Secondary end points were death, MI, and stent occlusion.

Purpose: To compare the effects of aggressive antiplatelet treatment with anticoagulation after implantation of a Wiktor stent on bleeding rates and stent thrombosis rates.

Population: 485 patients undergoing elective (58%) or unplanned (42%) coronary stenting.

Exclusion Criteria: Platelet count <150,000, bleeding disorders, recent (<6 months) gastrointestinal bleeding, recent stroke, angiographic evidence of thrombus at target site, and allergy to aspirin or ticlopidine.

Treatment: Antiplatelet therapy with aspirin, 100 to 325 mg/day, and ticlopidine, 250 mg twice daily for 6 weeks [first dose (500 mg) given in catheterization laboratory], or anticoagulation with heparin (target activated partial thromboplastin time, 2.0 to 2.5 times control) and then warfarin for 6 weeks (target international normalized ratio, 2.5 to 3.0). The anticoagulation group also received aspirin. All patients received heparin, 10,000-U bolus before the procedure.

Results: Successful stent implantation was achieved in 99%. The antiplatelet group had fewer bleeding and peripheral vascular complications (13.5% vs. 21%; OR, 0.6; $p = 0.03$). Major cardiac events in electively stented patients were less common in the antiplatelet group (2.4% vs. 9.9%; OR, 0.23; $p = 0.01$). Antiplatelet patients had a shorter average hospital stay (4.3 vs. 6.4 days; $p = 0.0001$).

119. Leon MB, et al.; for the Stent Anticoagulation Restenosis Study (STARS) Investigators. A clinical trial comparing three antithrombotic-drug regimens after coronary-artery stenting. *N Engl J Med* 1998;339:1665–1671.

Design: Prospective, randomized, open, multicenter study (54). The 30-day primary composite end point was death, MI, TLR, and angiographically evident thrombosis.

Purpose: To compare clinical outcomes for three antithrombotic regimens after elective coronary stenting.

Population: 1,653 patients who underwent successful stenting of a more than 60% stenosis in a native coronary artery with a diameter of 3 to 4 mm.

Exclusion Criteria: MI in prior 7 days, abciximab administration, and planned revascularization within 30 days.

Treatment: Aspirin, 325 mg daily; aspirin, 325 mg daily, and intravenous heparin followed by warfarin (target international normalized ratio, 2.0 to 2.5); or aspirin, 325 mg daily, and ticlopidine, 250 mg twice daily.

Results: Aspirin plus ticlopidine group had a significant reduction in the incidence of primary composite end points for aspirin and warfarin (0.5% vs. 2.7%) and for aspirin alone (3.6%; $p < 0.001$ for comparison of all three groups). Hemorrhagic and vascular surgical complications occurred less frequently with aspirin alone: 1.8% versus 5.5% (aspirin plus ticlopidine) and 6.2% (aspirin and warfarin) and 0.4% versus 2.0% and 2.0%. No significant differences were observed in the incidences of neutropenia or thrombocytopenia (overall incidence, 0.3%).

120. Bertrand ME, et al. Double-blind study of the safety of clopidogrel with and without a loading dose in combination with aspirin, compared with ticlopidine in combination with aspirin after coronary stenting: the Clopidogrel Aspirin Stent International Cooperative Study (CLASSICS). *Circulation* 2000;102:624–629.

Design: Prospective, randomized, double-blind, placebo-controlled, multicenter study. The primary end point was a composite of major peripheral bleeding complications, neutropenia, thrombocytopenia, or early discontinuation of the drug because of a noncardiac event. Secondary end point was cardiac events, consisting of cardiovascular death, MI, or TVR.

Purpose: To demonstrate that clopidogrel has an efficacy similar to and better tolerability than has ticlopidine.

Population: 1,020 patients who had undergone successful planned or unplanned coronary stenting (1 or 2 stents) in a single vessel (reference vessel diameter, more than 2.8 mm) with the use of any non–heparin-coated stent(s).

Exclusion Criteria: Included acute ST elevation MI; CK 2× normal or greater; stent(s) in left main coronary artery, vein grafts, or at a major bifurcation; oral anticoagulants, GP IIb/IIIa–receptor antagonists, or other antiplatelet agents, except for aspirin, in previous month (or required after the procedure); and percutaneous or surgical revascularization (PTCA, CABG) in the previous 2 months.

Treatment: Ticlopidine, 250 mg twice daily for 4 weeks; clopidogrel, 75 mg once daily for 4 weeks; or clopidogrel, 300 mg loading dose followed by 75 mg once daily (days 2 to 28). All patients received aspirin, 325 mg once daily.

Results: The clopidogrel groups had a significantly lower incidence of the primary composite end point, which consisted of major bleeding, neutropenia, thrombocytopenia, and early discontinuation of therapy: 2.9% (loading dose group) and 6.4% [clopidogrel, 75 mg/day (all clopidogrel patients, 4.6%) vs. 9.1% for ticlopidine ($p = 0.005$)]. No significant differences were seen among the three groups in the incidence of the secondary end point (0.9%, 1.5%, and 1.2% of patients, respectively).

Comments: Clopidogrel appears to have superior safety and tolerability compared with ticlopidine and acceptable efficacy in the prevention of MACEs after coronary stenting. Although this study was not developed to determine efficacy, the results support the use of clopidogrel as an alternative to ticlopidine after coronary stenting.

121. PCI-CURE (Clopidogrel in Unstable angina to prevent Recurrent ischemic Events); Mehta SR, et al. Effects of pretreatment with clopidogrel and aspirin followed by long-term therapy in patients undergoing percutaneous coronary intervention: the PCI-CURE study. *Lancet* 2001;358:527–533.

Design: Prospective, randomized, placebo-controlled, double-blinded, multicenter trial. Primary end point was 30-day composite of cardiovascular death, MI, or urgent TVR and cardiovascular death or MI to end of trial. Mean follow-up was 8 months.

Purpose: To determine if pretreatment with clopidogrel before PCI would be superior to placebo in preventing major ischemic events after PCI and if long-term treatment with clopidogrel for up to 1 year after PCI would result in additional benefit.

Population: 2,658 patients with mean age of 61 years and acute coronary syndromes who were hospitalized within 24 hours of onset of symptoms. ECG evidence of new ischemia (but <1-mm ST elevation) or elevated concentrations of cardiac enzymes (2× normal or more) were required.

Exclusion Criteria: Contraindications to antithrombotic or antiplatelet therapy, high bleeding risk, NYHA Class IV heart failure, need for oral anticoagulation, coronary revascularization in previous 3 months, and GP IIb/IIIa–receptor inhibitors in previous 3 days.

Treatment: Clopidogrel, 300 mg loading dose, or matching placebo followed by 75 mg clopidogrel, or matching placebo once daily for 3 to 12 months (mean, 9 months). Patients underwent PCI at a mean 10 days after randomization. All received aspirin, 75 to 325 mg once daily. The use of GP IIb/IIIa–receptor antagonists was discouraged but allowed during PCI.

Results: Before PCI, the clopidogrel group had a lower incidence of MI or refractory ischemia compared with placebo (12.% vs. 15.3%; RR, 0.76; p = 0.008). At 30 days after PCI, the clopidogrel group had a lower incidence in the primary composite outcome of cardiovascular death, MI, or urgent revascularization (4.5% vs. 6.4%; RR, 0.70; p = 0.03). Long-term administration of clopidogrel after PCI was associated with a lower rate of the composite end point (p = 0.03) and cardiovascular death or MI (p = 0.047). Including events before and after PCI, the clopidogrel group was associated with a 31% lower incidence of cardiovascular death or MI (8.8% vs. 12.6%; p = 0.002; see **Fig. 2.3**). Clopidogrel use was associated with similar rate of major bleeding compared with placebo.

122. Steinhubl SR, et al. Ticlopidine pretreatment before coronary stenting is associated with sustained decrease in adverse cardiac events: data from the Evaluation of Platelet IIb/IIIa Inhibitor for Stenting (EPISTENT) Trial. *Circulation* 2001;103:1403–1409.

Design: Nonrandomized, multicenter study. Primary composite end points were all-cause mortality, nonfatal MI, or urgent revascularization at 30 days, and at 1 year, all-cause mortality, MI, and TVR.

Purpose: To determine whether pretreatment with ticlopidine before coronary stenting results in a sustained reduction in adverse cardiac events.

Population: Included 1,603 patients enrolled in the EPISTENT trial who were randomized to either placebo or abciximab. Of these, 932 patients received pretreatment with ticlopidine before stenting, at the discretion of the investigator.

Exclusion Criteria: see EPISTENT trial.

Treatment: Abciximab (bolus and 12-hour infusion) and stenting, placebo and stenting, or abciximab and balloon angioplasty. Investigators were encouraged to treat all patients with ticlopidine according to their usual practice before stenting. All were pretreated with aspirin.

Results: Among patients randomized to placebo, ticlopidine pretreatment was associated with a significant decrease in death, MI, or TVR at 1 year (adjusted HR, 0.73; 95% CI, 0.54 to 0.98; p = 0.036). At 30-day follow-up, the primary end point had occurred in 13.4% of patients in the no-abciximab or ticlopidine group, 8.9% of patients in the placebo + ticlopidine group, 5.5% of patients in the abciximab/no-ticlopidine group (p = 0.028 vs. placebo and plus ticlopidine), and 5.2% of patients in the abciximab + ticlopidine group. The benefit of pretreatment with ticlopidine in the placebo group was primarily attributable to a lower incidence of MI (8.4% vs. 12.5%; p = 0.048). At 1 year, fewer primary events occurred in the placebo group in patients pretreated with ticlopidine compared with patients not pretreated with ticlopidine (20.7% vs. 28.5%; $p = 0.008$), whereas no difference was related to pretreatment with ticlopidine in the abciximab group (19.5% for abciximab + ticlopidine vs. 20.9% for abciximab/no ticlopidine). Controlling for patient characteristics and for the propensity to use ticlopidine, Cox regression model identified ticlopidine pretreatment as an independent predictor of the need for TVR at 1 year (hazard ratio, 0.62; 95% CI, 0.43 to 0.89; $p = 0.01$) in both placebo-treated and abciximab-treated patients. By multivariate modeling, however, the beneficial effect of ticlopidine on TVR was diminished by treatment with abciximab.

Comments: Duration of pretreatment with ticlopidine was uncertain. Beneficial effect of ticlopidine in placebo-treated group may have been due to an antiplatelet effect in aspirin-resistant patients.

123. Bhatt DL, et al. Meta-analysis of randomized and registry comparisons of ticlopidine with clopidogrel after stenting. J Am Coll Cardiol 2002;39:9–14.

Data were pooled and analyzed from published trials and registries comparing clopidogrel with ticlopidine in a total of 13,955 patients undergoing stenting. The pooled rate of MACEs was 2.10% in the clopidogrel group and 4.04% in the ticlopidine group. After adjustment for trial heterogeneity, the OR for ischemic events was lower with clopidogrel compared with ticlopidine (95% CI, 0.59 to 0.89; $p = 0.002$). The clopidogrel group also had a significantly lower mortality compared with the ticlopidine group (0.48% vs. 1.09%; OR, 0.55; 95% CI, 0.37 to 0.82; $p = 0.003$). The authors note that these findings may be due to the more rapid onset of an antiplatelet effect with the loading dose of clopidogrel, which was used in most of these studies, or to better patient compliance with clopidogrel therapy.

124. Hongo RH, et al. The effect of clopidogrel in combination with aspirin when given before coronary artery bypass grafting. J Am Coll Cardiol 2002;40:231–237.

This nonrandomized observational study of 224 consecutive patients undergoing non-emergency first-time CABG compared those with preoperative clopidogrel exposure within 7 days ($n = 59$) with those without exposure ($n = 165$). Groups had comparable baseline characteristics. The clopidogrel group had higher 24-hour mean chest tube output (1.2 L vs. 0.84 L; $p = 0.001$) and more transfusions of red blood cells (2.51 U vs. 1.74 U; $p = 0.036$), platelets (0.86 U vs. 0.24 U; $p = 0.001$), and fresh frozen plasma (0.68 U vs. 0.24 U; $p = 0.015$). Reoperation for bleeding was 10-fold higher in clopidogrel group (6.8% vs. 0.6%; $p = 0.018$). The clopidogrel group also had a trend toward less hospital discharge within 5 days (33.9% vs. 46.7%; $p = 0.094$).

125. Steinhubl SR, et al.; for the Clopidogrel in Unstable angina to Prevent Recurrent Events CREDO Investigators. Early and sustained dual oral antiplatelet therapy following percutaneous coronary intervention. JAMA 2002;288:2411–2420.

Design: Prospective, randomized, double-blind, placebo-controlled, multicenter study. Primary end points were death, MI, or stroke at 1 year and death, MI, or urgent TVR at 28 days in the per-protocol population.

Purpose: To evaluate long-term treatment (1 year) with clopidogrel after elective PCI and initiation of clopidogrel with a preprocedural loading dose, both in addition to aspirin therapy.

Population: 2,116 patients scheduled to undergo elective PCI or deemed at high likelihood of undergoing PCI.

Exclusion Criteria: Included contraindications to antithrombotic/antiplatelet therapy, failed PCI in previous 2 weeks, coronary anatomy not amenable to stenting or >50% left main stenosis, planned staged procedure, and administration of the following medications before randomization: GP IIb/IIIa inhibitors (within 7 days), clopidogrel (10 days), and thrombolytics (24 hours).

Treatment: Clopidogrel loading dose (300 mg) or placebo, 3 to 24 hours before PCI. All patients then received clopidogrel, 75 mg/day, through day 28. From day 29 through 12 months, loading dose patients received clopidogrel, 75 mg/day, and control patients received placebo. Both groups received aspirin throughout the study. GP IIb/IIIa inhibitors were administered in 45% of the per-protocol population. PCI was performed in 86%.

Results: At 1 year, long-term clopidogrel therapy was associated with a 26.9% relative reduction in death, MI, or stroke [8.5% vs. 11.5% (placebo); $p = 0.02$]. Although not a prespecified analysis, a further 37.4% relative reduction in major events occurred from day 29 to 1 year with clopidogrel ($p = 0.04$). At 28 days, clopidogrel pretreatment was associated with a nonsignificant 18.5% relative reduction in death, MI, or urgent TVR (6.8% vs. 8.3%; $p = 0.23$). However, in a prespecified subgroup analysis, those given clopidogrel at least 6 hours before PCI had a significant 38.6% RR reduction ($p = 0.05$) compared with no reduction with treatment <6 hours before PCI. Among those receiving a GP IIb/IIIa inhibitor and clopidogrel pretreatment, a 30% reduction in events was found [7.3% vs. 10.3% (no pretreatment, GP IIb/IIIa); $p = 0.12$]. A trend toward a higher incidence of major bleeding was found with clopidogrel (at 1 year, 8.8% vs. 6.7%; $p = 0.07$).

Comments: This trial, together with CURE and PCI-CURE, supports long-term use of clopidogrel plus aspirin post-PCI.

126. Sabatine MS, et al. Effect of clopidogrel pretreatment before percutaneous coronary intervention in patients with STEMI treated with fibrinolytics the PCI-CLARITY study. JAMA 2005;294:1224–1232.

This prospectively planned substudy of the CLARITY-TIMI 28 trial (see Chapter 4 for its complete details) evaluated the 1,863 patients in the original trial who underwent PCI following mandated angiography. All patients were initially randomized to either clopidogrel or placebo (in addition to aspirin and other medical therapies) at enrollment; they subsequently underwent angiography (2 to 8 days later) and all patients requiring PCI subsequently received clopidogrel regardless of initial randomization assignment. However, in patients initially randomized to clopidogrel (thus, having been on it for 2 to 8 days prior to PCI), there was a significant reduction in MI or stroke prior to PCI (4.0% vs. 6.2%; $p = 0.03$), as well as a reduction in cardiovascular death, MI, or stroke after PCI (3.6% vs. 6.2%; $p = 0.008$). In this group undergoing PCI following fibrinolysis for STEMI, pretreatment with clopidogrel on presentation, prior to PCI, significantly reduced 30-day rates of cardiovascular death, MI, or stroke (7.5% vs. 12.0%; $p = 0.001$), without excess rates of major or minor bleeding (2.0% vs. 1.9%; $p > 0.99$).

127. Mega JL, et al. Cytochrome P-450 polymorphisms and response to clopidogrel. N Engl J Med 2009;360:354–362.

Based on previous data suggesting variable clinical response to clopidogrel based on cytochrome P450 polymorphisms, the investigators of the TRITON-TIMI 38 trial (see Chapter 4) assessed clinical cardiovascular outcomes in patients with ACS, receiving clopidogrel, stratified by genotype. Among patients in the TRITON-TIMI 38 trial who were carriers of the CYP2C19 polymorphism, there was a relative increase over noncarriers of 53% in the primary end point, a composite of cardiovascular death, MI, or stroke (12.1% vs. 8.0%; $p = 0.01$). There was also, notably, a threefold increase in the risk of stent thrombosis in the carrier group (2.6% vs. 0.8%; $p = 0.02$). This represents one of the earliest studies to link pharmacogenomic status to clinical outcomes and surely the beginning of more specific tailoring of pharmacotherapy to genetic profile.

128. Kastrati A, et al.; for the Intracoronary Stenting and Antithrombotic Regimen–Rapid Early Action for Coronary Treatment (ISAR-REACT) Study Investigators. A clinical trial of abciximab in elective percutaneous coronary intervention after pretreatment with clopidogrel. N Engl J Med 2004;350:232–238.

Design: Randomized, double-blind, placebo-controlled trial. Primary end point was a composite of death, MI, or urgent TVR within 30 days.

Purpose: To compare abciximab versus placebo in stable patients undergoing elective PCI with clopidogrel pretreatment.

Population: 2,159 patients with stable CAD of low risk, undergoing elective PCI.

Exclusion Criteria: Recent MI (14 days), current ACS, positive troponin, or any of several other markers of higher risk.

Treatment: Abciximab infusion during PCI or placebo infusion; all patients were pretreated with 600 mg clopidogrel.

Results: There was no significant difference in rates of the primary end point between those who received abciximab and placebo (4% for abciximab vs. 4% placebo; $p = 0.82$). Bleeding end points were also roughly equivalent. The only significant difference between the groups was incidence of profound thrombocytopenia (1% for abciximab vs. 0% for placebo; $p = 0.002$).

129. Kastrati A, et al.; for the Intracoronary Stenting and Antithrombotic Regimen: Rapid Early Action for Coronary Treatment 2 (ISAR-REACT 2) Trial Investigators. Abciximab in patients with acute coronary syndromes undergoing percutaneous coronary intervention after clopidogrel pretreatment: the ISAR-REACT 2 randomized trial. JAMA 2006;295:1531–1538.

Design: Randomized, controlled, double-blind, multicenter international trial. Primary end point was a composite of death, MI, or urgent TVR within 30 days. Bleeding complications were secondary end points.

Purpose: To assess the utility of adding abciximab to clopidogrel load in patients undergoing PCI for NSTEMI.

Population: 2,022 patients with NSTEMI undergoing PCI.

Treatment: PCI with abciximab bolus and infusion or PCI with placebo; both groups received pretreatment with 600 mg of clopidogrel.

Results: Rates of the primary end point significantly favored the abciximab group (8.9% vs. 11.9%; $p = 0.03$). However, this effect was confined to those patients with an elevated troponin. Bleeding rates were no different in the two groups.

GLYCOPROTEIN IIB/IIIA INHIBITORS

130. Evaluation of 7E3 for the Prevention of Ischemic Complications (EPIC) Investigators. Use of a monoclonal antibody directed vs platelet glycoprotein IIb/IIIa receptor in high-risk percutaneous transluminal coronary angioplasty. N Engl J Med 1994;330:956–961.

Design: Prospective, randomized, double-blind, multicenter study. The 30-day primary composite end point was death, MI, CABG surgery, repeated PCI for acute ischemia, and stenting due to procedural failure or placement of an intra-aortic balloon pump.

Purpose: To determine whether the monoclonal antibody c7E3 Fab provides clinical benefit in patients undergoing coronary angioplasty or atherectomy.

Population: 2,099 high-risk patients, defined as having experienced acute MI with onset of symptoms within previous 12 hours, two episodes of postinfarct angina within previous 24 hours with ECG changes, or high-risk clinical or angiographic features, who underwent percutaneous intervention (PTCA, 90%; directional atherectomy, 5%; both, 5%).

Exclusion Criteria: Included bleeding diathesis, major surgery in prior 6 weeks, and stroke in prior 2 years.

Treatment: Abciximab, 0.25 mg/kg intravenous bolus (started 10 minutes before procedure) and then 10 μg/min infusion for 12 hours, or placebo. All patients received heparin (10,000- to 12,000-U bolus; target ACT, 300 to 350 seconds).

Results: Abciximab bolus plus infusion group had 35% fewer end points (death, MI, unplanned surgical revascularization, repeated percutaneous procedure, need for intra-aortic balloon pump): 12.8% versus 11.4% (bolus only; $p = 0.43$) and 8.3% (placebo; $p = 0.008$). A significant reduction was observed in the MI rate only: 5.2% versus 8.6% for placebo ($p = 0.013$). Abciximab was associated with more bleeding episodes: 14% versus 7% ($p = 0.001$). Follow-up studies have shown abciximab to be associated with persistent significant reductions at 6 months (27% vs. 35.1%; $p = 0.001$) and 3 years [41.1% vs. 47.4% (bolus only) and 47.2% (placebo); $p = 0.009$]. Three-year follow-up also showed that the subgroup of patients with an evolving MI or refractory unstable angina (28% of patients) had a significant 60% reduction in mortality rate (5.1% vs. 12.7%; $p = 0.01$).

Comments: Significant bleeding likely was due to high heparin dosing.

131. Integrilin to Minimize Platelet Aggregation and Coronary Thrombosis II (IMPACT II). Randomised placebo-controlled trial of effect of eptifibatide on complications of percutaneous coronary intervention: IMPACT-II. *Lancet* 1997;349:1422–1428 (editorial, 1409–1410).

Design: Prospective, randomized, double-blind, multicenter study. The 30-day primary composite end point was death, MI, unplanned surgical or repeated percutaneous revascularization, or stenting for abrupt closure.

Purpose: To determine the effectiveness of eptifibatide in reducing ischemic complications in patients undergoing nonsurgical coronary revascularization.

Population: 4,010 patients who underwent elective, urgent, or emergency percutaneous intervention (PTCA, 91% to 93%).

Exclusion Criteria: Bleeding diathesis, major surgery in prior 6 weeks, and any history of stroke.

Treatment: Eptifibatide, 135 μg/kg intravenous bolus (10 to 60 minutes before procedure) and then 0.5 or 0.75 μg/kg/min for 20 to 24 hours, or placebo.

Results: At 30 days, a nonsignificant reduction in the primary composite end point was observed: 9.2% (135/0.5 group) and 9.9% (135/0.75 group) versus 11.4% (placebo) ($p = 0.063, 0.22$). On-treatment analysis showed that the 135/0.5 group had a significant 22% reduction in composite primary end point (9.1% vs. 11.6%; $p = 0.035$). No significant differences in bleeding or transfusion rates were observed.

132. c7E3 Fab Antiplatelet Therapy in Unstable Refractory Angina (CAPTURE) Investigators. Randomized, placebo-controlled trial of abciximab before and during coronary intervention in refractory unstable angina: the CAPTURE study. *Lancet* 1997;349:1429–1435 (editorial, 1409–1410).

Design: Prospective, randomized, placebo-controlled, multicenter study. The 30-day primary end point was death, MI, or urgent intervention for recurrent ischemia.

Purpose: To assess whether abciximab given before and until briefly after PCI improves outcome in patients with refractory unstable angina.

Population: 1,265 patients with chest pain at rest with ST segment depression or elevation or abnormal T waves, with one or more episodes (rest pain and/or ECG changes) occurring more than 2 hours after the start of intravenous heparin and nitrate therapy.

Exclusion Criteria: Recent MI, persisting ischemia that required immediate intervention, and left main stenosis as shown by angiography.

Treatment: After angiography, patients were randomized to abciximab (0.25 mg/kg bolus and then 10 μg/min) or placebo for 18 to 24 hours before and 1 hour after PCI (balloon angioplasty with stenting only if necessary to maintain vessel patency). Goal ACT was 300 seconds.

Results: Trial was stopped early because of significant treatment effect (1,400 patients planned). The abciximab group had a 29% reduction in 30-day primary end points of death, MI, and ischemia requiring intervention (11.3% vs. 15.9%; $p = 0.012$). Most of this difference was due to fewer MIs (defined as CK or CK-MB three times the upper limit of normal (ULN) in two samples): 4.1% versus 8.2% ($p = 0.002$). MIs occurred less frequently before and after PTCA in abciximab patients (0.6% vs. 2.1%; $p = 0.029$; 2.6% vs. 5.5%; $p = 0.043$). Importantly, no difference in event rates was seen at 6 months (31% vs. 30.8%). A two-fold higher major bleeding rate was observed in the abciximab group (3.8% vs. 1.9%; $p = 0.043$). An ECG ischemia substudy (332 patients monitored from start of treatment to 6 hours after intervention) showed that the abciximab group had a lower incidence of two episodes of significant (≥ 1 mm) ST-segment deviation (5% vs. 14%; $p < 0.01$).

Comments: In contrast to other studies, patients given abciximab for a substantial period before intervention and only briefly afterward had a reduction in events during the 18- to 24-hour interval before intervention. Lack of long-term benefits is likely owing to lack of 12-hour postintervention infusion.

133. Evaluation in PTCA to Improve Long-term Outcome with Abciximab Glycoprotein IIb/IIIa Blockade (EPILOG) Investigators. Platelet glycoprotein IIb/IIIa receptor blockade and low-dose heparin during percutaneous coronary revascularization. N Engl J Med 1997;336:1689–1696 (editorial, 1748–1749).

Design: Prospective, randomized, double-blind, multicenter study. Thirty-day composite primary end point was death, MI, ischemia requiring urgent coronary bypass surgery, or repeated percutaneous coronary revascularization.

Purpose: To determine whether the clinical benefits of abciximab extend to all patients undergoing coronary intervention and to evaluate whether hemorrhagic complications are reduced by adjusting heparin dosing.

Population: 2,792 patients undergoing urgent or elective revascularization.

Exclusion Criteria: Acute MI or unstable angina with ECG changes in prior 24 hours, planned stenting or atherectomy, PCI in prior 3 months, anticoagulant therapy, and major surgery or bleeding in prior 6 weeks.

Treatment: Abciximab [0.25 mg/kg intravenous bolus (10 to 60 minutes before procedure) and then 0.125 μg/kg/min for 12 hours] plus heparin (100 U/kg bolus), abciximab plus heparin, 70 U/kg, or placebo plus heparin, 100 U/kg.

Results: Abciximab groups had lower 30-day incidences of death, MI, and urgent revascularization: 5.4% and 5.2% versus 11.7% (OR, 0.45, 0.43; both $p < 0.001$). Fewer large non–Q-wave MIs also were observed (CK five times normal): 2.5% and 2% versus 5.6% ($p < 0.001$). Similar major bleeding rates were observed, but abciximab plus standard heparin was associated with more minor bleeds [7.4% vs. 4% (low heparin); $p < 0.001$]. At 6 months, similar rates of repeated revascularization and a smaller reduction in composite end points were observed (death, MI, and any revascularization): 22.3% and 22.8% versus 25.8% ($p = 0.04$). One-year follow-up showed persistent benefit in abciximab groups (incidences of primary end points were 9.6% and 9.5% in abciximab plus low-dose heparin and abciximab plus standard heparin groups, respectively, vs. 16.1% in placebo group).

Comments: In an effort to reduce bleeding rates, sheaths were removed as soon as possible, and no routine postprocedural heparin was administered.

134. Randomized Efficacy Study of Tirofiban for Outcomes and Restenosis (RESTORE) Investigators. Effects of platelet GP IIb/IIIa blockade with tirofiban on adverse cardiac events in patients with unstable angina or acute MI undergoing coronary angioplasty. Circulation 1997;96:1445–1453.

Design: Prospective, randomized, double-blind, placebo-controlled, multicenter study. Primary composite end point was death, MI, CABG due to failed PTCA or recurrent ischemia, and repeated PTCA of target vessel due to ischemia or stenting for actual or threatened abrupt closure.

Purpose: To evaluate the effectiveness of tirofiban in patients undergoing high-risk coronary interventions.

Population: 2,139 patients seen within 72 hours of onset of symptoms with a 60% stenosis.

Exclusion Criteria: Included scheduled stenting or adjunctive rotablation.

Treatment: Tirofiban (10 μg/kg intravenous bolus over 3 minutes and then 0.15 μg/kg/min for 36 hours) or placebo. All patients were taking aspirin and heparin.

Results: For the initial procedure, PTCA was performed in 92% to 93% and atherectomy in 7% to 8% of patients. At 30 days, a similar incidence of primary composite end points was observed (10.3% vs. 12.2%; $p = 0.16$). If only urgent/emergency CABG and PTCA are included, the rates are 8% versus 10.5% ($p = 0.052$). However, the tirofiban group had significantly fewer events at 2 days and 7 days (RR, 0.62; $p = 0.005$; RR, 0.73; $p = 0.022$), mostly because of less reinfarction and repeated PTCA [at 2 days, 2.7% vs. 4.4% ($p = 0.039$) and 1.1% vs. 3.2% ($p = 0.001$); at 7 days, 3.6% vs. 5.3% ($p = 0.055$) and 2.7% vs. 4.4% ($p = 0.034$)]. Similar rates of major bleeding and thrombocytopenia were observed [5.3% vs. 3.7% ($p = 0.096$) and 1.1% vs. 0.9%].

135. Evaluation of Platelet IIb/IIIa Inhibitor for Stenting (EPISTENT) Investigators. Randomized placebo-controlled and balloon-angioplasty-controlled trial to assess safety of coronary stenting with use of platelet glycoprotein IIb/IIIa blockade. *Lancet* 1998;352:87–92.

Design: Prospective, randomized, double-blind, placebo-controlled multicenter study. Primary composite end point was death, MI, and urgent revascularization at 30 days.

Purpose: To evaluate the effects of platelet GP IIb/IIIa blockade with abciximab in conjunction with elective coronary stenting in patients with 60% coronary lesions.

Population: 2,399 patients with ischemic heart disease and suitable coronary artery lesions (e.g., stenosis ≥60%).

Exclusion Criteria: Unprotected left main stenosis, stroke within prior 2 years, PCI in past 3 months, systolic blood pressure (SBP) > 180 mm Hg, and diastolic blood pressure (DBP) > 100 mm Hg.

Treatment: Stent plus placebo, stent plus abciximab [0.25 mg/kg bolus up to 60 minutes before intervention and then 0.125 μg/kg/min (maximum, 10 μg/min) for 12 hours], or balloon angioplasty plus abciximab. All patients were given aspirin and heparin (70 U/kg and 100 U/kg boluses in abciximab and placebo groups, respectively). Ticlopidine administration before enrollment was encouraged.

Results: Stent plus abciximab group had more than 50% reduction in 30-day composite end points compared with the stent plus placebo group (5.3% vs. 10.8%; $p < 0.01$), whereas the balloon angioplasty plus abciximab group had a 36% reduction (6.9%; $p = 0.007$). Death and large MIs (defined as CK greater than five times normal) occurred less frequently in the abciximab groups [3.0% and 4.7% vs. 7.8% (placebo)]. However, the rates of Q-wave MI were similar (0.9% to 1.5%). No significant differences were seen in major bleeding complications (1.4% to 2.2%).

136. The ESPRIT Investigators. Novel dosing regimen of eptifibatide in planned coronary stent implantation (ESPRIT): a randomised, placebo-controlled trial. *Lancet* 2000;356:2037–2044.

Design: Prospective, randomized, double-blind, placebo-controlled, multicenter study. Primary end point was death, MI, urgent TVR, and thrombotic bailout GP IIb/IIIa inhibitor therapy within 48 hours. Secondary end point was a composite of death, MI, and urgent TVR at 30 days.

Purpose: To determine whether double-bolus dosing of eptifibatide can improve outcomes of patients undergoing coronary stenting.

Population: 2,064 patients scheduled to undergo stent implantation.

Exclusion Criteria: These included ongoing chest pain necessitating urgent PCI, MI in prior 24 hours, PCI in prior 90 days, or planned staged PCI within 30 days, stroke or transient ischemic attack (TIA) in prior month, bleeding diathesis, major surgery in prior 6 weeks, SBP > 200 mm Hg or DBP > 110 mm Hg, and platelet count < 100,000, Cr > 350 μM.

Treatment: Placebo or eptifibatide (two 180 μg/kg boluses 10 minutes apart and then 2 μg/kg/min for 18 to 24 hours). Bailout blinded GP IIb/IIIa receptor was available.

Results: The eptifibatide group had a significantly lower incidence of the primary composite end point (6.4% vs. 10.5%; $p = 0.0015$). This benefit was consistent across different components of the primary end point, including death/MI/TVR (RR, 0.65; 95% CI, 0.47 to 0.87), death/MI (RR, 0.60; CI, 0.44 to 0.82), and death (RR, 0.5; CI, 0.05 to 5.42). At 30 days, the eptifibatide group also had a reduction in the secondary end point of death, MI, and urgent TVR (6.8% vs. 10.5%; $p = 0.0034$). Eptifibatide group did have a higher incidence of major bleeding compared with placebo (1.3% vs. 0.4%; $p = 0.027$). No significant differences in major bleeding were found in the lowest tertile of ACT (ACT <244 seconds; 0.6% in both groups). At 6-month follow-across, the composite end point of death or MI had occurred in 7.5% of eptifibatide-treated patients and 11.5% of placebo-treated patients (RR, 0.63; 95% CI, 0.47 to 0.84; $p = 0.002$), whereas the composite of death, MI, or TVR had occurred in 14.2% and 18.2% of patients, respectively (RR, 0.75; 95% CI, 0.60 to 0.93). The 6-month mortality rate was 0.8% in the eptifibatide group and 1.4% in the placebo group (RR, 0.56; 95% CI, 0.24 to 1.34; $p = 0.19$). Kaplan–Meier survival curves appeared to separate over time, with most of the difference in mortality occurring between 30 days and 6 months (see JAMA 2001;285:2468–2473). At 1-year follow-up, the significant difference continued to persist (6.6% vs. 10.5%; $p = 0.015$), and a cost analysis found eptifibatide use associated with $1,407 per year of life saved (see JAMA 2002;287:618).

Comments: The persistent benefit observed at 6 and 12 months further supports the use of GP IIb/IIIa–receptor blockers as standard of care for patients undergoing stent implantation.

137. Topol EJ, et al.; for the TARGET Investigators. Comparison of two platelet glycoprotein IIb/IIIa inhibitors, tirofiban and abciximab, for the prevention of ischemic events with percutaneous coronary revascularization. N Engl J Med 2001;344:1888–1894.

Design: Prospective, randomized, double-blind, double-dummy, multicenter study. Primary end points: death, nonfatal MI, or urgent TVR at 30 days.

Purpose: To compare the safety and efficacy of the two GP IIb/IIIa inhibitors, tirofiban and abciximab.

Population: 5,308 patients scheduled for coronary stenting with >70% stenoses in either de novo or restenotic lesions in native coronary arteries or bypass grafts.

Exclusion Criteria: Cardiogenic shock, acute STEMI, serum creatinine 2.5 mg/dL or greater, high risk for bleeding or ongoing bleeding, and platelet count <120,000.

Treatment: Tirofiban (10 μg/kg bolus and then 0.15 μg/kg/min for 18 to 24 hours) or abciximab [0.25 mg/kg bolus and then 0.125 μg/kg/min (maximum, 10 μg/min) for 12 hours]. All received preprocedural aspirin (250 to 500 mg). Clopidogrel loading dose (300 mg) was given, when possible, 2 to 6 hours before PCI and then continued for 30 days (75 mg once daily). All were given initial heparin bolus of 70 U/kg, with a target ACT of 250 seconds.

Results: In both groups, 95% underwent stenting. The abciximab group had a significantly lower incidence of the primary composite end point of death, nonfatal MI, or urgent TVR compared with the tirofiban group (6.0% vs. 7.6%; $p = 0.038$). The abciximab group had fewer MIs (CK-MB, three times or more ULN or new Q waves; 5.4% vs. 6.9%; $p = 0.04$), whereas no significant differences were found between the two groups in 30-day mortality (0.4% vs. 0.5%; $p = 0.66$) or urgent TVR (0.7% vs. 0.8%; $p = 0.49$). Subgroup analysis showed superiority of abciximab in all subgroups, including age (younger than 65 or 65 years or older), gender, diabetes, and clopidogrel pretreatment. No significant differences were seen between the two groups in major bleeding complications or transfusions [0.7% (abciximab) vs. 0.9%; $p = $ NS], but tirofiban was associated with lower rates of minor bleeding episodes (2.8% vs. 4.3%; $p < 0.001$) and thrombocytopenia (<100,000/mm^3; 0.1% vs. 0.9%; $p < 0.001$). At 6 months, however, no significant difference was found between the groups in the incidence of the primary composite end point (14.8% vs. 14.3%; $p = 0.59$) (see *Lancet* 2002;360:355–360).

Comments: Two studies found the TARGET tirofiban dosing results in lower platelet inhibition levels compared those with abciximab, especially from 15 to 60 minutes after drug administration, which typically coincides with iatrogenic vessel injury (see *Am J Cardiol* 2002;89:647, 1293).

138. Karvouni E, et al. Intravenous glycoprotein IIb/IIIa receptor antagonists reduce mortality after percutaneous coronary interventions. *J Am Coll Cardiol* 2003;41:26–32.

The authors compiled 19 randomized, placebo-controlled trials of 20,137 patients undergoing PCI with and without glycoprotein IIb/IIIa inhibition. The primary outcome was mortality, with secondary outcomes including MI, composite cardiac events, and major bleeding. The analysis included trials of both PTCA and stenting, in the elective as well as urgent/emergent setting (for acute MI). Postprocedural heparin was used in approximately half of the trials. At 30 days, there was a significant reduction in mortality favoring the glycoprotein IIb/IIIa group (RR, 0.69; 95% CI, 0.53 to 0.90); this effect was persistent up to 6 months (RR, 0.79; 95% CI, 0.64 to 0.97). This was a homogeneous effect across trials, for patients with and without acute MI, and regardless of continuous heparin infusion. Notably, excess bleeding was observed only in trials in which the heparin infusion was continued postprocedure (RR, 1.70; 95% CI, 1.36 to 2.14).

139. Deibele AJ, et al. Intracoronary eptifibatide bolus administration during percutaneous coronary revascularization for acute coronary syndromes with evaluation of platelet glycoprotein IIb/IIIa receptor occupancy and platelet function: the Intracoronary Eptifibatide (ICE) Trial. *Circulation* 2010;121(6):784–791.

The investigators randomized 43 patients with ACS undergoing PCI to bolus, systemic eptifibatide versus intracoronary eptifibatide during catheterization. The primary end point was local coronary bed platelet GP IIb/IIIa saturation, as measured by coronary sinus sampling—this was significantly greater in the intracoronary group. Microvascular perfusion, as assessed by the TIMI frame count, also significantly favored the intracoronary eptifibatide group.

140. Valgimigli M, et al.; for the Multicentre Evaluation of Single High-Dose Bolus Tirofiban vs Abciximab with Sirolimus-Eluting Stent or Bare Metal Stent in Acute Myocardial Infarction Study (MULTISTRATEGY) Investigators. Comparison of angioplasty with infusion of tirofiban or abciximab and with implantation of sirolimus-eluting or uncoated stents for acute myocardial infarction: the MULTISTRATEGY randomized trial. *JAMA* 2008;299:1788–1799.

Design: Randomized, controlled trial, with open-label therapies in a 2 × 2 factorial design. Primary end point differed for each comparison: in the drug comparison, it was ST-segment resolution at 90 minutes (with a noninferiority margin); in the stent comparison, it was a composite of death, reinfarction, or TVR at 8 months.

Purpose: To compare certain reperfusion strategies for STEMI, with respect to adjunctive IIb/IIIA therapy and stent selection.

Population: 745 patients with STEMI or new LBBB in Italy, Spain, and Argentina.

Treatment: Abciximab infusion versus tirofiban infusion during PCI and BMS versus DES in PCI (2 × 2 factorial, open-label comparisons).

Results: There was no significant difference in the primary end point for the drug comparison, achieving the prespecified noninferiority margin (RR, 1.020; $p < 0.001$ for noninferiority). Furthermore, bleeding complications were similar in the two groups. However, MACEs at 8 months, the primary end point, significantly favored the DES group in the stent comparison (7.8% vs. 14.5%; $p = 0.004$). This was driven by a decrease in revascularization rates in the coated stent group.

THROMBIN INHIBITORS

141. Bittl A, et al.; Hirulog Angioplasty Study investigators (HAS). Treatment with bivalirudin (hirulog) as compared with heparin during coronary angioplasty for unstable or postinfarction angina. N Engl J Med 1995;333:764–769 (also see *Am Heart J* 2001;142:952–959).

Design: Prospective, randomized, double-blind, multicenter study. Primary composite end point was death in hospital, MI, abrupt vessel closure, or rapid clinical deterioration of cardiac origin. Follow-up period was 6 months.

Purpose: To evaluate whether bivalirudin is more effective than is heparin in reducing mortality and ischemic events in unstable or postinfarction angina patients undergoing angioplasty.

Population: 4,098 patients undergoing coronary angioplasty (PTCA) for unstable angina or postinfarct angina.

Treatment: Bivalirudin, 1.0 mg/kg bolus and then 2.5 mg/kg/h for 4 hours and 1.0 mg/kg/h for 14 to 20 hours, or heparin, 175 U/kg bolus and then 15 U/kg/h for 18 to 24 hours. Agents were started immediately before angioplasty, and doses were adjusted according to ACTs. All patients received aspirin (300 to 325 mg daily).

Results: Overall, no significant difference occurred between the groups in the incidence of the primary composite end point at 6 months (11.4% vs. 12.2%). At 7 days, however, fewer events were found in the bivalirudin group (6.2% vs. 7.9%; $p = 0.039$). Among postinfarction angina patients, bivalirudin was associated with a significant reduction in composite end points (9.1% vs. 14.2%; $p = 0.04$), although at 6 months, the cumulative rates of death, MI, and repeated revascularization were similar (20.5% vs. 25.1%; $p = 0.1$). Bivalirudin was associated with decreased bleeding (3.8% vs. 9.8%; $p < 0.001$).

142. REPLACE-2; Lincoff AM, et al. Bivalirudin and provisional glycoprotein IIb/IIIa blockade compared with heparin and planned glycoprotein IIb/IIIa blockade during percutaneous coronary intervention: the REPLACE-2 randomized trial. JAMA 2003;289:853–863.

This prospective, randomized, double-blind, triple-dummy, multicenter trial randomized 6,010 PCI patients to heparin plus a GP IIb/IIIa blocker (eptifibatide or abciximab) or to bivalirudin alone (0.75 mg/kg bolus plus 1.75 mg/kg/hr for duration of PCI) with the provisional addition of a GP IIb/IIIa blocker if needed in a double-blind, triple-dummy design. Provisional GP IIb/IIIa–blocker treatment was given to 7.2% of the bivalirudin group and 5.2% of the heparin and GP IIb/IIIa–blocker group. A nonsignificant reduction in death, MI, urgent revascularization at 30 days, and major in-hospital bleeding (primary end point) with bivalirudin was found compared with heparin plus GP IIb/IIIa blockers (9.2% vs. 10.0%; $p = 0.32$). Among the four components, the only significant difference between the groups was a significantly lower incidence of bleeding with bivalirudin (2.4% vs. 4.1%). The secondary triple end point (death, MI, urgent revascularization) showed a trend toward fewer events in the heparin plus IIb/IIIa–blocker group [7.1% vs. 7.6% (bivalirudin)]; the difference was driven by a nonsignificant excess of MI with bivalirudin (7.0% vs. 6.2%). A cost analysis found that use of bivalirudin was associated with a cost savings of $448 per patient.

143. Kastrati A, et al.; for the ISAR-REACT 3 Trial Investigators. Bivalirudin versus unfractionated heparin during percutaneous coronary intervention. N Engl J Med 2008;359:688–696.

Design: Prospective, randomized, double-blind, multicenter study. Primary composite end point of death, MI, urgent TVR for ischemia, or major bleeding at 30 days; this was designed as a net clinical benefit end point.

Purpose: To establish whether bivalirudin is superior to UFH in patients undergoing PCI after pretreatment with clopidogrel.

Population: 4,570 patients with stable or low-risk (normal cardiac markers) unstable angina undergoing PCI and pretreated with 600 mg clopidogrel at least 2 hours before PCI.

Treatment: Treatment during PCI with either bivalirudin or UFH.

Results: The primary end point occurred in 8.3% of patients in the bivalirudin group versus 8.7% in the UFH group ($p = 0.57$). The secondary end point of death, MI, or urgent TVR for ischemia occurred in 5.9% of the bivalirudin group compared with 5.0% in the UFH group ($p = 0.23$). Major bleeding occurred in 3.1% of patients receiving bivalirudin and 4.6% patients in the UFH group ($p = 0.008$). Thus, while there was no significant clinical benefit in terms of ischemic events, bivalirudin did reduce bleeding events in low-risk patients undergoing PCI.

See also the **HORIZONS-AMI** study in Chapter 4.

Special Situations

CHRONIC TOTAL OCCLUSIONS

144. Rubatelli P, et al. Gruppo Italiano di Studio sullo Stent nelle Occlusioni Coronariche (GISSOC). Stent implantation vs balloon angioplasty in chronic coronary occlusions: results from the GISSOC trial. J Am Coll Cardiol 1998;32:90–96.

This randomized study was composed of 110 patients who underwent successful PTCA of a chronically occluded vessel 3 mm in diameter. Patients were randomized to PS stenting and warfarin for 1 month or to no other therapy. Repeated angiography (at mean 9 months) revealed that the stent group had a larger mean LD (1.74 mm vs. 0.85 mm; $p < 0.001$), lower restenosis rate (32% vs. 68%; $p < 0.001$), and less reocclusion (8% vs. 34%; $p = 0.003$). The stent group also had less recurrent ischemia (14% vs. 46%; $p = 0.002$) and TLR (5.3% vs. 22%; $p = 0.038$), although hospitalization was prolonged.

145. Buller CE, et al.; Total Occlusion Study of Canada (TOSCA) Investigators. Primary stenting versus balloon angioplasty in occluded coronary arteries. Circulation 1999;100:236–242.

This prospective, multicenter, randomized trial of primary stenting (with heparin-coated PS stent) versus balloon angioplasty was composed of 410 patients with symptomatic nonacute total occlusion (TIMI grade 0/1 flow) of native coronary arteries. Randomization occurred after successful placement of a guide wire across the occlusion and was stratified by duration of occlusion ($\leq$6 weeks vs. more than 6 weeks/unknown). The crossover rate to the stent arm was 10%. The overall incidence of the primary end point, failure of sustained TIMI grade 3 flow at 6 months (confirmed by angiography), was significantly lower in the stent group (10.9% vs. 19.5%; $p = 0.024$). The stent group also had a lower restenosis rate (<50% diameter stenosis; 55% vs. 70%; $p < 0.01$) and less TVR at 6 months (8.4% vs. 15.4%; $p = 0.03$).

146. Hochman JS, et al.; for the Occluded Artery Trial (OAT) Investigators. Coronary intervention for persistent occlusion after myocardial Infarction. N Engl J Med 2006; 355:2395–2407.

Design: Prospective, randomized, multicenter trial with a primary end point composite of death, MI, or NYHA Class IV heart failure at 4 years.

Purpose: To determine the safety of the treatment of diffuse ISR.

Population: 2,166 patients with stable CAD who had total occlusion of an infarct-related artery 3 to 28 days after MI and who had high-risk features (EF < 50% or proximal occlusion). Patients in whom the infarct zone did not appear akinetic or dyskinetic were required to undergo stress testing prior to randomization—those with severe ischemia were excluded.

Treatment: PCI of infarct-related artery with stenting and optimal medical therapy or optimal medical therapy alone.

Results: At 4 years of follow-up, a primary end point event occurred in 17.2% of the PCI group and 15.6% of the medical therapy group (HR, 1.16; $p = 0.20$). Rates of recurrent, nonfatal MI were 6.9% in the PCI group and 5.0% in the medical therapy arm ($p = 0.08$): notably, only 6 (0.6%) reinfarctions were attributed to the assigned PCI procedure. Based on these data, PCI does not appear to benefit patients who have had an evolved infarct without residual ischemia.

BYPASS GRAFT LESIONS

147. Feyter PJ, et al. Balloon angioplasty for the treatment of lesions in saphenous vein grafts. J Am Coll Cardiol 1993;21:1539–1549.

This review estimates an initial success rate of 90% and restenosis rate of 42%. The poorest outcomes were seen in patients with chronic total occlusions, diffuse SVG disease, and presence of chronic graft thrombus.

148. Savage MP, et al.; Saphenous Vein de novo (SAVED). Stent placement compared with balloon angioplasty for obstructed coronary bypass grafts. N Engl J Med 1997; 338:740–747.

Design: Prospective, randomized, multicenter study. Primary end point was restenosis.

Purpose: To compare stent implantation with balloon angioplasty for the treatment of obstructive disease of venous bypass grafts.

Population: 220 patients with obstructed coronary bypass grafts.

Exclusion Criteria: MI in prior 7 days, ejection fraction <25%, diffuse disease that would require more than stents, and presence of thrombus.

Treatment: PS stent or balloon angioplasty.

Results: Stent group had higher procedural efficacy, defined as residual stenosis <50% without cardiac complications (92% vs. 69%; $p < 0.001$). However, the stent group had more hemorrhagic complications (17% vs. 5%; $p < 0.01$). Restenosis rates were not significantly different [37% (stent group) vs. 46%; $p = 0.24$], but the stent group had a lower incidence in the composite end points of freedom from death, MI, repeated bypass surgery, and TLR (73% vs. 58%; $p = 0.03$).

149. Vermeersch P, et al. Randomized double-blind comparison of sirolimus-eluting stent versus bare-metal stent implantation in diseased saphenous vein grafts: six-month angiographic, intravascular ultrasound, and clinical follow-up of the RRISC trial. J Am Coll Cardiol 2006;48(12):2423–2431.

Seventy-five patients with 96 SVG lesions were randomized to PCI with either BMS or SES, and all underwent angiography 6 months later for the primary end point of in-stent late lumen loss. Lumen loss at 6 months was significantly lower in the SES group (0.38 mm vs. 0.79 mm; $p = 0.001$). Additionally, TLR (5.3% vs. 21.6%; $p = 0.047$) and TVR (5.3% vs. 27%; $p = 0.012$) rates were significantly lower for SES; however, MACE events were similar at 6 months. Notably, in the long-term follow-up study, mortality at mean follow-up of 32 months was lower in the BMS group (29% vs. 0%; $p < 0.001$), and the 6-month advantage of SES for repeat revascularizations was lost [see DELAYED-RRISC, *J Am Coll Cardiol* 2007;50(3):261–267].

150. Brilakis ES, et al. A randomized controlled trial of a paclitaxel-eluting stent versus a similar bare-metal stent in saphenous vein graft lesions the SOS (Stenting of Saphenous Vein Grafts) trial. *J Am Coll Cardiol* 2009;53(11):919–928.

Not to be confused with another SOS trial, these investigators randomized 80 patients with 112 SVG lesions, in a controlled, multicenter trial, to either BMS or PES for their SVG disease. Primary end point was binary in-segment restenosis at 12 months (by angiography). This was dramatically lower in the PES group (9% vs. 51%; $p < 0.0001$); over 18 months, TLR was significantly lower, as well (5% vs. 28%; $p = 0.03$). There were also nonsignificant trends toward reduced target vessel failure and MI in the PES group, with similar mortality.

151. Rodés-Cabau J, et al. Comparison of plaque sealing with paclitaxel-eluting stents versus medical therapy for the treatment of moderate nonsignificant saphenous vein graft lesions: the moderate vein graft lesion stenting with the Taxus stent and intravascular ultrasound (VELETI) pilot trial. *Circulation* 2009;120(20):1978–1986.

The investigators randomized 57 patients with at least 1 SVG lesion of 30% to 60% to PCI with a PES or medical therapy alone, with IVUS and angiography at baseline and 12-month follow-up. Primary end points of the study were minimal SVG lumen by IVUS and changes in atheroma volume in disease-free SVG by ultrasound. At follow-up, patients in the medical therapy group had significant progression of disease within the index lesion compared with patients who received PES (22% vs. 0%; $p = 0.014$). Additionally, mean minimal lumen area also increased to a greater extent in the PES group ($p = 0.001$). At 12 months, incidence of MACE was 19% in the medical therapy group versus 3% in the PES group ($p = 0.091$).

SMALL VESSELS

152. Akiyama T, et al. Angiographic and clinical outcome following coronary stenting of small vessels. *J Am Coll Cardiol* 1998;32:1610–1618.

This analysis showed that stenting of small vessels is associated with poorer outcomes. A total of 1,298 consecutive patients with 1,673 lesions were identified; angiographic follow-up was done in 75%. Patients with smaller than 3-mm vessels versus 3 mm showed no difference in procedural success or subacute stent thrombosis rates (95.9% vs. 95.4%; 1.4% vs. 1.5%) but had a higher restenosis rate (32.6% vs. 19.9%; $p < 0.0001$) and a lower rate of event-free survival (63% vs. 71.3%; $p = 0.007$).

153. Savage MP, et al. Efficacy of coronary stenting versus balloon angioplasty in small coronary arteries: Stent Restenosis Study (STRESS) Investigators. *J Am Coll Cardiol* 1998;31:307–311.

Angiographic substudy of 331 STRESS I–II patients who had symptomatic CAD, de novo >70% stenosis in native coronary vessel, lesion length <15 mm, and reference vessel diameter <3.0 mm by QCA. Patients underwent PS stenting (170) or balloon angioplasty. Compared with angioplasty, stenting was associated with a larger postprocedural lumen diameter (2.26 mm vs. 1.80 mm; $p < 0.001$), and this advantage persisted at 6 months (1.54 mm vs. 1.27 mm; $p < 0.001$). The binary restenosis rates at 6 months were 34% for stenting and 55% for angioplasty ($p < 0.001$). At 1 year, the event-free (death, MI, or revascularization) survival rate was better with stenting (78% vs. 67%; $p = 0.019$), primarily because of a lower TLR rate with stenting (16.1% vs. 26.6%; $p = 0.015$).

154. Kastrati A, et al. A randomized trial comparing stenting with balloon angioplasty in small vessels in patients with symptomatic coronary artery disease. ISAR-SMART Study Investigators. *Intracoronary stenting or angioplasty for restenosis reduction in small arteries.* Circulation 2000;102:2593–2598.

Design: Prospective, randomized, multicenter study. Primary end point was the incidence of angiographic restenosis at 6 months.

Purpose: To assess whether, compared with PTCA, stenting of small coronary vessels is associated with a reduction of restenosis.

Population: 404 patients with symptomatic CAD with lesions in vessels with 2.0- to 2.8-mm diameter.

Exclusion Criteria: Included acute MI in previous 3 days, left main stenoses, and ISR.

Treatment: Stenting or PTCA. Adjunct therapy consisted of abciximab, ticlopidine, and ASA.

Results: In the PTCA group, 16.5% received at least one stent. Six-month angiographic restenosis rates were similar between the two groups [35.7% (stent) vs. 37.4% (PTCA); $p = 0.74$]. At 7 months, similar rates were found of death or MI (3.4% vs. 3.0%) and TVR (20.1% vs. 16.5%; $p = 0.35$).

Comments: In a prespecified subgroup analysis of the 98 (24%) patients with long lesions (15 mm), stenting was associated with a significant 41% relative reduction in restenosis compared with PTCA (35.6% vs. 60.6%; $p = 0.028$); however, 1-year TVR rates were not significantly different (see *Am J Cardiol* 2002;89:58).

155. Koning R, et al.; for the BESMART (BeStent in Small Arteries) Trial Investigators. Stent placement compared with balloon angioplasty for small coronary arteries: in-hospital and 6-month clinical and angiographic results. *Circulation* 2001;104: 1604–1608.

Design: Prospective, randomized, double-blind, multicenter study. Primary end point was angiographic restenosis rate at 6 months.

Purpose: To compare the results of balloon angioplasty with stenting in small arteries.

Population: 381 symptomatic patients with de novo focal lesions in small coronary vessels (<3.0 mm).

Exclusion Criteria: Ostial and/or bifurcation lesion, LVEF 30%, MI in previous 3 days, and contraindication to ASA or ticlopidine.

Treatment: Stent implantation or standard balloon angioplasty.

Results: Angiographic success rates were similar [97.6% (stent), 93.9% (PTCA)]. At follow-up angiography (obtained in 91%), the stent group had a significant 55% relative reduction in restenosis (21% vs. 47%; $p = 0.0001$). Repeated TLR was less frequent in the stent group (13% vs. 25%; $p = 0.0006$).

156. Doucet S, et al.; for the Stent In Small Arteries (SISA) Trial Investigators. Stent placement to prevent restenosis after angioplasty in small coronary arteries. *Circulation* 2001;104:2029–2033.

Design: Prospective, randomized, multicenter study. Primary end point was angiographic restenosis at 6 months (repeated angiography performed in 85.3%).

Purpose: To compare the effects of stenting and angioplasty in small vessels on restenosis rates and other major outcomes.

Population: 351 patients with stable angina, stabilized unstable angina, or documented silent ischemia with a de novo lesion and with reference vessel diameter between 2.3 mm and 2.9 mm.

Treatment: Balloon angioplasty (PTCA) alone or stent implantation.

Results: Angiographic success was achieved in 98.2% of stent patients versus 93.9% of PTCA patients ($p = 0.0065$). In the angioplasty group, 37 (20.3%) patients crossed over to stent implantation. Clinical success was higher in the stent group (95.3% vs. 87.9%; $p = 0.007$). No differences were found in major in-hospital cardiac complications including death (none), Q-wave MI (none), non–Q-wave MI (4.9% in the PTCA group vs. 1.8% in the stent group), CABG surgery (0.5% vs. 0.6%), and repeated angioplasty (2.7% vs. 0.6%). A trend toward fewer in-hospital events was seen in the stent group (3.0% vs. 7.1% in angioplasty group; $p = 0.076$), driven primarily by a lower incidence of non–Q-wave MI in the stent group. At 6 months, no significant differences were seen in the rates of angiographic restenosis [28% (stenting) vs. 32.9%] or TVR (17.8% vs. 20.3%).

DIABETES

157. Kip KE, et al. Coronary angioplasty in diabetic patients: the NHLBI PTCA Registry. Circulation 1996;94:1818–1825.

In this analysis of the 1985 to 1986 NHLBI Registry, 281 diabetic and 1,833 nondiabetic patients were studied. The diabetic group was older and had more triple-vessel coronary disease, atherosclerotic lesions, and comorbidities. At 9-year follow-up, diabetic patients had a twofold higher mortality rate (35.9% vs. 17.9%) and increased incidence of nonfatal MI (29% vs. 18.5%), CABG surgery (36.7% vs. 27.4%), and repeated PTCA (43.7% vs. 36.5%).

158. Van Belle E, et al. Effects of coronary stenting on vessel patency and long-term clinical outcome after percutaneous coronary revascularization in diabetic patients. J Am Coll Cardiol 2002;40:410–417.

A total of 314 diabetics undergoing stenting ($n = 157$) or balloon angioplasty ($n = 157$) were matched for gender, diabetes treatment regimen, stenosis location, reference diameter, and MLD. Other baseline characteristics were similar between groups. At 6 months, the stent group had a significantly lower restenosis rate (27% vs. 62%; $p < 0.0001$) and occlusion rate (4% vs. 13%; $p < 0.005$) than did the angioplasty group. The ejection fraction in the stent group remained unchanged at 6 months, whereas the angioplasty group had a significant decrease ($p = 0.02$). At 4-year follow-up, the stent group had lower rates of cardiac death and nonfatal MI (14.8% vs. 26.0%; $p = 0.02$) and revascularization (35.4% vs. 52.1%).

159. Sabaté M, et al.; for DIABETES Investigators. Randomized comparison of sirolimus-eluting stent versus standard stent for percutaneous coronary revascularization in diabetic patients: the diabetes and sirolimus-eluting stent (DIABETES) trial. Circulation 2005;112:2175–2183.

Design: Prospective, randomized, multicenter study. Primary end point was in-stent late lumen loss on angiographic restenosis at 9 months.

Purpose: To compare the effects of stenting with BMS versus SES in patients with diabetes.

Population: 160 patients with diabetes, 33% of whom were on insulin, with de novo coronary stenoses.

Treatment: PCI with BMS or SES.

Results: At 9-month angiography, in-stent late lumen loss was significantly less in the SES group (0.06 mm) compared with the BMS group (0.47 mm; $p < 0.001$), as were TLR rates (7.3% vs. 31.3%; $p < 0.001$) and MACE rates (11.3% vs. 36.3%; $p < 0.001$). Outcomes were similar between patients on insulin and those off insulin.

Comment: Long-term follow-up demonstrated persistent differences in rates of TLR and long-term safety of SES. However, they did observe stent thromboses in the SES group between 1 and 2 years, when patients had discontinued clopidogrel (see *Eur Heart J* 2007;28(16):1946–1952).

160. Lee S-W, et al. A randomized comparison of sirolimus- versus paclitaxel-eluting stent implantation in patients with diabetes mellitus (The DES-DIABETES [Drug-Eluting Stent in patients with DIABETES mellitus] Trial). *J Am Coll Cardiol* 2008;52:727–733.

Design: Prospective, randomized, multicenter study. Primary end point was ISR at 6 months.

Purpose: To compare the effects of stenting with PES versus SES in patients with diabetes.

Population: 400 patients with diabetes with native-vessel coronary stenoses.

Treatment: PCI with PES or SES.

Results: At 6-month angiographic follow-up, the SES had improved rates of ISR (3.4% vs. 18.2%; $p < 0.001$), in-segment restenosis (4.0% vs. 20.8%; $p < 0.001$), as well as 9-month TLR rates (2.0% vs. 7.5%; $p = 0.017$). The groups had similar rates of death or MI at 9 months.

Comment: Long-term follow-up demonstrated similar findings at 24 months, that is, rates of death or MI were similar, but SES continued to carry an advantage for TVR (5.5% vs. 12.0%; $p = 0.014$) and TLR (3.5% vs. 11.0%; $p = 0.004$) [see *J Am Coll Cardiol* 2009;53(9):812–813].

Complications

POSTINTERVENTION CK/CK-MB AND TROPONIN STUDIES

161. Abdelmeguid AE, et al. Significance of mild transient release of CK-MB fraction after percutaneous coronary interventions. *Circulation* 1996;94:1528–1536.

This retrospective analysis focused on 4,484 patients after PTCA or directional atherectomy. No elevations were detected in 3,776 patients; the CK level was 100 to 180 IU/L, and MB, >4% in 450 patients, and CK, 181 to 360 IU/L, and MB, more than 4% in 258 patients. CK-MB elevation predictors included atherectomy (OR, 4.1) and catheterization laboratory complications (OR, 2.6). At 3 years, the group with elevated CK and CK-MB had more MIs (RR, 1.3), cardiac deaths (RR, 1.3), and ischemic complications (death, MI, revascularization; 48.9% vs. 43.3% vs. 37.3%).

162. Kong TQ Jr, et al. Prognostic implication of CK elevation following elective coronary artery interventions. *JAMA* 1997;277:461–466.

This retrospective cohort study was composed of 253 consecutive patients with CK and CK-MB elevations and 120 patients without CK elevations. The CK elevation group had increased cardiac mortality ($p = 0.02$), highest if more than three times normal (RR, 1.05 per 100 U/L CK increase). The effect was independent of procedure type and outcome. Top mortality predictors were peak CK and ejection fraction (both $p < 0.001$).

163. Tardiff BE, et al. Clinical outcomes after detection of elevated cardiac enzymes in patients undergoing percutaneous intervention. *J Am Coll Cardiol* 1999;33:88–96.

This analysis of the IMPACT-II database showed that even small elevations in cardiac enzymes are associated with an increased short-term risk of adverse outcomes. No CK-MB elevation was seen in 1,779 (76%) patients, whereas levels were elevated to one to three times the ULN in 323 patients (13.8%), three to five times ULN in 3.6%, five to ten times ULN in 3.7%, and more than ten times ULN in 2.9%. For all devices, including stents, CK-MB elevations of any magnitude were associated with an increased incidence of the composite end point at 30 days and 6 months (at 6 months, normal CK-MB level was 20.2% to 27.3%; CK-MB, one to three times ULN, was 29.6% to 40.0%). The degree of risk correlated with the increase in enzymes, even for patients who had undergone successful procedures without abrupt closure. As seen in other studies, atherectomy performed in conjunction with angioplasty was associated with a greater incidence of postprocedural CK-MB elevations than was angioplasty alone ($p < 0.0001$).

164. Bonz AW, et al. Effect of additional temporary glycoprotein IIb/IIIa receptor inhibition on troponin release in elective percutaneous coronary interventions after pretreatment with aspirin and clopidogrel (TOPSTAR Trial). *J Am Coll Cardiol* 2002;40:662–668.

This prospective, randomized, double-blind, placebo-controlled, single-center study enrolled 109 patients with stable angina undergoing PCI. All were pretreated with a loading dose of clopidogrel (375 mg) and ASA (500 mg) 1 day before PCI. Patients were randomized to receive tirofiban (10 μg/kg bolus and then 0.15 μg/kg/min for 18 hours) or placebo. At 12, 24, and 48 hours after PCI, the tirofiban-treated patients had a lower incidence of troponin T release (12 hours, 40% vs. 63%; $p < 0.05$; 24 hours, 48% vs. 69%; $p < 0.05$; 48 hours, 58% vs. 74%; $p < 0.08$). At 9 months, the tirofiban group had a lower incidence of death, MI, and TVR (2.3% vs. 13.0%; $p < 0.05$). Future, larger studies are needed to confirm these findings, especially whether small troponin elevations with normal CK-MB levels are correlated with worse prognosis.

Also, see *Ann Clin Biochem* 2002;39:392–397: troponin I 2.0 or more seen in 27% and correlated with an increased incidence of recurrent angina, repeated PCI, coronary bypass surgery, and cardiac death at 2 years.

165. Ellis SG, et al. Death following CK-MB elevation after coronary intervention: identification of an early risk period: importance of CK-MB level, completeness of revascularization, ventricular function, and probable benefit of statin therapy. *Circulation* 2002;106:1205–1210.

This analysis examined 8,409 consecutive nonacute MI patients with successful PCI and no emergency surgery or Q-wave MI; average follow-up was 3.2 years. Post-PCI CK-MB was above normal on routine ascertainment in 17.2%. Patients were prospectively stratified into those with CK-MB one to five times or CK-MB more than five times normal. No patient with CK-MB one to five times normal died during the first week after PCI, and excess risk of early death for patients with CK-MB elevation occurred mostly in the first 3 to 4 months. The actuarial 4-month risk of death was 8.9%, 1.9%, and 1.2% for patients with CK-MB greater than five times, CK-MB one to five times, and CK-MB more than one time normal ($p < 0.001$). Incomplete revascularization ($p < 0.001$), CHF class ($p = 0.005$), and no statin treatment at hospital discharge ($p = 0.009$) were associated with death at 4 months.

166. Prasad A, et al. Prognostic significance of periprocedural versus spontaneously occurring myocardial infarction after percutaneous coronary intervention in patients with acute coronary syndromes: an analysis from the ACUITY (Acute Catheterization and Urgent Intervention Triage Strategy) trial. *J Am Coll Cardiol* 2009;54(5):477–486.

Investigators from the ACUITY trial (see Chapter 3) sought to assess the prognostic importance (if any) of periprocedural and/or spontaneous postprocedural MI in the 7,789 patients (56% of total) from the main trial who underwent an invasive strategy that included PCI for NSTEMI. They identified 466 (6.0%) periprocedural MIs and 200 (2.6%) spontaneous MIs unrelated to PCI. These patients had significantly higher rates of unadjusted 30-day mortality (5.0% vs. 3.2%; $p < 0.0001$) and 12-month mortality (16.0% vs. 6.0%; $p < 0.0001$). After risk adjustment, spontaneous MI (HR, 7.49; $p < 0.0001$), and not periprocedural MI, remained a significant predictor of mortality. However, these results are difficult to draw and solid conclusions form, given that all patients presented in the acute setting of high-risk non–ST segment elevation ACS.

STENT THROMBOSIS

167. Cutlip DE, et al. Stent thrombosis in the modern era: a pooled analysis of multi-center coronary stent clinical trials. *Circulation* 2001;103:1967–1971.

These combined results from six stent trials and associated registries included 6,186 patients who received at least one coronary stent and adjunctive therapy with aspirin and ticlopidine. At 30 days, 0.9% developed stent thrombosis (0.7% documented on angiography). Significant, procedural predictors of thrombosis in this cohort receiving BMS included persistent dissection, total stent length, and final lumen diameter.

168. Jeremias A, et al. Stent thrombosis after successful sirolimus-eluting stent implantation. *Circulation* 2004;109:1930–1932.

In this singe-center observational study of 652 patients undergoing PCI with SES, the investigators followed patients prospectively for a median of 100 days. In all, seven stent thromboses occurred during the follow-up period; these patients had significantly smaller final nominal balloon diameters (2.75 vs. 3.00 mm; $p = 0.04$) and over half (4/7) had discontinued antiplatelet therapy after the procedure. Of these seven patients with stent thrombosis, one died and five had resulting MIs.

169. Iakovou I, et al. Incidence, predictors, and outcome of thrombosis after successful implantation of drug-eluting stents. *JAMA* 2005;293:2126–2130.

In this multicenter, observational study in Europe, the investigators followed 2,229 patients who underwent PCI with either SES or PES. All patients received aspirin indefinitely and clopidogrel or ticlopidine for at least 3 months after SES and at least 6 months after PES. Primary outcomes of subacute thrombosis (up to 30 days following PCI) and late thrombosis (after 30 days) occurred in 0.6% and 0.7%, respectively, at 9-month follow-up. Overall, 0.8% of patients with SES and 1.7% with PES had stent thrombosis ($p = 0.09$). Significant, independent predictors of stent thrombosis in this cohort included premature antiplatelet therapy discontinuation (HR, 89.78; $p < 0.001$), renal failure (HR, 6.49; $p < 0.001$), bifurcation lesions (HR, 6.42; $p < 0.001$), diabetes (HR, 3.71; $p = 0.001$), and a lower EF (HR, 1.09; $p < 0.001$ for each 10% decrease).

170. Chechi T, et al. ST-segment elevation myocardial infarction due to early and late stent thrombosis: a new group of high-risk patients. *J Am Coll Cardiol* 2008;51:2396–2402.

In this retrospective study of 190 patients with STEMI, the authors identified 115 definite cases of stent thrombosis. All patients underwent primary PCI for their acute index event. Compared with patients that had STEMI from de novo coronary lesions, patients with stent thrombosis were less likely to get successful reperfusion ($p < 0.0001$), had higher distal embolization ($p = 0.01$), and were more likely to have in-hospital MACEs or major adverse cerebrovascular events ($p = 0.003$). However, among patients who survived to hospital discharge, 6-month outcomes were no different ($p = 0.7$).

OTHER COMPLICATIONS

171. Solomon R, et al. Effects of saline, mannitol, and furosemide on acute decreases in renal function induced by radiocontrast agents. *N Engl J Med* 1994;331:1416–1420.

Prospective, randomized study of 78 patients with chronic renal insufficiency (mean creatinine, 2.1 mg/dL) who underwent coronary angiography. Patients received 0.45% saline alone for 12 hours before and 12 hours after angiography, saline plus mannitol, or saline plus furosemide. Mannitol and furosemide were given just before angiography. An increase in the creatinine of 0.5 mg/dL or more after angiography was seen in 26%. The saline group had a lower incidence of elevated creatinine compared with the mannitol and furosemide groups (11% vs. 28% and 40%; $p = 0.05$). The mean increase in serum creatinine 48 hours after angiography was significantly greater in the furosemide group ($p = 0.01$) than in the saline group.

172. Kay J, et al. Acetylcysteine for prevention of acute deterioration of renal function following elective coronary angiography and intervention: a randomized controlled trial. *JAMA* 2003;289:553–558.

Prospective, randomized, double-blind, placebo-controlled trial of 200 patients with stable moderate renal insufficiency [creatinine clearance (CrCl), <60 mL/min] who underwent elective coronary angiography. Patients received oral acetylcysteine, 600 mg twice daily, or placebo, on the day before and the day of angiography. The acetylcysteine group had a significantly lower incidence of a >25% increase in serum creatinine level within 48 hours compared with placebo (4% vs. 12%; relative $p = 0.03$). Average serum creatinine also was lower in the acetylcysteine group (1.22 mg/dL vs. 1.38 mg/dL; $p = 0.006$). The benefit of acetylcysteine was present in all patient subgroups and persisted for at least 7 days.

173. Marenzi G, et al. *N*-acetylcysteine and contrast-induced nephropathy in primary angioplasty. N Engl J Med 2006;354(26):2773–2782.

Investigators randomized 354 consecutive patients with STEMI undergoing primary angioplasty to placebo, standard-dose, or high-dose *N*-acetylcysteine. In-hospital mortality was significantly higher among patients who developed contrast-induced nephropathy (26% vs. 1%; $p < 0.001$). Increase in creatinine of 25% or more occurred in 33% of patients receiving placebo, 15% in the standard-dose *N*-acetylcysteine, and 8% of the high-dose *N*-acetylcysteine group ($p < 0.001$).

174. ACT Investigators. Acetylcysteine for prevention of renal outcomes in patients undergoing coronary and peripheral vascular angiography main results from the randomized Acetylcysteine for Contrast-Induced Nephropathy Trial (ACT). *Circulation* 2011;124:1250–1259.

The investigators randomized 2,308 patients with at least 1 risk factor for contrast-induced acute kidney injury to acetylcysteine 1,200 mg (2 doses before and 2 after the procedure) versus placebo. The primary end point (contrast-induced acute kidney injury) occurred in 12.7% of each group (RR, 1.00; 95% CI, 0.81 to 1.25; $p = 0.97$).

175. Stone GW, et al.; for the CONTRAST Investigators. Fenoldopam mesylate for the prevention of contrast-induced nephropathy: a randomized controlled trial. JAMA 2003;290(17):2284–2291.

This prospective, randomized, multicenter study enrolled 315 patients with baseline CrCl of <60 cm³/min. Patients received fenoldopam (0.05 to 0.10 μg/kg/min) or placebo, starting 1 hour before angiography and continuing for 12 hours thereafter. There was no significant difference between the groups in primary end point of ≥2.5%. Serum creatinine increased in first 96 hours [33.6% (fenoldopam) vs. 30.1%; $p = 0.54$]. Additionally, there were no significant differences in death, new dialysis, or hospitalization at 30 days.

176. Merten GJ, et al. Prevention of contrast-induced nephropathy with sodium bicarbonate: a randomized controlled trial. JAMA 2004;291(19):2328–2334.

The investigators randomized 119 patients undergoing radiologic or interventional procedure requiring intravenous contrast (e.g., CT scans, angiography, etc.) to receive prehydration with either normal saline or iso-osmolar sodium bicarbonate. Regardless of randomization assignment, patients received 3 mL/kg/h for 1 hour prior to contrast and then 1 mL/kg/h during and 6 hours after the procedure. The primary end point of ≥25% increase in creatinine within 2 days occurred in 13.6% of patients in the normal saline group versus 1.7% of those receiving sodium bicarbonate ($p = 0.02$). Notably, patients in the sodium chloride group had nonsignificantly higher creatinine levels at baseline (1.89 vs. 1.71; $p = 0.09$); however, contrast loads were similar between the two groups.

177. Brar SS, et al. Sodium bicarbonate vs sodium chloride for the prevention of contrast medium–induced nephropathy in patients undergoing coronary angiography: a randomized trial. JAMA 2008;300(9):1038–1046.

The investigators randomized patients with moderate to severe chronic kidney disease (estimated GFR ≤60 mL/min per 1.73 m²) undergoing coronary angiography to either sodium bicarbonate or normal saline at similar volumes before, during, and after angiography. Additionally, patients had at least one of the following comorbidities: diabetes, CHF, HTN, or age >75 years. Rates of acute kidney injury (≥25% increase in creatinine within 4 days) were similar in the two groups (13.3% for sodium bicarbonate vs. 14.6% for normal saline; $p = 0.82$). Rates of death, dialysis, MI, or cerebrovascular events were also similar at 30 days.

178. Narins CR, et al. Relation between activated clotting time during angioplasty and abrupt closure. *Circulation* 1996;93:667–671.

This study correlated low ACTs with adverse outcomes. The analysis focused on 62 of 1,290 consecutive nonemergency angioplasty patients with in- or out-of-catheterization laboratory closure and 124 matched controls. Abrupt closure patients had a lower initial and minimum ACT (350 vs. 380 seconds; 345 vs. 370 seconds). High ACTs were not associated with more major bleeding complications.

179. Schaub F, et al. Management of 219 consecutive cases of postcatheterization pseudoaneurysm. *J Am Coll Cardiol* 1997;30:670–675.

This analysis focused on 219 patients with postcatheterization pseudoaneurysm. A compression bandage was reapplied in 132 patients with 32% success [more likely if small pseudoaneurysm (10 mm; 71% vs. 95%) and patient not anticoagulated (72% vs. 93%)]. Ultrasound-guided compression repair was undertaken in 124 patients (primary treatment modality in 49). The success rate was 84%, higher if preceded by reapplied bandage (89% vs. 76%; $p = 0.04$). Overall, surgical repair was necessary in only 7% of patients.

Coronary Restenosis

180. Belle EV, et al. Restenosis rates in diabetic patients. *Circulation* 1997;96:1454–1460 (editorial, 1374–1377).

This retrospective analysis showed an increased risk of restenosis among diabetic patients undergoing balloon angioplasty but not stenting. A total of 300 stented patients (one native-vessel procedure, no high-pressure balloon inflation; 19% diabetics) and 300 balloon angioplasty (PTCA) patients were analyzed. The PTCA group had a nearly two-fold higher restenosis rate (63% vs. 36%; $p = 0.0002$), whereas among stented patients, diabetics and nondiabetics had a similar rate of restenosis (25% vs. 27%). Editorial points out that these findings suggest that vascular remodeling (vs. neointimal proliferation) drives the excess in post-PTCA restenosis in diabetics. However, these findings contradict those of other studies that have shown no special benefit with stenting in diabetics. One possible explanation for the differences in results is that the lack of high-pressure balloon inflation in this stented population led to less vessel damage and subsequently less intimal proliferation (the latter may be especially important in the restenotic process in diabetics).

REPEAT PERCUTANEOUS CORONARY INTERVENTION FOR RESTENOSIS AFTER PERCUTANEOUS TRANSLUMINAL CORONARY ANGIOGRAPHY

181. Erbel R, et al. REST (Restenosis Stent Study). Coronary-artery stenting compared with balloon angioplasty for restenosis after initial balloon angioplasty. *N Engl J Med* 1998;339:1672–1678.

Design: Prospective, randomized, multicenter study. Primary end point was angiographic evidence of restenosis at 6 months.

Purpose: To determine whether coronary stenting, as compared with balloon angioplasty, reduces restenosis after prior successful balloon angioplasty.

Population: 383 patients with clinical and angiographic evidence of restenosis after successful balloon angioplasty.

Treatment: Standard balloon angioplasty or PS stent implantation; crossover to stenting was allowed if symptomatic dissection occurred that could not be managed with repeated balloon inflations.

Results: Stent group had a significantly lower restenosis rate (18% vs. 32%; $p = 0.03$) and less TVR (10% vs. 27%; $p = 0.001$). The difference resulted from smaller MLD in angioplasty (1.85 vs. 2.04 mm; $p = 0.01$). The stent group had better event-free survival at 250 days (84% vs. 72%; $p = 0.04$), but a nonsignificant increase was found in death and MI (at 6 months, 5.6% vs. 2.3%). Subacute thrombosis occurred more frequently in the stent group (3.9% vs. 0.6%).

Comments: These results are consistent with prior studies (35–38) that have shown a reduction in TVR but an excess of the hard end points of death and MI.

182. Alfonsa F, et al.; for the Restenosis Intra-stent: Balloon Angioplasty Versus Elective Stenting (RIBS) Investigators. A randomized comparison of repeat stenting with balloon angioplasty in patients with in-stent restenosis. *J Am Coll Cardiol* 2003;42:796–805.

Design: Prospective, randomized, multicenter study. Primary end point was recurrent ISR at 6 months.

Purpose: To compare the strategy of balloon angioplasty with restenting in patients with ISR.

Population: 450 patients with ISR more than 1 month out from prior stent placement.

Treatment: Balloon angioplasty or stent implantation.

Results: While immediate postprocedural mean luminal diameter was greater in the stenting group, at 6-month follow-up, binary restenosis rates were similar in the two groups (38% for stenting vs. 39% for balloon). Additionally, 1-year survival was similar in the two groups (77% for stent vs. 71% for balloon; $p = 0.19$). However, in the prespecified group of patients with larger vessels (≥ 3 mm), restenosis rates (27% vs. 49%; $p = 0.007$) and survival (84% vs. 62%; $p = 0.002$) favored the stenting group.

Comment: Long-term results with follow-up up to a median of 4.3 years confirmed the similar clinical outcomes in the two groups, as well as persistence of vessel diameter as a significant predictor of outcome (see *J Am Coll Cardiol* 2005;46:756–760).

183. Neumann FJ, et al. Effectiveness and safety of sirolimus-eluting stents in the treatment of restenosis after coronary stent placement (TReatment Of Patients with an In-STENT REstenotic Coronary Artery Lesion [TROPICAL]). *Circulation* 2005;111:2107–2111.

This prospective, multicenter registry followed 162 patients with ISR who were treated with PCI with SES. A 6-month follow-up angiography, in-lesion late loss was 0.08 mm, with a binary restenosis rate of 9.7%. These data supported the use of DES for ISR, leading to further clinical trials (see below).

184. Kastrati A, et al.; for the ISAR-DESIRE Study Investigators. Sirolimus-eluting stent or paclitaxel-eluting stent vs balloon angioplasty for prevention of recurrences in patients with coronary in-stent restenosis a randomized controlled trial. *JAMA* 2005;293:165–171.

Design: Prospective, randomized, multicenter study. Primary end point was recurrent ISR at 6 months, as compared between stent groups and balloon angioplasty.

Purpose: To compare the strategy of balloon angioplasty with restenting using DES in patients with ISR.

Population: 300 patients with ISR of a BMS in a native coronary artery segment.

Treatment: Balloon angioplasty or PCI with either SES or PES. All patients received a clopidogrel loading dose prior to procedure.

Results: At follow-up angiography 6 months later, binary restenosis occurred in 44.6% of patients who underwent balloon angioplasty, compared with 14.3% in the SES group ($p < 0.001$ vs. balloon) and 21.7% in the PES group ($p = 0.001$ vs. balloon). In a pre-specified comparison of SES and PES groups, restenosis ($p = 0.19$) and TVR rates (8% for SES vs. 19% for PES; $p = 0.02$) favored the SES group.

185. ISAR-DESIRE 2. Preliminary results presented at TCT 2009, San Francisco, CA.

In this subsequent study, 450 patients with ISR of prior SES were randomized to restent-ing with either PES or repeat SES. Late lumen loss at 1 year was similar in the two groups (0.40 for SES and 0.38 for PES), as were rates of the composite end point of death, MI, or stent thrombosis (6.1% for SES vs. 6.3% for PES; $p = NS$).

EFFECT OF STENT DESIGN

186. Kastrati A, et al. Intracoronary stenting and angiographic results: Strut Thickness Effect on Restenosis Outcomes (ISAR-STEREO) Trial. *Circulation* 2001; 103:2816–2821.

This prospective, randomized study of 651 patients examined whether stents with dif-ferent strut thickness result in similar restenosis rates and clinical outcomes. Patients receive either a thin-strut stent (ACS MULTI-LINK stent) or thick-strut stent (ACS MULTI-LINK DUET stent). At 30 days, urgent TVR was the same in the two groups (both 1.5%); mortality and MI rates also were similar. At 6-month follow-up angiography [obtained in 79% (thin strut) and 82%], the primary end point of restenosis was signifi-cantly lower in the thin-strut group compared with the thick-strut group (15% vs. 25.8%; $p = 0.003$). At 1-year follow-up, 8.6% of the thin-strut stent patients and 13.8% of the thick-strut stent patients required TVR because of restenosis-related ischemia ($p = 0.03$). This study shows that even small changes in stent design can result in different angio-graphic and clinical outcomes.

187. Pache J, et al. Intracoronary stenting and angiographic results: Strut Thickness Effect on Restenosis Outcome (ISAR-STEREO-2) Trial. *J Am Coll Cardiol* 2003;41:1283–1288.

This prospective, randomized study also evaluated the effect of stent strut thickness on restenosis rates in 611 patients with stenoses in native coronary arteries 2.8 mm or more in diameter. Patients received a thin-strut stent (50 mm thickness) or thick-strut stent (140 mm thickness). Vessel size, lesion length, MLD, and GP IIb/IIIa platelet inhibitor use were similar in both groups. At 6 months, QCA showed that the thin-strut group had a greater MLD and less late lumen loss compared with the thick-strut group, as well as a significantly lower binary restenosis rate (17.9% vs. 31.4%; $p < 0.001$). Clinical restenosis (TVR) also was significantly lower in the thin-strut group (12.3% vs. 21.9%; $p = 0.002$). Combined death and MI rates were similar at 1 year.

188. Briguori C, et al. In-stent restenosis in small coronary arteries: impact of strut thickness. *J Am Coll Cardiol* 2002;40:403–409.

Retrospective analysis of 821 patients who had successful stenting in small native ves-sels (3.0-mm reference diameter) and had angiographic follow-up available. The thin-strut group (<0.10 mm) included 400 patients with 505 lesions, whereas the thick-strut group had 421 patients with 436 lesions. The thin-strut group had a significantly lower restenosis rate compared with the thick-strut group (28.5% vs. 36.6%; $p = 0.009$). When three subgroups were defined (2.50 mm or smaller, 2.51 to 2.75 mm, and 2.76 to 2.99 mm), strut thickness influenced restenosis only in the 2.76- to 2.99-mm subgroup [23.5% (thin) vs. 37%; $p = 0.006$]. By logistic regression analysis, predictors of restenosis were stent length, strut thickness, and diabetes.

DRUG STUDIES

189. Schwartz L, et al. Aspirin and dipyridamole in the prevention of restenosis after PTCA. N Engl J Med 1988;318:1714–1719.

Prospective, randomized, double-blind, placebo-controlled, multicenter study of 376 patients undergoing coronary angioplasty. Patients received aspirin, 330 mg/day, and dipyridamole, 75 mg three times daily (started 24 hours before angioplasty), or placebo. Dipyridamole was given by continuous intravenous infusion (10 mg/h) from 16 hours before the procedure until 8 hours after. Among 249 patients who underwent follow-up angiography, similar restenosis rates [37.7% vs. 38.6% (placebo)] were observed. The drug therapy group had 77% fewer periprocedural Q-wave MIs (1.6% vs. 6.9%; $p = 0.01$).

190. Faxon DP, et al. Enoxaparin Restenosis after Angioplasty (ERA). Low molecular weight heparin in prevention of restenosis after angioplasty: results of enoxaparin restenosis (ERA) trial. Circulation 1994;90:908–914.

Prospective, randomized, double-blind, placebo-controlled, multicenter study of 458 patients who underwent successful angioplasty. Patient received enoxaparin, 40 mg s.c. once daily for 1 month, or placebo. At 6 months, restenosis rates were similar in the two groups [51% (placebo) vs. 52%; $p = 0.63$]. Clinical event rates also were similar, except for minor bleeding, which was more frequent in the enoxaparin group.

191. Weintraub WS, et al. Lack of effect of lovastatin on restenosis after coronary angioplasty. N Engl J Med 1994;331:1331–1337.

Prospective, randomized, double-blind, placebo-controlled, multicenter study of 404 patients undergoing successful elective coronary angioplasty of native coronary vessels. Patients received lovastatin, 40 mg twice daily, started 7 to 10 days before angioplasty, or placebo. At 6-month angiography (321 patients), no significant reduction between the groups in luminal diameter was noted (preangioplasty, 64% vs. 63%; at 6 months, 44% vs. 46%; $p = 0.50$).

192. Serruys PW, et al.; the HELVETICA Investigators. A comparison of hirudin with heparin in the prevention of restenosis after coronary angioplasty. N Engl J Med 1995;333:757–763.

Prospective, randomized, double-blind, multicenter study of 1,141 unstable angina patients in three groups. Group 1, heparin, 10,000-U bolus, continuous infusion for 24 hours and then s.c. placebo twice daily for 3 days; group 2, hirudin, 40 mg, i.v. infusion for 24 hours and then s.c. placebo twice daily for 3 days; group 3, same as group 2, except hirudin 40 mg s.c. twice daily for 3 days. Hirudin-treated patients had decreased early (96-hour) cardiac events (7.9% and 5.6% vs. 11%), but no significant differences were seen in the primary end point of event-free survival at 7 months (67.3%, 63.5%, 68%). Mean MLDs at 6-month follow-up angiography were 1.54, 1.47, and 1.56 mm, respectively ($p = 0.08$).

193. Subcutaneous Heparin and Angioplasty Restenosis Prevention Trial (SHARP). The SHARP trial: results of a multicenter randomized trial investigating the effects of high dose unfractionated heparin on angiographic restenosis and clinical outcome. J Am Coll Cardiol 1995;26:947–954.

Prospective, randomized, parallel-group, open-label, multicenter study of 339 patients who had undergone successful coronary angioplasty of de novo lesions. Patients received heparin, 12,500 U s.c. twice daily for 4 months, or no treatment. At follow-up angiography (mean, 4.2 months), no significant differences were found between treatment groups in change in mean lumen diameter.

194. Cairns JA, et al.; Enoxaparin MaxEPA Prevention of Angioplasty Restenosis (EMPAR). Fish oils and low-molecular-weight heparin for the reduction of restenosis after percutaneous transluminal coronary angioplasty. *Circulation* 1996;94:1553–1560.

Prospective, randomized, partially open, multicenter study of 814 patients undergoing elective angioplasty of de novo lesions. Patients received maxEPA, 18 capsules per day (5.4-g n-3 fatty acids), or placebo started a median 6 days before angioplasty and continued for 18 weeks. After sheath removal, 653 patients had one successfully dilated lesion and were randomized to enoxaparin, 30 mg s.c. twice daily or control (no treatment) for 6 weeks. At follow-up angiography (18 ± 2 weeks), no significant differences were observed in restenosis rates per patient and per lesion (fish oils, 46.5% vs. 39.7%; placebo, 44.7% vs. 38.7%; enoxaparin, 45.8% vs. 38.0%; control, 45.4% vs. 40.4%).

195. Karsch KR, et al. Reduction of Restenosis after PTCA: early Administration of Reviparin in a Double-Blind, Unfractionated Heparin and Placebo-Controlled Evaluation (REDUCE). Low-molecular weight heparin (reviparin) in percutaneous transluminal coronary angioplasty. *J Am Coll Cardiol* 1996;28:1437–1443.

Prospective, randomized, double-blind, multicenter study of 625 stable or unstable angina patients with single lesions suitable for elective PTCA. Patients received reviparin, 7,000 U, before PTCA, followed by 10,500 U over a 24-hour period, and then 3,500 U twice daily for 28 days, or heparin, 10,000 U over a 24-hour period, and then s.c. placebo. At 30 weeks, no significant differences were seen between groups in the primary composite end point of death, MI, reintervention, or CABG surgery [33.3% (reviparin) vs. 32%], loss of lumen diameter, and bleeding. The reviparin group had fewer acute events (3.9% vs. 8.2%; *p* < 0.03).

196. Bertrand ME, et al. Prevention of Restenosis by Elisor after Transluminal Coronary Angioplasty Trial (PREDICT). Effect of pravastatin on angiographic restenosis after coronary balloon angioplasty. *J Am Coll Cardiol* 1997;30:863–869.

Prospective, randomized, double-blind, placebo-controlled, multicenter study of 695 patients with total cholesterol, 200 to 310 mg/dL, undergoing elective angioplasty. Patients received pravastatin, 40 mg/day, or placebo for 6 months. No significant difference in mean lumen diameter was observed between the two groups [1.54 mm (pravastatin) vs. 1.54 mm; *p* = 0.21]. Late loss and net gain did not differ significantly between groups. Restenosis rates also were similar [39.2% (pravastatin) vs. 43.8%; *p* = 0.26].

197. Kastrati A, et al. Restenosis after coronary stent placement and randomized to a 4-week combined antiplatelet or anticoagulant therapy. *Circulation* 1997;96:462–467 (editorial, 383–385).

This analysis of 432 ISAR patients who underwent 6-month angiography showed no favorable effects on restenosis in patients receiving an antiplatelet regimen. Antiplatelet versus anticoagulant therapy showed no significant differences in restenosis rate (26.8% vs. 28.9%), mean luminal diameter (1.95 vs. 1.90 mm), late lumen loss (1.10 vs. 1.15 mm), or TVR (14.6% vs. 15.6%). The accompanying editorial points out that this analysis was poorly powered to detect a restenosis difference.

198. Dwens JA, et al. Usefulness of nisoldipine for prevention of restenosis after percutaneous transluminal coronary angioplasty (results of the nisoldipine in Coronary Disease in Leuven (NICOLE) study). *Am J Cardiol* 2001;87:28–33.

This randomized, double-blind, placebo-controlled, single-center trial enrolled 826 patients who underwent successful intervention in native coronary arteries. Patients were randomized to nisoldipine (20 mg/day for 2 weeks and then 40 mg/day for 3 years) or placebo. At 6 months, no significant difference was found between groups in MLD, initial gain, late loss, diameter stenosis, or binary restenosis. The nisoldipine group had a lower incidence of unscheduled coronary angiography (*p* = 0.006), CABG surgery (*p* = 0.012), and repeated target lesion PTCA (*p* = 0.017), which was likely driven by the lower incidence of recurrent angina in nisoldipine-treated patients (12% vs. 21%; *p* = 0.004).

199. Tsuchikane E, et al. Impact of cilostazol on restenosis after percutaneous coronary balloon angioplasty. *Circulation* 1999;100:21–26.

A total of 211 patients with 273 lesions who had successful PTCA were randomized to cilostazol (200 mg/day for 3 months) or aspirin (250 mg/day). At follow-up angiography (193 patients), the cilostazol group had significantly lower restenosis and TVRs compared with the aspirin group (17.9% vs. 39.5%; $p < 0.001$; 11.4% vs. 28.7%; $p < 0.001$).

200. Douglas JS, et al.; Cilostazol for Restenosis Trial (CREST) Investigators. Coronary stent restenosis in patientsm treated with cilostazol. *Circulation* 2005;112: 2826–2832.

Prospective, randomized, double-blind, placebo-controlled trial of cilostazol versus placebo to prevent ISR in 705 patients with recent BMS placement. Primary outcome of restenosis at 6 months was lower in the cilostazol group (22.0% vs. 34.5%; $p = 0.002$), an effect that was consistent in patients with diabetes as well as those with small vessels, long lesions, and LAD lesion sites. Clinical outcomes of bleeding, rehospitalization, TVR, MI, or death were similar in the two groups.

201. Lee SW, et al. Drug-eluting stenting followed by cilostazol treatment reduces late restenosis in patients with diabetes mellitus the DECLARE-DIABETES trial (A Randomized Comparison of Triple Antiplatelet Therapy With Dual Antiplatelet Therapy After Drug-Eluting Stent Implantation in Diabetic Patients). *J Am Coll Cardiol* 2008;51:1181–1187.

Prospective, randomized, multicenter trial of 400 patients with diabetes undergoing PCI with DES, randomized to cilostazol or placebo, in addition to standard dual antiplatelet therapy (aspirin and clopidogrel). After 6 months of therapy, in-stent and in-segment late loss were both significantly lower ($p = 0.025$ and $p = 0.031$, respectively). Binary restenosis rates were lower for cilostazol (8.0% vs. 15.6%; $p = 0.033$), as were 9-month TLR rates (2.5% vs. 7.0%; $p = 0.034$). There was a trend toward lower MACE rates as well (3.0% vs. 7.0%; $p = 0.066$).

202. Lee SW, et al. A randomized, double-blind, multicenter comparison study of triple antiplatelet therapy with dual antiplatelet therapy to reduce restenosis after drug-eluting stent implantation in long coronary lesions: results from the DECLARE-LONG II (Drug-Eluting Stenting Followed by Cilostazol Treatment Reduces Late Restenosis in Patients with Long Coronary Lesions) trial. *J Am Coll Cardiol* 2011;57(11):1264–1270.

Prospective, randomized, double-blind, multicenter trial enrolled 499 patients with stable angina or ACS and a native long coronary lesion ≥25 mm to either cilostazol or placebo in addition to dual antiplatelet therapy after receiving a drug-eluting stent. The primary end point was in-stent late loss at the 8-month follow-up angiography. The in-stent (0.56 ± 0.55 mm vs. 0.68 ± 0.59 mm; $p = 0.045$) and in-segment (0.32 ± 0.54 mm vs. 0.47 ± 0.54 mm; $p = 0.006$) late loss were significantly lower in the triple group than in the dual group.

203. Johansen O, et al. Coronary Angioplasty Restenosis Trial (CART). n-3 Fatty acids do not prevent restenosis after coronary angioplasty: results from the CART study. *J Am Coll Cardiol* 1999;33:1619–1626.

Prospective, randomized, double-blind, placebo-controlled study of 500 patients undergoing elective coronary angioplasty. Patients received n-3 fatty acids, 5.1 g/day, or corn oil (placebo) starting at least 2 weeks before and continued for 6 months after angioplasty. The restenosis rates were similar in the two groups (defined as MLD, <40%): 40.6% in the n-3 fatty acid group and 35.4% in the placebo group ($p = 0.21$).

204. Evaluation of Reopro and Stenting to Eliminate Restenosis (ERASER) Investigators. Acute platelet inhibition with abciximab does not reduce in-stent restenosis. *Circulation* 1999;100:799–806.

This prospective, multicenter, double-blind, placebo-controlled trial randomized 225 patients undergoing primary stent implantation to abciximab (12- or 24-hour infusion) or placebo. Target lesions were de novo 60% stenoses in native vessels with 3.0 mm to 3.5 mm diameter. At 6-month follow-up, no significant differences between groups were found in in-stent volume obstruction (primary end point).

205. Jorgensen B, et al. Restenosis and clinical outcome in patients treated with amlodipine after angioplasty: results from the Coronary AngioPlasty Amlodipine REStenosis Study (CAPARES). *J Am Coll Cardiol* 2000;35:592–599.

This prospective, randomized, double-blind, placebo-controlled, multicenter study enrolled 585 patients. Patients received amlodipine (5 to 10 mg/day) or placebo started 2 weeks before the procedure. Nonstudy calcium channel blockers were prohibited. Stenting was allowed only for bailout or unsatisfactory PTCA results (15.6%). At follow-up angiography, no significant differences were noted between groups in primary end point of mean loss in mean luminal diameter [0.30 mm (amlodipine) vs. 0.29 mm (placebo)]. At 4 months, the amlodipine group had a lower incidence of death, MI, CABG surgery, and repeated PTCA [9.4% vs. 14.5% (placebo group); $p = 0.049$]; this difference was primarily owing to fewer repeated PTCAs [3.1% vs. 7.3% (placebo group); $p = 0.02$].

206. Meneveau N, et al. Local delivery of nadroparin for the prevention of neointimal hyperplasia following stent implantation: results of the IMPRESS trial, a multicentre, randomized, clinical, angiographic and intravascular ultrasound study. *Eur Heart J* 2000;21:1767–1775.

Prospective, randomized, open-label, multicenter study of 250 patients who underwent PTCA followed by stenting. Patients were assigned to no local drug delivery (control group) or intramural delivery of nadroparin (2 mL of 2,500 anti-Xa units/mL). Local nadroparin delivery was not associated with an increase in stent thrombosis, coronary artery dissection, side-branch occlusion, distal embolization, or abrupt arterial closure. At 6-month angiography, no significant differences were noted between groups in primary end point of late loss in lumen diameter [0.84 mm (control) vs. 0.88 mm (nadroparin)] and binary restenosis rate [20% (control) vs. 24% (nadroparin)]. An IVUS substudy found that the average area of neointimal tissue within the stent was similar between the groups (2.86 mm vs. 2.90 mm). MACE rates also were similar.

207. Serruys PW, et al. Carvedilol for prevention of restenosis after directional coronary atherectomy: final results of the European Carvedilol Atherectomy Restenosis (EUROCARE) Trial. *Circulation* 2000;101:1512–1518.

This prospective, double-blind, randomized, placebo-controlled trial enrolled 406 patients; 377 underwent attempted DCA with a 50% diameter stenosis achieved in 89% without stent use. Patients received carvedilol, 25 mg twice daily, starting 24 hours before scheduled DCA and for 5 months after a successful procedure, or placebo. At follow-up angiography (mean, 6 months), no significant differences were seen between the placebo and carvedilol groups in MLD (1.99 mm vs. 2.00 mm) or angiographic restenosis (23.4% vs. 23.9%). TLR and event-free survival also were similar at 7 months (16.2% vs. 14.5%; 79.2% vs. 79.7%).

208. Neumann F, et al. Treatment of *Chlamydia pneumoniae* infection with roxithromycin and effect on neointima proliferation after coronary stent placement (ISAR-3): a randomised, double-blind, placebo-controlled trial. *Lancet* 2001;357:2085–2089.

Prospective, randomized, double-blind trial of 1,010 consecutive patients who underwent successful stenting. Patients received roxithromycin, 300 mg once daily for 28 days, or placebo. No difference was found between the groups in the primary end point of angiographic restenosis [31% (roxithromycin group) vs. 29%; $p = 0.43$] as well as TVR (19% vs. 17%; $p = 0.30$). Interestingly, in patients with high serum titers of C. *pneumoniae*, roxithromycin use was associated with a significantly lower restenosis rate [adjusted ORs at a titer of 1:512 were 0.44 (0.19 to 1.06) and 0.32 (0.13 to 0.81), respectively].

209. Holmes DR Jr, et al. Results of Prevention of REStenosis with Tranilast and its Outcomes (PRESTO) Trial. *Circulation* 2002;106:1243–1250.

Design: Prospective, randomized, placebo-controlled, double-blind, multicenter study. Primary composite end point of death, MI, or ischemia-driven TVR at 9 months.

Purpose: To determine whether tranilast reduces restenosis and major coronary events compared with placebo in patients undergoing successful PCI.

Population: 11,484 patients who underwent successful PCI and had no evidence of MI.

Treatment: Tranilast, 300 or 450 mg twice daily, for 1 or 3 months (four groups) or placebo.

Results: At 9 months, the incidence of the composite primary end point coronary was similar in the three groups (1-month tranilast group, 15.5%; placebo, 15.8%; 3-month tranilast group, 16.1%). In an angiographic substudy of 2,018 patients, the follow-up mean MLDs were similar (placebo, 1.76-mm group; tranilast, 1.72 to 1.78 mm); binary restenosis (>50%) rates also were similar (32% to 35%). In an IVUS substudy of 1,107 patients, plaque volume was not different between the placebo and tranilast groups (39.3 vs. 37.5 to 46.1 mm^3, respectively; $p = 0.16$ to 0.72).

Coronary Artery Bypass Graft Surgery

210. Eagle KA, et al. ACC/AHA 2004 guideline update for coronary artery bypass graft surgery: a report of the American College of Cardiology/American Heart Association Task Force on Practice Guidelines (Committee to Update the 1999 Guidelines for Coronary Artery Bypass Graft Surgery). *J Am Coll Cardiol.* 2004;44;e213–e310 Available at: http://www.acc.org/clinical/guidelines/cabg/cabg.pdf

211. Yusuf S, et al. Effect of coronary artery bypass graft surgery on survival: overview of 10-year results from randomised trials by the CABG Trialists Collaboration. *Lancet* 1994;344:563–570.

This review of data focuses on 1,324 patients assigned to CABG surgery and 1,325 patients who received medical management. The CABG group had a significantly lower mortality rate at 5 years (10.2% vs. 15.8%; OR, 0.61; $p = 0.0001$), 7 years (15.8% vs. 21.7%; OR, 0.68; $p < 0.001$), and 10 years (26.4% vs. 30.5%; OR, 0.83; $p = 0.03$). The risk reduction was most marked in patients with left main CAD and triple-vessel disease or single- or two-vessel disease [ORs, 0.32, 0.58 vs. 0.77 (two- and single-vessel disease)]. High-risk patients (defined as those with two of the following: severe angina, history of hypertension, prior MI, and ST-segment depression at rest) had a 29% mortality reduction at 10 years compared with a 10% reduction in patients at moderate risk and a nonsignificant trend toward higher mortality in low-risk patients [no risk factors (except ST depression) allowed].

212. Nwasokwa ON. Coronary artery bypass graft disease. *Ann Intern Med* 1995;123:528–545.

This thorough review of the literature showed only an approximate 50% patency of SVGs at 10 years after bypass surgery versus more than 90% patency achieved with IMA grafts. The use of IMA grafts leads to less frequent symptoms, better LV function, decreased need for reoperation, and improved survival. The role of antiplatelet agents in decreasing graft occlusion rates also is reviewed.

213. Pocock SJ, et al. Meta-analysis of randomised trials comparing coronary angioplasty with bypass surgery. *Lancet* 1996;346:1184–1189.

This analysis of data was derived from 3,771 patients in eight trials (CABRI, RITA, EAST, GABI, MASS, ERACI, Toulouse, Lausanne). The average follow-up period was 2.7 years. No differences were demonstrated in overall cardiac mortality between PTCA and CABG. However, CABG patients had 90% fewer 1st-year reinterventions

(3.3% vs. 33.7%) and less angina. A CABG was performed in 18% of PTCA patients within 1 year. The impact of longer follow-up is unknown (e.g., increased saphenous venous graft disease).

214. Roach G, et al. Adverse cerebral outcomes after coronary bypass surgery. N Engl J Med 1996;335:1857–1863.

This prospective study was composed of 2,108 patients, 6.1% with cerebral events: type I, 3.1% [focal injury or stupor or coma at hospital discharge (D/C); 55 of 66 had nonfatal strokes] or type II, 3% (deterioration in intellectual function, memory deficit, or seizures). Events were associated with increased in-hospital mortality [21% (type I) and 10% vs. 2%], longer hospital stay (25 days, 21 days, 10 days), and more patients discharged to intermediate or long-term care (47%, 30%, 8%). Type I predictors included proximal aortic atherosclerosis, history of neurologic disease, and age; type II predictors included age, hypertension, pulmonary disease, and alcohol consumption.

CORONARY ARTERY BYPASS GRAFT SURGERY VERSUS MEDICAL THERAPY

215. European Coronary Surgery Study (ECSS) Group. Long-term results of prospective randomised study of coronary artery bypass surgery in stable angina pectoris. Lancet 1982;320:1173–1180.

Design: Prospective, randomized, open study. Primary end point was all-cause mortality. Follow-up period was 5 to 8 years.

Purpose: To compare CABG surgery with initial medical management in patients with angina and multivessel CAD.

Population: 768 men aged ≤65 years with mild to moderate angina, ≥50% stenosis in two major vessels, and good LV function.

Treatment: CABG surgery or medical therapy.

Results: Surgery was beneficial in the total population (88.6% survival vs. 79.9% at 8 years), although most of the benefit was seen in patients with proximal LAD artery stenoses (10-year survival, 76% vs. 66%). No benefit was present if left main disease was present. Independent predictors of surgical benefit were abnormal rest ECG, ST depression 1.5 mm with exercise, peripheral vascular disease, and increased age.

216. Coronary Artery Surgery Study (CASS) Principal Investigators and their associates. Myocardial infarction and mortality in the CASS randomized trial. N Engl J Med 1984;310:750–758.

Design: Prospective, randomized, open, parallel-group study. Primary end point was all-cause mortality. Mean follow-up period was 6 years.

Purpose: To determine whether CABG surgery reduces mortality and MI rates in patients with mild angina and angiographically documented CAD.

Population: 780 patients aged ≤65 years with coronary artery stenosis ≥70%.

Exclusion Criteria: Prior CABG, unstable angina, and heart failure (NYHA Class III or IV).

Treatment: CABG surgery or medical therapy.

Results: Lower mortality trend was observed with CABG (1.1% per year vs. 1.6% per year), strongest in patients with EF ≤50% ($p = 0.085$) and triple vessel disease and EF ≤50% ($p = 0.063$). Among patients with triple vessel disease and EF of 35% to 49%, a significant mortality difference was found at subsequent follow-up [12% (CABG) vs. 35% mortality; $p = 0.009$]. At 10-year follow-up, CABG had been performed in 40% of medical patients, and no overall survival difference was noted (medical group, 79%; surgical group, 82%). However, the results of CABG were significantly better than medical therapy in patients with an EF <50% (79% vs. 61%; $p = 0.01$).

Comments: Long-term follow-up in 912 patients with left main equivalent disease (e.g., severe proximal LAD and left circumflex disease) showed that surgery prolongs life (13.1 vs. 6.2 years), but not if normal LV function is present (15-year survival, 63% vs. 54%; $p =$ NS), even with right coronary artery stenosis $\geq 70\%$ (see *Circulation* 1995;91:2335).

217. VA Coronary Artery Bypass Surgery Cooperative Study Group. Eleven year survival in Veterans Affairs randomized trial of coronary bypass surgery for stable angina. N *Engl J Med* 1984;311:1333–1339.

Design: Prospective, randomized, multicenter, open study. Primary end point was all-cause mortality. Average follow-up was 11.2 years.

Purpose: To compare CABG with medical therapy in patients with stable angina.

Population: 686 patients with stable angina pectoris of longer than 6-month duration.

Exclusion Criteria: MI in prior 6 months, unstable angina, DBP > 100 mm Hg, and uncompensated congestive heart failure.

Treatment: CABG surgery or medical therapy.

Results: Overall, a significant mortality difference was observed between groups at 7 years (77% survival in CABG group vs. 70%; $p = 0.043$) but not at 11 years (57% vs. 58%). Surgery was beneficial in the following subgroups: (a) triple-vessel disease plus LV dysfunction (per angiography), 50% versus 38% survival at 11 years ($p = 0.026$); (b) clinically high-risk patients (at least two of the following: resting ST depression, history of MI, history of hypertension), 49% versus 36% survival ($p = 0.015$); and (c) combined angiographic and clinically high risk, 54% versus 24% ($p = 0.005$). Patients with LV dysfunction (EF, <45%; end-diastolic pressure, more than 14 mm Hg; or any contraction abnormality) benefited from surgery at 7 years (survival, 74% vs. 63%; $p = 0.049$) but not at 11 years (53% vs. 49%).

Comments: Subsequent 18-year follow-up report showed no benefit of surgery, even in the high-risk subgroups. Overall, the benefits of surgery began to diminish after 5 years, a time course that parallels the development of graft disease.

CORONARY ARTERY BYPASS GRAFT SURGERY VERSUS PERCUTANEOUS TRANSLUMINAL CORONARY ANGIOGRAPHY

218. RITA Trial Participants. Coronary angioplasty vs coronary artery bypass surgery: the Randomised Intervention Treatment of Angina (RITA) trial. *Lancet* 1993;341:573–580.

Design: Prospective, randomized, multicenter study. Primary end point was death and MI. Mean follow-up period was 2.5 years.

Purpose: To compare bypass surgery with coronary angioplasty in patients in whom equivalent myocardial revascularization could be achieved by either treatment methods.

Population: 1,011 patients with multivessel coronary disease (55% with at least two diseases of the coronary arteries).

Exclusion Criteria: Left main disease, prior coronary angioplasty or bypass surgery, and significant valve disease.

Treatment: CABG surgery or PTCA.

Results: No difference was observed in the primary composite end point of death or MI at 5 years (8.6% vs. 9.8%; RR, 0.88; 95% CI, 0.59 to 1.29). CABG patients had a longer recovery but fewer additional measures. At 2 years, repeated angiography was performed in 7% versus 31% ($p < 0.001$), and revascularization or a primary event occurred in 11% versus 38% ($p < 0.001$). CABG patients also had less angina (22% vs. 31% at 2 years). A subsequent report showed that the PTCA group had a higher out-of-work rate at 2 years (26% vs. 22%) (see *Circulation* 1996;94:135).

219. Hamm CW, et al. German Angioplasty Bypass Surgery Investigation (GABI). A randomized study of coronary angioplasty compared with bypass surgery in patients with symptomatic multivessel coronary disease. *N Engl J Med* 1994;331:1037–1043.

Design: Prospective, randomized, multicenter study. Primary end point was freedom from angina at 1 year.

Purpose: To compare the clinical efficacy of bypass surgery with balloon angioplasty in patients with symptomatic multivessel CAD.

Population: 8,981 patients younger than 75 years were screened, and 359 were enrolled (total revascularization of at least two major vessels needed and feasible technically).

Exclusion Criteria: Totally occluded vessels, left main stenosis > 30%, MI in prior 4 weeks, and prior bypass or angioplasty.

Treatment: CABG surgery or PTCA.

Results: CABG group had longer hospitalization (19 vs. 5 days) and more MIs (8.1% vs. 2.3%; $p = 0.022$) owing to procedures. However, CABG patients had similar in-hospital mortality rates (2.5% vs. 1.1%), fewer interventions (6% vs. 44%; $p < 0.001$), and less angina at hospital discharge (7% vs. 18%; no difference at 1 year), and fewer patients were taking antianginal medications (12% vs. 22%; $p = 0.041$).

220. King SB, et al.; Emory Angioplasty vs Surgery Trial (EAST). A randomized trial comparing coronary angioplasty with coronary bypass surgery. *N Engl J Med* 1994; 331:1044–1050 (editorial, 1086–1087).

Design: Prospective, randomized, multicenter study. Composite primary end point was death, Q-wave MI, and large defect on thallium scan at 3 years.

Purpose: To compare outcomes of bypass surgery with angioplasty in patients with multivessel disease.

Population: 392 patients with two- or triple-vessel CAD (5,118 patients screened; 842 eligible).

Exclusion Criteria: Prior bypass surgery or coronary angioplasty, recent MI (<5 days), old chronic occlusions (more than 8 weeks), left main stenosis > 30%, and EF <25%.

Treatment: CABG surgery or PTCA.

Results: No significant difference was observed between groups in 3-year mortality (7.1% vs. 6.3%) or primary composite end points (28.8% vs. 27.3%). However, CABG patients required fewer repeated CAGB surgeries (1% vs. 22%; $p < 0.001$) and fewer angioplasties (13% vs. 41%; $p < 0.001$) and reported less angina (12% vs. 20%).

221. CABRI Trial Participants. First year results of CABRI (Coronary Angioplasty vs Bypass Revascularization Investigation). *Lancet* 1995;346:1179–1184.

Design: Prospective, randomized, multicenter, open study. Primary outcomes were 1-year mortality and symptom status (based on angina class) at 1 year.

Purpose: To compare bypass surgery with angioplasty in patients with multivessel coronary disease requiring intervention.

Population: 1,054 patients aged ≤75 years with multivessel disease and typical angina or unstable angina, 62% with Class III angina.

Treatment: CABG surgery or PTCA.

Exclusion Criteria: MI in prior 10 days, EF <35%, and prior PTCA or CABG.

Results: At 1-year follow-up, mortality rates were similar between groups (2.7% for CABG, 3.9% for PTCA). The CABG group had 81% fewer reinterventions (6.5% vs. 33.6%; $p < 0.001$) and 35% less angina, and patients were taking fewer medications. The 1-year mortality rate was highest in patients with grade IV angina or unstable angina (5% vs. 2.7%).

Comments: Complete revascularization was not required, and patients with total occlusions were not excluded.

222. Frye RL, et al.; Bypass Angioplasty Revascularization Investigation (BARI). Comparison of coronary bypass surgery with angioplasty in patients with multivessel disease. N Engl J Med 1996;335:217–225 (editorial, 275–276).

Design: Prospective, randomized, multicenter study. Primary end point was all-cause mortality. Follow-up period was 5.4 years.

Purpose: To compare outcomes of bypass surgery with angioplasty in patients with multivessel disease and severe angina or ischemia.

Population: 1,829 patients; 41% had triple-vessel CAD.

Treatment: CABG surgery or PTCA.

Results: CABG and PTCA groups had similar in-hospital mortality rates [1.3% (CABG) vs. 1.1%] and 5-year survival rates (89% vs. 86%; $p = 0.19$). The CABG group had more in-hospital Q-wave MIs (4.6% vs. 2.1%; $p < 0.01$) but had an 85% lower 5-year revascularization rate (8% vs. 54%) and 44% better 5-year survival in patients with diabetes (19% of enrolled patients; 81% vs. 66%; $p = 0.003$). The PTCA group had a 31% 5-year CABG rate.

Comments: Accompanying editorial reports that combining data from the BARI, EAST, and CABRI trials, CABG is associated with nonsignificant 14% mortality reduction (95% CI, +16% to −37%). A subsequent cost and quality-of-life analysis of 934 patients showed that the initial costs were 35% lower in the PTCA group but only 5% lower at 5 years ($56,000 vs. $58,900; $p = 0.047$). The cost of surgery was −$26,000 per year of life added, and surgical patients returned to work 5 weeks later but had better functional status at 3 years. Another analysis showed that more lesions were favorable for revascularization by CABG (92% vs. 78%; $p < 0.001$), especially 99% to 100% lesions (78% vs. 22%).

223. Rodriguez A, et al.; ERACI II Investigators. Argentine randomized study: coronary angioplasty with stenting versus coronary bypass surgery in patients with multiple-vessel disease (ERACI II): 30-day and one-year follow-up results. J Am Coll Cardiol 2001;37:51–58.

Design: Prospective, randomized, multicenter study. Primary end point: death, MI, repeated revascularization procedures, and stroke at 30 days.

Purpose: To compare PTCR with stent implantation with conventional CABG surgery in symptomatic patients with multivessel CAD.

Population: 450 patients with multivessel CAD (2,759 screened) and an indication for revascularization.

Treatment: PTCR (225 patients) or CABG (225 patients).

Results: At 30 days, the PTCR group had fewer major adverse events compared with the CABG group (3.6% vs. 12.3%; $p = 0.002$), including a significantly lower mortality (0.9% vs. 5.7%; $p < 0.013$). At follow-up (mean, 18.5 months), the PTCR had a persistent mortality benefit (3.1% vs. 7.5%; $p < 0.017$). However, as seen in prior trials of similar design, the PTCR group had a much higher revascularization rate than did the CABG group (16.8% vs. 4.8%; $p < 0.002$).

224. Serruys PW, et al.; for the Arterial Revascularization Therapies Study (ARTS) Group. Comparison of coronary-artery bypass surgery and stenting for the treatment of multivessel disease. N Engl J Med 2001;344:1117–1124.

Design: Prospective, randomized, parallel-group study. Primary end point: Freedom from death, MI, any cerebrovascular event, and any repeated coronary revascularization at 1 year.

Purpose: To compare coronary artery stenting with CABG surgery in patients with multivessel disease.

Population: 1,205 patients (average age, 61 years) who had not undergone bypass surgery or angioplasty with stable angina, unstable angina, or silent ischemia AND ≥2 de novo lesions in different vessels and territories that were amenable to stenting. The average interval between randomization and treatment was 27 days for patients in surgery group and 11 days for the stenting group.

Exclusion Criteria: LVEF 30% or less, overt congestive heart failure, history of cerebrovascular accident (CVA), transmural MI in previous week, severe hepatic or renal disease, diseased saphenous veins, neutropenia or thrombocytopenia, intolerance or contraindication to aspirin or ticlopidine, and need for major surgery.

Treatment: Stenting or CABG surgery (randomized *after* a cardiac surgeon and an interventional cardiologist concurred that the same extent of revascularization could be achieved with either technique). The average interval between randomization and treatment was 27 days for patients in the surgery group and 11 days for the stenting group. Fewer than 4% were treated with GP IIb/IIIa inhibitors.

Results: At 1 year, no significant differences were seen between the two groups in death, stroke, or MI. Surgery was associated with a higher event-free survival compared with stenting (87.8% vs. 73.8%; $p < 0.001$). This difference was due to primarily the much higher rate of repeated revascularization in the stenting group; among those without a stroke or MI, the incidence was 16.8% versus 3.5% in the surgery group. No significant difference was noted between the two groups in the incidence of death (2.8% vs. 2.5%), stroke (2.0% vs. 1.5%), or MI (4.0% vs. 5.3%). The costs for the initial procedure were $4,212 less per patient for the stenting group, but this difference narrowed to $2,973 per patient by 1-year follow-up. Among CABG patients, an elevated CK-MB was observed in 61%, and an increase to more than five times normal in 12%, and was an independent predictor of adverse clinical events. A subsequent report (see *Circulation* 2001;104:533) found that diabetics who underwent stenting had the lowest event-free survival (63.4% vs. 84.4% diabetes and CABG, 76.2% no diabetes and stenting, and 88.4% no diabetes plus CABG); this was owing to an increased incidence of repeated revascularization. A nonsignificant trend toward a lower mortality rate was seen in the diabetic CABG group compared with the diabetic stenting group (3.1% vs. 6.3%).

Comments: GP IIb/IIIa inhibitors were used infrequently in this trial; higher use may have decreased the 2.8% stent thrombosis rate and the 30% CK-MB release in the stent group. Outcomes in the modern era of GP IIb/IIIa inhibition, clopidogrel, and coated stents and with longer follow-up to detect late graft failure are not known.

225. Morrison DA, et al.; for the Investigators of the Department of Veterans Administration Affairs Cooperative Study 385, the Angina with Extremely Serious Operative Mortality Evaluation (AWESOME). Percutaneous coronary intervention vs. coronary artery bypass graft surgery for patients with medically refractory myocardial ischemia and risk factors for adverse outcomes with bypass: a multicenter, randomized trial. *J Am Coll Cardiol* 2001;38:143–149.

Design: Prospective, randomized, multicenter study. Primary end point was survival. Secondary end points were unstable angina, repeated hospitalization, repeated catheterization, and repeated revascularization with CABG or PCI.

Purpose: To compare PCI with CABG in high-risk patients with medically refractory MI.

Population: 554 patients (22,662 screened) with evidence of medically refractory MI and 1 or more of 5 high-risk clinical characteristics for CABG including prior open heart surgery, older than 70 years, LVEF <35, MI within 7 days, or intra-aortic balloon pump requirement.

Treatment: PCI or CABG surgery. The use of left IMA grafting increased from 57% in 1995 to 78% in 2000 (average, 70%), whereas stent use increased from 26% to 88% (average, 54%) and GP IIb/IIIa inhibitor use from 1% to 52% (average, 11%).

Results: The in-hospital and 30-day survival rates were 96% and 95%, respectively, for CABG and 99% and 97% for PCI. At 6-month follow-up, the small difference in survival rates was still present (90% for CABG and 94% for PCI), whereas at 3-year follow-up, survival rates were similar (79% for CABG and 80% for PCI; $p = 0.46$). No significant differences were noted between the groups in freedom from unstable angina [65% (CABG) vs. 59%; $p < 0.16$], whereas freedom from unstable angina and repeated revascularization was significantly better with CABG compared with PCI (61% vs. 48%; $p = 0.001$).

226. SoS (Stent or Surgery).; SoS Investigators. Coronary artery bypass surgery versus percutaneous coronary intervention with stent implantation in patients with multivessel coronary artery disease (the Stent or Surgery Trial): a randomised controlled trial. *Lancet* 2002;360:965–970.

Design: Prospective, randomized, open, multicenter study. Primary outcome measure was rate of repeat revascularization. Median follow-up was 2 years.

Purpose: To assess the effect of stent-assisted PCI versus CABG in multivessel CAD patients.

Population: 988 patients with symptomatic multivessel CAD.

Exclusion Criteria: Previous CABG or PCI, acute MI in prior 48 hours, intervention of valves, myocardium, great vessels, carotids, or aorta scheduled for index revascularization procedure.

Treatment: Angioplasty with stenting (PCI) or CABG surgery; in PCI arm, mean number of vessels treated was 2.2, with 78% of lesions receiving stents.

Results: The PCI group had a higher revascularization rate compared with the CABG group (21% vs. 6%; $p < 0.0001$). The incidence of death or MI at 2 years was similar in both groups (PCI 9%, CABG 10%), though the mortality rate was significantly lower in the surgery group (2% vs. 5%; $p = 0.01$).

Comments: Although the revascularization rate was higher in the stent arm, the rates were about half those seen in the BARI and EAST trials.

227. Diegeler A, et al. Comparison of stenting with minimally invasive bypass surgery for stenosis of the left anterior descending coronary artery. *N Engl J Med* 2002;347:561–566.

A total of 220 symptomatic patients with high-grade proximal LAD lesions of the coronary artery were randomized to minimally invasive surgery (thoracotomy; no cardiopulmonary bypass) or stenting. At 6 months, the surgery group had a lower incidence of MACEs, consisting of cardiac death, MI, and TLR, compared with the stenting group (15% vs. 31%; $p = 0.02$). The difference was primarily owing to higher TLR for restenosis after stenting (29% vs. 8%; $p = 0.003$), as the combined rates of death and MI did not differ significantly between groups [6% (surgery) vs. 3%; $p = 0.50$]. The surgery group had more patients free from angina after 6 months compared with the stenting group (79% vs. 62%; $p = 0.03$). It should be noted that the stent group did not receive GP IIb/IIIa inhibitors.

228. Bravata DM, et al. Systematic review: the comparative effectiveness of percutaneous coronary interventions and coronary artery bypass graft surgery. *Ann Intern Med* 2007;147:703–716.

The investigators combine results from 23 randomized studies of 5,019 patients undergoing PCI (both balloon angioplasty and stenting with BMS, only one small trial with DES) and 4,944 undergoing CABG. Over 10 years of follow-up, mortality difference between the two groups was <1%. Consistent with previous findings, procedure-related stroke incidence was higher for the CABG group (1.2% vs. 0.6%; $p = 0.002$); however, repeat revascularization rates heavily favored CABG (33% reduction at 5 years, $p < 0.001$; absolute 5-year rates of 46.1% after balloon angioplasty, 40.1% after stenting, and 9.8% after CABG). Relief of angina also favored CABG. Importantly, specific patient comorbidities possibly confounding data could not be assessed, and DES were used in a small minority of patients.

229. Daemen J, et al. Long-term safety and efficacy of percutaneous coronary intervention with stenting and coronary artery bypass surgery for multivessel coronary artery disease: a meta-analysis with 5-year patient-level data from the ARTS, ERACI-II, MASS-II, and SoS trials. *Circulation* 2008;118:1146–1154.

In a meta-analysis that included more stenting, the authors combined 4 randomized trials of 3,051 patients, following up at 5 years. Incidence of the primary end point, a composite of death, MI, and stroke, was similar (16.7% for PCI vs. 16.9% for CABG; $p = 0.69$); however, repeat revascularization rates strongly favored CABG (29.0% vs. 7.9%; $p < 0.001$). Heterogeneity analysis did not reveal differing effects in patients with diabetes. However, importantly, the four trials included were of bare-metal stenting; DES were not part of this meta-analysis.

230. Hlatky MA, et al. Coronary artery bypass surgery compared with percutaneous coronary interventions for multivessel disease: a collaborative analysis of individual patient data from ten randomised trials. *Lancet* 2009;373:1190–1197.

The authors combined data from 10 randomized trials, six of balloon angioplasty versus CABG, and four with bare-metal stenting versus CABG; mean follow-up was 5.9 years. Mortality between any PCI and CABG was similar (16% vs. 15%; $p = 0.12$); however, in the subset of patients with diabetes, mortality rates favored CABG (HR, 0.70; 95% CI, 0.56 to 0.87). Mortality also trended significantly to be lower as patient age increased ($p = 0.002$ for interaction). The authors conclude that patient-specific parameters should dictate which strategy they undergo, with the exception of older patients or those with diabetes in whom CABG may be more beneficial.

231. Hannan EL, et al. Long-term outcomes of coronary-artery bypass grafting versus stent implantation. *N Engl J Med* 2005;352:2174–2183.

In New York's cardiac registry, the authors identified patients with multivessel disease who underwent PCI with bare-metal stenting ($n = 22,102$) or CABG ($n = 37,212$) for revascularization. In this nonrandomized cohort, risk-adjusted survival rates significantly favored the CABG cohort, as stratified by disease: those with triple-vessel disease involving the proximal LAD had HR of 0.64 (95% CI, 0.56 to 0.74), and 0.76 (0.60 to 0.96) for patients with two-vessel disease involving the LAD, but not proximally. Repeat revascularization rates were higher for stenting (7.8% underwent subsequent CABG and 27.3% subsequent PCI) compared with the original CABG group (0.3% repeat CABG, 4.6% repeat PCI).

232. Hannan EL, et al. Drug-eluting stents vs. coronary-artery bypass grafting in multivessel coronary disease. *N Engl J Med* 2008;358:331–341.

In a follow-up study (see above), the authors identified patients in the New York cardiac registry who underwent either PCI with DES or CABG for multivessel CAD. This included 9,963 patients in the PCI group and 7,437 in the CABG group, with overall follow-up at approximately 18 months. In risk-adjusted analysis of patients with triple-vessel disease, overall survival rates favored the CABG group (94% vs. 92.7%; $p = 0.03$), as did survival free of MI (92.1% vs. 89.7%; $p < 0.001$). Similar distinctions were found in patients with two-vessel disease; overall survival favored CABG

(96% vs. 94.6%; $p = 0.003$), as did survival free of MI (94.5% vs. 92.5%; $p < 0.001$). In these observational data, mortality and MI rates favored CABG over PCI for patients with multivessel CAD.

233. Seung KB, et al. Stents versus coronary-artery bypass grafting for left main coronary artery disease (MAIN-COMPARE). N Engl J Med 2008;358:1781–1792.

The investigators compiled outcomes in patients with unprotected left main CAD who underwent either PCI ($n = 1,102$) or CABG ($n = 1,138$). In the PCI group, 318 (28.9%) received BMS and 784 (71.1%) received DES; mean follow-up overall was 1,017 days. There was no overall difference in rates of death (HR for stenting, 1.18; 95% CI, 0.77 to 1.80) or the composite of death, MI, or stroke (HR for stenting, 1.10; 95% CI, 0.75 to 1.62). Rates of TVR were significantly higher in the stenting group (HR, 4.76; 95% CI, 2.8 to 8.11). There was no difference in outcomes between patients who received BMS versus DES in the PCI group. These findings are persistent in long-term follow-up up to 3 years (see J Am Coll Cardiol 2009;54:853–859).

234. Serruys PW, et al.; for the SYNergy between percutaneous coronary intervention with TAXus and cardiac surgery (SYNTAX) Investigators. Percutaneous coronary intervention versus coronary-artery bypass grafting for severe coronary artery disease. N Engl J Med 2009;360:961–972.

Design: Prospective, randomized, multicenter study. Primary end point was a composite of death, stroke, MI, or repeat revascularization at 12 months, for noninferiority.

Purpose: To assess the effect of PCI with DES versus CABG in patients with triple-vessel CAD and/or left main disease.

Population: 1,800 patients with previously untreated triple-vessel CAD or left main CAD, whom both a cardiac surgeon and an interventional cardiologist had agreed were anatomically appropriate for either surgical or percutaneous revascularization.

Treatment: Complete revascularization of all vessels at least 1.5 mm in diameter with stenoses of at least 50%, either by PCI with stenting or by CABG.

Results: Results of the primary composite end point heavily favored the CABG group (12.4% vs. 17.8%; $p = 0.002$), driven predominantly by a surfeit of repeat revascularization in the PCI group (5.9% vs. 13.5%; $p < 0.001$). The trial failed to meet its noninferiority margin. However, rates of guideline-recommended therapies were more frequently used in the PCI group (e.g., aspirin, thienopyridine, statin, and ACE inhibitor use at discharge). At 12 months, rates of death or MI were similar; rates of stroke favored the PCI group (2.2% for CABG vs. 0.6% for PCI; $p = 0.003$).

Comments: Each patient's anatomy was scored for complexity, using the SYNTAX score; stratification of patients by the SYNTAX score may help determine which patients are more likely to benefit from CABG and which could be more appropriate for PCI (see Am J Cardiol 2007;99:1072–1081).

235. The BARI 2D Group. A randomized trial of therapies for type 2 diabetes and coronary artery disease. N Engl J Med 2009;360:2503–2515.

Design: Prospective, randomized, multicenter trial of patients with diabetes and CAD. Primary outcomes were death and a composite of death, MI, or stroke at 5 years.

Purpose: To assess the best management strategy for patients with type 2 diabetes and stable CAD.

Population: A total of 2,368 patients with type 2 diabetes and CAD who had not undergone revascularization in the previous 12 months were randomized following diagnostic angiography (ensuring they were suitable for either PCI or CABG but did not require urgent revascularization or have left main disease).

Treatment: Patients were randomized to either medical therapy or revascularization. Randomization was stratified by revascularization with PCI or CABG, and in a 2 × 2 factorial design, patients were also randomized to insulin sensitization or provisional insulin (to target HbA1c <7%). Overall, 763 were found to be suitable for CABG (378 randomized to CABG and 378 to medical therapy), while 1,605 were selected for PCI (798 received PCI and 807 medical therapy). Overall, 977 were randomized to insulin sensitization and 967 to provisional insulin.

Results: There was no difference in mortality at 5 years between medical therapy and revascularization (88.3% for revascularization and 87.8% for medical therapy; $p = 0.97$) and between insulin sensitization and provisional therapy (88.2% for insulin sensitization and 87.9% for provisional insulin; $p = 0.89$). Freedom from major adverse cardiovascular events also was not different among the groups (77.2% for revascularization vs. 75.9% for medical therapy; $p = 0.70$; 77.7% for insulin sensitization and 75.4% for provisional insulin; $p = 0.13$). However, when stratified by revascularization, patients who underwent CABG had lower rates of major adverse cardiovascular events than did those who received medical therapy (22.4% for CABG vs. 30.5% for medical therapy; $p = 0.002$); this effect was not detected in the PCI group. Rates of severe hypoglycemia were higher in the insulin-sensitization group, compared with provisional insulin (9.2% vs. 5.9%; $p = 0.003$).

Comments: Adding evidence to the results of the COURAGE trial (see above), these findings provided additional data to support the more limited use of PCI for revascularization. It should be noted that only a minority of eligible patients in the BARI 2D study received DES (35%) and thienopyridine therapy (21%).

236. Farkouh ME, et al.; for the FREEDOM Trial Investigators. Strategies for Multivessel Revascularization in Patients with Diabetes. N Engl J Med 2012;367:2375–2384.

Design: Prospective, randomized, multicenter trial of patients with diabetes and multivessel coronary disease. The primary endpoint was a composite of death, nonfatal MI, or nonfatal stroke.

Purpose: To evaluate the best revascularization strategy—CABG versus PCI—in patients with diabetes and multivessel coronary disease.

Population: 1900 patients with diabetes and angiographically confirmed multivessel CAD (83% with 3-vessel disease) with stenosis of more than 70% in two or more major epicardial vessels involving at least two separate coronary artery territories and without left main coronary stenosis at 140 centers from 2005 to 2010.

Treatment: Randomized to CABG versus PCI with drug-eluting stents. Dual antiplatelet therapy was recommended for at least 12 months.

Results: The primary outcome occurred in 205 (26.6%) patients in the PCI group and 147 patients (18.7%) in the CABG group ($p = 0.005$).

Comments: It is noteworthy that nearly 33,000 patients were screened for the study, yet only 1900 were randomized, calling into question the generalizability of the results.

GRAFT AND PATENCY

237. Loop FD, et al. Influence of the internal mammary graft on 10 year survival and other cardiac events. N Engl J Med 1986;314:1–6.

This retrospective analysis focused on 5,931 patients who underwent CABG from 1971 to 1979; 3,625 patients had SVGs only. IMA patients had better survival. Ten-year rates were 93.4% versus 88% ($p = 0.05$) for single-vessel disease, 90% versus 79.5% ($p < 0.0001$) for two-vessel disease, and 82.6% versus 71% ($p < 0.001$) for triple vessel disease. A Cox multivariate analysis was performed, and for the SVG group, the RR of death was 1.61; late MI RR, 1.14; hospitalization for cardiac events RR, 1.25; and cardiac reoperation RR, 2.0.

238. Cameron A, et al. Coronary bypass surgery with internal thoracic artery grafts: effects on survival over a 15-year period. N Engl J Med 1996;334:216–219 (editorial, 263–265).

This analysis focused on 5,637 CASS registry patients, including 749 patients who received arterial grafts. In multivariate analysis, internal thoracic artery patients had a 27% lower mortality rate at 15-year follow-up. Benefit was seen in all major subgroups, with the mortality difference widening over time. The accompanying editorial refers to specific situations in which internal thoracic artery grafting is contraindicated: radiation damage, extensive brachiocephalic atherosclerosis, and subclavian steal.

239. Fitzgibbon GM, et al. Coronary bypass graft fate and patient outcome: angiographic follow-up of 5065 grafts related to survival and reoperation in 1388 patients during 25 years. J Am Coll Cardiol 1996;28:616–626.

This retrospective analysis focused on 1,388 patients (mostly male veterans) who underwent surgery between 1969 and 1994; 91% of grafts were venous. SVG patency was 88% at early angiography, 81% at 1 year, 75% at 5 years, and 50% at 15 years. At 15 years, 44% had more than 50% stenoses. Arterial patency rates were significantly better: early 95% and late (5 years) 80%. Reoperative mortality (6.6% vs. 1.4% for isolated first CABG) and morbidity were mostly owing to vein graft atheroembolism.

240. Goldman S, et al. Predictors of graft patency 3 years after coronary artery bypass graft surgery. J Am Coll Cardiol 1997;29:1563–1568.

This retrospective analysis focused on 266 male VA patients with 656 grafts patent at 7 to 10 days. Multivariate analysis predictors of 3-year patency (related to operative technique vs. antiplatelet therapy) included total cholesterol ≤225 mg/dL ($p = 0.024$), no more than two proximal anastomoses ($p = 0.032$), vein preservation solution temperature ≤5°C ($p = 0.004$), and recipient artery diameter more than 1.5 mm ($p = 0.034$).

241. Lopes RD, et al. Endoscopic versus open vein-graft harvesting in coronary-artery bypass surgery. N Engl J Med 2009;361:235–244.

This was a retrospective pooled analysis of 3,000 patients in the PREVENT IV trial, a trial of vein graft treatment with E2F transcription factor decoy, edifoligide, in patients undergoing CABG. In the present study, the investigators assessed the primary outcome of vein graft failure (stenosis of at least 75%) at 12 to 18 months postoperatively. Though the method of vein harvesting was at the surgeon's discretion (nonrandomized), baseline characteristics between the two groups were similar. However, vein graft failure was higher in patients who underwent endoscopic vein harvesting, compared with those who underwent open harvesting (46.7% vs. 38.0%; $p < 0.001$). Clinical outcomes were also worse in the endoscopic group, with higher rates of death (7.4% vs. 5.8%; $p = 0.005$) or MI (9.3% vs. 7.6%; $p = 0.01$) and the composite of death, MI, or repeat revascularization (20.2% vs. 17.4%; $p = 0.04$). This study called into question the method of vein harvesting, and further, randomized data are needed.

242. Jones RH, et al.; for the STICH Hypothesis 2 Investigators. Coronary bypass surgery with or without surgical ventricular reconstruction. N Engl J Med 2009;360:1705–1717.

The investigators sought to test the hypothesis that surgical reduction of LV volume in patients with dilated, ischemic cardiomyopathy undergoing CABG would improve outcomes. They randomly assigned 1,000 patients with EF of ≤35% and CAD amenable to CABG and ventricular reconstruction to either routine CABG or CABG with LV reconstruction. At a median follow-up of 48 months, there was no difference in the primary outcome of death or cardiac hospitalization (59% for CABG alone vs. 58% for CABG plus reconstruction; $p = 0.90$). However, surgical reconstruction did significantly reduce end-systolic volume index by 19% (compared with 6%) for patients in that group; there was no difference in patients' symptoms.

243. Shroyer AL, et al.; for the Veterans Affairs Randomized On/Off Bypass (ROOBY) Study Group. On-pump versus off-pump coronary-artery bypass surgery. N Engl J Med 2009;361:1827–1837.

Design: Prospective, randomized, multicenter study. Primary end point was a composite of death, stroke, MI, or repeat revascularization at 12 months, for noninferiority.

Purpose: To assess the effect on complication rate of CABG without cardiopulmonary bypass (off-pump), compared with the use of cardiopulmonary bypass (on-pump). Primary outcome was a composite of death, repeat revascularization, or MI at 1 year after surgery.

Population: 2,203 patients undergoing CABG (urgently or electively).

Treatment: CABG surgery either on-pump or off-pump

Results: One year after surgery, rates of the composite primary outcome favored the on-pump group (7.4% vs. 9.9%; $p = 0.04$), while rates at 30 days showed a similar, nonsignificant trend (5.6% for on-pump vs. 7.0% for off-pump; $p = 0.19$). One source of the difference in clinical outcomes may be that fewer planned grafts were able to be placed in the off-pump group (17.8% incomplete revascularization rate vs. 11.1%; $p < 0.001$). Graft patency on follow-up angiography was also lower in the off-pump group (82.6% vs. 87.8%; $p < 0.01$). On neuropsychological testing, there were no differences in short-term outcomes.

Transcatheter Aortic Valve Replacement

244. Leon MB, et al. Transcatheter Aortic-Valve Implantation for Aortic Stenosis in Patients Who Cannot Undergo Surgery (PARTNER cohort B). N Engl J Med 2010;363:1597–1607.

Design: Prospective, randomized, multicenter trial. The primary end point was the rate of death from any cause.

Purpose: To evaluate the safety and efficacy of TAVR versus medical therapy in patients with severe aortic stenosis deemed inoperable candidates. Severe aortic stenosis was defined as an aortic valve area of <0.8 cm², a mean aortic valve gradient of 40 mm Hg or more, or a peak aortic jet velocity of 4.0 m/s or more.

Population: 358 patients with severe aortic stenosis deemed too high risk for surgery. All the patients had New York Heart Association (NYHA) Class II, III, or IV symptoms.

Major Exclusion Criteria: Bicuspid or noncalcified aortic valve, acute MI, significant CAD requiring revascularization, an LVEF < 20%, a diameter of the aortic annulus <18 mm or >25 mm, severe mitral or aortic regurgitation, a cerebrovascular event within the previous 6 months, and severe renal impairment.

Treatment: Transfemoral TAVR with a trileaflet bovine pericardial valve and a balloon-expandable, stainless steel support frame (Edwards SAPIEN) versus standard medical therapy.

Results: At 1 year, the rate of death from any cause was 30.7% with TAVR, as compared with 50.7% with standard therapy (HR with TAVR, 0.55; 95% CI, 0.40 to 0.74; $p < 0.001$). There were more strokes in the TAVR arm (5.0% vs. 1.1%; $p = 0.06$) as well as major vascular complications (16.2% vs. 1.1%; $p < 0.001$).

245. Smith CR, et al. Transcatheter versus Surgical Aortic-Valve Replacement in High-Risk Patients (PARNTER cohort A). N Engl J Med 2011;364:2187–2198.

Design: Prospective, randomized, multicenter trial. The primary end point was death from any cause at 1 year.

Purpose: To compare transfemoral or transapical TAVR with a balloon-expandable valve versus surgical aortic valve replacement in high-risk patients with severe aortic stenosis. Severe aortic stenosis was defined as an aortic valve area of <0.8 cm^2 plus either a mean valve gradient of at least 40 mm Hg or a peak velocity of at least 4.0 m/s.

Population: 699 patients with severe aortic stenosis and NYHA Class II or higher heart failure deemed high risk for surgery and STS score of at least 10%.

Major Exclusion Criteria: Bicuspid or noncalcified valve, CAD requiring revascularization, an LVEF < 20%, an aortic annulus diameter <18 mm or >25 mm, severe mitral or aortic regurgitation, a recent neurologic event, and severe renal impairment.

Treatment: Transfemoral (244 patients) or transapical (104 patients) TAVR with an Edwards SAPIEN balloon-expandable valve versus surgical aortic valve replacement.

Results: At 1 year, the rate of death from any cause was 24.2% in the TAVR group versus 26.8% in the surgical group ($p = 0.44$) (noninferiority $p = 0.001$). Rates of major stroke were 3.8% in the TAVR group and 2.1% in the surgical group at 30 days ($p = 0.20$) and 5.1% and 2.4%, respectively, at 1 year ($p = 0.07$).

246. Adams DH, et al. Transcatheter Aortic-Valve Replacement with a Self-Expanding Prosthesis (US CoreValve High Risk Trial). N Engl J Med 2014;370(19): 1790–1798.

Design: Prospective, randomized, multicenter noninferiority trial. The primary end point was death from any cause at 1 year, evaluated by noninferiority and superiority testing.

Purpose: To compare TAVR with CoreValve (Medtronic) self-expanding prosthesis versus surgical aortic valve replacement in high-risk patients with severe aortic stenosis. Aortic stenosis was defined as an aortic valve area of 0.8 cm^2 or less or an aortic valve index of 0.5 cm^2/m^2 or less and either a mean aortic valve gradient of more than 40 mm Hg or a peak aortic jet velocity of more than 4.0 m/s.

Population: 795 patients with severe aortic stenosis and NYHA Class II heart failure or higher deemed high risk for surgery, defined has having a risk of death within 30 days after surgery of 15% or more and a risk of death or irreversible complications within 30 days after surgery of <50% (determined by 2 surgeons and 1 interventional cardiologist).

Treatment: Iliofemoral or non-iliofemoral (subclavian or direct aortic) TAVR with a self-expanding CoreValve versus surgical AVR.

Results: The primary end point of the rate of death from any cause at 1 year was lower in the TAVR group than in the surgical group (14.2% vs. 19.1%), representing an absolute risk reduction of 4.9% ($p < 0.001$ for noninferiority; $p = 0.04$ for superiority). The rates of any stroke were 4.9% in the TAVR group and 6.2% in the surgical group at 30 days ($p = 0.46$) and 8.8% and 12.6%, respectively, at 1 year ($p = 0.10$). Permanent pacemaker implantation at 30 days was much more frequent in the TAVR group (19.8% vs. 7.1%; $p < 0.001$).

247. Abdel-Wahab M, et al. Comparison of Balloon-Expandable vs Self-expandable Valves in Patients Undergoing Transcatheter Aortic Valve Replacement (The CHOICE Trial). JAMA 2014;311(15):1503–1514.

Design: Prospective, randomized, multicenter trial. The primary end point was device success, which was a composite end point including successful vascular access and deployment of the device and retrieval of the delivery system, correct position of the device, intended performance of the heart valve without moderate or severe regurgitation, and only one valve implanted in the proper anatomical location.

Purpose: To evaluate TAVR with a balloon-expandable valve versus a self-expandable valve among high-risk patients with iliac arteries suitable for transfemoral access. Severe aortic stenosis was defined as aortic valve area ≤ 1.0 cm^2 or indexed aortic valve area ≤ 0.6 cm^2/m^2.

Population: 241 high-risk patients with severe aortic stenosis undergoing TAVR. High risk was defined as >75 years of age, logistic euroSCORE $\geq 20\%$, STS score of $\geq 10\%$, or contraindications to surgical AVR.

Treatment: TAVR with an Edwards SAPIEN XT balloon-expandable valve ($n = 121$) versus a Medtronic CoreValve self-expanding valve ($n = 12$).

Results: Device success occurred more frequently in the balloon-expandable group versus the self-expanding group (95.9% vs. 77.5%; RR 1.24; 95% CI, 1.12 to 1.37; $p < 0.001$). This difference was primarily driven by significantly more-than-mild aortic regurgitation in the self-expanding group (4.1% vs. 18.3%; RR, 0.23; 95% CI, 0.09 to 0.58; $p < 0.001$). Placement of a new permanent pacemaker was less frequent in the balloon-expandable valve group (17.3% vs. 37.6%, $p = 0.001$).

chapter 3

Unstable Angina/Non–ST Elevation MI

Christopher P. Cannon, Benjamin A. Steinberg, and Matthew W. Sherwood

EPIDEMIOLOGY

Each year in the United States, approximately 780,000 persons are admitted to hospitals for unstable angina and non–ST-elevation myocardial infarction (UA/NSTEMI), and 2 to 2.5 million worldwide. This incidence has been steadily falling over the past decade.

PATHOPHYSIOLOGY

UA/NSTEMIs are typically the result of nonocclusive coronary artery thrombus due to ruptured plaque(s). Other causes include vasoconstriction (e.g., Prinzmetal angina, microcirculatory angina), progressive mechanical obstruction, and secondary causes (e.g., tachycardia, fever, thyrotoxicosis, anemia, and hypotension) (**Fig. 3.1**).

Acute coronary syndrome (ACS) patients also have significant inflammation and plaque instability in nonculprit lesions and vessels, suggesting a widespread process. In an intravascular ultrasound study of ACS patients, plaque ruptures were evident in other lesions and vessels in more than 70% of cases (5). One study examined neutrophil myeloperoxidase (MPO) levels in several types of patients and found that the UA subset had evidence of widespread inflammation [i.e., right and left coronary circulations with low MPO levels (indicative of enzyme depletion due to neutrophil activation)].

CLASSIFICATION

Unstable Angina

Canadian Cardiovascular Society (CCS) classification of angina and Braunwald classification of UA (see *Circulation* 2000;102:118–122) are the most commonly used classifications systems. In the CCS scale, class I is angina only with strenuous

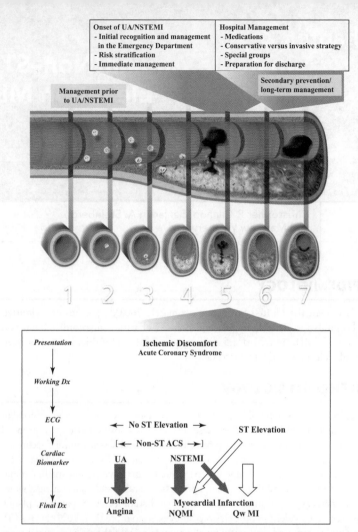

Figure 3.1 • Pathophysiology of acute coronary syndromes. **Top:** Schematic depiction of the progression of atherosclerotic CHD from natural endothelium with circulating lipids (frames 1 and 2), to deposition of lipids with formation of plaques (frames 3 and 4), leading to either unstable plaque rupture (frame 5) or stable, obstructive CHD (frames 6 and 7). **Bottom:** Clinical presentation of ACS, with correlation between ECG findings of "No ST Elevation" indicating only partial coronary occlusion, and "ST Elevation" indicating complete coronary occlusion yielding a Q-wave infarct. (Reprinted from **Anderson JL, et al.** ACC/AHA 2007 guidelines for the management of patients with unstable angina/non-ST-elevation myocardial infarction: a report of the American College of Cardiology/American Heart Association Task Force on Practice Guidelines (Writing Committee to Revise the 2002 Guidelines for the Management of Patients With Unstable Angina/Non-ST-Elevation Myocardial Infarction): developed in collaboration with the American College of Emergency Physicians, American College of Physicians, Society for Academic Emergency Medicine, Society for Cardiovascular Angiography and Interventions, and Society of Thoracic Surgeons. *J Am Coll Cardiol* 2007;50:e1–e157, with permission from Elsevier.)

activity, class II is slight limitation with vigorous activity, class III indicates marked limitation with normal activity, and class IV patients are unable to perform activities of daily living and have episodes of rest angina. The Braunwald system is multitiered; severity of angina consists of three classes: class I, new-onset (<2 months), severe, or accelerated, with no rest pain in the preceding 2 months; class II, subacute (angina at rest more than 48 hours to 1 month previously); and class III, acute (at least one episode in the preceding 48 hours). Patients also are assigned a clinical class as follows: class A, secondary UA (e.g., triggered by anemia, infection, thyrotoxicosis); class B, primary UA; class C, postinfarction UA [<2 weeks after documented myocardial infarction (MI)]. Class IIIB patients are further subdivided into troponin-negative and troponin-positive patients. The third tier of the system is intensity of therapy: (a) absence of or minimal therapy; (b) occurring in the presence of standard therapy for chronic stable angina (e.g., oral β-blockers, nitrates, calcium antagonists); and (c) occurring despite maximal therapy [oral therapy and intravenous (IV) nitroglycerin (NTG)].

Non–ST-Elevation Myocardial Infarction

One-third to one-half of patients in UA trials actually had an NSTEMI, defined as an elevation of cardiac markers of necrosis such as creatine kinase (CK)-MB or a troponin isoform.

CLINICAL AND LABORATORY FINDINGS

History and Symptoms

Chest discomfort typically occurs at rest or with increasing frequency and lasts 5 to 20 minutes but can last several hours. However, some patients, particularly women and those with diabetes, may experience atypical symptoms and may not have any chest discomfort. Temporary/incomplete relief may be provided by sublingual NTG.

Electrocardiogram

In UA/NSTEMI, ST-segment depression is seen in approximately 20% to 30% of cases, and transient ST-segment elevation in 2% to 5%; these changes are predictive of adverse outcomes. T-wave inversions occur in approximately 20%; if present in five or more leads, they are associated with higher risk. In NSTEMI patients, Q waves develop in 15% to 25%.

Cardiac Enzymes

CREATINE KINASE AND CREATINE KINASE-MB

These markers of myocardial necrosis are elevated in patients with NSTEMI. Both levels will typically increase approximately 6 hours after onset of ischemic symptoms and normalize within 48 to 72 hours.

TROPONINS T AND I

An elevated troponin in the appropriate clinical scenario is a qualifying crite-rion for MI. Because these markers are more sensitive than CK and CK-MB, the new MI definition will lead to higher MI rates, as one in three patients previously diagnosed with UA have had NSTEMI. In a meta-analysis of 21 published studies, the two types of troponins were found to be equally sensitive and specific. In one study of patients with rest pain, troponin T was detected in 39%, whereas CK-MB was elevated in fewer than 10%. Troponin levels begin to increase within 4 to 6 hours after symptom onset, remain ele-vated for several days, and thus are a reliable marker for diagnosing MI within the preceding 2 to 7 days. For the same reason, however, CK-MB levels are usually necessary to diagnose reinfarction within the first several days of an index infarction.

Later-generation assays of troponin, labeled high-sensitivity troponin (hsTroponin) have become available with significantly lower limits of detection. These tests are so sensitive, a small proportion of the general population will have detectable levels of troponin depending on the assay used. While several studies have demonstrated their clinical utility for risk stratification (88,89), no hsTroponin test is currently approved for clinical use.

MYOGLOBIN

Usefulness of myoglobin is limited by lack of cardiac specificity and period of brief elevation (<24 hours). However, in conjunction with other data, a nega-tive myoglobin can be helpful in ruling out MI.

ESTIMATION OF EARLY RISK AT PRESENTATION

The Thrombolysis in Myocardial Infarction (TIMI) risk score (TRS) consists of seven predictor variables (each worth one point): age older than 65 years, three or more coronary artery disease (CAD) risk factors, prior coronary ste-nosis of more than 50%, ST-segment deviation on initial electrocardiography (ECG), two or more anginal events in prior 24 hours, use of aspirin in prior 7 days, and elevated serum cardiac markers. With TIMI 11B and Efficacy and Safety of Subcutaneous Enoxaparin in Non–Q-Wave Coronary Events (ESSENCE) data, the event rate (death, new or recurrent MI, ischemia requir-ing urgent revascularization) at 14 days increased from 4.7%, with a TRS of 0 or 1, to 40.9% for a score of 6 or 7 (**Fig. 3.2**) (see *Am J Cardiol* 1999;83:1147–1151). This score has been validated in eight studies including the TIMI 3 Registry (see *Am J Cardiol* 2002;90:303), the Platelet Receptor Inhibition in Ischemic Syndrome Management in Patients Limited by Unstable Signs and Symptoms (PRISM-PLUS) study (see *Eur Heart J* 2002;23:223), and the Clopidogrel in Unstable Angina to Prevent Recurrent Events (CURE) trial (see *Circulation* 2002;106:1622), where a higher risk also predicted greater benefit from glycoprotein (GP) IIb/IIIa inhibition. In a prespecified analysis in Treat Angina with Aggrastat and Determine Cost of Therapy with an Invasive

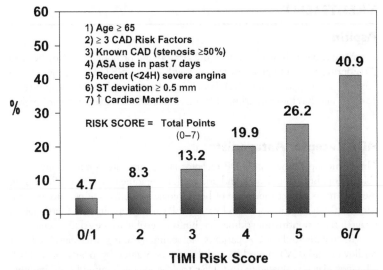

Figure 3.2 • **This risk score is derived from data on TIMI IIB and ESSENCE patients and shows a clear gradation of increasing risk with a higher risk score.** (Data from **Antman EM, et al.** The **TIMI Risk Score** for unstable angina/non–ST elevation MI. A method for prognostication and therapeutic decision making. JAMA 2000;284:835–842.)

or Conservative Strategy (TACTICS)-TIMI 18 trial, those with higher TRS were found to have a significantly greater benefit from an early invasive strategy, whereas those with TRS of 0 to 2 had similar outcomes with an invasive or conservative strategy. In summary, this score with broad applicability is easily calculated and identifies patients with different responses to treatments for UA/NSTEMI (62).

Boersma et al. (see *Circulation* 2000;101:2557) also developed a risk-estimation score based on analysis of Platelet Glycoprotein IIb/IIIa in Unstable Angina Receptor Suppression Using Integrilin Therapy (PURSUIT) trial data. The most important baseline features associated with death were age, higher heart rate (HR), lower systolic blood pressure (SBP), ST-segment depression, signs of heart failure, and elevated cardiac markers.

Lastly, a risk score to predict mortality was derived from the Global Registry of Acute Coronary Events (GRACE) registry of 15,007 patients in the derivation cohort (79). The model predicted 6-month mortality for patients with STEMI, NSTEMI, and UA based on nine clinical criteria: older age, history of MI, history of heart failure, tachycardia at presentation, hypotension at presentation, elevated initial creatinine, elevated initial biomarkers, ST-segment depression at presentation, and not having percutaneous coronary intervention (PCI) in-hospital. This score also could predict the risk of death or MI.

TREATMENT

Aspirin

Aspirin has been shown to reduce the risk of fatal or nonfatal MI by 50% to 70% during the acute phase in patients with UA or NSTEMI and by 50% to 60% at 3 months to 3 years (7,8). For chronic treatment, low-dose aspirin (e.g., 75 to 81 mg) has lower bleeding risk and similar efficacy compared with higher doses (11).

ADP Receptor Antagonists

Three thienopyridine-type ADP receptor antagonists are commercially available, ticlopidine, clopidogrel, and prasugrel; ticlopidine has largely fallen out of use, due to its higher incidence of hematologic side effects, especially neutropenia (<0.1% risk for clopidogrel vs. 1% risk with ticlopidine). A fourth agent, ticagrelor, is a nonthienopyridine that binds reversibly to the ADP receptor.

In an early study of UA patients, ticlopidine (250 mg twice daily) reduced cardiovascular (CV) mortality and reinfarction rates by nearly 50% (10). Clopidogrel was evaluated in the CURE trial, which randomized 12,662 patients with unstable or NSTEMI to aspirin alone or clopidogrel, 300-mg loading dose and 75 mg once daily, and aspirin (11). At follow-up (mean, 9 months), the clopidogrel group had a significant 20% reduction in CV death, MI, or stroke compared with the aspirin-only group. An initial loading dose of clopidogrel (300 mg) was given, and the event curves separated within 2 hours. The clopidogrel group had a higher incidence of major bleeding at 1 year (3.7% vs. 2.7%).

Based on these results, the American College of Cardiology (ACC)/American Heart Association (AHA) guidelines advocate dual antiplatelet therapy with an ADP receptor antagonist and aspirin for ideally a year, in patients with UA/NSTEMI whether managed with revascularization or medically.

Prasugrel was evaluated in the 13,608-patient TRITON-TIMI 38 trial, in which patients with ACS, including STEMI patients, as well as those with UA/NSTEMI (74% of the total) were planned for PCI, and most often had undergone angiography without pretreatment with clopidogrel (12). The overall results found that prasugrel significantly reduced the risk of CV death, MI, or stroke by 19%, from 12.1% for clopidogrel to 9.9% for prasugrel ($p < 0.001$). In UA/NSTEMI patients undergoing PCI, prasugrel significantly lowered rates of the primary endpoint (a composite of CV death, MI, or stroke) at 15 months, when compared to clopidogrel (9.9% vs. 12.1%, hazard ratio 0.82; $p = 0.002$). A subsequent study of prasugrel for pretreatment in the setting of non-STE ACS patients scheduled for a invasive approach showed no improvement in rates of CV death, MI, or stroke (13). However, pretreatment with prasugrel did result in an increase of major bleeding events (13) when compared to selective use of prasugrel in patients at the time of PCI. Additionally, the TRILOGY ACS trial (14) showed that in patients presenting with non-STE ACS in whom a medical management strategy was planned, prasugrel therapy, as compared with clopidogrel, did not improve CV outcomes and again resulted in an increased risk for major bleeding events. Thus, prasugrel is approved for use in ACS, but *only* at the time of PCI.

Ticagrelor was studied in the PLATO (PLATelet Inhibition and Patient Outcomes) trial of patients with ACS (both UA/NSTEMI and STEMI). The study compared ticagrelor to clopidogrel in the prevention of CV events in 18,624 patients admitted to the hospital with ACS, with or without ST-segment elevation. The primary endpoint was the composite of death from vascular causes, MI, or stroke at 1 year. The endpoint had occurred in 9.8% of patients receiving ticagrelor as compared with 11.7% of those receiving clopidogrel (hazard ratio 0.84; 95% CI, 0.77 to 0.92; $p < 0.001$). No significant differences in the overall rate of major bleeding rates were found between the two groups ($p = 0.43$), although ticagrelor was associated with a higher rate of major bleeding not associated with coronary artery bypass graft (CABG). Total mortality was reduced with ticagrelor, 4.5%, versus 5.9% with clopidogrel; $p < 0.001$. Benefit was seen both in patients managed with an invasive strategy as well as a conservative strategy (see *BMJ* 2011;342:d3527). As such, current guidelines recommend ticagrelor over clopidogrel in patients managed with either strategy (4).

PAR-1 RECEPTOR ANTAGONISTS

A novel antiplatelet agent, vorapaxar, has recently been studied as an adjunctive therapy to aspirin and a P2Y12 inhibitor for the prevention of thrombotic events post-ACS. This drug is an antagonist of the PAR-1 receptor on the platelet, one of the most potent receptors for platelet activation. In the TRACER trial (16) the addition of vorapaxar to standard of care therapy (dual antiplatelet therapy for the large majority) on admission for ACS resulted in similar rates of CV death, MI, stroke, and urgent revascularization over 2-year follow-up. In addition, patients on vorapaxar had significantly greater risk for major bleeding events compared with patients on standard therapy. This resulted in the rejection of application to the FDA for use of vorapaxar in the ACS setting.

Nonetheless, the drug has been recently approved in the secondary prevention of MI based on the TRA 2P-TIMI 50 trial (17). Since enrollment criteria were between 2 weeks and 1 year post MI, some patients would appear to benefit from vorapaxar in the post-ACS setting, although increased risk of bleeding needs to be considered (see Chapter 1).

Heparin

In a meta-analysis of six trials, unfractionated heparin (UFH) showed a strong trend toward reducing rates of reinfarction and recurrent ischemia when used with aspirin [odds ratio (OR), 0.67; 95% confidence interval (CI) 0.44 to 1.02] (21). Increased rates of adverse events have been identified with heparin therapy for >48 hours after admission for UA. After discontinuation of heparin infusion, a rebound phenomenon occurs, with patients at increased risk of reactivation of UA and MI (20).

Low-Molecular-Weight Heparins

The ESSENCE and TIMI IIB trials showed enoxaparin to be superior to UFH, resulting in 15% to 20% fewer major events (death, MI, and urgent revascularization) at 6 weeks (25,27). In the smaller EVET trial, enoxaparin was directly compared with another low-molecular-weight heparin (LMWH), tinzaparin; the enoxaparin group had a significantly lower incidence of recurrent UA or need for revascularization (see *J Am Coll Cardiol* 2001;37:365).

In the Fragmin during Instability in CAD (FRISC) trial (23), dalteparin (120 IU/kg subcutaneously twice daily for 6 days, and then 7,500 IU/day for 35 to 45 days) showed a significant reduction in death and MI at 6 days compared with placebo, whereas the Fragmin in Unstable Coronary Artery Disease (FRIC) trial showed equivalence between dalteparin and IV UFH (24). In FRISC II (26), extended use of dalteparin (120 IU/kg twice daily for 3 months) was associated with a significant reduction in death or MI at 30 days, but the reduction did not remain significant at 3 months. In the Fraxiparine in Ischemic Syndrome (FRAXIS) trial (28), Fraxiparine showed no benefit compared with UFH; this study enrolled many low-risk patients.

It is not clear why enoxaparin is the only agent with a clear benefit, but it does have a higher ratio of anti-factor Xa to antithrombin activity (3.8:1.0) than does dalteparin or Fraxiparine. The current ACC/AHA guidelines have a class Ia recommendation for either LMWH or UFH as treatment for UA/NSTEMI (**Fig. 3.2** and **Table 3.1**).

LMWH can be used in conjunction with GP IIb/IIIa inhibitors. In the Integrilin and Enoxaparin Randomized Assessment of Acute Coronary Syndrome Treatment (INTERACT) trial, 746 UA/NSTEMI patients receiving eptifibatide were randomized to heparin or enoxaparin, and the enoxaparin group had a significantly lower incidence of death and MI at 30 days (29). The A to Z study compared enoxaparin with UFH in a patient population that all received IIb/IIIa inhibitors and mainly involved a noninvasive approach. A total of 3,987 high-risk ACS patients, all of whom received aspirin and tirofiban, were randomized to enoxaparin or UFH; 60% of patients underwent angiography. The enoxaparin group had a 12% reduction in death, MI, or refractory ischemia compared to UFH (8.4% vs. 9.4%), which fulfilled the trial's noninferiority goal but did not demonstrate superiority ($p = 0.23$). Finally, the 10,000-patient SYNERGY trial compared the two agents in patients who were all going to the catheterization lab; enoxaparin was not superior, but was noninferior to heparin for death or MI at 30 days (see Chapter 2 for more details).

LMWHs stimulate platelets less than do UFHs and have a lower incidence, compared with UFH, of heparin-induced thrombocytopenia (HIT). However, these agents also are associated with a higher incidence of minor bleeding compared with UFH.

An alternative to both UFH and LMWHs is the pentasaccharide factor Xa inhibitor fondaparinux, which was evaluated most extensively in the Organization to Assess Strategies for Ischemic Syndromes (OASIS) 5 trial (31).

Table 3.1	Factors Associated with Appropriate Selection of Early Invasive Strategy or Ischemia-guided Strategy in Patients with NSTE-ACS

Immediate invasive (within 2 h)
 Refractory angina
 Signs or symptoms of HF or new or worsening mitral regurgitation
 Hemodynamic instability
 Recurrent angina or ischemia at rest or with low-level activities despite intensive
  medical therapy
 Sustained VT or VF

Ischemia-guided strategy
 Low-risk score (e.g., TIMI [0 or 1], GRACE [<109])
 Low-risk Tn-negative female patients
 Patient or clinician preference in the absence of high-risk features

Early invasive (within 24 h)
 None of the above, but GRACE risk score >140
 Temporal change in Tn (Section 3.4)
 New or presumably new ST depression

Delayed invasive (within 25–72 h)
 None of the above but diabetes mellitus
 Renal insufficiency (GFR < 60 mL/min/1.73 m^2)
 Reduced LV systolic function (EF < 0.40)
 Early postinfarction angina
 PCI within 6 mo
 Prior CABG
 GRACE risk score 109–140; TIMI score ≥2

From **Amsterdam E, et al.** 2014 AHA/ACC Guideline for the Management of Patients With Non-ST-Elevation Acute Coronary Syndromes: a Report of the American College of Cardiology/American Heart Association Task Force on Practice Guidelines. *Circulation* 2014;130:e344–e426. doi: 10.1161/cir.0000000000000134

The investigators randomized 20,078 patients with UA/NSTEMI to either enoxaparin or fondaparinux for the primary endpoint of death, MI, or recurrent ischemia at 9 days. There were no statistically significant differences in the primary endpoint (5.8% for fondaparinux vs. 5.7% for enoxaparin). However, the incidence of catheter-related thrombus in patients undergoing PCI on fondaparinux led to hesitation in using this agent as sole anticoagulant during PCI, and most interventionalists will switch to UFH.

Direct Thrombin Inhibitors

In the Global Utilization of Streptokinase and Tissue Plasminogen Activator for Occluded Coronary Arteries (GUSTO) IIb trial, hirudin use in patients with ACS (chest pain with ECG changes) resulted in a nonsignificant 11% reduction in death and MI at 30 days compared with heparin (39). In the OASIS-2 trial, medium-dose hirudin (0.4 mg/kg bolus and then 0.15 mg/kg/h) resulted in a nonsignificant 16% reduction in CD and MI at 7 days. A meta-analysis of the GUSTO IIb, TIMI 9B, OASIS 1, and OASIS 2 trials found that hirudin was associated with a significant 10% lower risk of death or MI at 35 days compared with heparin ($p = 0.015$) (42). Hirudin is currently indicated only for anticoagulation in patients with HIT, but these data show that additional trials of the direct antithrombins are warranted.

In addition to the data from the REPLACE-2 trial (see Chapter 2), bivalirudin was tested in the ACUITY trial, in which investigators randomized 13,819 patients with UA/NSTEMI undergoing invasive management to a heparin (UFH or LMWH) plus GP IIb/IIIa, bivalirudin plus GP IIb/IIIa, or bivalirudin alone. The primary endpoints included a composite of ischemic events, bleeding, and net clinical benefit (ischemia and bleeding combined). For the comparison of either heparin or bivalirudin (both with GP IIb/IIIa agents), the bivalirudin group had similar rates of ischemic and bleeding. When used without a GP IIb/IIa inhibitor, bivalirudin was associated with significantly less bleeding when compared to a heparin with GP IIb/IIIa inhibition. This trial specifically enrolled patients undergoing aggressive, early invasive management. Thus, the use of bivalirudin as part of early management in patients with UA/NSTEMI is a class I recommendation only for those undergoing an invasive strategy.

Factor Xa Inhibitors

Newer agents, such as factor Xa inhibitors have been studied in the ACS setting as well. The ATLAS 2 ACS TIMI 51 trial (43) evaluated the use of low-dose rivaroxaban in addition to mono- or dual antiplatelet therapy for the treatment of ACS (both STEMI and NSTE-ACS). The trial found that both the 5- and 2.5-mg doses of rivaroxaban were associated with modest benefit in terms of CV death, MI, and stroke, but also an increased risk of major bleeding events. The 2.5-mg dose of rivaroxaban was also associated with small absolute mortality benefit. The risk of fatal bleeding events was very low and similar in all treatment arms. Despite the modest benefit in this setting, rivaroxaban has not been approved by the FDA for use in patients with ACS. In a similar trial, the factor Xa inhibitor apixaban was associated with increased bleeding in ACS patients, when added to standard therapy (44). Additional trials using non–vitamin K oral anticoagulants are described in Chapter 6.

Glycoprotein IIB/IIIA Inhibitors

INTRAVENOUS AGENTS

The current ACC/AHA guidelines recommend (class IA) the use of either an IV GP IIb/IIIa antagonist or clopidogrel in UA/NSTEMI patients in whom catheterization and PCI are planned. Eptifibatide or tirofiban is preferred for "upstream" use (class IB); if it is only a short time to angiography, then abciximab can be used. Both clopidogrel and a GP IIb/IIIa may be used in some circumstances (class IIa). In patients being managed with a conservative strategy, a GP IIb/IIIa inhibitor could be considered (class IIb), but it would be also reasonable to add only if a patient developed recurrent ischemia (see **Table 3.1**):

1. Tirofiban: In the PRISM-PLUS trial (45), tirofiban, heparin, and aspirin resulted in decreased rates of death, MI, and refractory ischemia at 7 days compared with heparin alone, and death and MI were decreased by approximately 30% at 30 days.
2. Eptifibatide: In the large PURSUIT trial, eptifibatide showed an approximately 10% reduction in death and MI at 30 days (47).
3. Abciximab: The Evaluation of c7E3 for the Prevention of Ischemic Complications (EPIC), Evaluation in PTCA to Improve Long-term Outcome with Abciximab Glycoprotein IIb/IIIa Blockade (EPILOG), and c7E3 Fab Antiplatelet Therapy in Unstable Refractory Angina (CAPTURE) trials were interventional studies that enrolled some UA patients, and all showed substantial reductions (30% to 60%) at 30 days in the rates of death, MI, and ischemia-provoked intervention or revascularization (see Chapter 2). The 6-month results of the Evaluation of Platelet IIb/IIIa Inhibitor for Stenting (EPISTENT) trial, another interventional study comparing stenting alone versus stenting plus abciximab versus balloon angioplasty plus abciximab, showed a 10% absolute reduction in death and MI in the subgroup of patients with UA. However, the large GUSTO IV-ACS trial, which enrolled all ACS patients (7,800), abciximab was associated with no reduction in death or MI at 30 days compared with placebo, and the mortality rate was actually higher in the first 48 hours in the abciximab groups (51). Based on these results, abciximab is not recommended in ACS patients in whom PCI will be delayed. In the ISAR-REACT 2 trial, abciximab retained its benefit after the addition of clopidogrel in patients with ACS undergoing PCI, though the advantage was confined to those patients with elevated troponin (52).

The question of timing of administration of GP IIb/IIIa inhibitors was addressed in the 9,492-patient EARLY ACS trial (55). The investigators randomized patients undergoing invasive management of UA/NSTEMI to either early eptifibatide (12 hours or more prior to PCI) or provisional eptifibatide after angiography (but before intervention). For the primary outcome composite of death, MI, recurrent ischemia requiring revascularization, or thrombotic complication during PCI (requiring "bailout" therapy), there was no statistical difference between the early or delayed groups (9.3% for early vs. 10.0% in delayed group; $p = 0.23$). Bleeding rates were higher in patients receiving early eptifibatide. As such, routine early initiation of GP IIb/IIIa inhibition could not be recommended on the basis of this trial.

ORAL AGENTS

In contrast to the IV agents, several oral agents have shown an *increased* risk of death or bleeding events (see *Circulation* 2002;106:375; *Am J Med* 2002;112:647). The OPUS-TIMI 16 trial was terminated early because of an increased 30-day mortality in one of the orbofiban arms (48). In the SYMPHONY trial (49), sibrafiban was comparable to aspirin for major events but was associated with increased bleeding; these results prompted the early termination of the larger SYMPHONY II trial (50).

Thrombolytic Therapy

Thrombolytic therapy was not found to be beneficial in the TIMI 3 and the Unstable Angina Study Using Eminase (UNASEM) trials (56,57). Use was associated with increased bleeding and MI rates, and no benefit of adjunctive intracoronary thrombolytic therapy was observed during PTCA in the Thrombolysis and Angioplasty in Unstable Angina (TAUSA) trial (58).

Anti-Ischemic Medications

β-BLOCKERS

Limited randomized trial data are available on the use of β-blockers in specifically UA/NSTEMI. However, given the significant benefit demonstrated in STEMI, recent MI, heart failure, and stable angina, it is appropriate to extrapolate to UA/NSTEMI (see Chapter 4 for more details). They have been associated with lower mortality in patients undergoing PCI for ACS (see *J Interv Cardiol* 2003;16:299–305). Specific medication choices include metoprolol, propranolol, and atenolol. β-Blockers are contraindicated in the presence of marked first-degree atrioventricular (AV) block; any second- or third-degree block; severe bronchospastic lung disease; severe left ventricular dysfunction with evidence of acute congestive heart failure (CHF); relative bradycardia; or relative hypotension. The ACC/AHA guidelines added a class III recommendation that "It may be harmful to administer IV beta blockers to UA/NSTEMI patients who have contraindications to beta blockade (as noted above), signs of heart failure or low-output state, or other risk factors for cardiogenic shock, which include age >70 years, SBP < 120 mm Hg, sinus tachycardia >110 or HR < 60, presentation more than 6 hour after symptom onset."

NITRATES

Nitrates are useful for treating episodes of recurrent ischemia (reducing both left ventricular end-diastolic pressure and SBP). If no relief is gained from three sublingual NTG tablets, IV NTG should be started. If nitrates do not provide adequate relief or if acute pulmonary congestion is found, consider morphine administration. Nitrates are contraindicated if a patient has hypotension (particularly in cases of right-ventricular infarction) or has taken a PDE inhibitor (e.g., sildenafil [Viagra]) within 24 hours. Furthermore, there is a paucity of data demonstrating any improvement in clinical outcomes with nitrates, and, as such, current recommendations are for the use of nitrates to relieve ischemia, but they should *not* preclude use with proven therapies (such as β-blockers or ACE inhibitors).

CALCIUM CHANNEL BLOCKERS

Calcium channel blockers are as effective in relieving symptoms, but an overview of randomized trials showed no reduction in mortality or MI rates. Diltiazem confers a possible benefit in non–Q wave MI patients (majority with NSTEMI). In the Diltiazem Reinfarction Study, diltiazem use was associated with a significant reduction in in-hospital mortality (33). However, no overall benefit was observed by the Multicenter Diltiazem Postinfarction Trial Research Group, although a post hoc analysis showed benefit in patients without evidence of left ventricular dysfunction. Similar to the effect of nitrates, calcium channel blockers' benefit is largely confined to the reduction of ischemic discomfort and has not demonstrated a significant effect on clinical outcomes in UA/NSTEMI. Furthermore, clinicians should be aware of the potential for reflex tachycardia (and adverse events) in patients receiving dihydropyridine calcium channel blockers (particularly immediate-release nifedipine) in the absence of β-blockade.

3-HYDROXY-3-METHYLGLUTARYL COENZYME A REDUCTASE INHIBITORS (STATINS)

In the Myocardial Ischemia Reduction with Aggressive Cholesterol Lowering (MIRACL) study, 3,086 conservatively managed UA/NSTEMI patients were randomized to high-dose atorvastatin (80 mg once daily) or placebo (38). In the atorvastatin group, mean low-density lipoprotein (LDL) cholesterol decreased from 124 to 72 mg/dL, and a significantly lower incidence of death, nonfatal MI, cardiac arrest with resuscitation, or ischemia requiring rehospitalization was found. Data from the CHAMP study found that if a statin was started in hospital, 91% were taking a statin at 1 year versus only 10% if not given in-hospital, and 58% had an LDL <100 mg/dL versus only 6% prior to institution of the quality improvement program (see Am J Cardiol 2001;87:819). Increasing data favor the more aggressive use of higher-dose statins earlier in patients with ACS, particularly those undergoing invasive management (see J Am Coll Cardiol 2009;54:2290–2295). For more data on statins, see Chapter 1.

Invasive Strategy

With coronary angiography, multivessel disease is found in 40% to 50%, single-vessel disease in 30% to 35%, left main disease in 5% to 10%, and no critical obstruction in 10% to 20%.

The routine use of angiography and subsequent revascularization has been studied in numerous randomized trials, with the five most recent studies all showing a significant benefit associated with an invasive strategy. The first trial, TIMI 3B, showed that early angiography followed by revascularization (if indicated) did not reduce major cardiac events but did result in fewer hospital readmissions (59), whereas the Veteran Affairs Non–Q-wave Infarction Strategies in Hospital (VANQWISH) study, which enrolled medium- to high-risk patients, showed no benefit of an invasive strategy and a trend toward higher mortality

(60). The invasive group in the VANQWISH study had a high CABG operative mortality rate (12%). Both the TIMI 3B and VANQWISH trials were performed before GP IIb/IIIa inhibitors and coronary stenting was commonly used.

The FRagmin and Fast Revascularization during InStability in CAD study reported a significantly lower incidence of death or MI with an invasive strategy compared with a noninvasive strategy (at 6 months, 9.4% vs. 12.1%; $p = 0.031$) (61). A subgroup analysis showed that this benefit was restricted to men.

The TACTICS-TIMI 18 study enrolled 2,220 patients with at least one high-risk feature [ECG changes, elevated cardiac markers, or a history of CAD (prior catheterization, revascularization, or MI)] (62). Patients randomized to an early invasive strategy (routine catheterization within 4 to 48 hours and revascularization as appropriate) had a 22% lower incidence of death, nonfatal MI, and rehospitalization for an ACS at 6 months compared with a more conservative strategy (catheterization only if recurrent ischemia or abnormal stress test). Patients with an elevated troponin T had an even larger 39% reduction in the primary endpoint.

In the Randomised Intervention Trial of unstable Angina (RITA) 3 trial (63), 1,810 UA/NSTEMI patients were randomized to an early intervention or a conservative strategy. The intervention group had a 34% lower incidence of death, MI, or refractory angina at 4 months. Two other smaller randomized studies also found significant benefits with an early invasive strategy (TRUCS; see *Eur Heart J* 2000;21:1954; VINO, see *Eur Heart J* 2002;23:230).

The ICTUS trial tested the hypothesis of a "selectively invasive" strategy, randomizing 1,200 patients with NSTEMI at high risk (all patients had elevated troponin T and either ECG changes or a history of CAD) to either an early invasive strategy or a more conservative "selectively invasive" strategy whereby patients were taken to PCI only if they had refractory angina, hemodynamic or ECG instability, or significant ischemia on predischarge stress test (65). All patients received a contemporary in-hospital regimen, including aspirin, enoxaparin, and abciximab (at time of PCI); clopidogrel and aggressive lipid lowering were recommended. While the trial did not demonstrate any reduction in the primary endpoint of death, MI, or rehospitalization for angina within 1 year, it should be noted that nearly half of the patients in the "selectively invasive" arm underwent revascularization.

In summary, after extensive investigation of management strategy in the current era, the latest ACC/AHA guidelines stratify management approaches by immediate invasive, early invasive, delayed invasive, or "ischemia-guided" (previously "conservative") (**Fig. 3.2**). They consider an immediate invasive strategy a class I indication if any of the following high-risk features are present: (a) refractory angina or recurrent angina/ischemia at rest or low-level activity despite intensive therapy; (b) CHF signs or symptoms, new or worsening mitral regurgitation; (c) hemodynamic instability; or (d) sustained ventricular tachycardia (VT). With regard to timing of an early invasive strategy, the TIMACS trial compared early (median = 14 hours after randomization) with later (median = 50 hours) angiography. Overall, there was just a trend for reduction of the primary endpoint (death, MI, and stroke) in the group as a whole, but a significant reduction in patients with a high GRACE risk score. (See *N Engl J Med* 2009;360:2165–2175.) Thus, the highest-risk, most unstable patients should be sent to cardiac catheterization within 12 to 24 hours, whereas others can go within 2 to 3 days.

The success rate of PCI is 90% to 95%. Ischemic complications are reduced by concomitant administration of IV GP IIb/IIIa inhibitor (see earlier).

CORONARY ARTERY BYPASS GRAFT SURGERY

The operative mortality rate with CABG surgery is typically 3% to 4% in patients with refractory UA (vs. approximately 2% for patients with chronic stable angina). Improved survival has been demonstrated in patients with left main disease and three-vessel disease with significant left ventricular dysfunction (see Chapter 2). An intra-aortic balloon pump may be needed for stabilization before surgery.

NONINVASIVE EVALUATION

Exercise Treadmill Test

Treadmill testing should not be performed in the acute phase of UA/NSTEMI. In low-risk patients free of rest or low-level ischemia and CHF, the exercise treadmill test (ETT) can be performed after a minimum of 12 to 24 hours. In intermediate-risk patients, the wait should be at least 2 or 3 days. If the patient is high risk (e.g., ≥2-mm ST-segment depression), catheterization should be considered in place of ETT.

Exercise Treadmill Testing with Nuclear Imaging

The ACC/AHA guidelines have a class I recommendation for the following patient subsets: baseline ST-segment abnormalities, bundle branch block, left ventricular hypertrophy, intraventricular conduction delay, paced rhythm, pre-excitation, and digoxin effect. Imaging also adds sensitivity to low-level/nondiagnostic ETT tests. The size of perfusion defect(s) is predictive of mortality and major cardiac events.

Pharmacologic Stress Testing with Imaging

Pharmacologic stress testing with imaging is indicated in patients with severe physical limitations.

Echocardiography

In patients with chest pain but no ECG changes or an obscured ECG picture [left bundle branch block (LBBB), paced rhythm], echocardiography can be used to evaluate whether a wall-motion abnormality is present.

Coronary Computerized Tomography Angiography

In patients presenting with chest pain to the emergency department, but who are felt to have a low likelihood of actually having ACS, use of coronary computed tomography angiogram (CCTA) is now an option for "ruling out" coronary disease. Data from 368 patients in the ROMICAT trial demonstrated that in such low-risk patients (negative troponin and ECG), 64-slice coronary CTA (computed tomography angiogram) could effectively "rule out" patients for ACS during index hospitalization (69). The ROMICAT II trial extended these findings (70). In 1,000 patients evaluated in the emergency department for chest pain, the use of cardiac CT angiography, as compared with standard ED care, was associated with a shorter mean length of stay, a shorter mean time to diagnosis, and greater rates of direct discharge from the ED with no differences seen in periprocedural complications, major adverse cardiac events, or costs of care. Thus a normal CTA conferred extraordinary low risk for coronary disease, and can be used efficiently and effectively in the emergency department to speed care. However, in patients with coronary plaque or stenosis, further investigation is warranted.

PROGNOSIS AND BIOMARKERS

Unstable Angina

The hospital mortality rate is 1% to 2%; 1-year mortality rate, 7% to 10%; and 1-month reinfarction rate, approximately 5%. Twenty to twenty-five percent of patients are rehospitalized within 1 year. Recurrent ischemia is associated with a nearly threefold higher mortality.

Non–ST-Elevation Myocardial Infarction

The in-hospital mortality rate is 3% to 4%; reinfarction rate, 8% to 10%; and 1-year mortality rate, 10% to 15%. (The latter is similar to that of ST-elevation patients.)

Prior Aspirin Use (Aspirin Failures)

Prior aspirin use is associated with an increased risk of death or MI at 30 days.

Electrocardiography

A TIMI 3 Registry analysis showed an increased risk of death and MI at 1 year with LBBB on admission ECG [relative risk (RR), 2.8] and 0.5 mm of ST deviation (RR, 2.5). T-wave inversion alone was not associated with increased risk (98).

Troponin Levels

Troponin levels have been shown to provide substantial prognostic information. TIMI 3B and FRISC analyses showed a strong correlation between troponin T levels and adverse outcomes (84,85). In the FRISC trial, the benefit of LMWH over aspirin was limited to patients with elevated troponin T levels (84). In five trials (CAPTURE, PRISM, PRISM-PLUS, Paragon B, ISAR-REACT 2), the benefit of GP IIb/IIIa inhibition was magnified in patients with elevated troponin-T levels, with no benefit in troponin-negative patients (86). In the TACTICS-TIMI 18 trial, an elevated troponin level was associated with a 40% reduction in major cardiac events in the early invasive group versus conservative strategy group, whereas patients with normal levels (troponin I <0.1 ng/mL or troponin T <0.01 ng/mL) had no significant benefit from an early invasive strategy (87). The poor prognosis of elevated troponin even persisted in patients without significant angiographic CAD.

As noted above, more advanced troponin assays have been developed, with significantly lower limits of detection. Several studies have demonstrated their diagnostic and prognostic power in patients with ACS; however, none is currently approved.

C-Reactive Protein

Elevated levels of C-reactive protein (CRP) are found more commonly in patients with increased risk of mortality. Multiple analyses have shown an additive, yet separate, effect of CRP and troponin in predicting mortality (91–93).

B-Type Natriuretic Peptide

Brain (B-type) natriuretic peptide (BNP) is a neurohormone synthesized predominantly in ventricular myocardium.

A biomarker substudy of 2,525 ACS patients in the OPUS-TIMI 16 trial measured BNP in plasma samples at a mean of 40 ± 20 hours after the onset of symptoms (94). Baseline BNP level more than 80 pg/mL was significantly correlated with an increased risk of death, heart failure, and new or recurrent MI at 30 days and 10 months. Analysis of 1,676 TACTICS-TIMI 18 patients found similar findings; in addition, BNP was shown to add significant incremental prognostic information to troponin I measurement (95). Subsequent data from the A to Z trial demonstrated that serial, outpatient measurement of BNP following ACS predicted incidence of new heart failure or death (96).

REFERENCES

Review Articles and Pathophysiology

1. **Braunwald E.** Unstable angina: an etiologic approach to management. *Circulation* 1998;98:2219–2222.

   This editorial describes five different, though not mutually exclusive, causes of UA: (a) nonocclusive thrombus on preexisting plaques (most common); (b) dynamic obstruction (e.g., Prinzmetal variant angina, microcirculatory angina); (c) progressive mechanical obstruction; (d) inflammation and/or infection; and (e) secondary causes (e.g., fever, thyrotoxicosis, hypotension).

2. Libby P. Current concepts of the pathogenesis of the acute coronary syndromes. *Circulation* 2001;104:365–372.

This article provides a review of the underlying mechanisms of inflammation and acute thrombosis leading to ACSs. The article also addresses the myriad mechanisms by which agents such as statins and peroxisome proliferator-activated receptor (PPAR) agonists mitigate such processes.

3. Anderson JL, et al. ACC/AHA 2007 guidelines for the management of patients with unstable angina/non-ST-elevation myocardial infarction: a report of the American College of Cardiology/American Heart Association Task Force on Practice Guidelines (Writing Committee to Revise the 2002 Guidelines for the Management of Patients With Unstable Angina/Non-ST-Elevation Myocardial Infarction): developed in collaboration with the American College of Emergency Physicians, American College of Physicians, Society for Academic Emergency Medicine, Society for Cardiovascular Angiography and Interventions, and Society of Thoracic Surgeons. *J Am Coll Cardiol* 2007;50:e1–e157.

These guidelines provide a comprehensive approach to all aspects of risk assessment, and pharmacologic and interventional management for UA/NSTEMI.

4. Amsterdam E, et al. 2014 AHA/ACC Guideline for the Management of Patients With Non-ST-Elevation Acute Coronary Syndromes: a Report of the American College of Cardiology/American Heart Association Task Force on Practice Guidelines. *Circulation* 2014;130:e344–e426. 10.1161/cir.0000000000000134

This fully revised version of the guidelines highlighted the "ischemia-guided" approach with a focus on the continuum of ACS pathophysiology. Newer antithrombotic regimens, high-sensitivity troponins, and identification of high-risk patient populations are also addressed.

5. Rioufol G, et al. Multiple atherosclerotic plaque rupture in acute coronary syndrome: a three-vessel intravascular ultrasound study. *Circulation* 2002;106:804–808.

A total of 24 patients who underwent PCI after a first ACS with troponin-I elevation underwent intravascular ultrasound of the three major coronary arteries. Fifty plaque ruptures (mean, 2.08 per patient) were diagnosed by the association of a ruptured capsule with intraplaque cavity. Plaque rupture on the culprit lesion was seen in nine (37.5%) patients. At least one plaque rupture was found somewhere other than on the culprit lesion in 19 (79%) patients, and these lesions were in a different artery than the culprit artery in 70.8%. Thus, although one single lesion is clinically active at the time of ACS, the syndrome appears associated with overall coronary instability.

6. Thygesen K, et al. Joint ESC/ACCF/AHA/WHF Task Force for the Redefinition of Myocardial Infarction. Universal definition of myocardial infarction. *Eur Heart J* 2007;28:2525–2538.

With newer biochemical techniques and novel markers, the task force addresses the increasing specificity with which infarction can be detected. They update the definition to include the pathophysiologic basis, clinical scenario, as well as biochemical analysis for a complete assessment of myocardial necrosis.

Drugs and Studies

ASPIRIN

7. Lewis HD Jr, et al.; VA Cooperative Study. Protective effects of aspirin against acute MI and death in men with unstable angina. *N Engl J Med* 1983;309:396–403.

Design: Prospective, randomized, double-blind, placebo-controlled, multicenter study. Primary endpoint was death or MI at 12 weeks.

Purpose: To determine whether aspirin can decrease death and acute MI in patients with UA.

Population: 1,266 men with pain at rest, beginning within the previous month, and present within the last week and evidence of CAD, defined as one or more of the following: history of MI, ST depression ≥ 1 mm, angiogram showing 75% stenosis of at least one vessel, exercise test with ≥ 1-mm ST depression, and exertional angina relieved by NTG within 5 minutes.

Exclusion Criteria: Included new Q waves or ST elevation, elevated enzymes (more than twice normal level), severe heart failure (NYHA class IV), ventricular arrhythmia, oral anticoagulation, bleeding diathesis, allergy or intolerance to aspirin, recent aspirin ingestion (on more than 3 days of the previous 7), MI within the previous 6 weeks, bypass surgery in the previous 12 weeks, and cardiac catheterization in the prior week.

Treatment: Buffered aspirin, 324 mg once daily, or placebo for 12 weeks.

Results: At 12 weeks, the aspirin group had a 51% lower incidence of death and MI (5% vs. 10%; $p < 0.0005$), with both death and nonfatal MI being reduced by 51% (3.4% vs. 6.9%; $p = 0.005$; 1.6% vs. 3.3%; $p = 0.054$). No difference was observed in gastrointestinal symptoms or evidence of blood loss between the two treatment and placebo groups.

8. Cairns JA, et al. Aspirin, sulfinpyrazone, or both in unstable angina: results of a Canadian multicenter trial. *N Engl J Med* 1985;313:1369–1375.

Design: Prospective, randomized, double-blind, placebo-controlled, multicenter study. Primary endpoint was cardiac death and nonfatal MI. Mean follow-up period was 18 months.

Purpose: To evaluate the efficacy of aspirin, sulfinpyrazone, or both in the acute management of UA.

Population: 555 patients aged 70 years with evidence of myocardial ischemia (exertional angina, transient ST- or T-wave changes with pain, or relief with sublingual NTG in <10 minutes on at least three occasions in hospital) and unstable pain pattern (crescendo pain or pain 15 minutes in duration).

Exclusion Criteria: Included MI in preceding 12 weeks, contraindications to study medications, new Q waves on ECG, severe chest pain lasting 30 minutes or more, and elevated [more than twice the upper limit of normal (ULN)] enzymes (at least two of the following: serum aspartate aminotransferase, lactic dehydrogenase, CK), with positive CK-MB fraction or MB more than 5%.

Treatment: Aspirin, 325 mg four times daily; sulfinpyrazone, 200 mg four times daily; both; or neither.

Results: Aspirin groups had 51% less cardiac death and MI than did nonaspirin groups (8.6% vs. 17%; $p = 0.008$). The aspirin groups also had 71% lower all-cause mortality rates (3.0% vs. 11.7%; $p = 0.004$). Intention-to-treat analysis showed aspirin groups to have 30% lower rates of cardiac death and nonfatal MI ($p = 0.072$), 56% fewer cardiac deaths ($p = 0.009$), and 43% lower all-cause mortality rate ($p = 0.035$). Sulfinpyrazone showed no benefit for any outcome event.

9. Peters RJG, et al. Effects of aspirin dose when used alone or in combination with clopidogrel in patients with acute coronary syndromes: observations from the Clopidogrel in Unstable angina to prevent Recurrent Events (CURE) study. *Circulation* 2003;108:1682–1687.

Patients in the CURE trial of clopidogrel in UA/NSTEMI (see below) were randomized to clopidogrel or placebo, in addition to therapy with varying doses of aspirin (75 to 325 mg daily). While clopidogrel benefited patients in all groups of aspirin dosing, bleeding risk increased significantly with increasing aspirin dose, without observed benefit in reduced ischemic events. The authors conclude that optimal dosing of aspirin is 75 to 100 mg daily, regardless of clopidogrel use.

THIENOPYRIDINES

10. Balsano F, et al. Antiplatelet therapy with ticlopidine in unstable angina: controlled, multicenter clinical trial. *Circulation* 1990;82:17–26 (editorial, 296–298).

In this randomized trial, 652 patients received conventional therapy (without aspirin) or ticlopidine, 250 mg twice daily. At 6 months, the ticlopidine group had 46% fewer primary endpoints, consisting of vascular death or nonfatal MI (7.3% vs. 13.6%; $p = 0.009$). A 53% reduction in risk of fatal or nonfatal MI was found (5.1% vs. 10.9%; $p = 0.006$).

11. The Clopidogrel in Unstable Angina to Prevent Recurrent Events (CURE) Trial Investigators. Effects of clopidogrel in addition to aspirin in patients with acute coronary syndromes without ST segment elevation. *N Engl J Med* 2001;345:494–502.

Design: Prospective, randomized, double-blind, placebo-controlled, multicenter trial. Primary endpoint composite was CV death, MI, or stroke. Mean follow-up was 9 months (range, 3 to 12 months).

Purpose: To evaluate the efficacy and safety of the antiplatelet agent clopidogrel when given with aspirin in ACS without ST-segment elevation.

Population: 12,562 patients with UA or NSTEMI with ECG changes, positive serum cardiac markers, or history of CAD, and seen within 24 hours of symptom onset.

Exclusion Criteria: Age younger than 60 years, contraindication to antithrombotic therapy, ST elevation, high bleeding or CHF risk, oral anticoagulation, coronary revascularization in previous 3 months, and GP IIb/IIIa inhibitor in previous 3 days.

Treatment: Aspirin (75 to 325 mg once daily) and clopidogrel (300-mg loading dose, and then 75 mg once daily) or aspirin and placebo.

Results: The clopidogrel group had a 20% relative reduction in CV death, nonfatal MI, or stroke at 1 year compared with the placebo group (9.3% vs. 11.4%; $p < 0.001$). The clopidogrel group also had a significantly lower incidence of the primary composite endpoint or refractory ischemia (16.5% vs. 18.8%; RR, 0.86; $p < 0.001$; at 24 hours: 1.4% for clopidogrel vs. 2.1%; 34% RR reduction; $p = 0.002$). The incidence of in-hospital refractory or severe ischemia, heart failure, and revascularization procedures was also significantly lower with clopidogrel. The clopidogrel group experienced more major bleeding at 1 year than did the placebo group (3.7% vs. 2.7%; RR, 1.38; $p = 0.001$), but no significant excess of life-threatening bleeding occurred (2.1% vs. 1.8%; $p = 0.13$) or hemorrhagic strokes. Bleeding was lower in patients treated with aspirin, 75 to 100 mg once daily, compared with aspirin, 200 to 325 mg once daily (2.0% vs. 4.0%, respectively, in aspirin-only group; 2.6% vs. 4.9% in clopidogrel and aspirin group), indicating that bleeding appeared lower with clopidogrel and low-dose aspirin versus 325 mg of aspirin alone.

Comments: Benefits associated with clopidogrel occurred within 2 hours. The benefits were consistent in low-, intermediate-, and high-risk patients, as stratified by TRS (see *Circulation* 2002;106:1622).

12. Wiviott SD, et al.; for the TRITON-TIMI 38 Investigators. Prasugrel versus clopidogrel in patients with acute coronary syndromes. *N Engl J Med* 2007;357:2001–2015.

Design: Prospective, randomized, double-blind, active-controlled, multicenter, international study. The primary endpoint was a composite of CV death, reinfarction, or stroke at 15 months. The safety endpoint was bleeding.

Purpose: To compare a new thienopyridine, prasugrel, with clopidogrel in patients undergoing PCI for ACSs.

Population: 13,608 patients with moderate-to-high-risk ACSs and scheduled to undergo PCI; 10,074 patients had moderate-to-high-risk UA or NSTEMI, and 3,534 had STEMI.

Treatment: Clopidogrel (300-mg loading dose, followed by 75 mg daily) versus prasugrel (60-mg loading dose, followed by 10 mg daily).

Results: Prasugrel reduced the primary composite endpoint by an absolute 2.2% (9.9% vs. 12.1%; $p < 0.001$). However, major bleeding occurred in 2.4% of patients on prasugrel, versus 1.8% in the clopidogrel group ($p = 0.03$), and there was a similar increase in life-threatening bleeding (1.4% vs. 0.9%; $p = 0.01$).

Comment: Based heavily on this study, the FDA approved prasugrel for use in patients with high-risk ACSs *at the time of PCI*. However, they attached a black-box warning, advising physicians to consider a dose reduction (to 5 mg daily) in patients at a high risk of bleeding.

13. Montalescot G, et al.; on behalf of the ACCOAST Investigators. Pretreatment with prasugrel in non-ST-segment elevation acute coronary syndromes. N Engl J Med 2013;369(11):999–1010.

Design: Prospective, randomized, double-blind, active-controlled, multicenter, international study. The primary endpoint was a composite of CV death, MI, stroke, urgent revascularization, or glycoprotein IIb/IIIa inhibitor bailout at 7 days. The primary safety endpoint was TIMI major bleeding.

Purpose: To evaluate the efficacy and safety of pretreatment with prasugrel versus selective peri-PCI prasugrel therapy in patients with non-STE ACS who are intended to undergo an invasive treatment strategy.

Population: 4,033 patients hospitalized for ACS scheduled to undergo an invasive approach

Key Exclusion Criteria: STEMI patients, those with cardiogenic shock or cardiac arrest, patients with a recent history of severe bleeding, or those on oral anticoagulation.

Treatment: Prasugrel load of 30 mg at randomization with an additional 30 mg at time of PCI and then 10 mg daily versus prasugrel 60 mg at time of PCI and then 10 mg daily.

Results: Pretreatment with prasugrel resulted in similar efficacy and significantly more bleeding compared with selective peri-PCI treatment with prasugrel. The primary endpoint rates were 10% in prasugrel pretreated patients vs. 9.8% in prasugrel at time of PCI-treated patients (HR, 1.02; 95% CI, 0.84 to 1.25; $p = 0.81$). The primary safety endpoint occurred significantly more frequently in prasugrel pretreated patients (2.6% vs. 1.4%; $p = 0.006$) compared with the patients receiving prasugrel only in the PCI setting.

14. Roe MT, et al.; on behalf of the TRILOGY ACS Investigators. Prasugrel versus clopidogrel for acute coronary syndromes without revascularization. N Engl J Med 2012;367:1297–1309.

Design: Prospective, randomized, double-blind, active-controlled, multicenter, international study. The primary endpoint was a composite of CV death, MI, or stroke. The safety endpoint was total major bleeding.

Purpose: To evaluate the efficacy and safety of prasugrel versus clopidogrel in patients with non-STE ACS who undergo medical management without revascularization.

Population: 9,326 patients admitted with non–ST elevation ACS who were selected to receive medical management without plans for revascularization. Prespecified primary analyses included patients <75 years of age and those ≥75 years of age.

Exclusion Criteria: Patients with recent PCI or CABG, patients with history of stroke or TIA, patients on dialysis, or patients who are on concomitant oral anticoagulation therapy.

Treatment: Prasugrel 10 mg daily (in patients >75 years of age, 5 mg daily) versus clopidogrel 75 mg daily in addition to standard of care therapy.

Results: For patients <75 years old, the risk of primary endpoint events was similar in patients on prasugrel versus those on clopidogrel (13.9% vs. 16.0%; HR, 0.91; 95% CI, 0.79, 1.05; $p = 0.21$). Results were similar in the total group of patients including those ≥75 years of age (18.7% vs. 20.3%; HR 0.96; $p = 0.45$). Rates of non-CABG severe bleeding were also similar between treatment groups (1.1% vs. 1.0%; HR, 0.83; $p = 0.53$).

15. Wallentin L, et al.; for the PLATO Investigators. Ticagrelor versus clopidogrel in patients with acute coronary syndromes. N Engl J Med 2009;361:1045–1057.

Design: Prospective, randomized, double-blind, active-controlled, multicenter, international study. The primary endpoint was a composite of CV death, MI, or stroke through 12 months. The safety endpoint was total major bleeding.

Purpose: To compare the new reversible and direct-acting, oral P2Y12 receptor antagonist, ticagrelor with clopidogrel in patients with ACS.

Population: 18,624 patients hospitalized for ACS (with or without ST elevation) in the PLATO trial, treated with aspirin.

Treatment: Ticagrelor (180-mg loading dose, 90 mg twice daily thereafter) and clopidogrel (300- to 600-mg loading dose, 75 mg daily thereafter).

Results: Ticagrelor reduced the rate of CV death, MI, or stroke by 16%, from 11.7% for clopidogrel to 9.8% for ticagrelor, $p < 0.001$. Total mortality was also reduced from 5.9% for clopidogrel to 4.5% for ticagrelor, $p < 0.001$. No significant difference in the rates of major bleeding was found between the ticagrelor and clopidogrel groups (11.6% and 11.2%, respectively; $p = 0.43$), but ticagrelor had a higher rate of non–CABG-related bleeding (3.8% for clopidogrel vs. 4.5% for ticagrelor).

PAR-1 RECEPTOR ANTAGONISTS

16. Tricoci P, et al.; on behalf of the TRACER Investigators. Thrombin-receptor antagonist vorapaxar in acute coronary syndromes. N Engl J Med 2012;366(1):20–33.

Design: Prospective, randomized, double-blind, placebo-controlled, multicenter, international trial. The primary endpoint was a composite of CV death/MI/stroke/recurrent ischemia with hospitalization/urgent coronary revascularization at approximately 1 year. The safety endpoint was moderate or severe GUSTO bleeding.

Purpose: To assess the effect of the addition of a novel antiplatelet agent to dual antiplatelet therapy with aspirin and clopidogrel in patients with recent ACS.

Population: 12,944 patients recently hospitalized for ACS (biomarker positive or ECG changes) treated with dual antiplatelet therapy.

Exclusion Criteria: Patients on concurrent or anticipated oral anticoagulants, those with recent (30 days) significant bleeding.

Treatment: Vorapaxar 40-mg loading dose, followed by 2.5 mg daily versus placebo.

Results: Vorapaxar had little effect on the primary efficacy outcome of CV death/MI/recurrent ischemia compared with placebo (event rates 18.5% vs. 19.9%; $p = 0.07$), but was associated with increased risk for moderate or severe GUSTO bleeding (7.2% vs. 5.2%; HR, 1.35; 95% CI, 1.16–1.58; $p < 0.001$).

17. Morrow DA, et al. Vorapaxar in the secondary prevention of atherothrombotic events. N Engl J Med 2012;366:1404–1413. The TRA 2P-TIMI 50 Trial.

Design: Multicenter, international, prospective, randomized, double-blind, placebo-controlled trial. The primary endpoint was the composite of ischemic stroke, MI, or CV death at median follow-up of 30 months.

Purpose: To assess the safety and efficacy of adding vorapaxar to usual care in patients with stable atherothrombotic CV disease.

Population: 26,449 patients with a history of MI, ischemic stroke, or peripheral arterial disease.

Treatment: Vorapaxar 2.5 mg daily or placebo.

Results: There was a significant reduction in the primary endpoint for patients assigned to vorapaxar (9.3% vs. 10.5%; $p < 0.001$); however, after 2 years, the trial had stopped enrolling patients with a history of stroke, due to the risk of subsequent intracranial hemorrhage (ICH) observed. Overall, moderate or severe bleeding occurred in 4.2% of patients receiving vorapaxar, versus 2.5% receiving placebo ($p < 0.001$), and risk of ICH was significantly higher as well (1.0% vs. 0.5%; $p < 0001$).

UNFRACTIONATED HEPARIN AND WARFARIN

18. Theroux P, et al.; Montreal Heart Study. Aspirin, heparin, or both to treat acute unstable angina. N *Engl J Med* 1988;319:1105–1111.

Design: Prospective, randomized, double-blind, placebo-controlled, dual-center study. Major endpoints were death, MI, and refractory angina.

Purpose: To evaluate the usefulness of aspirin, IV heparin, and their combination in the early management of UA.

Population: 479 patients aged ≤75 years with accelerating pattern of chest pain occurring at rest or with minimal exercise, or pain lasting 20 minutes with the last episode in the previous 24 hours. Their ECG changes had to be consistent with ischemia; if absent, diagnosis had to be confirmed by two cardiologists. CK levels had to be less than twice the ULN.

Exclusion Criteria: Included regular use of aspirin, contraindications to heparin or aspirin, coronary angioplasty within the previous 6 months, and bypass surgery within the previous 12 months (or scheduled).

Treatment: Aspirin, 325 mg twice daily, or IV heparin, 1,000 U/h (given for average 6 days).

Results: Incidence of MI was significantly reduced in groups receiving aspirin [3% vs. 12% (placebo); $p = 0.01$], heparin (0.8%; $p < 0.001$), and aspirin plus heparin (1.6%; $p = 0.003$). No deaths occurred in these three treatment groups. Heparin was associated with a trend toward refractory angina compared with aspirin (RR, 0.47; 95% CI, 0.21 to 1.05; $p = 0.06$). Combination therapy was associated with more serious bleeding [3.3% vs. 1.7% (heparin alone)].

Comments: An additional 245 patients were randomized to either aspirin or heparin to allow an adequately powered comparison. A total of 484 patients was randomized to these two treatments, and the heparin group demonstrated a 78% lower MI rate at 5.7 ± 3.3 days (0.8% vs. 3.7%; $p = 0.035$). Only one death occurred (aspirin patient).

19. Wallentin LW, et al.; Research on Instability in CAD (RISC). Risk of MI and death during treatment with low dose aspirin and intravenous heparin in men with unstable coronary artery disease. *Lancet* 1990;336:827–830.

Design: Prospective, randomized, double-blind, placebo-controlled, 2 × 2 factorial, multicenter study. Primary endpoint was death and MI.

Purpose: To evaluate the efficacy of aspirin and/or heparin in acute treatment of unstable and non–Q-wave MI and to assess the long-term effects of aspirin compared with placebo in these patients.

Population: 796 men younger than 70 years with non–Q-wave MI or increasing angina within the previous 4 weeks, with the last episode of pain within 72 hours and ischemia on resting ECG or predischarge exercise test.

Exclusion Criteria: Included Q-wave MI, myocardial dysfunction due to prior MI, previous CABG surgery, LBBB or pacemaker, concurrent anticoagulant or aspirin therapy, and increased bleeding risk.

Treatment: Aspirin, 75 mg daily for 1 year, or placebo, and IV heparin boluses (10,000 U every 6 hours for four doses, and then 7,500 U every 6 hours for 4 days), or placebo alone.

Results: Trial was stopped early due to publication of ISIS-2 results (minimum follow-up reduced to 3 months vs. 12 months). Aspirin patients had a markedly reduced risk of MI and death at 5 days (OR, 0.43; $p = 0.033$), 1 month (OR, 0.31; $p < 0.0001$), and 3 months (OR, 0.36; $p < 0.0001$). No benefits were seen with heparin alone. The aspirin and heparin group had fewer events in the first 5 days [1.4% vs. 3.7% (aspirin alone); $p = $ NS; 5.5% (heparin alone); $p = 0.045$; 6.0% (both placebos); $p = 0.027$]. Gastrointestinal symptoms with aspirin became more frequent after 3 months.

20. Theroux P, et al. **Reactivation of unstable angina after the discontinuation of heparin.** **N Engl J Med 1992;327:141–145.**

This study demonstrated a clear rebound effect with discontinuation of heparin in patients not taking aspirin. Four hundred and three patients were randomized to IV heparin, aspirin, both, or neither, and completed 6 days of treatment without refractory angina or MI. After discontinuation of therapy, heparin-only patients had more frequent reactivation of UA or MI in the subsequent 96 hours: 14 of 107 patients versus only 5 patients in each of the other three groups ($p < 0.01$). Eleven of 14 of these reactivations required urgent interventions (thrombolysis, angioplasty, or bypass surgery) versus only 2 in the other groups combined ($p < 0.01$).

21. Oler A, et al. **Adding heparin to aspirin reduces the incidence of MI and death in patients with unstable angina: a meta-analysis.** **JAMA 1996;276:811–815.**

This meta-analysis was derived from 6 randomized trials enrolling 1,353 patients. Aspirin and heparin tended to be preferable to aspirin alone (RR of death and MI, 0.67; 95% CI, 0.44 to 1.02). Combination therapy also was associated with nonsignificant reduction in recurrent ischemia (RR, 0.82; 95% CI, 0.40 to 1.17). No difference in revascularization rates was observed (RR, 1.03; 95% CI, 0.74 to 1.43), whereas aspirin and heparin were associated with a nonsignificant increase in major bleeding (RR, 1.99; 95% CI, 0.52 to 7.65).

22. Organization to Assess Strategies for Ischemic Syndromes (OASIS) Investigators. **Comparison of the effects of two doses of recombinant hirudin compared with heparin in patients with acute myocardial ischemia without ST elevation.** *Circulation* **1997;96:769–777.**

Design: Prospective, randomized, open, multicenter study. Primary endpoint was CV death, MI, or refractory angina at 7 days.

Purpose: To compare the effects of a 3-day treatment with hirudin versus heparin on clinical outcomes in UA and NSTEMI patients.

Population: 909 patients with UA or suspected NSTEMI within 12 hours of the most recent episode of chest pain and with either ECG evidence of ischemia or previous objective documentation of CAD.

Treatment: UFH (5,000 IU bolus + 1,000 to 1,200 U/h), low-dose hirudin (0.2 mg/kg bolus and then 0.10 mg/kg/h infusion), or medium-dose hirudin (0.4 mg/kg bolus and then 0.15 mg/kg/h infusion) for 72 hours.

Results: At 7 days, CV death, new MI, or refractory angina (primary outcome) occurred in 6.5% in the heparin group, 4.4% in the low-dose hirudin group, and 3.0% in the medium-dose hirudin group ($p = 0.27$, heparin vs. low-dose hirudin; $p = 0.047$, heparin vs. medium-dose hirudin). The incidence of new MI was lower in the hirudin groups: 2.6% and 1.9% versus 4.6% ($p = 0.14$. heparin vs. low-dose hirudin; $p = 0.046$, heparin vs. medium-dose hirudin). An increase in ischemic events was seen in the low-dose hirudin group at around 24 hours after treatment cessation and at approximately 5 days in the medium-dose group, but the differences between hirudin and heparin persisted at 180 days.

LOW-MOLECULAR-WEIGHT HEPARINS

23. Wallentin L, et al. Fragmin during Instability in CAD (FRISC). Low molecular weight heparin during instability in coronary artery disease. *Lancet* 1996;347: 561–568.

Design: Prospective, randomized, double-blind, placebo-controlled, multicenter study. Primary endpoint was death or MI at 6 days.

Purpose: To evaluate whether subcutaneous dalteparin provides an additive benefit to that provided by aspirin and antianginal drugs in patients with UA or non–Q-wave MI.

Population: 1,506 patients (men aged 40 years, women more than 1 year after menopause) with chest pain in the previous 72 hours. All had newly developed or increasing angina or angina at rest during the previous 2 months or persisting chest pain with a suspicion of MI and ST depression ≥ 1 mm or T-wave inversion ≥ 1 mm in two adjacent leads without Q waves in ischemic leads.

Exclusion Criteria: Included increased bleeding risks.

Treatment: Dalteparin, 120 IU/kg subcutaneously twice daily for 6 days, and then 7,500 IU daily for 35 to 45 days; or placebo.

Results: At 6 days, the dalteparin group had a 63% lower rate of death and new MI (1.8% vs. 4.8%; $p = 0.001$); a nonsignificant reduction was observed at 40 days (8% vs. 10.7%; $p = 0.07$).

Comments: Subsequent analysis showed the additive value of troponin T to predischarge ETT in providing risk stratification.

24. Klein W, et al. Fragmin in Unstable Coronary Artery Disease (FRIC). Comparison of low molecular weight heparin with unfractionated heparin acutely and with placebo for 6 weeks in the management of unstable coronary artery disease. *Circulation* 1997;96:61–68.

Design: Prospective, randomized, partially open-label, parallel, multicenter study. Primary endpoint was death, MI, or recurrent angina.

Purpose: To compare the efficacy and safety of weight-adjusted subcutaneous dalteparin with UFH in the acute treatment of UA or non–Q-wave MI and the value of prolonged dalteparin compared with placebo in those initially given anticoagulants.

Population: 1,482 patients with chest pain in the preceding 72 hours and admission ECG with temporary or persistent ST depression ≥ 1 mV in at least two adjacent leads and/or temporary or persistent T-wave inversion ≥ 1 mm in two adjacent leads.

Exclusion Criteria: Included new Q waves, LBBB, indication for thrombolytic therapy, oral anticoagulation, diastolic blood pressure (DBP) >120 mm Hg or SBP <90 mm Hg, bleeding diathesis or recent surgery, and history of cerebrovascular event.

Treatment: Phase 1 (open label, days 1 to 6)—dalteparin, 120 IU/kg subcutaneously twice daily, or IV UFH. Phase 2 (double-blind, days 6 to 45)—dalteparin, 7,500 IU subcutaneously once daily, or placebo.

Results: In the first 6 days, no significant differences were observed between groups in death, MI, or recurrent angina [7.6% (heparin) vs. 9.3% (dalteparin); 95% CI, 0.84 to 1.66]; death and MI (3.6% vs. 3.9%); or revascularization (5.3% vs. 4.8%). For days 6 to 45, similar incidences of composite endpoints (both 12.3%) and revascularization [14.2% (placebo) vs. 14.3%] were observed. The dalteparin group had a higher phase 1 mortality rate (11 vs. 3 deaths; RR, 3.37; 95% CI, 1.01 to 11.24).

Comments: Lack of benefit with dalteparin may be due to the low ratio of anti-factor Xa to antithrombin activity (only 2.0).

25. Cohen M, et al. Efficacy and Safety of Subcutaneous Enoxaparin in Non-Q wave Coronary Events (ESSENCE). A comparison of low molecular weight heparin with unfractionated heparin for unstable coronary artery disease. N Engl J Med 1997;337:447–452 (editorial, 492–494).

Design: Prospective, randomized, double-blind, placebo-controlled, parallel-group, multi-center study. Primary endpoint was death, MI, or recurrent angina at 14 days.

Purpose: To compare the efficacy and safety of enoxaparin with UFH in patients with UA or non–Q-wave MI.

Population: 3,171 patients with rest pain 10 minutes in the preceding 24 hours accompanied by one of the following: (a) new ST depression ≥1 mm, transient ST elevation, or T-wave changes in at least two contiguous leads; (b) documented prior MI or revascularization procedure; or (c) noninvasive or invasive tests suggesting ischemic heart disease. Only about one-third had ST-segment changes on admission.

Exclusion Criteria: Included LBBB or pacemaker, persistent ST elevation, angina with an established precipitating cause (e.g., heart failure), contraindications to anticoagulation, and creatinine clearance <30 mL/min.

Treatment: Enoxaparin, 1 mg/kg subcutaneously twice daily, or UFH for 2 to 8 days (mean duration, 2.8 days).

Results: Enoxaparin group had a 16% lower rate of death, MI, and recurrent angina at 14 days (16.6% vs. 19.8%; $p = 0.019$); at 30 days, the benefit persisted (19.8% vs. 23.3%; $p = 0.016$). Enoxaparin also was associated with a lower 30-day revascularization rate (27% vs. 32.2%; $p = 0.001$). Similar rates of major bleeding were observed at 30 days (6.5% vs. 7.0%), but overall bleeding was higher in the enoxaparin group (18.4% vs. 14.2%; $p = 0.001$) because of injection-site ecchymoses.

26. FRagmin and Fast Revascularization during InStability in Coronary artery disease (FRISC II) Investigators. Long-term, low-molecular-mass heparin in unstable coronary artery disease: FRISC II prospective randomized multicenter study. Lancet 1999;354:701–707.

Design: Prospective, randomized, partially blinded parallel-group, multicenter study. Primary endpoint was death or MI at 3 months.

Purpose: To assess the effects of long-term treatment with dalteparin compared with a placebo in patients undergoing a noninvasive treatment strategy.

Population: 2,267 patients (median age, 67 years) with ischemic symptoms in the previous 48 hours accompanied by ECG changes (ST depression or T-wave inversion ≥0.1 mV) or elevated markers (e.g., CK-MB, more than 6 mg/L; troponin T, more than 0.10 mg/L).

Exclusion Criteria: Included angioplasty in previous 6 months, indication for or treatment with thrombolysis in past 24 hours, scheduled revascularization procedure.

Treatment: After 5 or more days of open-label dalteparin, patients randomized to subcutaneous dalteparin, 120 IU/kg twice daily, or placebo for 3 months.

Results: At 30 days, the dalteparin group had a significant reduction in death or MI (3.1% vs. 5.9%; $p = 0.002$), but at 3 months, the reduction was nonsignificant (6.7% vs. 8.0%; $p = 0.17$). A significant reduction was found in the 3-month incidence of death, MI, or revascularization (29.1% vs. 33.4%; $p = 0.031$), but this benefit did not persist at 6 months (38.4% vs. 39.9%; $p = 0.50$). Mortality was significantly reduced at 1 year (Lancet 2000;356:9).

27. Antman E; for the TIMI 11B Investigators. Enoxaparin prevents death and cardiac ischemic events in unstable angina/non–Q-wave MI: results of the TIMI 11B trial. Circulation 1999;100:1593–1601.

Design: Prospective, randomized, double-blind, placebo-controlled, multicenter study. Primary endpoint was death, MI, or urgent revascularization at 8 and 43 days.

Purpose: To evaluate the benefits of an extended course of enoxaparin compared with standard UFH for preventing death and cardiac events in patients with UA or non–Q-wave MI.

Population: 3,910 patients with ischemic discomfort at rest within the past 24 hours and ST-segment deviation or positive CK-MB or troponin.

Exclusion Criteria: Included planned revascularization within 24 hours, treatable cause of angina, evolving Q-wave MI, CABG surgery within 2 months, or PTCA within 6 months, UFH infusion for more than 24 hours before enrollment, history of HIT, contraindications to anticoagulation.

Treatment: Enoxaparin [1 mg/kg subcutaneously twice daily (acute phase), and then 60 mg (≥65 kg) or 40 mg (<65 kg) twice daily] during both acute (2 to 8 days) and chronic phases (through day 43) or IV UFH (acute phase only).

Results: Enoxaparin-treated patients had a significant 12% reduction in the primary composite endpoint of death, MI, or urgent revascularization at day 43 (17.3% vs. 19.7%; $p = 0.048$). This benefit was apparent by day 8 (12.4% vs. 14.5%; $p = 0.048$). During the first 72 hours and entire initial hospitalization, no difference was noted in the major bleeding rates between the treatment groups. However, long-term enoxaparin treatment was associated with an increase in the rate of major hemorrhage (spontaneous and instrumented; 2.9% vs. 1.5%; $p = 0.021$). At 1-year follow-up, a persistent significant benefit was associated with enoxaparin therapy (incidence of primary composite endpoint, 32.0% vs. 35.7%; $p = 0.022$; see J Am Coll Cardiol 2000;36:693).

Comments: When these results are pooled with the ESSENCE data, a significant reduction in death and MI is found at day 8 (4.1% vs. 5.3%), day 14 (5.2% vs. 6.5%), and day 43 (7.1% vs. 8.6%).

28. The FRAX.I.S. Study Group. Comparison of two treatment durations (6 days and 14 days) of a low molecular weight heparin with a 6-day treatment of UFH in the initial management of unstable angina or non-Q wave myocardial infarction: FRAXIS (FRAxiparine in Ischaemic Syndrome). *Eur Heart J* 1999;20:1553–1562.

This prospective, randomized, controlled study enrolled 3,468 patients with UA and non–Q-wave MI (angina within 48 hours and ST depression, T-wave inversion, or ST elevation not justifying thrombolysis). Patients received nadroparin for a short course (6 days) or long course (14 days) or UFH (6 ± 2 days). At 14 days, the incidence of the primary composite endpoint, consisting of CV death, recurrent angina, and recurrence of UA, was similar in the three treatment groups (heparin, 18.1%; short-course fraxiparine, 17.8%; long-course fraxiparine, 20%). A higher incidence of hemorrhage was seen in the long-course fraxiparine group [at 14 days, 3.5% vs. 1.6% (UFH) and 1.5% (short-course nadroparin)].

29. Goodman SG, et al.; for the Integrilin and Enoxaparin Randomized Assessment of Acute Coronary Syndrome Treatment (INTERACT) Trial Investigators. Randomized evaluation of the safety and efficacy of enoxaparin versus unfractionated heparin in high-risk patients with non-ST-segment elevation acute coronary syndromes receiving the glycoprotein IIb/IIIa inhibitor eptifibatide. *Circulation* 2003;107:238–244.

This prospective, randomized, open-label, multicenter trial enrolled 746 patients with ischemic chest discomfort without ST-segment elevation. Patients received UFH or enoxaparin. All aspirin (160-mg loading dose and then 80 to 325 mg/day) and the GP IIb/IIIa inhibitor eptifibatide (180-μg/kg IV bolus, and then 2.0 μg/kg/min for 48 hours), cardiac catheterization, and/or coronary revascularization decisions were left to the discretion of the investigator. The incidence of the primary endpoint, non-CABG TIMI major bleeding at 96 hours, occurred less frequently in the enoxaparin group than in the UFH group (1.8% vs. 4.6%; $p = 0.03$). The enoxaparin group also had a significantly lower incidence of death and nonfatal MI at 30 days (5.0% vs. 9.0%; $p = 0.031$). Limitations of this study include the open-label design and the long time to coronary revascularization (median, 101 hours vs. 21 hours in TACTICS-TIMI 18). The ongoing SYNERGY trial is examining the same issue among 8,000 patients treated with GP IIb/IIIa inhibitors.

30. Blazing MA, et al.; for the A to Z Investigators. Safety and efficacy of enoxaparin vs unfractionated heparin in patients with non-ST-segment elevation acute coronary syndromes who receive tirofiban and aspirin: a randomized controlled trial. JAMA 2004;292:55–64.

This prospective, randomized, open, multicenter trial enrolled 3,987 high-risk ACS patients (ST-segment changes or positive cardiac marker). All patients received aspirin and tirofiban: 60% of patients underwent angiography; crossover from enoxaparin to UFH in the catheterization lab was allowed. Patients were randomized to enoxaparin (1 mg/kg every 12 hours) or weight-adjusted UFH. The enoxaparin had a nonsignificant 12% reduction in death, MI, or refractory ischemia compared to UFH (8.4% vs. 9.4%; $p = 0.23$); however, the trial was designed to demonstrate noninferiority, and this goal was met.

31. The Fifth Organization to Assess Strategies in Acute Ischemic Syndromes Investigators. Comparison of fondaparinux and enoxaparin in acute coronary syndromes (OASIS 5). N Engl J Med 2006;354:1464–1476.

Design: Prospective, randomized, double-blind, double-dummy, multicenter, international trial. The primary endpoint was a composite of death, reinfarction, or refractory ischemia at 9 days. Patients were also followed for major bleeding and clinical outcomes out to 6 months.

Purpose: To compare efficacy and safety of fondaparinux versus enoxaparin, with regard to ischemic and bleeding outcomes, in patients with ACSs.

Population: 20,078 patients within 24 hours of symptoms of cardiac ischemia and at least two of the following—age ≤ 60 years, elevated troponin or CK-MG, or ECG changes indicative of ischemia.

Key Exclusion Criteria: Patients with contraindications to heparins, recent hemorrhagic stroke, severe renal insufficiency, or additional indications for anticoagulation.

Treatment: Fondaparinux 2.5 mg once daily (until discharge or for 8 days, whichever came first), or enoxaparin 1 mg/kg twice daily (for 2 to 8 days, or until the patient was clinically stable; enoxaparin was dose-reduced for patients with mild–moderate renal insufficiency).

Results: Similar rates of the primary endpoint were observed in each treatment group (5.8% for fondaparinux vs. 5.7% for enoxaparin; hazard ratio for fondaparinux 1.01; 95% CI, 0.90 to 1.13). This satisfied the noninferiority margin. However, rates of major bleeding at 9 days were significantly lower in the fondaparinux group (2.2% vs. 4.1%; $p < 0.001$). When bleeding was included, the composite clinical benefit endpoint of MACE and/or bleeding favored fondaparinux (7.3% vs. 9.0%; $p < 0.001$). Furthermore, mortality rates at 30 and 180 days were significantly lower in the fondaparinux group ($p = 0.02$ and 0.05, respectively).

32. Peterson JL, et al. Efficacy and bleeding complications among patients randomized to enoxaparin or unfractionated heparin for antithrombin therapy in non–ST-segment elevation acute coronary syndromes: a systematic overview. JAMA 2004;292:89–96.

The investigators combined the primary data from the ESSENCE, A to Z, SYNERGY, TIMI 11B, ACUTE II, and INTERACT trials, culminating in an analysis of 21,946 patients with NSTEMI randomized to UFH or enoxaparin, followed for clinical endpoints at 30 days. Mortality was equal between the two groups (3.0% for each); however, there was a significant reduction in the composite endpoint of death or MI at 30 days (10.1% vs. 11%; OR, 0.91; 95% CI, 0.83 to 0.99), favoring the enoxaparin group. Within 7 days, rates of major bleeding or blood transfusions were similar.

ANTI-ISCHEMIC MEDICATIONS

33. Gibson RS, et al.; Diltiazem Reinfarction Study Group. Diltiazem and reinfarction in patients with non–Q-wave MI. *N Engl J Med* 1986;315:423–429.

Design: Prospective, randomized, double-blind, multicenter study. Primary endpoint was reinfarction at 14 days.

Purpose: To determine whether diltiazem would reduce the incidence of early reinfarction in patients recovering from a non–Q-wave MI.

Population: 576 patients with non–Q-wave MI [elevated CK-MB and either ischemic pain for 30 minutes or ST-segment deviation (elevation or depression ≥1 mm or T-wave inversions in at least two leads)].

Exclusion Criteria: Included new Q waves, HR < 50 beats/min, advanced heart block, cardiogenic shock or sustained SBP < 100 mm Hg, coronary bypass surgery in the past 3 months, therapy with a calcium channel blocker.

Treatment: Randomized at 24 to 72 hours to diltiazem, 90 mg every 6 hours, or placebo.

Results: Diltiazem patients had a significantly lower 14-day reinfarction rate (5.2% vs. 9.3%; $p = 0.03$) and 50% less refractory angina (3.5% vs. 6.9%; $p = 0.03$). No significant difference was observed in mortality rates (3.1% vs. 3.8%). Adverse reactions were common in the diltiazem group [overall, 24% vs. 6% (AV block, 6% vs. 2%; SBP < 90 mm Hg, 8% vs. 2%)], but only 4.9% of the diltiazem patients stopped therapy because of the adverse effects.

34. Interuniversity Nifedipine/Metoprolol Trial (HINT) Research Group. Early treatment of unstable angina in the coronary care unit: a randomised, double blind, placebo controlled comparison of recurrent ischaemia in patients treated with nifedipine or metoprolol or both. *Br Heart J* 1986;56:400–413.

This prospective, randomized, double-blind, placebo-controlled, multicenter trial enrolled 515 patients with UA, of whom 338 were not pretreated with a β-blocker. In patients not pretreated with a β-blocker, no significant differences were found between the three groups (nifedipine, metoprolol, or both) in the incidence of recurrent ischemia or MI at 48 hours. However, a trend was seen toward a higher incidence of MI in the nifedipine group (RR, 1.51; 95% CI, 0.87 to 2.74). In patients already taking a β-blocker, the addition of nifedipine was beneficial (RR, 0.68; 95% CI, 0.47 to 0.97). These results suggest that in patients not taking previous β-blockade, metoprolol has a beneficial short-term effect on UA, and that nifedipine alone may be detrimental.

35. Doucet S, et al. Randomized trial comparing intravenous nitroglycerin and heparin for treatment of unstable angina secondary to restenosis after coronary artery angioplasty. *Circulation* 2000;101:955.

This prospective, randomized, double-blind, single-center study enrolled 200 patients hospitalized for UA within 6 months after angioplasty alone (no stenting). Patients received IV NTG, heparin, their combination, or placebo for 63 ± 30 hours. Recurrent angina occurred less frequently in the NTG groups [42.6% (NTG alone), 41.7% (NTG + heparin) vs. 75% (placebo and heparin-alone groups); $p < 0.003$]. Refractory angina requiring angiography occurred less often with NTG (4.3%, 4.2%, 22.9%, and 29.2%, respectively; $p < 0.002$). No deaths or MIs were found. These results suggest that smooth muscle cell proliferation and increased vasoreactivity are more important roles than thrombus formation in restenosis-related UA.

36. Emery M, et al.; for the GRACE Investigators. Patterns of use and potential impact of early beta-blocker therapy in non-ST-elevation myocardial infarction with and without heart failure: the Global Registry of Acute Coronary Events. *Am Heart J* 2006; 152:1015–1021. PMID: 17161045.

In an effort to identify the benefit of β-blockers in NSTEMI, the investigators assessed data from 7,108 patients with NSTEMI in the GRACE registry. In 76% of patients without contraindications, β-blocker therapy was initiated within 24 hours of presentation (more frequently in Killip I vs. III; $p < 0.001$). In multivariable analysis, such early therapy correlated with lower in-hospital mortality for patients with NSTEMI; this benefit appeared more robust for those with Killip II/III versus those with Killip I. The lower mortality persisted for 6 months for the entire NSTEMI cohort.

37. Ambrosio G, et al.; for the GRACE Investigators. Chronic nitrate therapy is associated with different presentation and evolution of acute coronary syndromes: insights from 52 693 patients in the Global Registry of Acute Coronary Events. *Eur Heart J* 2009;31:430–438.

The investigators sought to assess whether prior nitrate therapy afforded protection against subsequent ischemic events in 52,693 patients with ACS (41% with STEMI, 59% with UA/NSTEMI) in the GRACE registry. In all, 2,138 (80%) were not on prior nitrates (naïve) and 10,555 (20%) had been on chronic nitrates prior to admission; after adjustment for clinical factors, chronic nitrate use significantly predicted presentation with UA/NSTEMI, as opposed to STEMI (OR, 1.36; $p < 0.0001$). Levels of cardiac biomarkers were also significantly lower in the chronic nitrate group ($p < 0.0001$ for all). The findings suggest, though observational, that chronic nitrate use may mitigate the severity of acute coronary events.

38. Schwartz GG, et al.; Myocardial Ischemia Reduction with Aggressive Cholesterol Lowering (MIRACL) Study Investigators. Effects of atorvastatin on early recurrent ischemic events in acute coronary syndromes: the MIRACL study: a randomized controlled trial. *JAMA* 2001;285:1711–1718.

Design: Prospective, randomized, double-blind, placebo-controlled, multicenter trial. Primary composite endpoint was death, nonfatal acute MI, cardiac arrest with resuscitation, or recurrent symptomatic MI with objective evidence and requiring emergency rehospitalization.

Purpose: To determine whether treatment with high-dose atorvastatin initiated 24 to 96 hours after an ACS reduces death and nonfatal ischemic events.

Population: 3,086 conservatively managed patients with UA/NSTEMI. Patients had chest pain for more than 15 minutes at rest or with minimal exertion in the previous 24 hours and a change from a previous pattern of angina, new or dynamic ST- or T-wave changes, or new wall-motion abnormality, or positive noninvasive test; troponin or CK-MB less than twice the ULN for UA, or more than twice the ULN for non–Q-wave MI.

Exclusion Criteria: Included serum cholesterol more than 270, Q-wave MI in the prior 4 weeks, CABG surgery in the prior 3 months, PCI in the prior 6 months, LBBB or paced rhythm, lipid-lowering drugs other than niacin at doses >500 mg daily, vitamin E unless at doses of <400 IU daily, liver dysfunction [alanine aminotransferase (ALT) greater than twice the ULN], and insulin-dependent diabetes.

Treatment: Atorvastatin, 80 mg once daily, or matching placebo, in addition to standard therapy.

Results: The atorvastatin group had a significantly lower incidence of the composite primary endpoint compared with the placebo group (14.8% vs. 17.4%; RR, 0.84; $p = 0.048$). No significant differences were found between the groups in death, nonfatal MI, or cardiac arrest, although the atorvastatin group had less symptomatic recurrent ischemia with objective evidence and requiring emergency rehospitalization (6.2% vs. 8.4%; $p = 0.02$) and fewer strokes (12 vs. 24 events; $p = 0.045$). In the atorvastatin group, mean LDL cholesterol level decreased from 124 mg/dL (3.2 mM) to 72 mg/dL (1.9 mM). Abnormal liver transaminases (more than three times ULN) were more common in the atorvastatin group than in the placebo group (2.5% vs. 0.6%; $p < 0.001$); no cases of rhabdomyolysis were observed.

DIRECT THROMBIN INHIBITORS

39. Topol EJ, et al. Global Utilization of Strategies to Open Occluded Arteries (GUSTO IIb): a comparison of recombinant hirudin with heparin for the treatment of acute coronary syndromes. N Engl J Med 1996;335:775–782.

Design: Prospective, randomized, double-blind, multicenter study. Primary endpoint was death or nonfatal MI (or reinfarction) at 30 days.

Purpose: To compare the clinical effectiveness of hirudin with that of heparin in patients with all types of ACS.

Population: 12,142 patients with chest pain in the prior 12 hours accompanied by persistent ST elevation or depression ≥0.5 mm ($n ≥ 4,131$) or T-wave inversion ($n ≥ 8,011$).

Exclusion Criteria: Included oral anticoagulation, active bleeding, history of stroke, serum creatinine more than 2.0 mg/dL, contraindication to heparin, and SBP more than 200 mm Hg or DBP more than 110 mm Hg.

Treatment: Patients were randomized to heparin or hirudin [0.1 mg/kg IV bolus, and then 0.1 mg/kg/h (vs. 0.6, and then 0.2 in GUSTO IIa)].

Results: At 30 days, the hirudin group had a nonsignificant 11% reduction in death and MI (8.9% vs. 9.8%; $p = 0.06$). Post hoc analysis showed that the hirudin group had a significant reduction in death and MI at 24 hours (1.3% vs. 2.1%; $p = 0.001$). Hirudin patients had more moderate (but not severe) bleeds (8.8% vs. 7.7%). Patients with ST elevation were younger and had fewer cardiac risk factors but a higher 30-day mortality rate (6.1% vs. 3.8%).

40. Organization to Assess Strategies for Ischemic Syndromes (OASIS-2) Investigators. Effects of recombinant hirudin (lepirudin) compared with heparin on death, MI, refractory angina, and revascularization procedures in patients with acute myocardial ischaemia without ST elevation: a randomised trial. Lancet 1999;353:429–438 (editorial, 423–424).

Design: Prospective, randomized, multicenter, double-blind, double-dummy study. Primary endpoint was CV death or new MI at 7 days.

Purpose: To evaluate whether hirudin is superior to heparin in reducing major cardiac events in patients with UA or suspected NSTEMI.

Population: 10,141 patients aged 21 to 85 years with UA (abnormal ECG required if younger than 60 years) or suspected acute MI without ST elevation.

Exclusion Criteria: Included PTCA within the prior 6 months, planned thrombolysis or primary PTCA, and history of stroke in the prior year.

Treatment: Heparin, 5,000-U bolus, and then 15 U/kg/h for 72 hours, or hirudin, 0.4-mg/kg bolus, and then 0.15 mg/kg/h for 72 hours.

Results: Hirudin group had a nonsignificant 16% RR reduction in CV death and MI at 7 days (3.6% vs. 4.2%; $p = 0.077$). The hirudin group also had a significant 18% RR reduction in CV death, MI, and refractory angina at 7 days (5.6% vs. 6.7%; $p = 0.0125$). Most of the differences between the groups were observed during the first 72 hours: CV death or MI RR, 0.76 ($p = 0.039$), and CV death, MI, and refractory angina RR, 0.78 ($p = 0.019$). The hirudin group had an excess of major bleeding (1.2% vs. 0.7%; $p = 0.01$) but no excess of life-threatening bleeds.

41. Stone GW, et al.; for the ACUITY Investigators. Bivalirudin for patients with acute coronary syndromes. N Engl J Med 2006;355:2203–2216.

Design: Prospective, randomized, multicenter, open-label trial. Primary endpoint was CV death or new MI at 7 days. Multiple primary endpoints at 30 days included a composite of ischemic events (death, MI, or ischemia-driven revascularization), bleeding events, and net clinical benefit (a composite of ischemia and bleeding).

Purpose: To establish noninferiority (and possibly superiority, predefined) of bivalirudin as antithrombotic agent in moderate to high-risk patients with UA/NSTEMI undergoing PCI, as compared with UFH.

Population: 13,819 patients with UA/NSTEMI who had at least one of the following—significant ECG changes, elevated levels of troponin or CK-MB, known history of CAD, or all four remaining variables of the TRS (age >65, recent aspirin use in past 7 days, UA two or more times over 24 hours, and three or more cardiac risk factors).

Exclusion Criteria: STEMI, recent major bleeding.

Treatment: There were three treatment groups—heparin with GP IIb/IIIa inhibitor, bivalirudin with GP IIb/IIIa inhibitor, or bivalirudin alone.

Results: For the comparison of groups that received GP IIb/IIIa inhibitors, there was no significant difference in ischemic events (7.7% for bivalirudin plus GP IIb/IIIa vs. 7.3% for heparin plus GP IIb/IIIa), bleeding (5.3% vs. 5.7%), or net clinical events (11.8% vs. 11.7%), meeting the noninferiority margins for all three. As compared to heparin with GP IIb/IIIa inhibitor, bivalirudin alone also demonstrated noninferior rates of the composite ischemia endpoint (7.8% for bivalirudin vs. 7.3% for heparin with GP IIb/IIIa; $p = 0.32$), and significantly lower rates of bleeding (3.0% vs. 5.7%; $p < 0.001$), with significant net clinical benefit (10.1% vs. 11.7%; $p = 0.02$).

42. The Direct Thrombin Inhibitor Trialists' Collaborative Group. Direct thrombin inhibitors in acute coronary syndromes: principal results of a meta-analysis based on individual patients' data. *Lancet* 2002;359:294–302.

This meta-analysis included 35,970 patients from 11 randomized trials that enrolled 200 or more patients and assigned up to 7 days of treatment with a direct thrombin inhibitor or heparin and had a 30-day or longer follow-up. Compared with heparin, direct thrombin inhibitors were associated with a lower risk of death or MI at the end of treatment [4.3% vs. 5.1%; OR, 0.85 (95% CI, 0.77 to 0.94); $p = 0.001$] and at 30 days [7.4% vs. 8.2%; 0.91 (0.84 to 0.99); $p = 0.02$]. This was driven by fewer MIs [2.8% vs. 3.5%; 0.80 (0.71 to 0.90); $p < 0.001$]. Subgroup analyses revealed a benefit of direct thrombin inhibitors on death or MI in both ACS and PCI trials. A reduction in death or MI was evident with hirudin and bivalirudin but not with univalent agents (argatroban, efegatran, inogatran). Compared with heparin, an increased risk of major bleeding was found with hirudin, but a reduction with bivalirudin.

FACTOR XA INHIBITORS

43. Mega JL et al.; on behalf of the ATLAS ACS 2–TIMI 51 Investigators. Rivaroxaban in patients with a recent acute coronary syndrome. *N Engl J Med* 2012;366(1):9–19.

Design: Prospective, randomized, double-blind, placebo-controlled, multi-center, international trial. The primary efficacy endpoint was the composite of CV death, MI, or stroke. The primary safety endpoint was non–CABG-related TIMI major bleeding.

Purpose: To evaluate with addition of low dose factor Xa inhibitor anticoagulation to standard of care dual antiplatelet therapy for secondary prevention of adverse CV events in patients with recent ACS.

Population: 15526 patients recently admitted with ACS (STE and non-STE).

Key Exclusion Criteria: Patients with poor renal function (<30 Cr Cl) or with recent GIB history or history of ICH.

Treatment: Rivaroxaban 2.5 mg daily, 5 mg daily, or placebo.

Results: The addition of low-dose rivaroxaban compared with placebo was associated with a reduced rate of the primary endpoint (8.9% vs. 10.7%; HR, 0.84; 95% CI, 0.74 to 0.96; $p = 0.008$). However, rates of the primary safety endpoint were increased with rivaroxaban versus placebo (2.1% vs. 0.6%; HR, 3.96; 95% CI, 2.46 to 6.38; $p < 0.001$).

On further analyses based on rivaroxaban dosing, the greatest efficacy benefit was seen with the 2.5-mg dose, while this dose also had lower rates of TIMI minor bleeding as compared with the 5-mg dose (0.9% vs. 1.6%; $p = 0.046$).

44. Alexander JH, et al. Apixaban with antiplatelet therapy after acute coronary syndrome. N Engl J Med 2011;365:699–708. The APPRAISE-2 Trial.

Design: Multicenter, international, prospective, randomized, double-blind, placebo-controlled trial. The primary endpoint was the composite of ischemic stroke, MI, or CV death; the primary safety endpoint was TIMI major bleeding. Median follow-up was 241 days.

Purpose: To assess the safety and efficacy of adding apixaban to usual care in patients with ACS.

Population: 7,392 patients with ACS and at least 2 additional risk factors for ischemic outcomes.

Treatment: Apixaban 5 mg twice daily or placebo.

Results: The trial was terminated prematurely due to an increased risk of major bleeding in the apixaban group (1.3% vs. 0.5%; HR, 2.59; $p = 0.001$), without a reduction in ischemic events. Importantly, there were more intracranial and fatal bleeding events in the apixaban group. A primary efficacy endpoint event occurred in 7.5% of patients assigned to apixaban, versus 7.9% assigned placebo (HR, 0.95; $p = 0.51$).

Comment: Many have speculated that the APPRAISE-2 results are not that different from the ATLAS ACS-TIMI 51 results, given the higher relative dose of apixaban.

GLYCOPROTEIN IIB/IIIA INHIBITORS

45. Platelet Receptor Inhibition in Ischemic Syndrome Management in Patients Limited by Unstable Signs and Symptoms (PRISM-PLUS) Investigators. Inhibition of the platelet glycoprotein IIb/IIIa receptor with tirofiban in unstable angina and non–Q-wave myocardial infarction. N Engl J Med 1998;338:1488–1497 (editorial, 1539–1541).

Design: Prospective, randomized, double-blind, multicenter study. Primary endpoint was death, MI, or refractory ischemia at 7 days.

Purpose: To investigate the clinical efficacy of tirofiban, a short-acting, nonpeptide GP IIb/IIIa inhibitor, in the prevention of acute ischemic events in patients with UA and non–Q-wave MI.

Population: 1,915 patients with prolonged anginal pain or repetitive episodes of angina at rest or during minimal exercise in the previous 12 hours and new ST–T changes [$\geq$1-mm elevation or depression, $\geq$3-mm T-wave inversion on at least three limb leads or precordial leads (excluding V_1), or pseudonormalization $\geq$1 mm] or an elevated CK or CK-MB.

Exclusion Criteria: Included ST elevation longer than 20 minutes, thrombolysis in the previous 48 hours, angioplasty in the past 6 months, or CABG surgery in the previous month, stroke in the prior year, active bleeding or high bleeding risk, history of thrombocytopenia or platelet count <150,000, and creatinine more than 2.5 mg/dL.

Treatment: (a) Tirofiban, 0.6 μg/kg/min for 30 minutes, and then 0.15 μg/kg/min and placebo heparin; (b) tirofiban, 0.4 μg/kg/min for 30 minutes, and then 0.1 μg/kg/min, plus heparin; or (c) heparin plus placebo tirofiban.

Results: The tirofiban-plus-heparin group had a significant reduction compared with the heparin-alone group in the 7-day composite endpoints (12.9% vs. 17.9%; RR, 0.68; $p = 0.004$). This difference persisted at 30-day and 6-month follow-up (18.5% vs. 22.3%; $p = 0.03$; 27.7% vs. 32.1%; $p = 0.02$). The tirofiban-plus-heparin group also had a significant reduction in death or MI at 7 and 30 days (4.9% vs. 8.3%; $p = 0.006$; 8.7% vs. 11.9%; $p = 0.03$).

Comments: Benefit was seen regardless of treatment strategy—medical therapy group with 25% reduction in death or MI at 30 days, PCI group with 34% reduction, and CABG group with 30% reduction. The troponin substudy also showed that the combination of tirofiban plus heparin reduced infarct size, as measured by peak troponin. Angiographic study (1,491 patients) found a lower thrombus burden with tirofiban + heparin compared with heparin alone (OR, 0.65; $p = 0.002$) and higher TIMI grade 3 flow rate (82% vs. 74%).

46. Platelet Receptor Inhibition in Ischemic Syndrome Management (PRISM) Study Investigators. A comparison of aspirin plus tirofiban with aspirin plus heparin for unstable angina. N Engl J Med 1998;338:1498–1505 (editorial, 1539–1541).

Design: Prospective, randomized, multicenter study. Primary endpoint was death, MI, and refractory ischemia at 48 hours.

Purpose: To compare IV tirofiban with IV UFH for the treatment of UA in patients receiving aspirin.

Population: 3,232 patients with rest or accelerating chest pain within 24 hours of randomization and at least one of the following criteria: (a) ST depression ≥ 1 mm in at least two contiguous leads, transient (<20 minutes) ST elevation, or T-wave inversion; (b) elevated cardiac enzymes; and (c) history of MI, revascularization more than 6 months earlier, coronary surgery more than 1 month earlier, positive exercise or pharmacologic stress test result, or more than 50% stenosis on prior angiogram.

Exclusion Criteria: Included thrombolytic therapy in previous 48 hours, creatinine >2.5 mg/dL, increased bleeding risks, history of thrombocytopenia, SBP more than 180 mm Hg, and DBP more than 110 mm Hg.

Treatment: Tirofiban, 0.6 μg/kg/min for 30 minutes, and then 0.15 μg/kg/min through 48 hours, with placebo heparin, or UFH (5,000-U bolus, and then 1,000 U/h for 48 hours, adjusted if necessary based on aPTT at 6 and 24 hours). All patients were taking aspirin, 300 to 325 mg daily.

Results: Tirofiban group had a 32% reduction in the composite primary endpoints at 48 hours—3.8% vs. 5.6% (RR, 0.67; $p = 0.01$). At 30 days, a similar frequency of composite endpoints was observed (15.9% vs. 17.1%; $p = 0.34$). At 7 days, the tirofiban group had a significantly lower mortality rate (2.3% vs. 3.6%; $p = 0.02$) and tended toward a reduction in death and MI (5.8% vs. 7.1%; $p = 0.11$). Tirofiban was associated with increased thrombocytopenia (1.1% vs. 0.4%; $p = 0.04$). Identical major bleeding rates were observed (0.4%). At 30 days, death or MI occurred in 13.0% of troponin I–positive patients compared with 4.9% for troponin I–negative patients ($p < 0.0001$), and 13.7% compared with 3.5% for troponin T ($p < 0.001$) see Ref. 85. In troponin I–positive patients, tirofiban substantially lowered the risks of death [adjusted hazard ratio 0.25 (95% CI, 0.09 to 0.68); $p = 0.004$] and MI [hazard ratio 0.37 (0.16 to 0.84); $p = 0.01$].

47. Platelet Glycoprotein IIb/IIIa in Unstable Angina Receptor Suppression Using Integrilin Therapy (PURSUIT) Trial Investigators. Inhibition of platelet glycoprotein IIb/IIIa with eptifibatide in patients with acute coronary syndromes. N Engl J Med 1998;339:436–443.

Design: Prospective, randomized, double-blind, placebo-controlled, multicenter study. Primary endpoint was death or nonfatal MI at 30 days.

Purpose: To determine if the addition of eptifibatide to heparin and aspirin provides additional benefit in patients with ACSs without ST elevation.

Population: 10,948 patients with ischemic chest pain lasting 10 minutes in the prior 24 hours (median, 11 hours) and ECG changes (transient or persistent ST-segment depression more than 0.5 mm, transient ST-segment elevation more than 0.5 mm, or T-wave inversion more than 1 mm within 12 hours before or after chest pain), or serum CK-MB above the ULN.

Exclusion Criteria: Included persistent ST elevation more than 1 mm, SBP more than 200 mm Hg or DBP more than 100 mm Hg, major surgery within the prior 6 weeks, nonhemorrhagic stroke in the prior 30 days, or any history of hemorrhagic stroke, renal failure, planned used of thrombolytic or GP IIb/IIIa inhibitors, and thrombolysis in the prior 24 hours.

Treatment: Eptifibatide, 180-μg/kg bolus, and then 1.3 or 2.0 μg/kg/min for 72 hours (up to 96 hours if intervention was near the end of a 72-hour period), or placebo; 1.3-μg/kg/min infusion was dropped after 3,218 patients enrolled. No protocol-mandated strategy of catheterization and revascularization was undertaken.

Results: Eptifibatide was associated with a 9.6% relative reduction in death or MI at 30 days (14.2% vs. 15.7%; p = 0.04); this effect was apparent by 72 hours. Among patients undergoing early (<72 hours) PCI, eptifibatide was associated with a 32% benefit. Eptifibatide was associated with increased major bleeding (10.6% vs. 9.1%; p = 0.02) and higher transfusion rates (11.6% vs. 9.2%; RR, 1.3; 95% CI, 1.1 to 1.4). The eptifibatide group also had more cases of profound thrombocytopenia (platelet count <20,000): RR, 5.0 (nine vs. two patients; 95% CI, 1.3 to 32.4). Eptifibatide was not associated with increased incidence of bleeding in those undergoing CABG surgery. Stroke occurred in 79 (0.7%) patients, 66 of whom were nonhemorrhagic, and no significant differences in stroke rates were found between patients who received placebo and those assigned high-dose eptifibatide.

48. Cannon CP, et al. Oral glycoprotein IIb/IIIa inhibition with orbofiban in patients with unstable coronary syndromes (OPUS-TIMI 16) trial. *Circulation* 2000;102: 149–156.

Design: Prospective, randomized, double-blind, multicenter study. Primary endpoint was death, MI, recurrent ischemia requiring rehospitalization, urgent revascularization, or stroke.

Purpose: To determine whether prolonged oral GP IIb/IIIa inhibition with orbofiban provides additional reduction in recurrent ischemic events.

Population: 10,288 patients with ACS defined as ischemic rest pain within 72 hours and one or more of the following—new ST-segment deviation of 0.5 mm or more, T-wave inversion of 3 mm or more in three leads or LBBB, positive cardiac markers, or (for the first 3,000 patients only) history of MI, PCI, CABG surgery, coronary stenosis of 50% or more, age 65 years or older, and a history of angina or positive stress test, prior peripheral arterial or cerebrovascular disease, or diabetes mellitus.

Exclusion Criteria: Included increased bleeding risks (prior ICH, peptic ulcer within 6 months, etc).

Treatment: Orbofiban, 50 mg twice daily (50/50 group); orbofiban, 50 mg twice daily for 30 days followed by 30 mg orbofiban twice daily (50/30 group), or placebo.

Results: Trial was terminated early because of increased 30-day mortality in the 50/30 orbofiban group. At 10 months, mortality was 3.7% in the placebo group versus 5.1% in the 50/30 group (p = 0.008) and 4.5% in the 50/50 group (p = 0.11). No differences were found between the three groups in the incidence of the primary composite endpoint (22.9%, 23.1%, and 22.8%, for the placebo, 50/30, and 50/50 groups, respectively). The orbofiban groups had a significantly higher incidence of major or severe bleeding (but not ICH) compared with placebo [3.7% (50/30) and 4.5% (50/50) vs. 2.0%)].

49. Sibrafiban versus aspirin to yield maximum protection from ischemic heart events post-acute coronary syndromes (SYMPHONY) Investigators. Comparison of sibrafiban with aspirin for prevention of cardiovascular events after acute coronary syndromes: a randomised trial. *Lancet* 2000;355:337–345.

Design: Prospective, randomized, double-blind, multicenter study. Primary endpoint was death, MI, or severe recurrent ischemia at 90 days.

Purpose: To compare the efficacy, safety, and tolerability of long-term administration of the oral GP IIb/IIIa inhibitor sibrafiban with aspirin in ACS.

Population: 9,233 patients seen within 7 days of an ACS, clinically stable for 12 hours or more, and Killip class 1 or 2.

Exclusion Criteria: Serious illness, predisposition to bleeding, major surgery, previous stroke or ICH, thrombocytopenia, renal failure, treatment with oral anticoagulants, antiplatelet agents, or NSAIDs.

Treatment: Aspirin, 80 mg, low-dose sibrafiban (LDS; 4.5 or 3 mg, depending on creatinine and body weight), high-dose oral sibrafiban (6, 4.5, or 3 mg depending on creatinine and body weight). All were taken every 12 hours.

Results: No differences were found between the three groups in the incidence of the primary composite endpoint [9.8% (aspirin), 10.1% (LDS), 10.1% (high-dose sibrafiban, HDS); OR for aspirin vs. both the LDS and HDS, 1.03; 95% CI, 0.87 to 1.21]. Death or MI rates also were similar (7.0%, 7.4%, and 7.9%, respectively). Large MIs (CK-MB more than five times the ULN) occurred less frequently in the aspirin group (37.4%) than in the sibrafiban groups [45.3% (low dose), 49.7% (high dose)]. The aspirin group had a significantly lower incidence of bleeding (13.0% vs. 18.7% and 25.4%), whereas major bleeding occurred in 3.9%, 5.2%, and 5.7%, respectively.

50. SYMPHONY II Investigators. Randomized trial of aspirin, sibrafiban, or both for secondary prevention after acute coronary syndromes. *Circulation* 2001;103:1727–1733.

Design: Prospective, randomized, double-blind, multicenter study. Primary endpoint was death, MI, and severe recurrent ischemia.

Purpose: To assess whether longer treatment (12 to 18 months) with LDS in combination with aspirin or HDS alone was more effective for secondary prevention than is aspirin alone.

Population: Same inclusion criteria as SYMPHONY I; 6,671 patients completed a median of 90 days of follow-up (original design, 8,400 patients).

Exclusion Criteria: See SYMPHONY I.

Treatment: Aspirin alone (80 mg twice daily), LDS + aspirin, or HDS. Average time from qualifying event to first dose was 94 hours (range, 63 to 132 hours).

Results: Study terminated after SYMPHONY I results were reported. No difference was noted between the three groups in the incidence of the primary composite endpoint (aspirin, 9.3%; LDS + aspirin, 9.2%; HDS, 10.5%). The HDS group had a higher incidence of death or MI compared with the aspirin-alone group (6.1% vs. 8.6%), whereas major bleeding occurred more frequently in the LDS + aspirin group compared with the aspirin-alone group (5.7% vs. 4.0%).

Comments: Some evidence suggests that the increased thrombosis seen with oral GP IIb/IIIa inhibitors is due to enhanced receptor activity during the hours when the drugs are less active or not available.

51. Simoons ML; GUSTO IV-ACS Investigators. Effect of glycoprotein IIb/IIIa receptor blocker abciximab on outcome in patients with acute coronary syndromes without early coronary revascularisation: the GUSTO IV-ACS randomised trial. *Lancet* 2001;357:1915–1924.

Design: Prospective, randomized, open, multicenter study. Primary endpoint was death or MI at 30 days.

Purpose: To study the effect of the GP IIb/IIIa blocker abciximab in ACS patients not undergoing early revascularization.

Population: 7,800 patients with UA or NSTEMI. Eligible if chest pain longer than 5 minutes within the last 24 hours, 0.5 mm or more ST-segment depression, OR positive troponin T or I.

Exclusion Criteria: Included ST elevation or new LBBB, PCI within the past 2 weeks, planned PCI/CABG in the next 30 days, active bleeding or bleeding disorder, or other risk factor for bleeding.

Treatment: Abciximab for 24 hours, or abciximab for 48 hours, or placebo. All received aspirin and either UFH or LMWH.

Results: No significant differences were observed between the groups in the incidence of death or MI at 30 days (abciximab for 24 hours, 8.2%; abciximab for 48 hours, 9.1%; placebo, 8.0%; p = NS). No differences were noted among those with a positive troponin or in any other subgroups. The mortality rate was actually higher in first 48 hours in both abciximab groups compared with the placebo group [0.7% and 0.9% vs. 0.3%; ORs, 2.3 (p = 0.048) and 2.9 (p = 0.007)]. In particular, no benefit was seen in patients with increased cardiac troponin T or I concentrations at enrollment, although these patients had a strongly increased risk of subsequent events. Bleeding rates were low but were higher with abciximab, particularly in the 48-hour group. Thrombocytopenia also was more common in the abciximab groups.

52. Kastrati A, et al. Abciximab in patients with acute coronary syndromes undergoing percutaneous coronary intervention after clopidogrel pretreatment: the ISAR-REACT 2 randomized trial. JAMA 2006;295(13):1531–1538.

Design: Prospective, randomized, placebo-controlled, international, multicenter trial. Primary endpoint was death, MI, or urgent TVR at 30 days.

Purpose: To study the effect of the GP IIb/IIIa blocker abciximab in UA/NSTEMI patients undergoing PCI with clopidogrel adjunctive therapy.

Population: 2,022 patients with UA or NSTEMI (roughly 50% with elevated troponin) who received aspirin and clopidogrel prior to undergoing PCI (roughly half received DES).

Exclusion Criteria: Included ST elevation or new LBBB, hemodynamic instability, increased risk of bleeding (e.g., recent stroke), and concomitant malignancy shortening life expectancy.

Treatment: Abciximab infusion for 12 hours or placebo; both groups received heparin infusion.

Results: There was a significant reduction in the primary endpoint in the abciximab group (8.9% vs. 11.9%; p = 0.03); however, this difference was absent in patients without elevated troponin levels. Major bleeding, minor bleeding, and need for transfusion did not differ between the two groups.

53. Roffi M, et al. Platelet glycoprotein IIb/IIIa inhibitors reduce mortality in diabetic patients with non-ST-segment-elevation acute coronary syndromes. *Circulation* 2001;104:2767–2771.

This meta-analysis examined patients enrolled in six large GP IIb/IIIa inhibitor trials (PRISM, PRISM-PLUS, PARAGON A, PARAGON B, PURSUIT, GUSTO IV). Among the 6,458 diabetic patients, GP IIb/IIIa inhibitor use was associated with a significantly lower 30-day mortality compared with no GP inhibition (4.6% vs. 6.2%; OR, 0.74; 95% CI, 0.59 to 0.92; p = 0.007). The largest benefit was seen in the subgroup of 1,279 diabetic patients who underwent PCI during the index hospitalization; they had a 70% lower mortality with GP inhibitor use (1.2% vs. 4.0%; OR, 0.30; 95% CI, 0.14 to 0.69; p = 0.002). In contrast, among the 23,072 nondiabetic patients, no survival benefit was associated with GP inhibitor use (3.0% in both groups). The interaction between GP IIb/IIIa inhibition and diabetic status was statistically significant (p = 0.036).

54. Boersma E, et al. Platelet glycoprotein IIb/IIIa inhibitors in acute coronary syndromes: a meta-analysis of all major randomised clinical trials. *Lancet* 2002;359: 189–198.

This meta-analysis examined the same six trials (see preceding) that randomized 31,402 ACS patients to various GP IIb/IIIa inhibitors versus placebo or control. The meta-analysis of all endpoints was performed by using Cochrane–Mantel–Haenszel, Breslow–Day, and Kaplan–Meier methods. The 30-day pooled incidence of death or MI showed a significant absolute reduction of 1% with GP inhibitor use [10.8% vs. 11.8% (placebo or control); OR, 0.91; $p = 0.015$). A significant benefit also was seen at 5 days (5.7% vs. 6.9%; OR, 0.84; $p = 0.0003$). The benefits were seen in all important subgroups, such as age, diabetics, and prior cardiac history. GP IIb/IIIa inhibitor use was associated with an increased risk of bleeding (OR, 1.62), but no increased rate of ICH or stroke was seen. Gender difference favored treatment of men with GP IIb/IIIa inhibitors, but women benefited when controlled for baseline troponin. No benefit is apparent with GP inhibitor use when patients do not have a positive troponin test.

55. Giugliano RP, et al.; for the EARLY-ACS Investigators. Early versus delayed, provisional eptifibatide in acute coronary syndromes. *N Engl J Med* 2009;360(21): 2176–2190.

Design: Prospective, randomized, placebo-controlled, international, multicenter trial. Primary endpoint was death, MI, urgent TVR, or the requirement of bolus "thrombotic bailout" therapy during PCI at 96 hours.

Purpose: To study the effect of early versus provisional GP IIb/IIIa blocker administration in patients with UA/NSTEMI undergoing PCI.

Population: 9,492 patients with high-risk UA/NSTEMI undergoing PCI within 1 calendar day of randomization. Patients were high risk if they had at least two of the following: significant ECG changes, elevated troponin or CK-MB, and age >60 years.

Exclusion Criteria: Increased bleeding risk.

Treatment: Early, routine treatment with eptifibatide or placebo; following angiography, provisional administration of eptifibatide at the investigator's discretion (those who previously received eptifibatide got placebo bolus, and then open-label infusion; those who received placebo early got eptifibatide bolus, and then open-label infusion). If no provisional therapy was requested prior to PCI, and the operator detected a thrombotic complication of PCI after the guidewire crossed the lesion, they could request a "bailout" kit containing study drug assignment opposite that of the initial assignment (if the "bailout" kit was requested for any of the seven predefined thrombotic complications, this was considered a primary endpoint event by the Clinical Events Committee).

Results: There was no significant difference in rates of the primary endpoint at 96 hours, between patients receiving early routine eptifibatide (9.6%) and delayed, provisional administration (10.0%; $p = 0.23$). At 30 days, rates of death or MI were also similar, though with a trend toward the "early" group (11.2% for early eptifibatide vs. 12.3% for delayed; $p = 0.08$). TIMI major hemorrhage was 2.6% versus 1.8% (OR, 1.42; $p = 0.02$) and bleeding defined according to the GUSTO criteria, moderate bleeding was 6.8% in the early eptifibatide group versus 4.3% in the provisional eptifibatide group; OR, 1.60 ($p < 0.001$). GUSTO severe bleeding rates were similar, but minor bleeding and red cell transfusions were higher in the "early" group.

Conclusion: Early, routine administration of eptifibatide, as compared with provisional usage, in patients with UA/NSTEMI going to PCI did not significantly improve outcomes at 96 hours or 30 days, and there was a significant increase in major bleeding.

THROMBOLYTICS

56. Bar FW, et al.; Unstable Angina Study Using Eminase (UNASEM). Thrombolysis in patients with unstable angina improves the angiographic but not clinical outcome: results of UNASEM, a multicenter, randomized, placebo-controlled, clinical trial with anistreplase. *Circulation* 1992;86:131–137.

Prospective, randomized, double-blind, placebo-controlled, multicenter study of 159 patients aged 30 to 70 years with angina of recent onset (<4 weeks) or of the crescendo type with the last episode within 12 hours of admission and ischemic ST changes (ST depression, ≥1 mm; T-wave inversion, ≥2 mm). After coronary angiography, patients were randomized to anistreplase, 30 U over 5 minutes, or placebo; repeated angiography was performed at 12 to 28 hours. All patients were given heparin and aspirin, 300 mg/day (started after second catheterization). The anistreplase group had a significant decrease in stenosis diameter between the first and second angiograms [11% (from 70% to 59%) vs. 3% (from 66% to 63%); $p = 0.008$]. No difference was observed in clinical outcome between the groups (e.g., infarct size, MI rate), but more bleeding complications occurred with anistreplase (32% vs. 11%; $p = 0.001$).

57. Thrombolysis in Myocardial Ischemia (TIMI 3A) Investigators. Early effects of tissue-type plasminogen activator (tPA) added to conventional therapy on the culprit coronary lesion in patients presenting with ischemic cardiac pain at rest: results of the TIMI 3A trial. *Circulation* 1993;87:38–52.

Design: Prospective, randomized, open, parallel-group, multicenter study. Primary endpoint was 10% reduction of stenosis and improvement of two TIMI flow grades.

Purpose: To evaluate the effects of tPA added to conventional therapy on the culprit coronary lesion in patients with UA or non–Q-wave MI.

Population: 306 patients aged 22 to 75 years with chest pain at rest lasting 5 minutes to 6 hours and accompanied by ECG changes or documented CAD.

Exclusion Criteria: Included CABG surgery, MI in the prior 21 days, PTCA in the prior 6 months, cardiogenic shock, and oral anticoagulation requirement.

Treatment: Front-loaded tPA (maximum, 80 mg) or placebo plus conventional antianginal therapy. All patients received heparin (5,000-U bolus and infusion for 18 to 48 hours) and aspirin, 325 mg daily.

Results: The tPA group had more frequent improvement of TIMI flow by two grades or reduction of stenosis by 20% on repeated angiography at 18 to 48 hours (15% vs. 5%; $p = 0.003$). The tPA benefit was most marked in patients with thrombus-containing lesions (36% vs. 15%; $p < 0.01$) and non–Q-wave MI (33% vs. 8%; $p < 0.005$).

Comments: Only modest angiographic improvement was observed.

58. Ambrose JA, et al.; Thrombolysis and Angioplasty in Unstable Angina (TAUSA). Adjunctive thrombolytic therapy during PTCA for ischemic rest angina. *Circulation* 1994;90:69–77.

Design: Prospective, randomized, double-blind, multicenter study.

Purpose: To assess the role of intracoronary urokinase during angioplasty for UA or postinfarction rest angina.

Population: 469 patients aged ≤80 years with ischemic rest pain accompanied by ST-segment or T-wave changes and an angiogram demonstrating 70% stenosis.

Exclusion Criteria: Included normal baseline ECG, blood pressure >180/110, prior stroke, recent (within fewer than 10 days) major surgery, bleeding diathesis, and active GI or GU bleeding.

Treatment: Intracoronary urokinase (250,000 or 500,000 U) or placebo. All patients received aspirin and heparin.

Results: No significant differences in incidence of post-PTCA thrombi were observed [13.8% (urokinase) vs. 18%; p = NS], but the urokinase group had a higher acute closure rate (10.2% vs. 4.3%; p < 0.02; most of the difference was in the 500,000-U group) and more adverse outcomes (ischemia, MI, CABG surgery; 6.3% vs. 2.9%; p < 0.02).

Comments: Possible explanations of adverse effects of urokinase include increased hemorrhagic dissection, lack of intimal sealing, and procoagulant or platelet-activating effects.

59. Thrombolysis in MI (TIMI 3B). Effects of tissue plasminogen activator and a comparison of early invasive and conservative strategies in unstable angina and non–Q-wave MI. *Circulation* 1994;89:1545–1556.

Design: Prospective, randomized (2 × 2 factorial design), double-blind, placebo-controlled, multicenter study. Primary endpoint was death, MI, or failure of treatment at 6 weeks (for tPA comparison), and death, MI, or positive ETT (for strategy comparison).

Purpose: To evaluate the use of thrombolytic therapy in UA and non–Q-wave MI and to compare an early invasive with a conservative strategy.

Population: 1,473 patients aged 21 to 76 years within 24 hours of ischemic discomfort at rest consistent with UA or non–Q-wave MI.

Exclusion Criteria: Included treatable cause of UA, MI in the prior 21 days, coronary angiography in the prior 30 days, PTCA within 6 months, history of CABG, SBP higher than 180 mm Hg or DBP higher than 100 mm Hg, and contraindication to thrombolysis.

Treatment: tPA, 0.8 mg/kg over a 90-minute period (maximum, 80 mg; mean, 63 mg), including one-third of dose as an IV bolus (up to 20 mg); or placebo. The early invasive strategy involved catheterization 18 to 48 hours after randomization, and revascularization, if feasible. Conservative strategy allowed catheterization for recurrent ischemia at rest with ECG changes or other failure of medical therapy.

Results: No difference was observed between invasive and conservative strategies in combined primary endpoints (16.2% vs. 18.1%), but the early invasive strategy was associated with a shorter hospital stay and lower incidence of rehospitalization. tPA was not shown to be beneficial and may be harmful (e.g., four ICHs vs. none with placebo; p = 0.06).

Comments: One-year results showed similar death and nonfatal reinfarction rates between tPA and placebo (12.4% vs. 10.6%; p = 0.24) and early invasive versus early conservative groups (10.8% vs. 12.2%; p = 0.42). The early invasive group had a higher revascularization rate (64% vs. 58%; p < 0.001), primarily because of more PTCAs (39% vs. 32%), but fewer readmissions (26% vs. 33%; p < 0.001).

Invasive versus Conservative Management

60. Boden WE, et al.; for the Veteran Affairs Non–Q-Wave Infarction Strategies in Hospital (VANQWISH) Trial Investigators. Outcomes in patients with acute non–Q-wave MI randomly assigned to an invasive as compared with a conservative strategy. *N Engl J Med* 1998;338:1785–1792 (editorial, 1838–1839).

Design: Prospective, randomized, controlled, multicenter study. Primary endpoint was death or MI.

Purpose: To compare a conservative with an invasive strategy on the incidence of clinical outcomes in non–Q-wave MI.

Population: 920 patients with an evolving MI characterized by no Q waves on serial ECGs and CK-MB more than 1.5 times the ULN.

Exclusion Criteria: Persistent or recurrent ischemia at rest despite intensive medical therapy, severe heart failure despite IV diuretics and/or vasodilators, and serious coexisting conditions.

Treatment: Patients were assigned within 24 to 72 hours to invasive strategy (routine angiography followed by revascularization, if feasible) or conservative strategy [medical therapy, noninvasive testing (radionuclide left ventriculography and symptom-limited ETT with thallium scintigraphy), and invasive procedures only in a setting of spontaneous or inducible ischemia]. All patients received aspirin (325 mg daily) and diltiazem (180 to 300 mg/day).

Results: Only 9% were excluded secondary to high-risk ischemic complications. Only 29% of the conservative group (vs. 64% in TIMI 3B) underwent catheterization within 30 days. At follow-up (average, 23 months), the two groups had a similar incidence of death and MI [152 events (invasive, 32.9%) vs. 139 (conservative, 30.3%); $p = 0.35$]. The conservative group showed a nonsignificant trend toward lower mortality (hazard ratio, 0.72; 95% CI, 0.51 to 1.01). Fewer patients treated conservatively had death plus MI at hospital discharge (36 vs. 15 patients; $p = 0.004$; 21 vs. 6; $p = 0.007$), at 1 month (48 vs. 26; $p = 0.012$; 23 vs. 9; $p = 0.021$), and at 1 year (111 vs. 85; $p = 0.05$; 58 vs. 36; $p = 0.025$). The invasive group had a higher CABG surgery mortality rate [11.6% vs. 3.4% (11 vs. 3 patients in the conservative group)].

61. FRagmin and Fast Revascularization during InStability in coronary artery disease (FRISC II) Investigators. Invasive compared with noninvasive treatment in unstable coronary artery disease: FRISC II prospective randomized multicenter study. *Lancet* 1999;354:708–715.

Design: Prospective, randomized, partially open (strategy assignment), multicenter study. Primary endpoint was death or MI at 6 months.

Purpose: To compare an early invasive with a noninvasive strategy in patients with unstable coronary disease in addition to optimal background antithrombotic medication.

Population: 2,457 patients with ischemic symptoms in the previous 48 hours accompanied by ECG changes (ST depression or T-wave inversion ≥ 0.1 mV) or elevated markers (e.g., CK-MB >6 mg/L; troponin T >0.10 mg/dL).

Exclusion Criteria: See Ref. 22.

Treatment: Early invasive or noninvasive treatment strategy (coronary angiography within 7 days performed in 96% and 10%, and revascularization in first 10 days, in 71% and 9%). Patients also received dalteparin or placebo for 3 months.

Results: The invasive group had a significantly lower incidence of death or MI at 6 months [9.4% vs. 12.1% (noninvasive group); $p = 0.031$]. A significant decrease in MI alone was noted (7.8% vs. 10.1%; $p = 0.045$), whereas the reduction in mortality was nonsignificant (1.9% vs. 2.9%; $p = 0.10$). Subgroup analysis showed that these benefits were restricted to men (RRs of death or MI at 6 months, 0.64 in men and 1.26 in women, respectively). Invasive strategy also was associated with 50% lower recurrent angina and hospital readmission rates. At 1-year follow-up, a persistent reduction in the incidence of death or MI was seen in the invasive group (10.4% vs. 14.1%; RR, 0.74; $p = 0.005$); 52% of the noninvasive group had undergone coronary angiography (see *Lancet* 2000;354:9).

62. Cannon CP, et al.; for the Treat Angina with Aggrastat and Determine Cost of Therapy with an Invasive or Conservative Strategy (TACTICS)-TIMI 18 Investigators. Comparison of early invasive versus early conservative strategies in patients with unstable angina and non-ST elevation myocardial infarction treated with early glycoprotein IIb/IIIa inhibition. N *Engl J Med* 2001;344:1879–1887.

Design: Prospective, randomized, multicenter study. Primary endpoint composite of death, nonfatal MI, and rehospitalization for an ACS at 6 months.

Purpose: To compare an early invasive strategy with an early conservative strategy in patients with UA and NSTEMI treated with early GP IIb/IIIa inhibition.

Population: 2,220 patients with UA and NSTEMI who had one or more of the following—ECG changes, elevated levels of cardiac markers, or a history of CAD (prior cardiac catheterization, revascularization, or MI).

Exclusion Criteria: Included persistent ST elevation, secondary angina, PTCA or CABG within 6 months, history of GI bleeding, platelet disorder, thrombocytopenia or hemorrhagic cerebrovascular disease, nonhemorrhagic stroke or transient ischemic attack (TIA) within 1 year, severe CHF or cardiogenic shock, serum creatinine >2.5 mg/dL, treatment with abciximab within 96 hours, or current long-term treatment with ticlopidine, clopidogrel, or warfarin.

Treatment: Early invasive strategy (routine catheterization within 4 to 48 hours and revascularization as appropriate), or more conservative strategy [catheterization only if the patient had objective evidence of recurrent ischemia (ECG changes, positive markers) or an abnormal stress test]. All patients were treated with aspirin, heparin, and tirofiban, 0.4 μg/kg/min for 30 minutes.

Results: At 6 months, the early invasive strategy had a significantly lower incidence of the primary endpoint compared with the conservative strategy (15.9% vs. 19.4%; OR, 0.78; $p = 0.025$). The early invasive group also had a lower rate of death or nonfatal MI at 6 months (7.3% vs. 9.5%; OR, 0.74; $p < 0.05$). The invasive strategy provided a significantly greater benefit in the patients with baseline ST-segment changes (p for interaction ≥0.006). In patients with a troponin T level >0.01 ng/mL, a 39% relative reduction in the primary endpoint with the invasive strategy was noted, compared with the conservative strategy ($p < 0.001$), whereas patients with a troponin T level of 0.01 ng/mL or more had similar outcomes with either strategy. In a prespecified analysis that used the TRS (see JAMA 2000;284:835), the benefits of the invasive strategy were observed in intermediate- and high-risk patients (75% of the study population).

63. Fox KAA, et al.; for the Randomized Intervention Trial of unstable Angina (RITA) Investigators. Interventional versus conservative treatment for patients with unstable angina or non–ST-elevation myocardial infarction: the British Foundation RITA 3 randomised trial. *Lancet* 2002;360:743–751.

Design: Prospective, randomized, open, multicenter trial. Coprimary endpoints were death, MI, or refractory angina at 4 months and death or MI at 1 year. Median follow-up was 2 years.

Purpose: To determine whether routine early angiography with myocardial revascularization (as clinically indicated) is better than a conservative strategy in UA/NSTEMI patients.

Population: 1,810 patients with non–ST-elevation ACS.

Exclusion Criteria: Included probable evolving MI, CK or CK-MB twice the ULN before randomization, planned PCI within 72 hours, MI in the previous month, PCI in the previous year, or CABG at any time.

Treatment: Early intervention (angiography with PCI if indicated) or conservative strategy [ischemia- or symptom-driven angiography (performed in 48% at 1 year)]. Antithrombin agent in both groups was enoxaparin. Approximately 25% received a GP IIb/IIIa inhibitor.

Results: At 4 months, the early intervention group had a 34% lower incidence of death, MI, or refractory angina compared with the conservative strategy group (9.6% vs. 14.5%; $p = 0.001$). This benefit was primarily driven by a 53% reduction in refractory angina in the intervention group. Refractory angina required occurrence of ischemic pain, at rest or with minimal exertion, despite maximal medical treatment, associated with ECG changes, and prompting revascularization within 24 hours. At 1 year, the incidence of death or MI was similar in both groups (7.6% vs. 8.3%; $p = 0.58$). Using the ESC/ACC MI definition, death or MI at 1 year was reduced (12.5% vs. 17.1%; $p = 0.007$). The interventional group had a significant reduction in symptoms of angina and use of antianginal medications ($p < 0.0001$).

64. Neumann F-J, et al. Evaluation of prolonged antithrombotic pretreatment ("cooling-off" strategy) before intervention in patients with unstable coronary syndromes. A randomized controlled trial (ISAR-COOL). JAMA 2003;290:1593–1599.

Design: Prospective, randomized, controlled trial. Primary endpoint was a composite of death or MI at 30 days.

Purpose: To determine whether prolonged antithrombotic treatment prior to PCI is beneficial in patients undergoing PCI for UA/NSTEMI.

Population: 410 patients with UA/NSTEMI with *either* ST-segment depression or elevated levels of troponin.

Treatment: All patients received the same antithrombotic regimen—heparin infusion (with bolus), aspirin, clopidogrel (with load), and tirofiban infusion (with bolus). Patients in the immediate-intervention group went to PCI within 6 hours, whereas the prolonged group went to PCI at 3 to 5 days following presentation (unless they exhibited refractory ischemia or hemodynamic instability or met the primary endpoint).

Results: Patients in the prolonged pretreatment group had significantly higher rates of the primary endpoint at 30 days (11.6% vs. 5.9%; $p = 0.04$). The surplus of events occurred prior to catheterization, as there was no difference in the rates of events following catheterization. Delay of intervention for antithrombotic pretreatment is not beneficial in patients with moderate-risk UA/NSTEMI.

65. de Winter RJ, et al.; for the Invasive versus Conservative Treatment in Unstable Coronary Syndromes (ICTUS) Investigators. Early invasive versus selectively invasive management for acute coronary syndromes. N Engl J Med 2005;353:1095–1104.

Design: Prospective, randomized, multicenter, controlled trials. Primary endpoint was death, MI, or rehospitalization for angina.

Purpose: To identify the reduction in mortality, if any, of an early invasive strategy (compared with a "selectively" invasive strategy) for patients with UA/NSTEMI at moderate risk.

Population: 1,200 patients with UA/NSTEMI including elevated troponin levels and *either* significant ECG changes or known history of CAD.

Treatment: All patients received aspirin, enoxaparin, and abciximab (at the time of PCI). Clopidogrel and aggressive lipid-lowering therapy was recommended. Randomization was to either early invasive strategy of angiography within 24 to 48 hours or "selectively" invasive strategy where patients were treated medically and underwent angiography *only* if they had refractory symptoms, hemodynamic or ECG instability, or clinically significant ischemia on the predischarge stress test.

Results: There was no difference in rates of the primary endpoint between the early and selectively invasive groups (22.7% for early vs. 21.2% for selective; $p = 0.33$). Importantly, 53% of patients assigned to the selectively invasive strategy underwent catheterization during the index hospitalization. One-year mortality was identical between the two groups (2.5%), but rates of recurrent MI favored the selectively invasive group (15% for early vs. 10.0% for selective; $p = 0.005$). Patients in the selectively invasive group had a higher rate of rehospitalization (7.4% vs. 10.9%; $p = 0.04$).

66. O'Donaghue M, et al. Early invasive vs. conservative treatment strategies in women and men with unstable angina and non–ST-segment elevation myocardial infarction: a meta-analysis. JAMA 2008;300(1):71–80.

The authors combined data from eight trials (TIMI 3B, MATE, VANQWISH, FRISC II, TACTICS-TIMI 18, VINO, RITA 3, ICTUS) of invasive versus conservative strategies in patients with UA/NSTEMI (including 3,075 women and 7,075 men), and compiled patient-level data for rates of death, MI, or rehospitalization for ACS at 12 months. The benefit of invasive strategy was not significant in women (21.1% vs. 25.0%; OR, 0.81; 95% CI, 0.65 to 1.01) but did reach significance for men (21.2% vs. 26.3%; OR, 0.73; 95% CI, 0.55 to 0.98), without significant heterogeneity between sexes ($p_{interaction}$ = 0.26). However, when restricted to women with elevated troponin or CK-MB, the benefit of invasive strategy was statistically significant (OR, 0.67; 95% CI, 0.50 to 0.88). The authors conclude that the data support the most recent guideline recommendations for consideration of a conservative strategy in low-risk women.

67. Montalescot G, et al.; for the ABOARD Investigators. Immediate vs. delayed intervention for acute coronary syndromes: a randomized clinical trial. JAMA 2009; 302(9):947–954.

Design: Prospective, randomized, multicenter trial. Primary endpoint was the peak troponin I during hospitalization. Secondary endpoint was a composite of death, MI, or urgent revascularization at 1 month.

Purpose: To identify the optimal timing of intervention in patients with UA/NSTEMI.

Population: 352 patients with UA/NSTEMI and a TRS of 3 or more.

Treatment: Invasive strategy undergoing intervention either immediately or the next business day (between 8 and 60 hours after enrollment).

Results: The groups differed in time from randomization to sheath insertion by approximately 20 hours (70 minutes for immediate intervention vs. 21 hours for delayed intervention), and roughly half of patients who underwent PCI received DES. There was no significant difference in the primary endpoint of peak troponin I (median 2.1 for immediate vs. 1.7 for delayed; $p = 0.70$). Clinical events of the composite secondary endpoint also were not statistically different (13.7% vs. 10.2%; $p = 0.31$). Individual rates of death, MI, urgent revascularization, recurrent ischemia, or major bleeding at 1 month all were similar in the two groups.

68. Gluckman TJ, et al. A simplified approach to the management of non–ST-segment elevation acute coronary syndromes. JAMA 2005;293:349–357.

The authors performed a review of the literature and guidelines for the management of UA/NSTEMI, and then refined a simplified approach to each patient. They base their approach on the initial risk stratification of patients to identify those most likely to benefit from an early invasive strategy, and then use the "ABCDE" mnemonic for subsequent therapies: "A" for antiplatelet therapy, anticoagulation, and ACE-I/ARB; "B" for β-blockade and blood pressure control; "C" for cholesterol treatment and cigarette smoking cessation; "D" for diabetes management and diet; and "E" for exercise.

Noninvasive Assessment and Prognosis

69. Hoffmann U, et al. Coronary computed tomography angiography for early triage of patients with acute chest pain: the ROMICAT (Rule Out Myocardial Infarction using Computer Assisted Tomography) trial. J Am Coll Cardiol 2009;53:1642–1650.

In 368 patients in the emergency department with chest pain of low risk (negative troponin, nonischemic ECG), the investigators performed 64-slice coronary CTA prior to admission. Results were not disclosed, and they were subsequently treated as per routine and followed up for outcomes of ACS during index hospitalization or MACEs at

6 months. Freedom from CAD on CTA was highly and negatively predictive of events, with both sensitivity and negative predictive values for AS of 100%. They found that coronary plaque and stenosis on CTA not only independently predicted ACS but also predicted ACS incrementally over the TRS ($p < 0.0001$).

70. Hoffman U, et al. Coronary CT angiography versus standard evaluation in acute chest pain. N Engl J Med 2012;367:299–308. ROMICAT II

In 1,000 patients evaluated in the emergency department for chest pain, the use of cardiac CT angiography, as compared with standard ED care, was associated with a shorter mean length of stay (23 hours vs. 31 hours; $p < 0.001$). The use of cardiac CT angiography was also associated with a shorter mean time to diagnosis (10 hours vs. 19 hours; $p < 0.001$) and greater rates of direct discharge from the ED (47% vs. 12%; $p < 0.001$) compared with standard of care, but led to greater cumulative exposure to radiation (14 mSv vs. 5.3 mSv; $p < 0.001$. Compared with standard of care, there were no differences seen in periprocedural complications (0.4% vs. 0%; $p = 0.25$), major adverse cardiac events (0.4% vs. 1.2%; $p = 0.18$), or costs of care ($4,026 vs. $3,874; $p = 0.75$).

CLINICAL OR GENERAL ANALYSES

71. Armstrong PW, et al. Acute coronary syndromes in the GUSTO-IIb trial: prognostic insights and impact of recurrent ischemia. Circulation 1998;98:1860–1868.

Recurrent ischemia was approximately 50% more common in non–ST-elevation patients than in ST-elevation patients (35% vs. 23%; $p < 0.001$). This may explain why the non–ST-elevation group had a lower mortality rate at 30 days (3.8% vs. 6.1%; $p < 0.001$) but a similar rate by 1 year (8.8% vs. 9.6%). Compared with UA patients, NSTEMI patients had higher rates of reinfarction at 6 months (9.8% vs. 6.2%) and higher 6-month and 1-year mortality rates (8.8% vs. 5.0%; 11.1% vs. 7.0%).

72. Farkouh ME, et al. A clinical trial of a chest-pain observation unit for patients with unstable angina. N Engl J Med 1998;339:1882–1888.

This community-based, prospective study of 424 UA patients showed that a chest pain observation unit located in the emergency department can be safe, effective, and result in cost savings. Patients with rest angina lasting longer than 20 minutes, new-onset angina on exertion (CCS class 3 or higher), and postinfarction angina were eligible. High-risk patients were excluded (e.g., ST-segment depression in several ECG leads). Eligible patients were randomized to routine hospital admission (monitored bed on cardiology service) or admission to the chest pain observation unit. No significant difference was found in the rate of cardiac events between the two groups (OR for chest pain observation unit group, 0.50; 95% CI, 0.20 to 1.24). At 6 months, chest pain observation unit patients had used less resources ($p = 0.003$ by rank-sum test).

73. Stone PH, et al. Influence of race, sex and age of management of unstable angina and non–Q-wave MI (TIMI 3 registry). JAMA 1996;275:1104–1112.

This prospective analysis of 3,318 patients showed disparities in care among blacks, women, and the elderly. Compared with nonblacks, blacks were less likely to be treated with intensive anti-ischemic therapy and to undergo invasive procedures (RR, 0.65; $p < 0.001$). However, of those who had angiography (45% of blacks and 61% of nonblacks), blacks had less extensive and severe coronary stenoses. Blacks also had less recurrent ischemia. Women also were less likely to receive intensive anti-ischemic therapy and to undergo angiography (RR, 0.71; $p < 0.001$) and had less severe and extensive coronary disease; however, they had a similar risk of experiencing an adverse cardiac event by 6 weeks. Elderly patients (older than 75 years) received less aggressive therapy and had less-frequent angiography (RR, 0.65; $p < 0.001$) and fewer revascularization procedures (RR, 0.79; $p = 0.002$) despite having more extensive disease. At 6 weeks, the elderly had a higher incidence of adverse cardiac events (RR, 1.91; $p < 0.001$).

74. Vaccarino V, et al. Sex and racial differences in the management of acute myocardial infarction, 1994 through 2002. N Engl J Med 2005;353:671–682.

In the National Registry of Myocardial Infarction from 1994 to 2002, investigators reviewed 598,911 patients with acute MI. After multivariable adjustment, significant differences persisted in rates of reperfusion therapy (RR for white women 0.97, black men 0.91, black women 0.89, compared with white men) and angiography (0.91, 0.82, 0.76, respectively). Significant differences for use of aspirin and β-blockers in unadjusted rates were no longer significant in multivariable analysis. The only significant difference in mortality was for the comparison of black women to white men (RR, 1.11). These results were unchanged over the time period studied.

75. Popescu I, et al. Differences in mortality and use of revascularization in black and white patients with acute MI admitted to hospitals with and without revascularization services. JAMA 2007;297:2489–2495.

In a study of 1,215,924 Medicare beneficiaries admitted with acute MI, the authors analyzed outcomes by race, including adjusted rates of revascularization at 30 days, mortality at 1 year, and transfer to a hospital with revascularization services (for patients presenting to hospitals without revascularization services). In adjusted analyses, the investigators found that black patients admitted with acute MI were less likely to be transferred for revascularization (hazard ratio, 0.78; $p < 0.001$) and less likely to undergo revascularization in hospitals with (hazard ratio, 0.71; $p < 0.001$) and without revascularization available (hazard ratio, 0.68; $p < 0.001$). In the first 30 days, adjusted rates of mortality were lower for black patients ($p < 0.001$), but were higher in intervals up to 1 year ($p < 0.001$).

76. Berger JS, et al. Sex differences in mortality following acute coronary syndromes. JAMA 2009;302(8):874–882.

In a pooled sample of 11 randomized, clinical trials of ACS, the investigators assessed 30-day mortality rates of 136,247 patients by gender. Overall, 38,048 (28%) were women; 102,004 (26% women) had STEMI, 14,466 (29% women) had NSTEMI; and 19,777 (40% women) had UA. Overall, unadjusted 30-day mortality rates were 9.6% for women and 5.3% for men (OR, 1.91; 95% CI, 1.83 to 2.00). After multivariable analyses, this difference was no longer significant (OR, 1.06; 95% CI, 0.99 to 1.15). There was a significant interacting between gender and type of ACS ($p < 0.001$): in adjusted analyses, STEMI mortality rates were higher for women (OR, 1.15; 95% CI, 1.06 to 1.24), whereas NSTEMI and UA mortality rates were lower for women (OR, 0.77; 95% CI, 0.63 to 0.95 and OR, 0.55; 95% CI, 0.43 to 0.70, respectively). In further analyses of angiographic data in a subset of 35,128 patients, there were no significant differences in mortality between sexes or interaction with ACS type after multivariable analyses with adjustment for angiographic variables included. The authors conclude to suggest that angiographic differences in presentation between men and women could likely explain differences in mortality rates after ACS.

77. Donahoe SM, et al. Diabetes and mortality following acute coronary syndromes. JAMA 2007;298(7):765–775.

The investigators pooled 11 randomized trials of ACS from 1997 to 2006, to analyze outcomes in 62,036 patients with and without diabetes. In all, 46,577 had STEMI, 15,459 had UA/NSTEMI, and 10,613 (17.1%) had diabetes. Outcomes included mortality at 30 days and 1 year. After adjustment for other characteristics, diabetes predicted significantly higher 30-day mortality from UA/NSTEMI (OR, 1.78; 95% CI, 1.24 to 2.56) and STEMI (OR, 1.40; 95% CI, 1.24 to 1.57). Patients with diabetes at initial presentation also had higher 1-year mortality for both UA/NSTEMI (hazard ratio, 1.65; 95% CI, 1.30 to 2.10) and STEMI (hazard ratio, 1.22; 95% CI, 1.08 to 1.38). An interesting finding when comparing mortality rates is that diabetes associated with UA/NSTEMI appeared to portend a similar 1-year prognosis as STEMI without diabetes.

78. Antman EM, et al. The TIMI Risk Score for unstable angina/non–ST elevation MI. A method for prognostication and therapeutic decision making. JAMA 2000; 284:835–842.

This retrospective analysis of the TIMI IIB and ESSENCE trials (see references) developed a simple risk score that has broad applicability, is easily calculated, and identifies patients with different responses to treatments for UA/NSTEMI. The test cohort was the 1,957 TIMI IIB patients who received UFH, whereas the three validation cohorts were the UFH group from ESSENCE and both enoxaparin groups. Outcomes were TRS for developing at least one component of the primary endpoint (all-cause mortality, new or recurrent MI, or ischemia requiring urgent revascularization at 14 days). The seven TRS predictor variables were age older than 65 years, more than three CAD risk factors, prior coronary stenosis of more than 50%, ST-segment deviation on initial ECG, more than two anginal events in the prior 24 hours, use of aspirin in the prior 7 days, and elevated serum cardiac markers. As the TRS increased in the test cohort, event rates increased: 4.7% for a score of 0/1; 8.3% for 2; 13.2% for 3; 19.9% for 4; 26.2% for 5; and 40.9% for 6/7 ($p < 0.001$ by χ^2 for trend). The pattern of increasing event rates with increasing TRS was confirmed in all three validation groups ($p < 0.001$). The enoxaparin groups had a slower rate of increase in event rates with an increasing TRS.

79. Eagle KA, et al.; for the GRACE Investigators. A validated prediction model for all forms of acute coronary syndrome: estimating the risk of 6-month postdischarge death in an international registry. JAMA 2004;291:2727–2733.

In 17,142 patients with ACS enrolled in the GRACE registry from 1999 to 2002, investigators developed a simple regression model for mortality at 6 months. For all forms of ACS, the model included nine characteristics of presentation: age, history of MI, history of CHF, increased pulse, decreased SBP, elevated serum creatinine, elevated cardiac biomarkers, ST-segment depression on electrocardiogram, and not having in-hospital PCI. The c statistic for the development model was 0.81. It was subsequently validated in another GRACE cohort of 7,638 patients admitted from 2002 to 2003 (c statistic 0.75). Six-month mortality rates between the two cohorts were similar (4.8% in development cohort vs. 4.7% in validation cohort). Additionally, the GRACE score was also validated in a Canadian cohort, which implemented it to predict in-hospital mortality in patients with ACS (see Am Heart J 2009;158:392–399).

80. Yan AT, et al. Risk scores for risk stratification in acute coronary syndromes: useful but simpler is not necessarily better. Eur Heart J 2007;28:1072–1078.

In a prospective Canadian registry of 1,728 patients with UA/NSTEMI, the investigators calculated for each patient his or her PURSUIT risk score, TRS, and GRACE risk score. Each demonstrated decent predictive value for the endpoint of in-hospital mortality (c statistics 0.68 for TIMI, 0.80 for PURSUIT, and 0.81 for GRACE, all $p < 0.001$), as well as 1-year mortality (c statistics 0.69, 0.77, 0.79, respectively, all $p < 0.0001$). Significant predictive advantage was identified for the PURSUIT and GRACE risk scores over the TRS ($p < 0.04$ for each comparison to the TRS for both in-hospital and 1-year mortality rates).

Biomarkers

REVIEW ARTICLES AND MULTIMARKER STUDIES

81. Sabatine MS, et al. Multimarker approach to risk stratification in non-ST elevation acute coronary syndromes: simultaneous assessment of troponin I, C-reactive protein, and B-type natriuretic peptide. Circulation 2002;105:1760–1763.

In analysis of 450 patients with ACS in the OPUS-TIMI 16 trial, the investigators measured troponin I, CRP, and BNP. With each additional biomarker elevation, they identified significant increases in the risk of the composite endpoint of death, MI, or CHF ($p = 0.01$ for the trend). This was consistent up to 10 months. The assessment of risk by these three biomarkers was then validated with similar results in 1,635 patients in the TACTICS-TIMI 18 trial.

82. Eggers KM, et al. Prognostic value of biomarkers during and after non-ST-segment elevation acute coronary syndrome. *J Am Coll Cardiol* 2009;54:357–364.

In 877 patients with UA/NSTEMI in the FRISC study, the authors measured CRP, BNP, and troponin I and estimated glomerular filtration rate (GFR) at randomization, 6 weeks, and 6 months. At randomization, BNP was the strongest predictor of mortality at 5 years (adjusted hazard ratio, 1.7; $p < 0.001$). Predictive value of CRP was increased later in follow-up.

TROPONINS

83. Hamm CW, et al. The prognostic value of serum troponin T in unstable angina. *N Engl J Med* 1992;327:146–150 (editorial, 192–194).

This prospective, multicenter analysis focused on 109 consecutive UA patients (84 with rest angina and 25 with accelerated or subacute angina) who had CK, CK-MB, and troponin T sampled every 8 hours for 2 days after hospital admission. Troponin T was detected (range, 0.20 to 3.64 μg/L) in 39% of the 84 patients with rest angina; only 3 of these patients had an elevated CK-MB (1 of the 3 with negative troponin T). Positive troponin-T patients had high event rates, with MI occurring in 30%, and in-hospital death in 15%. In contrast, only 1 of the 51 patients with rest angina and a negative troponin T had an MI ($p < 0.001$), and this patient died ($p = 0.03$). Troponin T was not detected in any of the 25 patients with accelerated or subacute angina.

84. Lindahl B, et al. Relation between troponin T and the risk of subsequent cardiac events in unstable coronary artery disease. *Circulation* 1996;93:1651–1657.

This prospective analysis of 976 FRISC patients showed that 5-month rates of cardiac death and MI correlate with troponin T. In the first quintile (maximum troponin T in first 24 hours <0.06 μg/L), the incidence of death and MI was 4.3%; the second quintile (0.06 to 0.18 μg/L), 10.5%; the top three quintiles, 16.1%. In multivariate analysis, independent predictors of death and MI included troponin T (other predictors were age, hypertension, number of antianginal drugs, and rest ECG changes). A subsequent analysis showed that the dalteparin group had a lower rate of death and MI only if troponin T was ≥0.1 μg/L (7.4% vs. 14.2%; $p < 0.01$).

85. Antman E, et al. Cardiac-specific troponin I levels to predict the risk of mortality in patients with acute coronary syndromes. *N Engl J Med* 1996;335:1342–1349 (editorial, 1388–1389).

This analysis focused on 1,404 TIMI 3B patients. Troponin I was elevated (≥0.4 ng/mL) in 573 patients and associated with a significantly increased 42-day mortality rate (3.7% vs. 1.0%; $p < 0.001$). Each 1-ng/mL increase in troponin I was associated with a mortality increase: ≤0.4, 1%; 0.4 to 0.9, 1.7%; 1 to 1.9, 3.4%; 2 to 4.9, 3.7%; 5 to 8.9, 6%; and ≥9, 7.5%. If no CK-MB elevation was present (948 patients), a troponin I elevation was still associated with increased mortality: 2.5% vs. 0.8% (RR, 3.0; 95% CI, 0.97 to 9.2).

86. Hamm CW, et al. Benefit of abciximab in patients with refractory unstable angina in relation to serum troponin T levels. *N Engl J Med* 1999;340:1623–1629.

This analysis focused on 890 CAPTURE trial patients with UA who had serum samples drawn at the time of randomization to abciximab or placebo. Patients with postinfarction angina were excluded. Among placebo-treated patients, the incidence of death or nonfatal MI at 6 months was threefold higher in patients with elevated troponin-T levels (more than 0.1 ng/mL; 23.9% vs. 7.5%; $p < 0.001$), whereas no difference was found among abciximab-treated patients (9.5% vs. 9.4%). The lower incidence of death or MI in elevated troponin-T patients receiving abciximab compared with placebo (RR, 0.32; $p = 0.002$) was owing to the significant reduction in MI rate (OR, 0.23; $p < 0.001$). In patients without elevated troponin-T levels, no significant benefit was associated with abciximab treatment.

87. Morrow DA, et al.; for the TACTICS-TIMI 18 Investigators. Ability of minor elevations of troponin I and T to predict benefit from an early invasive strategy in patients with unstable angina and non-ST elevation myocardial infarction: results from a randomized trial. JAMA 2001;286:2405–2412.

This prospective study obtained baseline troponin-level data in 1,821 ACS patients (of 2,220 total). An elevated cTnI level (0.1 ng/mL or greater; $n \geq 1,087$) was associated with a significant reduction in death, MI, or rehospitalization for ACS at 6 months with the invasive versus conservative strategy (15.3% vs. 25.0%; OR, 0.54; 95% CI, 0.40 to 0.73). Low-level cTnI elevations (0.1 to 0.4 ng/mL) also were associated with a benefit of an invasive strategy (30-day incidence of composite endpoint, 4.4% vs. 16.5%; OR, 0.24; 95% CI, 0.08 to 0.69). Patients with cTnI levels <0.1 ng/mL had no significant benefit from an early invasive strategy (16.0% vs. 12.4%; OR, 1.4; 95% CI, 0.89 to 2.05; $p < 0.001$ for interaction). Similar results were observed with cTnT. Furthermore, even in patients without significant CAD on angiography, elevated troponin in patients presenting with ACS predicted a high risk for death or reinfarction (see *J Am Coll Cardiol* 2005;45:19–24).

HIGH-SENSITIVITY TROPONINS

88. Keller T, et al. Sensitive troponin I assay in early diagnosis of acute myocardial infarction. N Engl J Med 2009;361:868–77.

In 1,818 patients presenting with suspected ACS, the investigators measured high-sensitivity troponin I, in addition to traditional troponin T and other biomarkers, at baseline, 3, and 6 hours. The sensitive troponin demonstrated the best diagnostic accuracy at baseline (AUC 0.96 vs. 0.85), and was consistent across time points irrespective of chest pain onset. They conclude that high-sensitivity troponin I is better for early diagnosis of acute MI.

89. Reichlin T, et al. Early diagnosis of myocardial infarction with sensitive cardiac troponin assays. N Engl J Med 2009; 361:858–867.

In an analysis of 4 different high-sensitivity Troponin assays, the investigators studied 718 patients presenting with symptoms of ACS. For early diagnosis of the 123 confirmed acute MI cases. the hsTroponin assays performed significantly better, with AUC measurements of 0.95 to 0.96 versus 0.90 for the standard assay. The difference was more dramatic among patients presenting within 3 hours of symptoms (AUC 0.92 to 0.93 for hsTroponin vs. 0.76 for the standard assay).

INFLAMMATORY MARKERS

90. Haverkate F, et al. Production of C-reactive protein and risk of coronary events in stable and unstable angina. Lancet 1997;349:362–366.

This analysis focused on 2,121 outpatients with angina (1,030 unstable, 743 stable, 348 atypical); all had baseline angiography. At 2-year follow-up, patients with CRP in the fifth quintile (more than 3.6 mg/L) had a twofold higher risk of a coronary event. Thus, acute-phase responses are probably not due to myocardial necrosis.

91. Morrow DA, et al. C-reactive protein is a potent predictor of mortality independent of and in combination with troponin T in acute coronary syndromes: a TIMI-11 substudy. J Am Coll Cardiol 1998;31:1460–1465.

A total of 437 UA/non–Q-wave MI patients had quantitative CRP and rapid troponin-T assays performed. CRP was higher among patients who died than in survivors (7.2 vs. 1.3 mg/dL; $p = 0.0038$). Patients with CRP = 1.55 mg/dL and an early positive troponin-T assay result (≥10 minutes) had the highest mortality rates, followed by those with either CRP = 1.55 or early positive troponin-T assay results, whereas those with a low CRP and negative troponin-T assay results were at very low risk (9.10% vs. 4.65% vs. 0.36%; $p = 0.0003$).

92. James SK, et al.; for GUSTO-IV-ACS Investigators. Troponin and C-reactive protein have different relations to subsequent mortality and myocardial infarction after acute coronary syndrome: a GUSTO-IV substudy. *J Am Coll Cardiol* 2003;41: 916–924.

The investigators measured baseline levels of troponin T and CRP in 7,108 patients in the GUSTO IV trial, and assessed outcomes at 30 days. Both biomarkers significantly and independently predicted mortality in multivariable analysis. Troponin T elevation also helped predict recurrent MI, whereas CRP did not.

93. Schiele F, et al. C-reactive protein improves risk prediction in patients with acute coronary syndromes. *Eur Heart J* 2009;31:290–297.

The investigators measured the GRACE risk score in 1,408 patients with ACS, and then added CRP to the prediction model for the outcome of 30-day mortality. CRP significantly improved the GRACE risk score model (c statistic from 0.795 to 0.823) and was an independent predictor of mortality.

B-TYPE NATRIURETIC PEPTIDE

94. de Lemos JA, et al. The prognostic value of B-type natriuretic peptide in patients with acute coronary syndromes. *N Engl J Med* 2001;345:1014–1021.

This substudy of 2,525 ACS patients in the OPUS-TIMI 16 trial measured BNP in plasma samples obtained at mean of 40 ± 20 hours after the onset of symptoms. Baseline BNP level was significantly correlated with the risk of death, heart failure, and new or recurrent MI at 30 days and 10 months. The unadjusted rate of death increased in a step-wise fashion among patients in increasing quartiles of baseline BNP levels ($p < 0.001$). This mortality association was significant in the major patient subgroups [STEMI ($p = 0.02$), NSTEMI ($p < 0.001$), and UA ($p < 0.001$)]. After risk-factor adjustment, the ORs for death at 10 months in the second, third, and fourth quartiles of BNP were 3.8 (95% CI, 1.1 to 13.3), 4.0 (95% CI, 1.2 to 13.7), and 5.8 (95% CI, 1.7 to 19.7).

95. Morrow DA, et al. Evaluation of B-type natriuretic peptide for risk assessment in unstable angina/non-ST-elevation myocardial infarction: B-type natriuretic peptide and prognosis in TACTICS-TIMI 18. *J Am Coll Cardiol* 2003;41:1264–1272.

The investigators measured BNP, in addition to troponin I, in 1,676 patients with UA/NSTEMI in the TACTICS-TIMI 18 trial. At a cutoff of 80 pg/mL, patients with elevated BNP above that threshold had a higher rate of death at 7 days (2.5% vs. 0.7%; $p = 0.006$). At 6 months, elevated BNP predicted mortality (8.4% vs. 1.8%; $p < 0.0001$), and this remained significant in multivariable analysis including clinical predictors, as well as troponin I level. Risk of developing CHF was also significantly higher in the elevated BNP at 30 days (5.9% vs. 1.0%; $p < 0.0001$).

96. Morrow DA, et al.; for the A to Z Investigators. Prognostic value of serial B-type natriuretic peptide testing during follow-up of patients with unstable coronary artery disease. JAMA 2005;294:2866–2871.

In a substudy of the A to Z trial, the investigators sought to identify the utility of serial measurements of BNP in patients following any ACS. In 4,497 patients with UA/NSTEMI or STEMI, they measured BNP prior to discharge, at 4 months, and at 12 months to assess its prognostic significance for death or new CHF at 2 years. At each time period, elevated BNP (>80 pg/mL) was significantly associated with elevated risk of death or new CHF. Patients with newly elevated BNP at 4 months were at increased risk of the primary outcome, whereas those whose BNP levels normalized from discharge to 4 months had only modestly increased risk (compared with patients who had normal BNP at both visits). The authors conclude that serial measurements of BNP could provide improved prognostic ability, as well as potentially facilitate clinical decision making.

SPECIFIC TESTS: ANGIOGRAPHY, ECG, AND HOLTER

97. Dewood MA, et al. Coronary arteriographic findings soon after non-Q wave MI. *N Engl J Med* 1986;315:417–423.

In this angiography study, 341 non–Q-wave MI patients were divided into three groups: angiography at ≤24, 24 to 72, and more than 72 hours for 7 days. Frequency of total occlusion and visible collateral vessels both increased with time [26% at ≤24 hours vs. 42% at ≥72 hours ($p < 0.05$); 27% vs. 42% ($p < 0.05$)]. The subtotal occlusion rate decreased with time.

98. Cannon CP, et al. The electrocardiogram predicts one year outcome of patients with unstable angina and non–Q-wave MI: results of TIMI 3 Registry Ancillary Study. *J Am Coll Cardiol* 1997;30:133–140.

This prospective study focused on 1,416 patients, 14.3% with new ST deviation ≥1 mm; 21.9% had isolated T-wave inversion, and 9% had LBBB. The incidence of death and MI at 1 year was 11% in the group with ST changes [$p < 0.001$ (vs. no ST deviation)], 6.8% with T-wave inversion, and 8.2% without ECG changes. Two high-risk groups were identified: one with LBBB [22.9%; RR, 2.80 (multivariate analysis)] and the other with 0.5-mm ST changes (16.3%; RR, 2.45).

99. Al-Khatib SM, et al. Sustained ventricular arrhythmias among patients with acute coronary syndromes with no ST-segment elevation. *Circulation* 2002;106:309–312.

Data analyzed from 26,416 patients in GUSTO-IIb, PURSUIT, PARAGON-A, and PARAGON-B trials. Independent predictors of in-hospital ventricular fibrillation included prior MI, prior hypertension, chronic obstructive pulmonary disease, and ST-segment changes at presentation. In-hospital VT was predicted by prior MI, COPD, and ST changes. In Cox proportional-hazards modeling, in-hospital VF and VT were independently associated with markedly higher rates of 30-day mortality (hazard ratio, 23.2; 95% CI, 18.1 to 29.8, for VF; and hazard ratio, 7.6; 95% CI, 5.5 to 10.4, for VT) and 6-month mortality (hazard ratio, 14.8; 95% CI, 12.1 to 18.3, for VF; and hazard ratio, 5.0; 95% CI, 3.8 to 6.5, for VT). After exclusion of heart failure patients, those in cardiogenic shock, and those who died within 24 hours of enrollment, these differences remained significant.

chapter 4
ST Elevation Myocardial Infarction

Christopher P. Cannon, Benjamin A. Steinberg, and Justin M. Dunn

EPIDEMIOLOGY

According to the Heart Disease and Stroke Statistics 2014 Update, an estimated 720,000 US patients will have an acute myocardial infarction (AMI) in 2014 (1), of which approximately 25% to 40% will have ST elevations on the initial electrocardiogram (ECG) (2). The proportion of AMIs that were ST elevation myocardial infarctions (STEMIs) has been decreasing, with one study analyzing over 46,000 hospitalizations showing a decrease from 47% in 1999 to 22.9% in 2008 (4). Mortality due to STEMI has also declined. A recent analysis of the Atherosclerosis Risk in Communities (ARIC) Study revealed that from 1987 to 2008 in patients with STEMI aged 35 to 74 years, the overall 28-day age- and gender-adjusted case fatality decreased from 8.9% to 5.4% (5). Approximately 30% to 35% of STEMIs occur in women.

PATHOGENESIS

STEMI is the result of atherosclerosis, plaque rupture, and consequent thrombotic coronary artery occlusion in more than 90% of patients. Inflammation appears to play a role in plaque rupture (6). Extent of damage is related to the site and duration of occlusion and the presence or absence of adequate collateral supply. Nonatherosclerotic causes include emboli (atrial fibrillation, endocarditis), cocaine, trauma/contusion, arteritis, spasm, and dissection. Non-STEMIs are typically a manifestation of the same pathophysiologic process, but the result is a nonocclusive thrombus (see Chapter 3). Approximately two-thirds of MIs occur in plaques with <50% underlying stenosis (7), though this concept is being challenged by more recent data (8,9).

Diagnosis

The revised 2007 joint ESC/ACCF/AHA/WHF criteria defining MI were again revised in 2012, as the third universal definition of MI (10). The updated criteria require detection of a characteristic rise and/or fall in cardiac biomarkers (including at least one value >99th percentile upper reference limit), as well as at least one of the following: symptoms of ischemia, new or presumed new significant ST-segment T-wave changes or new left bundle branch block (LBBB), development of pathologic Q waves, imaging evidence of new loss of viable myocardial tissue or new regional wall motion abnormality, or identification of an intracoronary thrombus by angiography or autopsy. Alternatively, sudden, unexpected cardiac death accompanied by either significant ECG changes (new ST elevation or LBBB) or thrombotic coronary occlusion on angiography or autopsy can also define an MI. Separate definitions for periprocedural MI [in the setting of percutaneous coronary intervention (PCI) or coronary artery bypass graft (CABG)] and MI due to ischemic imbalance have also been formally outlined and further refined in this update.

Chest Pain

The pain of MI is often described as chest pressure and typically lasts for more than 30 minutes (11–14). In one study, the probability of MI (or unstable angina) was very low if (a) the pain was sharp or stabbing, (b) the pain was reproducible by palpation or was pleuritic or positional, and (c) the patient had no history of angina or MI.

Electrocardiography

Early ECG may show only hyperacute T waves. ST elevation of 1 mm or more in two contiguous leads is highly sensitive but also can be seen in left ventricular (LV) hypertrophy, early repolarization, and pericarditis. Confirmed, new LBBB should raise strong clinical suspicion of MI in the appropriate clinical setting (15).

With right ventricular (RV) infarction, ST elevation is seen in the V_4R lead with a sensitivity of approximately 90% and specificity of approximately 80% (192). With posterior infarction, precordial ST-segment depression is seen in leads V_1 and V_2 and/or ST elevation in leads V_7 to V_9 (16,17).

Echocardiography

Echocardiography is useful if the ECG results have been nondiagnostic and in patients with suspected aortic dissection. Areas of abnormal wall motion are typically observed in patients with AMI, especially those with transmural involvement.

Biomarkers

Creatine kinase (CK)-MB, troponin I (TnI), and troponin T (TnT) exceed normal ranges within 4 to 8 hours, and levels peak at 24 hours (CK-MB peak occurs sooner with successful thrombolysis). CK-MB levels normalize by 48 to

72 hours, whereas TnI remains elevated for up to 7 to 10 days and TnT for up to 14 days, allowing detection of MI days before but reducing their value in the diagnosis of recurrent MI within this time frame. TnI and TnT are cardiac specific, and levels strongly correlate with mortality (19–21). Serial troponin checks also contribute to risk stratification (22). Please see Chapter 3 for further discussion on the emergence of high-sensitivity troponin assays. Myoglobin peak levels are reached earlier (within 1 to 4 hours), with a rapid increase indicative of successful reperfusion (*J Am Coll Cardiol* 1999;34:739–747). Myoglobin also has an excellent negative predictive value (18) yet is much less specific for cardiac injury than troponin.

TREATMENT

Aspirin

In the second International Study of Infarct Survival (ISIS-2) (27), aspirin (162 mg chewed, to ensure rapid therapeutic blood levels) use was associated with a 23% lower mortality rate, as well as significantly fewer reinfarctions and strokes (**Table 4.1**). Aspirin and thrombolytic therapy have an additive benefit (42% lower mortality rate in ISIS-2). A large analysis by the Antithrombotic Trialists' Collaboration (ATT) found that aspirin reduces the risk of nonfatal stroke, nonfatal MI, or vascular mortality by 25% to 32% in patients at high risk of occlusive vascular events (29). The most recent ACC/AHA guidelines recommend 162 to 325 mg loading dose prior to PCI in STEMI and 81 to 325 mg

Table 4.1	Treatment of ST Elevation Myocardial Infarction		
Beneficial	**Limited Data or No Benefit**	**Special Situations**	**Harmful**
Aspirin	Nitrates	Oral anticoagulation	Nifedipine
P2Y12 inhibitors	Magnesium	Vasopressors	Other antiarrhythmics
β-Blockers	Verapamil	Diuretics	
ACE inhibitors/ ARBs	Adenosine	Insulin	
Thrombolytics		Intra-aortic balloon pump	
Primary PCI		Surgery	
GP IIb/IIIa inhibitors		Aldosterone inhibition	
Antithrombins		Amiodarone	

PCI, percutaneous coronary intervention; ACE, angiotensin-converting enzyme; ARB, angiotensin II receptor blocker; GP, glycoprotein.

daily maintenance dose indefinitely. The 81-mg dose is preferred, primarily based on data from the CURRENT-OASIS 7 trial, which found that low-dose aspirin (75 to 100 mg) was similar in efficacy to higher-dose aspirin (300 to 325 mg) but with less bleeding risk (30). If a patient has an aspirin allergy, clopidogrel (75 mg daily) can be substituted because it showed a slight benefit compared with aspirin in more than 8,000 patients with a recent MI (CAPRIE trial; see Chapter 1).

P2Y12 Inhibitors

Clopidogrel blocks platelet activation by inhibiting the ADP receptor. Its efficacy in STEMI was demonstrated in the Clopidogrel as Adjunctive Reperfusion Therapy (CLARITY)–Thrombolysis in Myocardial Infarction (TIMI) 28 study, in which 3,491 patients with STEMI were randomized to clopidogrel or placebo, in addition to fibrinolysis and contemporary therapies (32). Patients receiving clopidogrel had a significantly lower rate of the composite end point of infarct artery occlusion on angiography (within 48 to 192 hours) or death or recurrent MI before angiography (15.0% vs. 21.7%, $p < 0.001$). At 30 days, there was also a significant 20% reduction in adverse clinical events without a significant increase in bleeding events. Data from the Clopidogrel and Metoprolol in Myocardial Infarction Trial (COMMIT) confirmed these findings, with a significant reduction in total mortality seen as well, thus expanding clopidogrel's application to patients who received either fibrinolysis or no reperfusion therapy (33).

Prasugrel is a more potent P2Y12 inhibitor, which was compared with clopidogrel in the TRITON–TIMI 38 trial. This trial randomized 13,608 moderate- to high-risk ACS patients undergoing PCI to prasugrel or clopidogrel; 3,534 patients had STEMI (34; see also Chapter 3). The primary end point of CV death, nonfatal MI, or nonfatal stroke occurred less frequently in the prasugrel arm at 30 days and at 15-month follow-up [10 vs. 12.4%; HR, 0.79 (95% CI, 0.65 to 0.97); $p = 0.02$] as well as less definite or probable stent thrombosis. However, it should be noted that a loading dose of 300 mg of clopidogrel was used rather than 600 mg, which is the current recommended loading dose. In the overall trial, bleeding was more common in the prasugrel arm. However, in the subgroup of STEMI patients, bleeding rates were similar between the two groups except for patients undergoing CABG.

Ticagrelor is a reversible P2Y12 inhibitor, which also has been shown to be beneficial in ACS patients, including patients with STEMI undergoing primary PCI. It was primarily studied in the PLATO trial (see Chapter 3), in which 35% of the 18,624 patients with ACS presented with STEMI. The primary end point of MI, stroke, or CV death occurred less frequently in the ticagrelor arm, but there was no significant difference in bleeding. All-cause mortality, definite stent thrombosis, and MI were also significantly less frequent in the ticagrelor arm.

The 2013 ACC/AHA STEMI Guidelines recommend a loading dose of any of the three approved P2Y12 inhibitors (all class I) as early as possible in patients presenting with STEMI, then continued for 1 year in patients who receive a stent [BMS (bare metal stent) or drug-eluting stent (DES)]. Given the increased bleeding risk, prasugrel received a class III recommendation (harm) in patients with a prior stroke or transient ischemic attack (TIA).

Cangrelor is an ADP receptor antagonist that is administered intravenously. The potential benefit of this agent was studied in the CHAMPION trials, most recently the CHAMPION-PHOENIX trial (35). This large trial randomized 11,145 patients undergoing urgent or elective PCI to cangrelor versus clopidogrel (300 or 600 mg). Cangrelor significantly reduced the number of ischemic events [OR 0.78 (95% CI, 0.66 to 0.93) p = 0.005] with no significant increase in severe bleeding. It is not currently approved in the United States, however.

β-Blockers

Early randomized trials showed mortality benefits with timolol, propranolol, and metoprolol (36,37,42). In the large ISIS-1 trial (39), use of atenolol was associated with a 15% mortality benefit. In the TIMI IIB trial (40), immediate initiation of β-blockade was shown to be superior to delayed initiation (at 6 to 8 days). A meta-analysis of randomized trials (most completed before the widespread use of thrombolysis and aspirin) showed a 13% mortality reduction with early initiation of a β-blocker agent. However, even delayed therapy provides substantial benefit, as shown in the early placebo-controlled trials (36,37). β-Blockade also was associated with a decreased incidence of cardiac rupture and ventricular fibrillation (VF) (43). One analysis showed that the benefits of β-blockade are independent of thrombolytic and angiotensin-converting enzyme (ACE) inhibitor use.

However, in the largest trial of early β-blockade in acute MI, the COMMIT trial enrolled 45,852 patients within 24 hours of suspected acute MI and randomized to early metoprolol (intravenously then oral) or placebo (there was also an antiplatelet agent randomization in the trial, as discussed elsewhere). β-Blockade did not reduce the incidence of the primary end point, a composite of death, reinfarction, or cardiac arrest; however, it did reduce the rates of reinfarction and VF at the expense of increased risk of cardiogenic shock. The trial underscored the need for attentive hemodynamic evaluation and monitoring prior to the use of β-blockade in patients with acute MI, and this impact was highlighted in the most recent guidelines (44). The 2013 ACC/AHA STEMI Guidelines state, "It is reasonable to administer IV β-blockers at the time of presentation to patients with STEMI and no contraindications to their use who are hypertensive or have ongoing ischemia" (class IIa).

The METOCARD-CNIC trial supports the use of IV β-blockers prior to reperfusion in certain patients presenting with STEMI without contraindications to β-blockers (45). This trial randomized 270 patients with anterior STEMI and a planned early reperfusion strategy to IV metoprolol versus control. The results suggest that patients who present with STEMI and Killip class <III may have a significantly smaller infarct size (p = 0.012) if treated with IV metoprolol prior to reperfusion.

Metoprolol was the agent used in the COMMIT and METOCARD-CNIC trials. Carvedilol, which is both a β and an α antagonist, has also shown significant promise in AMI patients and is now indicated for use in post-MI patients with LV dysfunction. In the CAPRICORN trial (41), which enrolled 1,959 patients with an ejection fraction (EF) of 40% or less, long-term use of carvedilol was associated with a 23% relative reduction in all-cause mortality compared with placebo. These beneficial effects are additive to those provided by ACE inhibitors.

Contraindications to the use of β-blockers include signs of HF, evidence of a low output state, increased risk for cardiogenic shock, or other contraindications to use of β-blockers (PR interval more than 0.24 seconds, second- or third-degree heart block, active asthma, or reactive airway disease).

Angiotensin-converting Enzyme Inhibitors

Early initiation of ACE inhibition was found to decrease mortality in two large placebo-controlled trials. In Gruppo Italiano per lo Studio della Sopravvivenza nell' Infarto Miocardico (GISSI-3) (52), use of lisinopril was associated with a 12% mortality reduction, whereas in ISIS-4 (53), use of captopril was associated with a 7% mortality reduction (greatest benefit in those with anterior MI). Among patients with LV dysfunction, mortality was reduced by approximately 20% to 30% by oral ACE inhibition [Survival and Ventricular Enlargement (SAVE), Acute Infarction Ramipril Efficacy (AIRE), and Trandolapril Cardiac Evaluation (TRACE) trials (49,51)]. Intravenous administration was used in the Cooperative New Scandinavian Enalapril Survival Study (CONSENSUS II) and was deemed harmful (50). A meta-analysis of 15 trials with more than 100,000 patients showed a 7% relative risk reduction (RRR), with the majority of benefit seen in anterior MIs (1.2% absolute mortality benefit vs. 0.1% for inferior MIs) (48). Approximately one-third of the benefit of ACE inhibition is seen in the first few days after MI. Based on these data, current class I indications are as follows: (a) within 24 hours with anterior ST elevation or evidence of congestive heart failure (CHF) and (b) left ventricular ejection fraction (LVEF) <40% or evidence of CHF during or after recovery.

Results from trials of angiotensin II receptor blockers (ARBs) confirm that ACE inhibitors should remain first-line therapy in high-risk AMI patients. For example, in the OPTIMAAL study (54), losartan was compared with captopril in 5,477 MI patients within 10 days of presentation, and a nonsignificant trend toward an increased incidence of mortality was found with losartan (18.2% vs. 16.4%, $p = 0.069$). In patients who cannot tolerate ACE inhibitors, ARBs appear beneficial. The large VALIANT study evaluated valsartan compared with or in addition to captopril in 14,703 post-MI patients complicated by heart failure and/or LV dysfunction. There was no difference among all three groups (valsartan alone, captopril alone, or valsartan and captopril) in the primary end point of death from any cause at median follow-up of 2 years. The combination of valsartan and captopril did increase the rates of adverse events (55). This finding, combined with other trials showing parity of ARB with ACE inhibitors, has led the 2009 ACC/AHA STEMI guideline–focused update to add ARB as an equally suitable choice as ACE inhibitor for STEMI patients (3).

Aldosterone Antagonism

Based on the results of the Eplerenone Post-Acute Myocardial Infarction Heart Failure Efficacy and Survival Study (EPHESUS, see Chapter 5), aldosterone antagonists are now a class I indication in STEMI patients already receiving an ACE inhibitor and a β-blocker with an EF $\leq$40% and either symptomatic heart failure or diabetes. Post hoc analysis of this trial suggests that starting eplerenone within the first 7 days of the MI had the greatest impact on all-cause mortality, sudden cardiac death, and cardiovascular mortality/hospitalization.

Thrombolytic Therapy

Thrombolytic therapy confers a 20% to 25% mortality benefit in patients with STEMI. Time to treatment is important: a 6.5% absolute mortality benefit if given in the first hour versus 2% to 3% if given after 1 to 6 hours (**Fig. 4.1**) (57). No benefit results if thrombolytic therapy is given after 12 hours (77). The largest absolute benefit is seen in those with anterior MI and in patients presenting with LBBB as manifestation of AMI (**Fig.4.2**). Combination

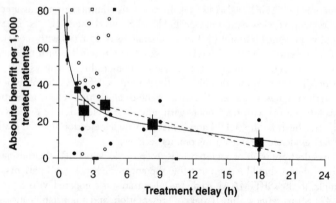

Figure 4.1 • Absolute 35-day mortality reduction versus treatment delay. ●, Information from trials included in FTT analysis, which found a linear relation between treatment delay and absolute mortality benefit (*dotted line*); ○, information from additional trials; □, data beyond scale of *x/y* cross; ■, average effects in six time-to-treatment groups. (Areas of squares are inversely proportional to variance of absolute benefit described.) The analysis by Boersma et al. of randomized trials with 100 or more patients (50,246 patients) yielded a nonlinear regression curve (*solid line*), suggesting greatest benefit with time saved early after symptom onset (Reprinted from Boersma E, et al. Early thrombolytic treatment in acute myocardial infarction: reappraisal of the golden hour. *Lancet* 1996;348(9030):771–775).

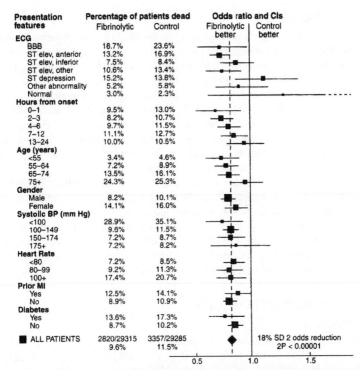

Presentation features	Percentage of patients dead		Odds ratio and CIs	
	Fibrinolytic	Control	Fibrinolytic better	Control better
ECG				
BBB	18.7%	23.6%		
ST elev, anterior	13.2%	16.9%		
ST elev, inferior	7.5%	8.4%		
ST elev, other	10.6%	13.4%		
ST depression	15.2%	13.8%		
Other abnormality	5.2%	5.8%		
Normal	3.0%	2.3%		
Hours from onset				
0–1	9.5%	13.0%		
2–3	8.2%	10.7%		
4–6	9.7%	11.5%		
7–12	11.1%	12.7%		
13–24	10.0%	10.5%		
Age (years)				
<55	3.4%	4.6%		
55–64	7.2%	8.9%		
65–74	13.5%	16.1%		
75+	24.3%	25.3%		
Gender				
Male	8.2%	10.1%		
Female	14.1%	16.0%		
Systolic BP (mm Hg)				
<100	28.9%	35.1%		
100–149	9.6%	11.5%		
150–174	7.2%	8.7%		
175+	7.2%	8.2%		
Heart Rate				
<80	7.2%	8.5%		
80–99	9.2%	11.3%		
100+	17.4%	20.7%		
Prior MI				
Yes	12.5%	14.1%		
No	8.9%	10.9%		
Diabetes				
Yes	13.6%	17.3%		
No	8.7%	10.2%		
ALL PATIENTS	2820/29315	3357/29285		18% SD 2 odds reduction
	9.6%	11.5%		2P < 0.00001

0.5   1.0   1.5

Figure 4.2 • Mortality differences during days 0 to 35 subdivided by presentation features in a collaborative overview of nine thrombolytic trials. Absolute mortality rates are shown for the fibrinolytic and control groups in the center portion of the figure for each of the clinical features at presentation listed on the left side of the figure. The ratio of the odds of death in the fibrinolytic group to that in the control group is shown for each subdivision (■), along with its 99% confidence interval (*horizontal line*). The summary OR at the bottom of the figure corresponds to an 18% proportional reduction in 35-day mortality and is highly statistically significant. The absolute reduction is nine deaths per 1,000 patients treated with thrombolytic agents (Reprinted from Fibrinolytic Therapy Trialists' (FTT) Collaborative Group. Indications for fibrinolytic therapy in suspected acute myocardial infarction: collaborative overview of early mortality and major morbidity results from all randomised trials of more than 1000 patients. *Lancet* 1994;343(8893):311).

regimens including reduced-dose thrombolytics have also been tested but are generally not recommended (see below, "Intravenous Glycoprotein IIb/IIIa Inhibitors")

INDICATIONS FOR THROMBOLYSIS

It is a class I indication to administer fibrinolytic therapy to patients with STEMI and onset of symptoms within 12 hours if it is anticipated that primary PCI cannot be performed within 120 minutes of first medical contact.

CONTRAINDICATIONS

Contraindications include substantial active bleeding (excluding menses), aortic dissection (known or suspected), intracranial neoplasm/aneurysm/arteriovenous malformation, significant head/facial trauma within 3 months, intracranial or intraspinal surgery in the prior 2 months, severe uncontrolled hypertension, any prior hemorrhagic stroke, or any stroke within the prior 3 months.

Relative contraindications include nonhemorrhagic stroke more than 3 months earlier, active peptic ulcer disease, oral anticoagulant use, pregnancy, prolonged (>10 min) cardiopulmonary resuscitation (CPR), SBP ≥180 mm Hg or diastolic BP ≥110 mm Hg, dementia, major surgery <3 weeks, noncompressible vascular punctures, and internal bleeding within 2 to 4 weeks.

Advanced age is not a contraindication (class IIa if older than 75 years). These patients have increased complications (especially intracranial hemorrhage) but a substantial absolute mortality reduction.

Prehospital administration has been shown to confer a benefit in several trials (76,78). A systematic overview showed a significant 17% mortality reduction. The magnitude of benefit correlates with time saved; in the ER-TIMI 19 trial, the median time saved was 32 minutes (80).

COMMON FIBRINOLYTIC AGENTS

Streptokinase

Intravenously, streptokinase (SK) regimens proved superior to placebo in the trial of the GISSI-1 (18% lower mortality) (73) and ISIS-2 (25% lower mortality) (**Table 4.2**) (74). SK was comparable with tissue plasminogen activator (tPA) in GISSI-2 and ISIS-3 (62,63) but was inferior to it in the Global Utilization of Strategies to Open Occluded Arteries (GUSTO-I) study (see the section "Tissue Plasminogen Activator") (64). This agent is routinely used in certain parts of the world because of its lower cost; however, it is a less specific thrombolytic agent (not fibrinolytic).

Tissue Plasminogen Activator

A clear mortality benefit with tPA compared with placebo was shown in the Anglo-Scandinavian Study of Early Thrombolysis (ASSET) (75). When compared with SK in the large GISSI-2 and ISIS-3 trials, mortality rates were similar. However, the front-loaded tPA regimen was not used, and tPA was given without heparin or with subcutaneous (s.c.) heparin. The now standard front-loaded regimen (15-mg bolus, then 50 mg over a 30-minute period, and 35 mg over the final 60 minutes) was shown to achieve earlier patency with better TIMI grade 3 flow at 60 and 90 minutes. This also was demonstrated in TIMI-4 (66) and the GUSTO angiography substudy (65).

In the GUSTO-I trial (64), the tPA and intravenous heparin group had the best outcome: 6.3% 30-day mortality versus 7.2% and 7.4% in the SK groups (p < 0.001). The greatest benefit was seen in those patients with large anterior MIs.

Table 4.2	Characteristics of Commonly Used Fibrinolytic Agents				
Agent	**Dosage**	**90-Minute TIMI Grade 3 Flow**	**Heparin**	**Allergy**	**Cost**
SK	1.5 million U over 60 min	30%–35%	No	Yes	Low
tPA	15-mg bolus, 0.75 mg/kg over 30 min, and then 0.5 mg/kg over 60 min (maximum, 100 mg)	54%–60%	Yes	No	High
TNK	Bolus over 5–10 min (30 mg if <60 kg, 35 mg if 60–69 kg, 40 mg if 70–79 kg, 45 mg if 80–89 kg, 50 mg if ≥90 kg)	~60%	Yes	No	High
rPA	10 + 10 U given 30 min apart	~60%	Yes	No	High

TIMI, Thrombolysis in Myocardial Infarction; tPA, tissue plasminogen activator; TNK, tenecteplase; rPA, reteplase (from Refs. **Gruppo Italiano per lo Studio della Streptochinasi nell'Infarto Miocardico (GISSI-2)**. GISSI-2: a factorial randomised trial of alteplase vs. streptokinase and heparin vs. no heparin among 12,490 patients with acute MI. *Lancet* 1990;336:65–71; **ISIS-3 Collaborative Group**. A randomised comparison of streptokinase versus tissue plasminogen activator versus anistreplase and of aspirin and heparin versus aspirin alone among 41,299 cases of suspected acute MI. *Lancet* 1992;339:753–770; **Cannon CP, et al.; TIMI-4.** Comparison of front-loaded recombinant tissue plasminogen activator, anistreplase and combination thrombolytic therapy for acute MI. *J Am Coll Cardiol* 1994;24:1602–1610.)

Reteplase

A double-bolus regimen of reteplase (rPA) was approved for use by the U.S. Food and Drug Administration (FDA) based on demonstrated equivalence to SK in the International Joint Efficacy Comparison of Thrombolytics (INJECT) trial (67). In the RAPID II angiographic trial (68), rPA showed better TIMI grade 3 flow at 90 minutes compared with front-loaded tPA (60% vs. 45%, $p = 0.01$); however, mortality was similar to that with tPA in the large GUSTO-III study (69).

Tenecteplase

Tenecteplase (TNK) is a single-bolus thrombolytic that achieves TIMI grade 3 flow similar to or slightly higher than that of tPA alone. The Assessment of the Safety and Efficacy of a New Thrombolytic: TNK (ASSENT-2) trial enrolled 16,949 patients and showed TNK to be statistically equivalent to tPA alone (30-day mortality rates, 6.17% and 6.15%) (71). A potential benefit of TNK is ease of administration (single bolus). [In GUSTO-I, incorrect dosing of tPA was associated with higher mortality (7.7% vs. 5.5% for correct dosing, $p < 0.0001$).] Intracranial hemorrhage rates were similar, whereas noncerebral bleeding occurred less frequently with TNK (26.4% vs. 29.0%).

PROGNOSTIC INDICATORS

1. Early infarct-related artery (IRA) patency. Ninety-minute patency (TIMI grade 2 or 3 flow) correlates strongly with outcome: greater than twofold higher 1-year mortality rate in those with persistent occlusion at 90 minutes in TIMI 1 and similar findings in subsequent studies (233). Subsequent analyses showed TIMI grade 3 flow to be associated with significantly better outcomes than TIMI grade 2 flow (233,234,236). The corrected TIMI frame count (CTFC), which treats flow as a continuous variable, appears to provide an even more accurate prognostic assessment (237).

2. Microvascular reperfusion. The TIMI myocardial perfusion (TMP) grade classification is as follows: TMP grade (TMPG) 1 indicates presence of myocardial blush but no clearance from the microvasculature (blush or a stain was present on the next injection); TMPG 2 blush clears slowly (blush is strongly persistent and diminishes minimally or not at all during three cardiac cycles of the washout phase); and TMPG 3 indicates that blush begins to clear during washout (blush is minimally persistent after three cardiac cycles of washout). Analyses of angiographic cine films from the TIMI 10B (thrombolysis) (238) and ESPRIT trials (PCI trial, see Chapter 2) demonstrate that a TMPG 0/1 is associated with frequent adverse outcomes even in patients with optimal epicardial flow (TIMI grade 3), whereas the lowest mortality is seen in patients with both TMPG 3 and TIMI 3 flow. In a multivariate model, TIMI flow, TMPG, and TIMI frame count were all predictors of mortality (239).

3. Time to treatment. Lower mortality is achieved with early administration of thrombolytic agents, especially within the first "golden" hour (40). The latest guidelines recommend that when chosen as the primary reperfusion strategy, fibrinolytics should be administered within 30 minutes of hospital arrival.

4. Reocclusion. A 4% to 10% incidence is observed at 2 to 4 weeks. Although approximately 50% of cases are not accompanied by clinical reinfarction or ischemia (i.e., silent), reocclusion is associated with a more than twofold higher mortality rate (261). Revascularization appears to be helpful in these cases.

5. Reinfarction is associated with a two- to threefold higher mortality rate.

Percutaneous Coronary Intervention

PRIMARY ANGIOPLASTY

The 2013 updated AHA/ACC class I indications for primary PCI are as follows: (a) within 12 hours or after 12 hours if ischemic symptoms persist and (b) in patients with STEMI and cardiogenic shock or acute severe heart failure irrespective of the time delay from MI onset (see the section "Cardiogenic Shock") (**Fig. 4.3**).

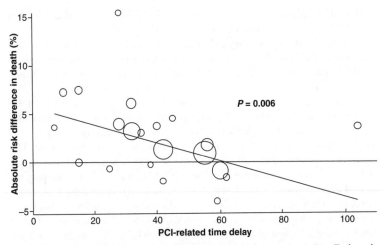

Figure 4.3 • Relationship between timing of PCI and absolute mortality. Each circle represents a study of varying size, with a weighted meta-regression (*solid line*) demonstrating higher absolute risk reduction in all-cause mortality with lower PCI-related time delay. It is based on these data, in part, that door-to-balloon timing benchmarks were established (From Nallamothu BK, Bates ER. Percutaneous coronary intervention versus fibrinolytic therapy in acute myocardial infarction: is timing (almost) everything? *Am J Cardiol* 2003;92:824–826).

Procedural Volume

Substantial data on operator and hospital volume have now been accumulated. Primary PCI performed in high-volume hospitals (57 or more cases/year) was associated with a 44% lower in-hospital mortality reduction compared with that in low-volume hospitals. As for hospital volume, one large analysis of 62,299 patients found that primary PCI was superior to thrombolytic therapy for treatment of acute STEMI at hospitals with intermediate (17 to 48 procedures/year) and high volume (>49 per year), whereas no significant mortality difference was found between the treatments at low-volume hospitals (112). Another analysis of 98,898 Medicare patients found that those admitted to hospitals in the lowest quartile of volume of invasive procedures had a 17% higher in-hospital mortality rate compared with patients at highest-volume-quartile hospitals [hazard ratio, 1.17; 95% confidence interval (CI), 1.09 to 1.26; $p < 0.001$] (111).

Primary Angioplasty versus Thrombolysis

PCI had a lower associated mortality rate in the Primary Angioplasty in MI (PAMI) trial (2.6% vs. 6.5%) (112), and a nonsignificant trend toward lower mortality was observed in the larger GUSTO-IIb trial (90). However, no mortality difference was found in a subsequent study of 19 Seattle hospitals (89).

A meta-analysis of 10 trials through 1997 showed a significant mortality benefit of primary angioplasty compared with thrombolysis: odds ratio (OR), 0.66 (95% CI, 0.46 to 0.94) (83). An updated meta-analysis of 23 studies published in 2003 confirmed that primary PCI had lower short-term mortality than did thrombolytic therapy (7% vs. 9%) (84).

More recent studies compared primary PCI with thrombolysis, including two that included facilities without PCI capability (i.e., transfer required for the PCI group). In the second Danish Trial in Acute MI (DANAMI-2), primary PCI was associated with a 45% lower incidence of death, reinfarction, or disabling stroke, primarily because of less reinfarction [1.6% vs. 6.3% (tPA)] (93). In PRAGUE-2, primary PCI was associated with a nonsignificant mortality reduction compared with SK (6.8% vs. 10%); however, a significant mortality reduction was seen in those seen at 3 to 12 hours (6% vs. 15.3%) (94). The rapid transfer and door-to-balloon times in these two trials are likely not typical of the usual community setting. In the Air PAMI study, all enrolled patients arrived in hospitals without on-site PCI; despite long transfer delays, the emergency transfer for the primary PCI group had a nonsignificant 38% reduction in major events compared with on-site thrombolysis (91). Finally, in the Atlantic Cardiovascular Patient Outcomes Research Team (C-PORT) study, sites without preexisting primary PCI programs had one installed (without on-site surgery) and involved high-volume, experienced operators and catheterization teams. The primary PCI group had significantly lower incidence of death, recurrent MI, or disabling stroke compared with those given tPA (92).

In summary, primary PCI is superior to thrombolysis for STEMI when performed at experienced centers that can achieve a short door-to-balloon time.

Rescue Angioplasty

Rescue angioplasty has been defined as PCI carried out very early (1 to 2 hours) after failed thrombolytic therapy—that is, in patients who have evidence of not achieving reperfusion of the IRA usually diagnosed by persistent ST elevation and chest pain. Several trials have shown that rescue PCI is superior to conservative therapy or repeat thrombolysis (87,109,110). The ACC/AHA 2013 guidelines give a class IIa recommendation (level of evidence B) for a strategy of coronary angiography with intent to perform rescue PCI as reasonable for patients in whom fibrinolytic therapy has failed.

Routine PCI (After Thrombolysis) Versus Delayed or Conservative Management

A significant evolution of interventional approaches has led to changes in recommendations for early PCI following fibrinolysis. Early trials performed in the mid-1980s showed immediate PCI to be associated with increased bleeding and an overall trend toward increased mortality [Thrombolysis and Angioplasty in MI (TAMI), TIMI-2A, and European Cooperative Study Group (ECSG-4)] (95,96). In addition, routine *delayed* angioplasty following fibrinolysis was not seen to improve mortality or reinfarction rates in older studies [TIMI IIB and the Should We Intervene Following Thrombolysis (SWIFT) study] (40,98).

However, given the advances in interventional approaches and antithrombotic therapy, the approach was revisited. Observational data from recent trials suggested a potential benefit of early PCI (106). Now several randomized trials have shown benefit of early PCI. The GRACIA trial compared routine angiography within 24 hours of thrombolysis with an ischemia-guided approach (105) and showed that the routine invasive group had a significantly lower incidence of death, reinfarction or revascularization (0.8% vs. 3.7%, p = 0.003). The CARESS-in-AMI trial also found benefit of early transfer in high-risk STEMI patients (103), as did the Trial of Routine Angioplasty and Stenting after Fibrinolysis to Enhance Reperfusion in Acute Myocardial Infarction (TRANSFER-AMI, 107). Approximately 1,000 patients with STEMI who received fibrinolytic therapy and were then transferred for PCI within 6 hours had a significant reduction in the composite end point of death, reinfarction, recurrent ischemia, new/worsening CHF, or cardiogenic shock at 30 days, when compared to patients who received fibrinolytic therapy alone (11.0% vs. 17.2%; relative risk (RR) 0.64; p = 0.0004) (107). No mortality benefit was seen, but a reduction in recurrent MI and ischemia was seen. The Norwegian Study on District Treatment of ST-Elevation Myocardial Infarction (NORDISTEMI) had similar results to the TRANSFER-AMI trial. This study randomized 266 patients with STEMI treated with fibrinolytics to immediate transfer for angiography/PCI versus transfer only for a rescue indication or for deteriorating clinical status. There was no significant difference in the composite primary end point of death/reinfarct/stroke/new ischemia between the two groups [27.3% in the conservative arm versus 20.9% in the early invasive arm, HR, 0.72 (95% CI, 0.44 to 1.18), p = 0.18]; however, there was a significant decrease in death/reinfarct/stroke in the early invasive arm [15.9% vs. 6.0%, HR, 0.36 (95% CI, 0.16 to 0.81), p = 0.01] (108). It is a class IIa (B) recommendation in the 2013 guidelines to routinely transfer patients to a PCI-capable facility for PCI 3 to 24 hours after fibrinolysis. Due to increased bleeding risk, catheterization within 3 hours of fibrinolysis should be reserved for patients with failed fibrinolysis and significant myocardial jeopardy.

FACILITATED PERCUTANEOUS CORONARY INTERVENTION

Given the benefit of primary PCI, the concept of combining fibrinolysis and immediate PCI was pursued as a way to achieve earlier reperfusion but retain the benefits of primary PCI. Following small observational analyses, several randomized trials were conducted comparing facilitated PCI to primary PCI. (The section above showed that early PCI following fibrinolysis was superior to fibrinolysis.)

In 2006, the Assessment of the Safety and Efficacy of a New Treatment Strategy with Percutaneous Coronary Intervention (ASSENT-4 PCI) trial patients were randomized to receive TNK and immediate PCI (approximately 1 hour) versus primary PCI. Despite a planned enrollment of 4,000 patients for the primary end point of death, CHF, or shock within 90 days, the trial was stopped early due to a higher in-hospital mortality in the facilitated PCI group (6% vs. 3%, p = 0.0105) (101). A meta-analysis published simultaneously, and including this trial, combined 17 trials and 4,504 patients and concluded that there was no benefit to facilitated PCI compared with primary PCI, and that such regimens including full-dose thrombolytics should not be used (86).

However, additional data on alternative regimens for facilitated PCI came from the Facilitated Intervention with Enhanced Reperfusion Speed to Stop Events (FINESSE) study, randomizing patients with STEMI to primary PCI versus PCI facilitated with either abciximab only or abciximab in combination with half-dose reteplase. Neither of the comparator regimens demonstrated any improvement in rates of the primary outcome, a composite of death, VF (>48 hours from randomization), cardiogenic shock, or CHF within 90 days (9.8% vs. 10.5% vs. 10.7% in the combination-facilitated, PCI group, abciximab-facilitated group, and primary PCI group, respectively, $p = 0.55$) (see also *Eur Heart J* 2007;28:1545–1553) (102). As such, the current guidelines recommend against the use of a strategy of routine immediate PCI following lysis (<2 to 3 hours).

Cardiogenic Shock

The Should We Emergently Revascularize Occluded Coronaries for Cardiogenic Shock (SHOCK) trial found that emergency revascularization (ERV; balloon angioplasty or bypass surgery) did not result in improved 30-day survival (primary end point) compared with aggressive medical management [e.g., thrombolysis, intra-aortic balloon pump (IABP)] (198). However, at 6 months, mortality was lower with ERV (50.3% vs. 63.1%, $p = 0.027$). Among patients younger than 75 years, ERV was significantly better than medical therapy (30-day mortality, 41% vs. 57%, $p < 0.01$; 6 months, 48% vs. 69%, $p < 0.01$). In the nonrandomized SHOCK Registry, however, elderly patients had a substantial survival benefit as well. Based on these results, the 2013 ACC/AHA guidelines consider primary PCI (or CABG) a class I indication in suitable patients with cardiogenic shock due to pump failure (rather than a mechanical complication) after STEMI, irrespective of the time delay from MI onset.

Stenting in STEMI

Before the identification of an effective antiplatelet regimen to prevent stent thrombosis, stent use was typically avoided in the patients with AMI. However, several studies then showed that stenting in AMI was safe and efficacious (114,115). The STAT and STOPAMI-2 trials demonstrated superior outcomes with stenting compared with fibrinolytic therapy (117,118). The larger Stent PAMI study compared primary PTCA (percutaneous transluminal coronary angioplasty) alone with heparin-coated Palmaz–Schatz stenting in 900 patients (116). At 6 months, stenting was associated with a significant reduction in the 6-month composite primary end point (12.6% vs. 20.1%, $p < 0.01$), primarily because of a lower rate of ischemia-driven target vessel revascularization (TVR; 7.7% vs. 17%; $p < 0.001$). The Controlled Abciximab and Device Investigation to Lower Late Angioplasty Complications (CADILLAC) trial enrolled 2,082 patients and compared PTCA alone, PTCA plus abciximab, stenting alone, and stenting plus abciximab in 2,082 patients (152). At 6 months, the stent groups had a lower incidence of death, reinfarction, disabling stroke, and ischemia-driven TVR [11.5% (stent alone) and

10.2% vs. 20% (PTCA alone) and 16.5% (PTCA plus abciximab)]. As in Stent PAMI, the benefit was owing to a lower TVR rate benefit, whereas no difference in mortality rates was found. These lower TVR rates are the result of the lower restenosis rates seen with PTCA compared with angioplasty alone.

The 2003 meta-analysis of 23 intervention trials (a minority of the trials did not use stents) identified a significant, absolute 2% reduction in short-term death for patients receiving primary PCI (7% vs. 9%, p = 0.0002) (84). Subsequent analysis of data from the National Registry of Myocardial Infarction (NRMI) demonstrated significantly improved outcomes in patients treated at hospitals with greater specialization of primary PCI. In summary, these data demonstrate that in experienced centers, stent implantation should be considered the preferred reperfusion strategy (81).

The release in 2004 of the first DES saw a significant increase in their use for STEMI, despite an indication limited to elective, nonurgent PCI (see Chapter 2). Thus, while multiple retrospective and observational studies of off-label DES use in acute MI yielded mixed results, randomized trials demonstrated noninferior short-term outcomes with DES and potentially fewer repeat procedures over the long term (121,122). The 2013 Updated ACC/AHA guidelines give a class I indication to placement of a DES or BMS during primary PCI. The guidelines do specify, however, that BMS should be used in patients with high bleeding risk, anticipated invasive procedures in the next 12 months, or inability to adhere to a 12-month course of dual antiplatelet therapy (DAPT). In fact, DES is given a class III indication (harm) in patients who cannot comply with DAPT for 12 months. The guidelines suggest, however, that DES is the preferred stent in STEMIs due to lower restenosis rates compared with BMS.

Antithrombotic Regimens

HEPARIN

Intravenous heparin should be used in conjunction with tPA, or rPA or TNK [GUSTO data show the optimal partial thromboplastin time (PTT) range to be 50 to 70 seconds]. Heparin is also optimal if the patient is not receiving a thrombolytic agent. A meta-analysis of prethrombolytic trials showed an approximately 20% mortality benefit (*N Engl J Med* 1992;327:248–254). Another meta-analysis of trials comprising approximately 70,000 patients showed borderline benefit when used with thrombolytics (6% lower mortality, p = 0.03). Subcutaneous administration showed no benefit in reducing death or reinfarction (ISIS-3 and GISSI-2) (62,63). Heparin (with or without a GP IIb/IIIa inhibitor) is also one of the two recommended anticoagulants used during primary PCI (the other being bivalirudin; see below).

ENOXAPARIN

Low molecular weight heparins have now been evaluated in several studies and appear safe and efficacious in the acute STEMI setting. In the Assessment of the Safety and Efficacy of a New Thrombolytic Regimen (ASSENT)-3 trial, those treated with enoxaparin and TNK had significantly fewer major events compared with the unfractionated heparin (UFH) and TNK group (11.4% vs. 15.4%, $p < 0.001$); bleeding events were similar in both groups. In the smaller ENTIRE-TIMI 23 trial, TIMI grade 3 flow rates were similar between enoxaparin- and UFH-treated patients (128). However, among patients receiving full-dose TNK, the enoxaparin group had a lower incidence of death or recurrent MI at 30 days (4.4% vs. 15.9%, $p = 0.005$). The Enoxaparin and Thrombolysis Reperfusion for Acute Myocardial Infarction Treatment (ExTRACT)–TIMI 25 study compared enoxaparin to UFH in 25,056 patients with STEMI who received thrombolytics. There was a significant, absolute 2.1% reduction in the primary end point of death or nonfatal, recurrent MI at 30 days (12.0% vs. 9.9%, $p < 0.001$) (129).

In the Acute Myocardial Infarction Treated with Primary Angioplasty an Intravenous Enoxaparin or Unfractionated Heparin to Lower Ischemic and Bleeding Events at Short- and Long-Term Follow-Up (ATOLL) trial, 910 STEMI patients undergoing primary PCI were randomized to enoxaparin versus heparin as the anticoagulant during primary PCI. There was no statistically significant difference in the primary composite end point of death/MI complications/procedural failure/major bleeding between the two groups [34% in the UFH group vs. 28% in the enoxaparin group; RR, 0.83 (95% CI, 0.68 to 1.01); $p = 0.06$], though there was a trend toward benefit with enoxaparin (132).

FONDAPARINUX

Fondaparinux is a synthetic pentasaccharide antithrombin, which selectively inhibits factor Xa. The Organization for the Assessment of Strategies for Ischemic Syndromes (OASIS) 6 trial randomized 12,092 patients with STEMI to either fondaparinux or control (either placebo or UFH depending on whether UFH was contraindicated). At 30 days, the composite primary end point of death or reinfarction was significantly reduced in the fondaparinux group (11.2% vs. 9.7%, $p = 0.008$), a finding that later was isolated to only those patients who did not undergo PCI. Patients who received PCI derived no benefit from fondaparinux. Based on these studies, use of fondaparinux is an acceptable class IIa recommended alternative for patients with STEMI not receiving reperfusion therapy. However, currently, this is an off-label use in the United States; the drug's Canadian label does provide an indication for STEMI, as well as UA/NSTEMI.

DIRECT THROMBIN INHIBITORS

Trials using hirudin showed no significant advantage over heparin (134). In the Hirulog Early Perfusion/Occlusion (HERO) trial (135), hirulog showed better TIMI grade 3 flow compared with SK. In the larger HERO-2 trial (17,073 patients), bivalirudin was compared with UFH in patients receiving SK (136). No mortality difference occurred between the two groups. The bivalirudin group had a 30% reduction in the reinfarction rate, but it also was associated with an increased bleeding rate. In the Harmonizing Outcomes with Revascularization

and Stents in Acute Myocardial Infarction (HORIZONS-AMI) trial, bivalirudin, as compared with heparin plus glycoprotein IIb/IIIA inhibitors, reduced net
clinical events at 30 days, including major bleeding and ischemic cardiovascular
events (139).

The European Ambulance Acute Coronary Syndrome Angiography
(EUROMAX) trial compared bivalirudin to UFH or enoxaparin +/− provisional
GP IIb/IIIa inhibitors in 2,218 STEMI patients transported for primary PCI.
The results suggest that bivalirudin is superior to the heparin-based strategy with
a significantly better 30-day risk of death or major bleeding (140). The most
recent guidelines give bivalirudin a class I recommendation for anticoagulation
in primary PCI. However, data from the How Effective are Antithrombotic
Therapies in Primary PCI (HEAT-PPCI) trial found UFH to be superior to
bivalirudin in primary PCI, with significantly higher rates of MACE [RR, 1.52
(95% CI, 1.1 to 2.1); $p = 0.01$] and definite or probable stent thrombosis [RR,
3.91 (95% CI, 1.6 to 9.5); $p = 0.001$] seen in the bivalirudin group (141).

ORAL ANTICOAGULANTS

In the Aspirin/Anticoagulants Following Thrombolysis with Eminase in
Recurrent Infarction (AFTER) trial, patients treated with warfarin acutely had
similar cardiac outcomes compared with aspirin-treated patients, but warfarin
was associated with an increased incidence of bleeding (144). In the Warfarin,
Aspirin, Reinfarction Study (WARIS), a 24% lower mortality rate versus placebo was observed (15.5% vs. 20.3%, $p = 0.03$) (142). Based on these data, it
was recommended that warfarin could be used in aspirin-intolerant patients. It
also should be considered in those at high risk of LV thrombus formation (large
anterior MI, EF <20%) or with atrial fibrillation. In one analysis of 11 studies,
anticoagulation was associated with 68% lower rate of embolization (269).

Several studies examined warfarin plus aspirin with various intensities
of anticoagulation. In the large Combination Hemotherapy and Mortality
Prevention (CHAMP) study, lower-intensity anticoagulation [international
normalized ratio (INR), 1.5 to 2.5] plus aspirin had outcomes similar to
those with aspirin alone, whereas major bleeding occurred more frequently
with combination therapy (146). In the Antithrombotics in the Prevention
of Reocclusion in Coronary Thrombolysis (APRICOT)-2 trial, aspirin plus
moderate-intensity warfarin (goal INR, 2.0 to 3.0) was associated with less
reocclusion compared with aspirin alone (15% vs. 28%, $p = 0.02$), as well as
a lower incidence of death, reinfarction, or revascularization (14% vs. 34%,
$p < 0.01$) (149). No increased incidence of bleeding events was observed.
In the Antithrombotics in the Secondary Prevention of Events in Coronary
Thrombosis-2 (ASPECT-2) study, high-dose oral anticoagulation alone (target
INR, 3.0 to 4.0) and the combination of aspirin and moderate-dose anticoagulation (target INR, 2.0 to 3.0) resulted in a lower incidence of death, MI,
or stroke compared with low-dose aspirin (80 mg once daily) (147). Bleeding
rates were similar in all groups. The Warfarin, Aspirin, Reinfarction Study-2
(WARIS-2) examined high-intensity anticoagulation (INR, 2.8 to 4.2) as well

as moderate-dose anticoagulation (INR, 2.0 to 2.5) plus low-dose aspirin and low-dose aspirin alone (75 mg/day) (148). Both warfarin groups had a lower incidence of death, nonfatal MI, and stroke compared with aspirin alone. The warfarin plus aspirin group also had a significantly lower mortality than did aspirin alone (p = 0.003). However, the warfarin groups had more major bleeding, but these rates were relatively low (0.58/100 and 0.52/100 patient-years vs. 0.15/100 patient-years for aspirin).

More contemporary oral anticoagulants, such as oral factor Xa inhibitors, have been studied in patients with ACS. The results in ACS and atrial fibrillation are described in Chapters 3 and 6, respectively. In summary, no direct, oral anticoagulant is approved or guideline recommended as adjunctive therapy in patients with STEMI.

INTRAVENOUS GLYCOPROTEIN IIB/IIIA INHIBITORS

Use in Primary PCI

The ReoPro and Primary PTCA Organization and Randomized Trial (RAPPORT) showed that abciximab use in conjunction with primary PTCA resulted in a significant reduction in death, MI, and urgent revascularization at 30 days (see also EPIC and GUSTO-III subgroup analyses). The Abciximab Before Direct Angiography and Stenting in MI Regarding Acute and Long-Term Follow-Up (ADMIRAL) trial showed that abciximab use in conjunction with stenting resulted in a nearly 50% reduction in the incidence of death, MI, and urgent revascularization (151). The larger CADILLAC trial compared PTCA alone, PTCA plus abciximab, stenting alone, or stenting plus abciximab (152). At 6 months, death, reinfarction, disabling stroke, and ischemia-driven TVR occurred in 20.0% of the PTCA-alone group, 16.5% with PTCA plus abciximab, 11.5% with stenting, and 10.2% with stenting plus abciximab (p < 0.001). The differences in the incidence of this composite end point were primarily owing to varying TVR rates (15.7% with PTCA alone, 13.8% with PTCA 1 abciximab, 8.3% with stenting, and only 5.2% with stenting 1 abciximab; p < 0.001).

A 2007 meta-analysis of the ISAR-2, ADMIRAL, and ACE studies combined 1,101 patients with STEMI undergoing primary PCI and randomized to abciximab or placebo, for a primary end point of death or reinfarction at 3 years of follow-up (153). The abciximab group had a significantly lower event rate at 3 years (12.9% vs. 19.0%, p = 0.008), without significant increase in bleeding.

However, data comparing abciximab (a monoclonal antibody) to small-molecule IIb/IIIa inhibitors have been less definitive. Several studies comparing these agents have failed to demonstrate a significant difference in outcomes (154–156). Subsequent meta-analyses have also failed to demonstrated significant differences among them. Thus, the newest guidelines give the use of any IIb/IIIa inhibitor in certain settings of STEMI a class IIa recommendation, with a level of evidence of "A" for abciximab and "B" for both tirofiban and eptifibatide.

Glycoprotein IIb/IIIa Inhibition Plus Reduced-Dose Thrombolysis

Reduced-dose thrombolysis in conjunction with i.v. glycoprotein IIb/IIIa administration has been intensely evaluated. TIMI-14 found that a combination of abciximab and tPA (15-mg bolus and then 35 mg over a 60-minute period) resulted in better TIMI grade 3 flow at 60 and 90 minutes compared with tPA alone (72% vs. 43%, $p = 0.0009$; 77% vs. 62%, $p = 0.02$) (157). The Strategies for Patency Enhancement in the Emergency Department (SPEED) trial evaluated a regimen of abciximab plus reteplase (158). TIMI grade 3 flow rates were 54% with abciximab and reteplase, 5 U + 5 U, compared with 47% reteplase only (10 U + 10 U, $p = 0.32$).

The ASSENT-3 trial evaluated abciximab and TNK as well as comparing UFH and enoxaparin (72). The half-dose TNK and abciximab group had a lower incidence of death, in-hospital MI, or in-hospital refractory ischemia compared with full-dose TNK and UFH (11.1% vs. 15.4%) and similar to TNK and enoxaparin (11.4%). Of concern, the abciximab group had nearly twice the risk of major hemorrhage compared with the UFH group (4.3% vs. 2.2%, $p = 0.0002$; enoxaparin group, 3.0%, $p = $ NS vs. UFH).

The 16,558-patient GUSTO-V trial (159) compared standard-dose reteplase (two 10-U boluses, 30 minutes apart) with half-dose reteplase (two 5-U boluses) and full-dose abciximab. No significant differences were seen between the two groups in 30-day mortality. The combination-therapy group had significantly lower rates of death and reinfarction (7.4% vs. 8.8%, $p = 0.0011$) and reinfarction (at 7 days, 2.3% vs. 3.5%) but was associated with higher rate of nonintracranial bleeding complications. Thus, this strategy is not routinely used for the acute treatment of STEMI.

Other Therapies

NITRATES

Nitrates are indicated for relief of persistent pain and treatment of heart failure or hypertension (sublingual or i.v. nitroglycerin). A meta-analysis of data on approximately 2,000 patients treated in the pre-reperfusion era demonstrated a 35% mortality reduction with nitrate use. However, in the large GISSI-3, ISIS-4, and CCS-1 trials (52–54), routine use of i.v. and oral nitrates after MI conferred no mortality benefit. As such, current recommendations are for use of nitrates to relieve symptoms of ischemia and treat hypertension or heart failure; their use should not supersede that of agents proven to improve clinical outcomes, such as β-blockers and ACE inhibitors. Nitrates should not be used in patients with inferior MI complicated by RV involvement (reduces preload) or in patients with recent (24 to 72 hours) $5'$-phosphodiesterase inhibitors (e.g., sildenafil).

CALCIUM CHANNEL BLOCKERS

Nifedipine has been associated with increased mortality [Trial of Early Nifedipine in Acute MI (TRENT) and Secondary Prevention Reinfarction Israel Nifedipine Trials I and II (SPRINT-I and SPRINT-II)] (165,168). In the

Multicenter Diltiazem Post-Infarction Trial (MDPIT) (166), diltiazem was deemed harmful in those with pulmonary congestion and low EF (41% increase in cardiac events). A meta-analysis performed in 1993 of 24 trials of all types of calcium channel blockers showed a nonsignificant 4% increase in mortality (176). Verapamil appears to be safe; a meta-analysis of verapamil studies showed a significant 19% lower reinfarction rate and nonsignificant 7% mortality reduction (169). These agents should be considered only in patients with clear contraindication(s) to β-blockade and with good LV function. They are not routinely used for the acute treatment of STEMI.

ANTIARRHYTHMICS

Prophylactic use of lidocaine appears to be harmful, with a meta-analysis showing a 12% higher mortality rate (177). In the Cardiac Arrhythmia Suppression Trials (CAST I and II) (172), the routine use of type I agents (e.g., encainide, flecainide, moricizine) was associated with significantly higher all-cause mortality rates. However, lidocaine can be used in patients who have had ventricular tachycardia (VT) or VF.

In the Basel Antiarrhythmic Study of Infarct Survival (BASIS) (171), amiodarone in patients with complex ventricular ectopy was associated with 61% lower 1-year mortality rates ($p < 0.05$). However, in two large trials [the European MI Amiodarone Trial (EMIAT) and Canadian Amiodarone MI Arrhythmia Trial (CAMIAT) (174,175)], when given to patients with frequent ventricular ectopy and LV dysfunction, amiodarone (vs. placebo) showed no overall mortality benefit, although arrhythmic deaths were decreased. The Survival with Oral D-sotalol (SWORD) trial showed 65% increased mortality with D-sotalol (173).

MAGNESIUM

Initial studies suggested a mortality benefit [second Leicester Intravenous Magnesium Intervention Trial (LIMIT-2) (179)], and an early meta-analysis showed 54% lower mortality. However, in the ISIS-4 megatrial (180), magnesium had no mortality benefit and was associated with excess hypotension. Proponents of magnesium argued that it could be beneficial in high-risk patients and perhaps when given before thrombolytic therapy to prevent reperfusion injury. However, the large 6,213-patient National Heart, Lung, and Blood Institute (NHLBI)-sponsored MAGIC trial examined these hypotheses and found no benefit associated with magnesium administration (181). Thus, current guidelines recommend *against* the routine use of intravenous magnesium in STEMI patients that do *not* have significant electrolyte abnormalities or ventricular arrhythmias.

GLUCOSE–INSULIN–POTASSIUM

Aggressive serum glucose control in diabetics with insulin drip resulted in a significant mortality benefit in the Diabetic Insulin–Glucose Infusion in Acute MI (DIGAMI) trial (182). Follow-up studies have included combination glucose–insulin–potassium (GIK) therapy. A meta-analysis of nine randomized, placebo-controlled, prethrombolytic era trials with 1,932 patients (all prethrombolytic era) found that GIK was associated with lower hospital mortality (16.1% vs. 21%; OR, 0.72; p = 0.004). A 48% reduction was seen in the four trials using high-dose GIK (to suppress free fatty acid levels maximally). The OASIS-6 GIK trial of 2,748 STEMI patients found no benefit to GIK (overall mortality 10.8% for GIK vs. 10.4% controls at 6 months, p = 0.72). When combined with the CREATE-ECLA trial (185), there was a nonsignificant trend toward *harm* in the GIK group (9.7% mortality in GIK vs. 9.3% in the control at 30 days, p = 0.33). Thus, GIK infusions are not routinely used for care of STEMI.

INTRA-AORTIC BALLOON PUMP

Intra-aortic balloon pump placement appears useful in the treatment of cardiogenic shock (trend toward lower mortality in GUSTO-I) (174) and after emergency catheterization [IABP Trial (199)]. Contraindications include the presence of aortic regurgitation, thoracic or abdominal aortic pathology (aneurysm, dissection), and severe peripheral vascular disease. Vascular complications occur in 5% to 20% of cases (199–201). The IABP-SHOCK II trial randomized 600 STEMI patients with cardiogenic shock to IABP or no IABP and found no significant difference in 30-day mortality between the two groups [RR, 0.96 (95% CI, 0.79 to 1.17); p = 0.69]. The 2013 STEMI guidelines give a class IIa recommendation to using IABP in patients with STEMI and cardiogenic shock who do not quickly stabilize with pharmacologic therapy.

RIGHT VENTRICULAR INFARCTION

Right ventricular infarction is typically caused by right coronary artery occlusion proximal to the acute marginal branch and is associated with 20% to 50% of inferior MIs (192–196).

Diagnosis

1. Triad of hypotension, clear lung fields, and elevated jugular venous pressure are highly specific but only 25% sensitive.
2. Hemodynamics: right atrial pressure is more than 10 mm Hg and within 1 to 5 mm Hg of pulmonary capillary wedge pressure (73% sensitivity, 100% specificity).
3. ECG: ST elevation is present in lead V_4R (80% to 100% sensitivity, 80% to 100% specificity) and resolves quickly. In one study, ST elevation resolved in 48% of patients within 10 hours. RBBB and complete heart block may be observed.
4. Echocardiography: typical features are RV dilatation, RV wall asynergy, and abnormal interventricular septal motion. Tricuspid regurgitation, ventricular septal defect (VSD), and/or early pulmonary valve opening also may be seen.

Complications

High-degree AV block is present in up to 50% of patients and atrial fibrillation in up to one-third. A high incidence of pericarditis is seen, mostly because of transmural involvement of the thin-walled right ventricle. Less common complications include rupture of the interventricular septum, RV free wall rupture (FWR), pulmonary embolism, right atrial infarction, and right-to-left shunting across a patent foramen ovale.

Treatment

Diuretics and nitrates should be avoided (i.e., to not decrease preload). Beneficial measures include:

1. Volume loading (2 to 4 L of normal saline is commonly needed)
2. Inotropic support (dobutamine) if volume does not improve cardiac output
3. Temporary wire placement if complete heart block develops and AV sequential pacing if hemodynamics are poor
4. Cardioversion if atrial fibrillation is present
5. Thrombolysis significantly reduces mortality (194)

Unsuccessful PCI is associated with high mortality [58% vs. 2% in one study (195)].

COMPLICATIONS OF STEMI

Early

1. Pump failure/cardiogenic shock: incidence, 3% to 7%; most common if more than 40% of myocardium involved; hospital mortality is very high: 50% to 70%; prompt IABP insertion can be useful as a bridge to revascularization.
2. Postinfarct angina: more frequent after thrombolysis than after primary PCI
3. Reinfarction: more frequent after thrombolysis and, if non–Q-wave MI, should be treated as initial MI with medical therapy and intervention
4. Arrhythmias:
   a. VT: incidence, 5%; associated with larger infarcts/LV dysfunction; nonsustained VT (NSVT) occurring beyond 24 to 48 hours after MI portends poorer prognosis (218) and is an indication for an EP study and implantable cardioverter defibrillator (ICD) implantation.
   b. VF: declining incidence (now <1%); primary VF occurs in 85% to 90% of cases in the first 24 hours, 60% in the first 6 hours; secondary VF: occurs at 1 to 4 days, often associated with pump failure/shock and poor prognosis (40% to 60% in-hospital mortality).
   c. Asystole: associated with high mortality; transcutaneous or transvenous pacing is indicated.

d. Atrial fibrillation (252): incidence, 5% to 15%; treated with anticoagulation, rate control (β-blockers, calcium channel blockers, digoxin), cardioversion if hemodynamically unstable, or amiodarone if multiple episodes occur

e. Heart block: common with inferior MI (increased vagal tone, AV node ischemia), first-degree heart block typically progresses to Mobitz I and then to third degree; anterior MI (His–Purkinje system affected), BBB progresses to Mobitz II and then third degree (advanced block associated with mortality rate of >40%); temporary pacer indicated for high-degree block that develops via Mobitz II mechanism or bifascicular block

f. Accelerated idioventricular rhythm: occurs more frequently in patients with early reperfusion; temporary pacing is not indicated.

g. Premature ventricular contractions: incidence approximately 75%; routine suppression with lidocaine associated with increased mortality

h. Sinus tachycardia: if it persists, may signify evolving CHF

5. Cholesterol embolization: more common with thrombolytic therapy

Intermediate

1. LV thrombus: incidence, 4% to 20%; most common in anterior MI; treatment, anticoagulation (usually warfarin for 3 to 12 months); decreases the risk of embolization (296); primary prevention, consider anticoagulation if EF is <30% to 35%

2. Myocardial rupture: causes a higher percentage of deaths in patients undergoing thrombolysis [12% vs. 6% (253)]; risk factors include first MI, female gender, age older than 60 years, no LV hypertrophy, hypertension, and possibly thrombolysis after 12 hours [while primary PTCA appears protective (256)]:

a. Free wall: incidence approximately 5%; lower risk after thrombolysis and with use of β-blockers; although most die immediately, treatment includes emergency pericardiocentesis and fluids, followed by immediate surgical repair.

b. Septum: incidence, 0.5% to 2.0%; new murmur with palpable thrill in up to 90%; surgical mortality, 20% to 30% (higher if inferior MI and/or cardiogenic shock) versus 80% to 90% with medical therapy (272)

c. Papillary muscle: incidence approximately 1%; murmur is only 50%; occurs primarily with inferior MIs; posteromedial papillary muscle affected more often (six times) than anterolateral; best treatment is surgery (mortality, approximately 10%).

3. Fibrinous pericarditis: most common after Q-wave MI; treated with aspirin and analgesics, and the guidelines also include use of colchicine and/or acetaminophen in cases refractory to aspirin (2).

Late

1. Ventricular aneurysm: usually does not rupture, but often complicated by mural thrombi and severe CHF; treated with surgical resection if complicated by CHF, severe arrhythmias, and thromboemboli; primary prevention is early ACE inhibition.

2. Pseudoaneurysm: contained rupture of myocardium; surgical resection usually recommended.
3. Dressler syndrome (late pericarditis): usually occurs at 4 to 6 weeks; incidence, approximately 1%; treated with NSAIDs (if they fail, steroids).
4. Sudden cardiac death is increased in patients with reduced EF. The MADIT 2 Trial showed a 31% reduced mortality at 2 years with prophylactic ICD implantations in patients with EF < 30% (see Chapter 6).

PROGNOSIS AND RISK STRATIFICATION AFTER MYOCARDIAL INFARCTION

The majority of hospitalized patients with MI are at low risk for adverse outcomes. Age is a strong predictor of outcome. In a multivariate analysis of GUSTO-I data, mortality ranged from 1.1% in those younger than 45 years to 20.5% in those older than 75 (242). Other factors associated with mortality included lower SBP, higher Killip class, elevated HR, and anterior infarct. These five factors contributed to approximately 90% of prognostic information (**Fig. 4.4**). Another analysis of 3,339 TIMI-2 patients identified a low-risk group (26%; none of eight risk factors) that had a 6-week mortality rate of 1.5%. Patients with one risk factor (age 70 years, female gender, diabetes, prior MI, anterior MI, atrial fibrillation, SBP < 100 mm Hg, HR > 100 beats/min) had a 6-week mortality rate of 5.3% ($p < 0.001$), whereas those with four risk factors had a 17.2% mortality rate (**Fig. 4.5**).

Psychosocial predictors of adverse outcomes include depression (245) and living alone (244). Finally, an analysis of more than 8,000 Medicare patients showed that MI patients treated by cardiologists fared better than those treated by other types of physicians (247).

Uncomplicated STEMI

In patients treated with primary PCI, early hospital discharge has been shown to be safe and more cost effective. LVEF should be measured in all patients with STEMI; it is a class I indication. Catheterization should be considered for risk stratification if the EF is <40%. If the EF is 40% or higher, the TIMI IIB study observed no difference in outcome between an early conservative approach when the patient undergoes an exercise treadmill test (ETT) and an early invasive approach with routine angiography. Accordingly, the ACC/AHA guidelines recommend an early conservative approach to risk stratification. If the result of the ETT is positive for ischemia, or patient has rest pain, the patient should undergo cardiac catheterization. For a small MI, the patient should usually have a submaximal predischarge ETT. If results of this test are negative, medical therapy should be continued, with repeated symptom-limited ETT after several weeks. If the results are positive, catheterization is usually warranted for stratification (99). *An ETT is not required if complete revascularization has been performed.*

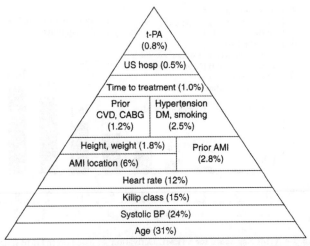

Figure 4.4 • Influence of clinical characteristics on 30-day mortality after myocardial infarction (MI) in patients treated with thrombolytic agents based on GUSTO-I data. Although much attention has been paid to optimizing thrombolytic regimens, the choice of the agent is far less important than are certain clinical variables with respect to mortality. This pyramid depicts the importance of such clinical characteristics, as calculated from a regression analysis in the GUSTO trial. Numbers in parentheses represent the proportion of risk for 30-day mortality associated with the particular characteristics. AMI, acute myocardial infarction; BP, blood pressure; CVD, cardiovascular disease; DM, diabetes mellitus; tPA, tissue-type plasminogen activator; US hosp, patients treated in a US hospital. A more recently developed clinical score, the TIMI risk score, was derived based on an analysis of 11,114 patients from the InTIME II trial (207). Ten baseline variables accounted for 97% of the predictive capacity of the model. These included age older than 75 years (3 points); age 65 to 74 years (2 points); diabetes, hypertension, or angina (1 point); SBP <100 mm Hg (3 points); heart rate more than 100 beats/min (2 points); Killip class II to IV (2 points); weight <67 kg (1 point); anterior STEMI or LBBB (1 point); and time to treatment more than 4 hours (1 point). The risk score showed a more than 40-fold graded increase in mortality (<1% with a score of 0 vs. 35.9% for score more than 8) (see **Fig. 4.5**). This scoring system was then applied to 84,029 STEMI patients in NRMI-3, and it showed a similar strong prognostic capacity with a graded increase in mortality with increasing TIMI risk score (range of 1.1% to 30.0%; $p < 0.001$ for trend) (208). The risk score was equally predictive in those treated with thrombolytic therapy or primary PCI (Modified from Braunwald EB. *Heart disease.* Philadelphia, PA: WB Saunders, 1997:1218, with permission).

Complicated Course

Examples of a complicated course include severe heart failure, cardiogenic shock, failed thrombolysis, recurrent ischemia, and VT or VF after 48 hours. Treatment is composed of catheterization and PCI or CABG surgery, as indicated; for late VT/VF, electrophysiologic testing with possible defibrillator implantation should be considered.

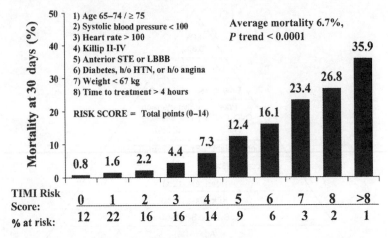

Figure 4.5 • TIMI risk score for STEMI. Derivation set based on InTIME II data. Ten baseline variables accounted for 97% of the predictive capacity of the model and composed the TIMI risk score. These included age older than 75 years (3 points); age 65 to 74 years (2 points); diabetes, hypertension, or angina (1 point); systolic blood pressure < 100 mm Hg (3 points); heart rate > 100 (2 points); Killip class II to IV (2 points); weight <67 kg (1 point); anterior ST elevation myocardial infarction or LBBB (1 point); and time to treatment >4 hours (1 point). The risk score showed a > 40-fold graded increase in mortality (<1% with a score of 0 vs. 35.9% for score >8) (Adapted from Morrow DA, et al. Evaluation of the time saved by pre-hospital initiation of reteplase for ST-elevation myocardial infarction: results of the Early Retavase-Thrombolysis in Myocardial Infarction (ER-TIMI) 19 trial. *J Am Coll Cardiol* 2002;40:71–77).

Specific Tests

1. ETT: submaximal test (70% predicted maximal HR or 5 to 6 METS) can be performed at days 3 to 5, or a symptom-limited test can be performed at days 14 to 21 (often as a prelude to initiation of rehabilitation program). This test has an excellent safety record: 0.03% mortality in one review of 151,949 tests (220). The strongest predictors of poor outcome are limited exercise duration and hypotension. ST depression was predictive of death in only 43% of studies in one large overview. If no predischarge ETT is performed, it is associated with a poor prognosis (221).

2. ETT with nuclear imaging may be used in patients who have baseline ECG abnormalities or who require localization of ischemia to guide planned PCI. Positive test results lead to angiography and revascularization, which reduce the future cardiac event rate.

3. Pharmacologic nuclear stress imaging is indicated in those who cannot exercise. It also is preferred to dobutamine stress echocardiography in those who had significant arrhythmia(s) (especially VT) and/or with marked hypertension.

4. Echocardiography is useful in the assessment of LV function (225), which often guides decisions about the need for catheterization, coronary bypass surgery (mortality benefit if EF < 35%; and three-vessel disease is present), prolonged ACE inhibition therapy, ICD implantation, and long-term anti-coagulation. End-systolic volume may be a stronger predictor of survival than is LVEF (226).

5. Pharmacologic stress echocardiography is performed by using agents such as dobutamine, adenosine, and dipyridamole and typically is performed in higher risk patients (226,227).

REFERENCES

General Review Articles and Guidelines

1. **Go AS, et al.** Heart disease and stroke statistics—2014 update: a report from the American Heart Association. *Circulation* 2014;129:e28–e292.

2. **O'Gara PT, et al.** 2013 ACCF/AHA guideline for the management of ST-elevation myocardial infarction: a report of the American College of Cardiology Foundation/ American Heart Association Task Force on Practice Guidelines. *Circulation* 2013;127:e362–e425.

This update to the STEMI guidelines was intended to be more concise and "user friendly" than previous versions. It provides a more global and comprehensive emphasis, with more focus on symptom recognition, early ECG interpretation in the field, hypothermia in cardiac arrest, and postprocedural care such as cardiac rehab.

3. **Kushner FG, et al.** 2009 focused updates: ACC/AHA guidelines for the management of patients with ST-elevation myocardial infarction (updating the 2004 guideline and 2007 focused update) and ACC/AHA/SCAI guidelines on PCI (updating the 2005 guideline and 2007 focused update): a report of the American College of Cardiology Foundation/American Heart Association Task Force on Practice Guidelines. *J Am Coll Cardiol* 2009;54:2205–2241.

This focused update to the STEMI guidelines largely addressed the timing of and role for GP IIb/IIIa inhibitors in patients with STEMI undergoing primary PCI. The committee also includes recommendations for the newest thienopyridine, prasugrel, and anticoagulant bivalirudin.

Epidemiology

4. **Yeh RW, et al.** Population trends in the incidence and outcomes of acute myocardial infarction. *N Engl J Med* 2010;362:2155–2165.

This study analyzed 46,086 hospitalizations for MI in the community-based Kaiser Permanente Northern California health system, limiting to patients aged 30 or older, to assess modern trends in MI incidence and outcomes. They found a significant decrease in the incidence of all types of MI since 2000, especially STEMIs. They also noted a significant increase in revascularization rates and a significant decrease in 30-day mortality in all types of MI.

5. **Newman JD, et al.** Trends in myocardial infarction rates and case fatality by anatomical location in four United States communities, 1987 to 2008 (from the Atherosclerosis Risk in Communities Study). *Am J Cardiol* 2013;112:1714–1719.

The ARIC Study is a prospective epidemiologic surveillance study sponsored by the NHLBI following patients in 4 US communities (Forsyth County, NC; Jackson, MS; suburban Minneapolis, MN; Washington County, MD). It was designed to investigate the causes and clinical outcomes of atherosclerosis. The Cohort component began in 1987 and has followed approximately 4,000 patients aged 45 to 64 from each community with semiannual exams. The community surveillance component investigates the long-term trends in hospitalized MI and CHD deaths in approximately 470,000 patients aged 35 to 84.

Pathogenesis

6. Libby P. Mechanisms of acute coronary syndromes and their implications for therapy. N Engl J Med 2013;368:2004–2013.

In this Mechanisms of Disease Review Article, Dr. Peter Libby discusses the natural progression of atherosclerosis and the mechanisms underlying the acute complications of atherosclerosis leading to acute coronary syndromes. He discusses the role of lowering LDL, the negative effects of inflammation, the benefits of statins, and the possible therapeutic implications of new mechanistic insights.

7. Little WC, et al. Can coronary angiography predict the site of a subsequent myocardial infarction in patients with mild-to-moderate coronary artery disease? Circulation 1988;78:1157–1166.

In this retrospective observational study, the authors reviewed 29 patients with a confirmed diagnosis of MI and a coronary angiogram after the MI as well as prior to the MI, though this time period ranged from 4 to 2,298 days prior to the MI. They found that 66% of the patients had the MI in a vessel with a stenosis <50% on their previous angiogram, and only one patient in this study had an MI in a lesion with a >70% lesion on prior angiography.

8. Stone GW, et al. A prospective natural-history study of coronary atherosclerosis. N Engl J Med 2011;364:226–235.

This prospective trial (the PROSPECT trial) of 697 patients presenting with acute coronary syndrome used angiography and intravascular ultrasound (IVUS) to evaluate the culprit lesion after PCI and also evaluated the other major nonculprit coronary arteries. They then monitored the patients for major adverse cardiac events (MACE) with a median follow-up of 3.4 years and categorized the events as occurring in the original culprit or nonculprit lesion. The overall cumulative MACE rate was 20.4% and 3-year follow-up, with events related to the culprit lesion in 12.9% of patients and a nonculprit lesion in 11.6% of patients. Though the nonculprit lesions leading to MACE were frequently mild by angiography, this study found that most of these lesions were characterized by a plaque burden ≥70%, a thin-cap fibroatheroma on IVUS, and a minimal lumen area (MLA) ≤4.0 mm^2.

9. Mancini GB, et al. Angiographic disease progression and residual risk of cardiovascular events while on optimal medical therapy: observations from the COURAGE trial. Circ Cardiovasc Interv 2011;4:545–552.

In this angiographic substudy of the COURAGE trial (see Chapter 2), 489 patients had symptom-driven follow-up coronary angiograms. Of the 130 patients who underwent angiography due to the diagnosis of MI/acute coronary syndrome, 31% had index lesions that were <50% on the original angiogram, but 51% had index lesions that were ≥50% on the original angiogram. In fact, the only independent angiographic risk factor for MI/ACS was the number of nonrevascularized lesions originally ≥50% diameter stenosis, not the number of lesions originally <50% diameter stenosis or any other angiographic parameter.

Diagnosis

10. Thygesen K, et al. ESC/ACCF/AHA/WHF expert consensus document, third universal definition of myocardial infarction. *Circulation* 2012;126:2020–2035.

This update to the 2007 document on the universal definition of MI augmented the 2nd task force definitions from 2007 by addressing the newer high-sensitivity troponin assays, MI related to procedures such as TAVR and mitral clip, and differentiation of recurrent MI from reinfarction.

CHEST PAIN AND SYMPTOMS

11. Douglas PS, et al. The evaluation of chest pain in women. N *Engl J Med* 1996;334:1311–1315.

This review article discusses the major determinants of coronary artery disease (CAD) in women [chest pain (quality and incidence), hormonal status, diabetes, peripheral vascular disease], as well as intermediate determinants (hypertension, smoking, lipoproteins) and minor determinants (age older than 65 years, obesity, sedentary lifestyle, family history). The review concludes with a discussion of diagnostic testing.

12. Goldman L, et al. Prediction of the need for intensive care in patients who come to emergency departments with chest pain. N *Engl J Med* 1996;334:1498–1504.

This study was composed, in part, of a derivation set (10,682 patients) used to identify clinical predictors of major complications: ST elevation or Q waves, other ECG changes indicating myocardial ischemia, low SBP, pulmonary rales above bases, or an exacerbation of known ischemic heart disease. The validation set (4,676 patients) stratified patients into four groups with risk of major complications ranging from 0.15% to 8%. After 12 hours, the probability was updated based on whether the patient had a complication or confirmed MI. Patients with intermediate events (e.g., heart block, pulmonary edema without hypotension, recurrent ischemia not requiring CABG or PTCA within 72 hours) or confirmed MI had 3.5% to 7.5% risk of a major event per 24-hour period. Authors recommended intensive care unit (ICU) admission in this group. Echocardiographic, serum marker, or stress imaging data were not incorporated into this risk stratification algorithm.

13. Panju AA, et al. Is this patient having a myocardial infarction? JAMA 1998;280:1256–1263.

Case-based discussion of history, physical, and ECG findings that are suggestive of the diagnosis of MI. Likelihood ratios are provided for these features; the most powerful predictors (or nonpredictors) of MI include new ST elevation (likelihood ratio range of 5.7 to 53.9), new Q wave (5.3 to 24.8), chest pain radiating to both arms simultaneously (7.1), positional chest pain (0.3), chest pain reproduced by palpation (0.2 to 0.4), pleuritic chest pain (0.2), and a normal ECG (0.1 to 0.3).

14. Lee TH, et al. Evaluation of the patient with acute chest pain. N *Engl J Med* 2000;342(16):1187–1195.

This review focuses on the evaluation of chest pain related to cardiac ischemia, highlighting the most useful tests, expected cardiac marker trends, and emergent management. Algorithms are provided for the safe "rule out" of patients without immediate evidence of cardiac injury, as well as helpful aids and guidelines for admitting such patients and identifying those at high risk for short-term morbidity and mortality.

ELECTROCARDIOGRAPHY

15. Sgarbossa EB, et al. Electrocardiographic diagnosis of evolving acute MI in the presence of left bundle branch block. N *Engl J Med* 1996;334:481–487 (editorial, 528–529).

Three ECG criteria were derived from an analysis of 131 GUSTO patients: (a) ST elevation of 1 mm concordant with QRS complex; (b) ST depression of 1 mm in V_1, V_2, or V_3; and (c) ST elevation of 5 mm discordant with QRS. ORs for confirmed MI were 25.2, 6.0, and 4.3. If the index score was 3 (a, $n = 5$ patients; b, $n = 3$ patients; c, $n = 2$ patients), sensitivity was 78% and specificity 90%. However, sensitivity was only 36% in the validation group of 45 patients. The authors assert that the low sensitivity is an intrinsic property of ST elevation. The reported sensitivity and specificity depend on a 50% prevalence of MI (i.e., high index of suspicion of MI necessary). A retrospective cohort analysis of 83 patients with LBBB and symptoms suggestive of MI found that the sensitivity of this algorithm was only 10%.

16. Zimetbaum PJ, Josephson ME. Use of the electrocardiogram in acute myocardial infarction. N Engl J Med 2003;348:933–940.

This review mainly focuses on the identification of ST elevations, the common distributions, and their anatomically correlating infarct territories. Prognostic signs on the ECG are reviewed, as are the common conduction diseases and sequelae of acute MI. The guidelines for temporary and permanent pacing, as well as a review of tachyarrhythmias, are also discussed.

17. Wang K, et al. ST-segment elevation in conditions other than acute myocardial infarction. N Engl J Med 2003;349:2128–2135.

The article discusses first the features of ST-segment elevation that are both typical and atypical for ischemia versus normal variants in healthy patients. The authors go on to discuss such identification in LBBB, as well as alternative causes of ST-segment elevation, such as pericarditis, myocarditis, hyperkalemia, Brugada syndrome, arrhythmogenic RV cardiomyopathy, pulmonary embolus, Prinzmetal angina, and postcardioversion ST-segment elevation. Examples of ECGs are provided.

BIOMARKERS

18. deWinter RJ, et al. Value of myoglobin, troponin T and CK-MB in ruling out an acute MI in the emergency room. Circulation 1995;92:3401–3407.

This prospective analysis focused on 309 consecutive patients with chest pain. At 3 to 6 hours after symptoms, myoglobin yielded the best negative predictive value (89% at 4 hours). The negative predictive value of CK-MB reached 95% at 7 hours. The markers were found to increase fastest with large MIs.

19. Stubbs P, et al. Prognostic significance of admission troponin T concentration in patients with MI. Circulation 1996;94:1291–1297.

This prospective study was composed of 240 patients showing any detectable TnT on admission associated with worse prognosis (median follow-up, 3 years). Admission TnT of 0.2 ng/mL was associated with a higher risk of subsequent cardiac death ($p = 0.0002$) and death plus MI ($p = 0.00006$). Most of this excess risk was confined to those with ST-segment elevation on admission ECG.

20. Ohman EM, et al. Cardiac troponin T levels for risk stratification in acute myocardial ischemia. N Engl J Med 1996;335:1333–1341.

This analysis focused on 801 GUSTO-IIa patients, of whom 72% had an MI. An elevated TnT (>1 ng/mL) was associated with a threefold higher 30-day mortality rate (11.9% vs. 3.9%, $p < 0.001$). Overall, the top mortality predictors were an elevated TnT (χ^2, 21; $p < 0.001$), ECG category (ST change or T-wave inversion; χ^2, 14; $p = 0.003$), and CK-MB (χ^2, 11; $p = 0.004$). TnT was still predictive in a model incorporating all three of these factors (χ^2, 9.2; $p = 0.027$). Proposed explanations of the increased mortality with elevated TnT included (a) later presentation; (b) higher cases of reocclusion, which is known to be associated with increased mortality; and (c) larger infarcts (also earlier release) in patients who died. TnT also had predictive prognostic value, even in patients with ST elevation.

21. Antman E, et al. Cardiac-specific TnI levels to predict the risk of mortality in patients with acute coronary syndromes. N Engl J Med 1996;335:1342–1349.

This analysis focused on 1,404 TIMI IIIB patients. TnI was elevated (0.4 ng/mL or more) in 573 patients and associated with a significantly increased 42-day mortality rate (3.7% vs. 1.0%, $p < 0.001$). Even after adjustments for ST depression and age of 65 years or older (the two independent mortality predictors), each 1-ng/mL increase in TnI was associated with a mortality increase: 0.4 or less, 1%; 0.4 to 0.9, 1.7%; 1 to 1.9, 3.4%; 2 to 4.9, 3.7%; 5 to 8.9, 6%; and 9, 7.5%. TnI provided more prognostic information in patients with a late presentation (>6 to 24 hours): mortality 4% (TnI, 0.4 ng/mL or more) versus 0.4% (relative risk, 9.5). In contrast, in patients seen early, the relative risk was only 1.8 (3.1% vs. 1.7%, p = NS). If no CK-MB elevation was present (948 patients), a TnI elevation was still associated with increased mortality: 2.5% versus 0.8% (relative risk, 3.0; 95% CI, 0.97 to 9.2). The elevated TnI group had more ST deviation and less stenosis on angiography at 18 to 48 hours after symptom onset. However, few had angiography within hours of symptom onset.

22. Newby LK, et al. Value of serial TnT measures for early and late risk stratification in patients with acute coronary syndromes. Circulation 1998;98:1853–1859.

This GUSTO-IIa substudy of 734 patients showed the usefulness of the addition of later cardiac TnT (cTnT) samples. All patients had cTnT samples drawn at baseline, 8 hours, and 16 hours. At baseline, 260 patients were cTnT positive (>0.01 ng/mL), 323 became positive later, and 151 remained negative. The mortality rates were 10% in the baseline-positive group, 5% in the late-positive group, and none in negative patients; thus, late-positive patients are at intermediate risk. After adjustment for baseline characteristics, any positive cTnT result predicted 30-day mortality. Only age and ST-segment elevation were stronger predictors than baseline cTnT. Most of the mortality difference between cTnT-positive and TnT-negative patients occurred in the first 30 days.

23. Steen H, et al. Cardiac troponin T at 96 hours after acute myocardial infarction correlates with infarct size and cardiac function. J Am Coll Cardiol 2006;48: 2192–2194.

The authors correlate a single measurement of TnT 96 hours after STEMI/NSTEMI (23 STEMI, 21 NSTEMI) with contrast-enhanced magnetic resonance imaging (CE-MRI) of myocardial scar. Linear regression correlation coefficients were excellent for STEMI (r = 0.910), and less so, but still significant, for NSTEMI (r = 0.575).

PREHOSPITAL AND EMERGENCY DEPARTMENT EVALUATION

24. Kontos MC, et al. Comparison of myocardial perfusion imaging and cardiac troponin I in patients admitted to the emergency department with chest pain. Circulation 1999;99:2073–2078.

This study was composed of 620 patients considered at low to moderate risk for acute coronary syndromes who underwent gated single-photon emission Tc sestamibi imaging and serial measurements of CK, CK-MB, and TnI over an 8-hour period. The incidence of MI was 9%, significant CAD was demonstrated in 13%, and revascularization was performed in 9%. Perfusion imaging was more sensitive but less specific than TnI in identifying patients who were revascularized [sensitivity, 81% vs. 26% (TnI, 1.0 ng/mL); specificity, 74% vs. 96%].

25. Carstensen S, et al. Field triage to primary angioplasty combined with emergency department bypass reduces treatment delays and is associated with improved outcome. Eur Heart J 2007;28:2313–2319.

The investigators randomized 301 Australian patients with STEMI to either ECG and triage in the field by emergency medical services (EMSs) (with then the option of going to a center offering primary PCI) or ECG and triage at the nearest emergency department. Not only did patients triaged in the field have lower symptom-to-balloon times (154 minutes vs. 249 minutes, $p < 0.001$) and peak creatinine kinase levels (in early presenting patients only, 1,435 vs. 2,320, $p = 0.009$) but also overall in-hospital mortality was significantly reduced for patients triaged in the field (1.9% vs. 7.3%, $p = 0.046$).

26. LeMay MR, et al. A citywide protocol for primary PCI in ST-segment elevation myocardial infarction. N Engl J Med 2008;358:231–240.

The authors demonstrate the results of a citywide, integrated system by which all patients with STEMI are referred from the field to specialized centers for primary PCI in the city of Ottawa. Compared with patients referred from emergency departments for primary PCI at another institution, those referred from the field had lower door-to-balloon times (median 69 minutes vs. 123 minutes, $p < 0.01$) and more commonly achieved door-to-balloon times of <90 minutes (79.7% vs. 11.9%, $p < 0.001$). While this was not a randomized trial (and the populations were not equivalent), clinical outcomes were similar with a trend toward lower in-hospital mortality for those referred directly from the field (3.0% vs. 5.7%, $p = 0.30$).

Treatment

ASPIRIN

27. Second International Study of Infarct Survival (ISIS-2). Randomised trial of intravenously streptokinase, oral, both, or neither among 17,187 cases of suspected acute MI. Lancet 1988;332:349–360.

This large trial clearly demonstrated the additive benefit of thrombolytic therapy and aspirin administration. Patients were randomized to SK, 1.5 million U over 60 minutes; and/or aspirin, 162.5 mg; or placebo. The SK and aspirin-alone groups had 25% and 23% lower 5-week vascular mortality, respectively [9.2% vs. 12.0% (placebo), $p < 0.00001$; 9.4% vs. 11.8%, $p < 0.00001$]. The SK and aspirin groups had a larger 42% mortality reduction (8% vs. 13.2%). Combination therapy also was effective in patients with LBBB (mortality, 14% vs. 27.7%). Aspirin reduced nonfatal reinfarction and stroke rates (1.0% vs. 2.0%; 0.3% vs. 0.6%).

28. Roux S, et al. Effect of aspirin on coronary reocclusion and recurrent ischemia after thrombolysis: a meta-analysis. J Am Coll Cardiol 1992;19:671–677.

This analysis of 32 studies (19 randomized, 13 nonrandomized) from 1980 to 1990 showed the impressive benefits of aspirin. In these studies, 3,209 of 4,930 patients were treated with aspirin. Among the 1,022 patients who underwent angiography, aspirin use was associated with a 56% lower reocclusion rate (11% vs. 25%, $p < 0.001$) and fewer recurrent ischemic events (25% vs. 41%, $p < 0.001$). This protective effect of aspirin was similar in trials with either SK or recombinant tPA (rtPA).

29. Antithrombotic Trialists' Collaboration. Collaborative meta-analysis of randomized trials of antiplatelet therapy for prevention of death, myocardial infarction, and stroke in high risk patients. BMJ 2002;324(7329):71–86.

This analysis was a collaborative meta-analysis of 287 randomized trials involving over 200,000 high-risk patients. 135,000 patients were involved in studies comparing an antiplatelet agent to control, and 77,000 patients were involved in studies comparing different antiplatelet agents. The primary outcome measure was "serious vascular event." The analysis found that aspirin (or another oral antiplatelet agent) is protective in patients with AMI or ischemic stroke, unstable or stable angina, previous myocardial infarction, stroke or cerebral ischemia, peripheral arterial disease, or atrial fibrillation. In addition, the analysis found aspirin doses of 75 to 150 mg to be effective for long-term use with the caveat that in acute settings an initial loading dose of at least 150 mg aspirin may be needed.

30. Mehta SR, et al. (CURRENT OASIS 7 Investigators). Dose comparisons of clopidogrel and aspirin in acute coronary syndromes. *N Engl J Med* 2010;363:930–942.

Design: Prospective, randomized, multicenter, international, 2 × 2 factorial design. The primary outcome is the composite of death from cardiovascular causes, myocardial (re)infarction, or stroke up to 30 days. The primary safety outcome is major bleeding.

Purpose: To evaluate the safety of (a) a higher loading and initial maintenance dose of clopidogrel compared with the standard-dose regimen and (b) high-dose aspirin compared with low-dose aspirin.

Population: 25,086 patients with ST or non–ST-segment elevation ACS managed with an early invasive strategy.

Exclusion Criteria: Increased risk of bleeding or active bleeding, known allergy to clopidogrel or aspirin.

Treatment: Clopidogrel high-dose regimen (600-mg loading dose on day 1 followed by 150 mg once daily on days 2 to 7, followed by 75 mg once daily on days 8 to 30) compared with the standard-dose regimen (300-mg loading dose on day 1, followed by 75 mg once daily on days 2 to 30) and high-dose aspirin (300 to 325 mg daily) versus low-dose aspirin (75 to 100 mg daily).

Results: In the overall population, there was no difference in the primary outcome between the two clopidogrel groups (4.2% in the double-dose group vs. 4.4% in the standard-dose group, p = 0.30), but there was an increase in major bleeding in the higher-dose group (2.5% vs. 2.0%, p = 0.01). In addition, there was no significant difference between higher and lower dose aspirin with respect to the primary outcome (4.2% in the high-dose group vs. 4.4% in the low-dose group, p = 0.61) and major bleeding (2.3% vs. 2.3%, p = 0.90).

31. Berger JS, et al. Initial aspirin dose and outcome among ST-elevation myocardial infarction patients treated with fibrinolytic therapy. *Circulation* 2008;117:192–199.

Combining data from the Global Utilization of Streptokinase and Tissue Plasminogen Activator for Occluded Coronary Arteries (GUSTO-I) and Global Use of Strategies to Open Occluded Coronary Arteries (GUSTO-III) trials (n = 48,422 STEMI patients), the investigators assessed both ischemic and bleeding events in patients, stratified by aspirin dose, and adjusted for previously identified risk factors for morbidity and mortality. In adjusted analyses, mortality did not differ between patients receiving 162-mg aspirin versus 325-mg aspirin. However, after adjustment, 325-mg dosing was associated with significantly more moderate/severe bleeding (OR 1.14, p = 0.003). Importantly, this was limited to patients receiving lysis; no primary PCI patients were included.

P2Y12 INHIBITORS

32. Sabatine MS, et al.; For the CLARITY-TIMI 28 Investigators. Addition of clopidogrel to aspirin and fibrinolytic therapy for myocardial infarction with ST-segment elevation. *N Engl J Med* 2005;352:1179–1189.

Design: Prospective, randomized, double-blind, international, multicenter study. The primary end point was a composite of occluded IRA on angiography or death or recurrent MI before angiography (at 48 to 192 hours).

Purpose: To determine the effect of clopidogrel on infarct artery reperfusion in patients with STEMI receiving fibrinolysis.

Population: 3,491 patients aged 18 to 75 years old, with STEMI, presenting with 12 hours of symptom onset, treated with fibrinolytic therapy.

Exclusion Criteria: Use of clopidogrel within the last 7 days, any contraindication to fibrinolytic therapy, prior CABG.

Treatment: Clopidogrel (300-mg load, followed by 75 mg daily) or placebo.

Results: Clopidogrel reduced the incidence of the primary end point (15.0% vs. 21.7%, $p < 0.001$). At 30 days, rates of clinical adverse events (a composite of cardiovascular death, recurrent MI, or urgent recurrent revascularization) were also reduced in the clopidogrel group (11.6% vs. 14.1%, $p = 0.03$). There was no increase in major bleeding.

33. COMMIT (ClOpidogrel and Metoprolol in Myocardial Infarction Trial) Collaborative Group. Addition of clopidogrel to aspirin in 45,852 patients with acute myocardial infarction: randomized placebo-controlled trial. *Lancet* 2005;366:1607–1621.

Design: Prospective, randomized, placebo-controlled, multicenter study. There were two prespecified coprimary end points at discharge or over a treatment period of 4 weeks (whichever came sooner): (a) a composite of death, reinfarction, or stroke and (b) death from any cause.

Purpose: To determine the benefit, if any, of adding clopidogrel to aspirin in the treatment of STEMI.

Population: 45,852 patients admitted within 24 hours of acute MI, with ST elevation, LBBB, or ST depression (7% of the trial population) on ECG.

Exclusion Criteria: Patients scheduled for primary PCI (clopidogrel would be indicated).

Treatment: Clopidogrel 75 mg daily or placebo.

Results: Clopidogrel reduced the incidence of the composite primary end point (9.2% vs. 10.1%, $p = 0.002$), as well as overall mortality (7.5% vs. 8.1%, $p = 0.03$). There was no increase in overall bleeding detected (0.58% vs. 0.55%, $p = 0.59$) or in the subgroups of those who received fibrinolytic therapy or older than 70 years of age. Importantly, these results were consistent across a wide and diverse range of subgroups analyzed, without any heterogeneity.

Comments: There was also a β-blocker arm of this study, reported below.

34. Montalescot G, et al.; for the TRITON-TIMI 38 Investigators. Prasugrel compared with clopidogrel in patients undergoing percutaneous coronary intervention for ST-elevation myocardial infarction (TRITON-TIMI 38): double-blind, randomised controlled trial. *Lancet* 2009;373:723–731.

The authors examine the subset of patients with STEMI from the TRITON-TIMI 38 trial, which included all spectra of ACS (see Chapter 3 for the complete trial details). Briefly, the trial compared the newest thienopyridine, prasugrel, with clopidogrel in 13,608 patients with ACS. Of these, 3,534 patients presented with STEMI (approximately 26%), the vast majority of whom underwent primary PCI (>95%). Roughly one-third received a DES. The primary end point of a composite of cardiovascular death, MI, or stroke at 15 months was significantly lower in the prasugrel group (6.5% vs. 9.5%, $p = 0.0017$), compared to clopidogrel. Consistently, the composite outcome of cardiovascular death, MI, or urgent TVR was also reduced at 30 days ($p = 0.0205$) and 15 months ($p = 0.025$). Overall, bleeding rates were similar, with the exception being patients who subsequently underwent CABG and had higher bleeding in the prasugrel group ($p = 0.0033$).

35. Bhatt DL, et al. Effect of platelet inhibition with cangrelor during PCI on ischemic events (CHAMPION-PHOENIX). *N Engl J Med* 2013;368:1303–1313.

Design: Prospective, randomized, double-blind, placebo-controlled trial. Primary efficacy end point was a composite rate of death from any cause, MI, ischemia-driven revascularization, or stent thrombosis in the 48 hours after randomization. Primary safety end point severe GUSTO bleeding not related to CABG at 48 hours.

Purpose: To evaluate the efficacy of an IV ADP receptor antagonism with cangrelor versus clopidogrel in patients undergoing PCI.

Population: 11,145 patients ≥18 years of age who require PCI (for ACS or stable angina, approximately 18% STEMI) and who had not received pretreatment with platelet inhibitors.

Treatment: Cangrelor bolus of 30 μg/kg and an infusion of 4 μg/kg versus 600 mg or 300 mg of clopidogrel prior to PCI.

Results: The primary end point occurred in 4.7% of the cangrelor patients versus 5.9% of the clopidogrel patients [OR, 0.78 (95% CI, 0.66 to 0.93); p = 0.005]. GUSTO severe bleeding occurred in 0.16% of the cangrelor patients and in 0.11% of the clopidogrel patients [OR, 1.50 (95% CI, 0.53 to 4.22); p = 0.44].

Comments: The FDA advisory panel advised against approval of cangrelor for the indication of reducing thrombotic events in patients undergoing PCI. This was partly due to the two previous CHAMPION trials (CHAMPION-PCI and CHAMPION-PLATFORM), which investigated the drug in patients with ACS undergoing PCI. They were both stopped early after analyses suggested that neither trial could show a benefit of cangrelor. However, approval consideration is ongoing for this and other indications, including bridging patients with coronary stents on dual antiplatelet therapy who need coronary bypass surgery based on the results of the BRIDGE trial (see JAMA 2012;307(3):265–274).

β-BLOCKERS

36. Norwegian Multicenter Group. Timolol-induced reduction in mortality and reinfarction in patients surviving acute MI. N Engl J Med 1981;304:801–807.

Design: Prospective, randomized, double-blind, placebo-controlled, multicenter study. The mean follow-up period was 17 months. The primary end point was all-cause mortality.

Purpose: To evaluate the efficacy of long-term β-blockade after MI.

Population: 1,884 patients randomized at 7 to 28 days after AMI meeting at least two of the following criteria: (a) chest pain longer than 15 minutes, acute pulmonary edema, or cardiogenic shock; (b) pathologic Q waves and/or ST elevation followed by T-wave inversion in at least two leads; or (c) elevated serum markers.

Exclusion Criteria: HR <50 beats/min; severe CHF; second- or third-degree AV block; SBP <100 mm Hg.

Treatment: Timolol, 10 mg twice daily, or placebo.

Results: Timolol group had a 39% lower mortality rate (13.3% vs. 21.9%, p < 0.001) and a 28% lower reinfarction rate (14.4% vs. 20.1%, p < 0.001).

Comments: Six-year follow-up showed a persistent mortality benefit of timolol (26.4% vs. 32.3%, p = 0.003).

37. β-Blocker Heart Attack Trial (BHAT) Research Group. A randomized trial of propranolol in patients with acute MI. JAMA 1982;247:1707–1714.

Design: Prospective, randomized, double-blind, placebo-controlled, multicenter study. The mean follow-up period was 25 months. The primary end point was all-cause mortality.

Purpose: To evaluate if long-term propranolol administration after MI reduces mortality.

Population: 3,837 patients younger than 70 years enrolled 5 to 21 days after an AMI.

Exclusion Criteria: Marked bradycardia, current β-blocker therapy, history of severe heart failure or asthma, and planned cardiac surgery.

Treatment: Propranolol, 60 to 80 mg, three times daily or placebo.

Results: Propranolol group had 26.5% lower mortality (7.2% vs. 9.8%, $p < 0.005$), 28% fewer sudden cardiac deaths (3.3% vs. 4.6%, $p < 0.05$), and 23% fewer major cardiac events (nonfatal MI plus fatal coronary disease). Serious side effects were infrequent.

Comments: Post hoc analysis showed that the benefit of propranolol was restricted to a high-risk group of 383 patients—43% mortality reduction ($p < 0.01$).

38. The Metoprolol in Acute MI (MIAMI) Trial Research Group. Metoprolol in acute MI (MIAMI): a randomised placebo-controlled international trial. *Eur Heart J* 1985;6:199–226.

Design: Prospective, randomized, double-blind, placebo-controlled, multicenter study. The primary end point was all-cause mortality.

Purpose: To evaluate whether metoprolol administration after MI reduces mortality.

Population: 5,728 patients younger than 75 years, seen within 24 hours of onset of symptoms (average, 7 hours).

Exclusion Criteria: Current treatment with β-blockers or calcium antagonists and HR 65 beats/min or less.

Treatment: Metoprolol, 15 mg i.v. and then 200 mg/day orally, or placebo.

Results: Metoprolol group had a nonsignificant 13% mortality reduction at 15 days (4.3% vs. 4.9%). The high-risk subgroup (meeting at least three of the following criteria: older than 60 years, prior MI, ECG consistent with MI, previous angina, CHF, diabetes, taking digoxin or diuretics) had 29% lower mortality.

39. ISIS-1 Collaborative Group. Randomised trial of intravenous atenolol among 16,107 cases of suspected acute MI. *Lancet* 1986;328:57–65.

Design: Prospective, randomized, open, parallel-group, multicenter study. The primary end point was vascular mortality at 7 days.

Purpose: To determine the effects of atenolol in MI patients on 7-day vascular mortality.

Population: 16,107 patients seen within 12 hours (average, 5 hours) of AMI who were not taking β-blockers or verapamil.

Exclusion Criteria: HR <50 beats/min, SBP <100 mm Hg, second- or third-degree heart block, severe heart failure, and bronchospasm.

Treatment: Atenolol, 5 to 10 mg i.v., over a 5-minute period, followed by 100 mg/day orally for 7 days. No placebo was given to controls.

Results: Atenolol group had a 15% lower 7-day vascular mortality rate (3.89% vs. 4.57%, $p < 0.04$). Most of mortality difference occurred in the first 24 hours. At 1 year, the benefit persisted, with an 11% vascular mortality reduction (10.7% vs. 12.0%, $p < 0.01$). After year 1, nonsignificant excess of vascular deaths was found in the atenolol group (179 vs. 145, $p = 0.07$).

Comments: A later analysis showed that the benefit of atenolol in the first 24 hours was primarily owing to a lower rate of pulseless electrical activity (PEA), reflecting less cardiac rupture.

40. Roberts R, et al.; for the TIMI-IIB Investigators. Immediate vs. deferred β-blockade following thrombolytic therapy in patients with acute MI: results of TIMI II-B. *Circulation* 1991;83:422–437.

Design: Prospective, randomized, open, parallel-group, multicenter study. The primary end point was predischarge LVEF.

Purpose: To compare immediate intravenously versus deferred (started on day 6) β-blocker in AMI patients treated with rtPA.

Population: 1,434 patients aged 75 years or younger seen within 4 hours of chest pain and with 1 mm or greater ST elevation in at least two contiguous ECG leads and having no contraindications to β-blockade. Low-risk subgroup is defined as an absence of all the following: history of MI, anterior ST elevation, rates greater than one-third up lung fields, SBP <100 mm Hg or cardiogenic shock, HR more than 100 beats/min, atrial fibrillation or flutter, and age 70 years or older.

Exclusion Criteria: HR <55 beats/min, SBP consistently <100 mm Hg, severe first-degree or advanced heart block, and wheezing or significant COPD.

Treatment: Immediate β-blockade group received metoprolol, 5 mg i.v., for three doses (given within 2 hours of rtPA) and then 50 to 100 mg twice daily. The deferred β-blockade group received metoprolol, 50 mg twice daily on day 6, followed by 100 mg twice daily. All patients received aspirin, heparin (i.v. for 5 days and then s.c. every 12 hours), and lidocaine (1.0 to 1.5 mg/kg and then 2.0 to 4.0 mg/min for 24 hours).

Results: No significant differences in mortality or LVEF were observed at discharge, but the subgroup of low-risk patients receiving β-blockade had a lower rate of death and nonfatal reinfarction (5.4% vs. 13.7%, $p = 0.01$), as well as less recurrent chest pain (18.8% vs. 24.1%, $p < 0.02$).

41. Dargie HJ. Effect of carvedilol on outcome after myocardial infarction in patients with left-ventricular dysfunction: the CAPRICORN randomised trial. *Lancet* 2001;357:1385–1390.

Design: Prospective, randomized, placebo-controlled, multicenter trial. The primary end point was all-cause mortality or CV-related hospital admission.

Purpose: To investigate the long-term efficacy of carvedilol on morbidity and mortality in patients with LV dysfunction after AMI treated according to current evidence-based practice.

Population: 1,959 patients with AMI and LVEF of 40% or less.

Treatment: Carvedilol (6.25 mg once daily titrated to 25 mg twice daily over 4 to 6 weeks) or placebo.

Results: No significant difference was observed between the carvedilol and placebo groups in the incidence of the primary end point [35% vs. 37%; hazard ratio, 0.92 (95% CI, 0.80 to 1.07)]. However, all-cause mortality was significantly lower in the carvedilol group [12% vs. 15%; hazard ratio, 0.77 (95% CI, 0.60 to 0.98); $p = 0.03$]. The carvedilol group also had lower rates of cardiovascular mortality, nonfatal MI, and all-cause mortality or nonfatal MI.

42. Hjalmarson A, et al. Effect on mortality of metoprolol in acute MI. *Lancet* 1981;2:823–827.

A total of 1,395 patients with chest pain lasting 30 minutes or longer and ECG changes were randomized at an average of 11 hours from onset of symptoms to 15 mg i.v. and then 100 mg twice daily or placebo. MI was confirmed in 69.6% of patients. The metoprolol group had a 36% lower 90-day mortality rate (5.7% vs. 8.9%, $p < 0.03$).

43. Ryden L, et al. A double-blind trial of metoprolol in acute MI: effects on ventricular arrhythmias. *N Engl J Med* 1983;308:614–618.

A total of 1,395 patients with suspected MI were given metoprolol, 15 mg i.v., 50 mg every 6 hours for 2 days, and then 100 mg twice daily for 3 months. Antiarrhythmic drugs were given only for VF and sustained VT. Only 58% of patients had a definite MI. The metoprolol group had less VF (0.9% vs. 2.4%, $p < 0.05$) and less lidocaine use ($p < 0.01$).

44. COMMIT (ClOpidogrel and Metoprolol in Myocardial Infarction Trial) Collaborative Group. Early intravenous then oral metoprolol in 45,852 patients with acute myocardial infarction: randomised placebo-controlled trial. *Lancet* 2005;366:1622–1632.

Design: Prospective, randomized, placebo-controlled, multicenter study. There were two prespecified coprimary end points at discharge or over a treatment period of 4 weeks (whichever came sooner): (a) a composite of death, reinfarction, or cardiac arrest and (b) death from any cause.

Purpose: To determine the benefit, if any, of adding β-blockade (metoprolol) to contemporary regimens for acute MI.

Population: 45,852 patients admitted within 24 hours of acute MI, with ST elevation, LBBB, or ST depression (7% of the trial population) on ECG.

Treatment: Metoprolol (up to 15 mg intravenously then 200 mg oral daily) or placebo.

Results: Similar rates of primary outcome events were observed in the metoprolol and placebo groups (9.4% for metoprolol vs. 9.9% for placebo, $p = 0.1$). While metoprolol did reduce rates of reinfarction (2.0% vs. 2.5%, $p = 0.001$) and VF (2.5% vs. 3.0%, $p = 0.001$), more patients in the metoprolol group developed cardiogenic shock (5.0% vs. 3.9%, $p < 0.00001$), predominantly in the first 24 hours of hospitalization.

Comments: The benefits of metoprolol were observed in hemodynamically stable patients, later in their course, while the adverse effects of metoprolol were seen early in the course of patients who were unstable hemodynamically. Thus, the trial highlighted the benefits and, more importantly, the pitfalls of β-blockade in acute MI in patients with evidence of heart failure or hemodynamic instability at presentation. See above for results of the clopidogrel arm of this trial.

45. Ibanez B, et al. Effect of early metoprolol on infarct size in ST-segment elevation myocardial infarction patients undergoing primary percutaneous coronary intervention: the Effect of Metoprolol in Cardioprotection During an Acute Myocardial Infarction (METOCARD-CNIC) trial. *Circulation* 2013;128:1495–1503.

Design: Multicenter, prospective, randomized, blinded-end point, parallel, stratified study.

Purpose: To evaluate early intravenous β-blocker treatment versus control in STEMI patients undergoing primary PCI. The primary end point was infarct size by MRI.

Population: 270 patients aged 18 or older presenting with anterior STEMI.

Exclusion Criteria: Killip class III or IV, systolic BP <120 mm Hg, heart rate <60 bpm, PR interval >240 ms, and active treatment with a β-blocker.

Treatment: IV metoprolol 5 mg, up to 3 doses, versus control. All patients received oral metoprolol within 24 hours.

Results: Infarct size at 5 to 7 days was 25.6 g in the β-blocker group versus 32 g in the control group ($p - 0.012$). LVEF 1 week after STEMI was also significantly increase by IV metoprolol. MACE rates were similar between the two groups within 24 hours.

Comments: This trial was small, but it essentially evaluated the subset of patients from the COMMIT trial who did not have poor outcomes with beta blockers in that trial, that is, patients with Killip class <III. It does not provide a definitive answer, but it does provide further evidence that in certain STEMI patients without evidence of significant hemodynamic compromise, pre-reperfusion IV metoprolol may reduce infarct size.

ANGIOTENSIN-CONVERTING ENZYME INHIBITORS
Reviews and Meta-Analyses
46. Latini R, et al.; for the Meeting Participants. ACE inhibitor use in patients with myocardial infarction: summary of evidence from clinical trials. *Circulation* 1995;92:3132–3137.

This report is the result of a meeting of experts in Berlin in 1994, which included the investigators from the CONSENSUS, AIRE, SAVE, SOLVD, ISIS-4, GISSI-3, and V-HeFT trials, as well as additional experts. The resulting manuscript reviews the overall data on ACE inhibitors in CAD, with particular focus on acute MI. They support the aggressive use of ACE inhibitors, particularly in the early phase of acute MI and in patients with impaired LV function.

47. ACE Inhibitor MI Collaborative Group. Indications for ACE inhibitors in the early treatment of acute MI: systematic overview of individual data from 100,000 patients in randomized trials. *Circulation* 1998;97:2202–2212.

This meta-analysis was composed of four randomized trials (CONSENSUS II, GISSI-3, ISIS-4, and CCS-1), 98,496 total patients, in which ACE inhibitors were started within 36 hours of AMI. ACE inhibition was associated with a 7% reduction in 30-day mortality (7.1% vs. 7.6%, $p < 0.004$). Most of the benefit was observed within the 1st week of treatment. The greatest mortality benefit was seen in high-risk groups (e.g., anterior MI; Killip class 2 to 3; HR, 100 beats/min at entry). ACE inhibition also was associated with a reduction in nonfatal cardiac failure (14.6% vs. 15.2%, $p = 0.01$) but led to more frequent hypotension (17.6% vs. 9.3%, $p < 0.01$) and renal dysfunction (1.3% vs. 0.6%, $p < 0.01$).

48. Domanski MJ, et al. Effect of angiotensin converting enzyme inhibition on sudden cardiac death in patients following acute MI. *J Am Coll Cardiol* 1999;33:598–604.

The results of this meta-analysis of 15 trials with 15,134 patients suggest that part of the benefit of ACE inhibition in AMI is related to a reduction in risk of sudden cardiac death. The majority of deaths (87%) were cardiovascular, of which 38.2% were deemed sudden cardiac deaths. Overall, ACE inhibitor therapy was associated with significant reductions in overall mortality [OR, 0.83 (95% CI, 0.71 to 0.97)], cardiovascular death [OR, 0.82 (95% CI, 0.69 to 0.97)], and sudden cardiac death [OR, 0.80 (95% CI, 0.70 to 0.92)].

Studies
49. Pfeffer MA, et al.; on behalf of the Survival and Ventricular Enlargement (SAVE) Investigators. Effect of captopril on mortality and morbidity in patients with left ventricular dysfunction after MI. *N Engl J Med* 1992;327:669–677.

Design: Prospective, randomized, double-blind, placebo-controlled, multicenter study. The mean follow-up period was 42 months. The primary end point was all-cause mortality.

Purpose: To determine the effect of captopril on mortality and morbidity when started 3 to 16 days after MI in patients with LV dysfunction.

Population: 2,231 patients aged 21 to 80 years with an EF of 40% or less but no overt heart failure.

Exclusion Criteria: Requirement or contraindication to ACE inhibition, creatinine >2.5 mg/dL, and unstable post-MI course.

Treatment: Captopril initiated 3 to 16 days after MI and titrated from 12.5 mg, three times daily, to 25 mg, three times daily, by hospital discharge (and later 50 mg, three times daily if tolerated) or placebo.

Results: Captopril group had the following risk reductions—19% lower all-cause mortality (20% vs. 25%, $p = 0.019$), 21% lower cardiovascular mortality ($p = 0.014$), 25% fewer recurrent MIs (11.9% vs. 15.2%, $p = 0.015$), and 22% less severe heart failure requiring hospitalization ($p = 0.019$). No difference was observed in deterioration of 9% in EF as measured by repeated radionuclide ventriculography at mean 36 months (13% vs. 16%, $p = 0.17$). Overall, captopril was associated with a 14% reduction in composite ischemic index of recurrent MI, revascularization, and unstable angina ($p = 0.047$).

50. Swedeberg K, et al.; on behalf of the Cooperative New Scandinavian Enalapril Survival Study (CONSENSUS II) Group. Effects of early administration of enalapril on mortality in patients with acute MI. *N Engl J Med* 1992;327:678–684.

Design: Prospective, randomized, double-blind, placebo-controlled, multicenter study. Average follow-up period was 188 days. The primary end point was all-cause mortality rate.

Purpose: To evaluate the effect on mortality of early i.v. administration of enalapril in AMI patients.

Population: 6,090 patients within 24 hours of symptom onset and one of the following—ST elevation in at least two contiguous leads, new Q waves, or elevated serum enzymes.

Exclusion Criteria: Included BP <105/65 mm Hg, history of adverse reaction to or requirement for ACE inhibition, and severe valvular stenosis.

Treatment: Intravenously enalaprilat, 1 mg, over a 2-hour period (stopped if BP decreased below 90/60 mm Hg). Oral enalapril was begun at 6 hours (initial dose, 2.5 mg, and increased up to 20 mg/day) or placebo.

Results: Trial was terminated early by the safety committee. No significant mortality difference was observed at 180 days: 10.2% (placebo) versus 11.0% (enalapril). Enalapril was associated with more frequent hypotension (BP <90/50 mm Hg): 12% versus 3% ($p < 0.001$).

51. Acute Infarction Ramipril Efficacy (AIRE) Study Investigators. Effect of ramipril on mortality and morbidity of survivors of AMI with clinical evidence of heart failure. *Lancet* 1993;342:821–828.

Design: Prospective, randomized, double-blind, parallel-group, placebo-controlled, multicenter study. Average follow-up period was 15 months. The primary end point was all-cause mortality.

Purpose: To evaluate whether ramipril started 3 to 10 days after MI reduces mortality in patients whose course is complicated by heart failure.

Population: 2,006 patients with a definite AMI and clinical evidence of heart failure at any point after MI.

Exclusion Criteria: Heart failure due to valvular disease, unstable angina, contraindications to ACE inhibition, and severe and resistant heart failure.

Treatment: Ramipril, 2.5 mg twice daily for 2 days and then 5 mg twice daily if tolerated.

Results: All-cause mortality was significantly lower in the ramipril group—27% risk reduction (17% vs. 23%, $p = 0.002$). Ramipril patients also had a 30% lower risk of sudden death ($p = 0.011$) and a 19% risk reduction in combined end points consisting of death, severe heart failure, MI, and stroke ($p = 0.008$). No significant difference was observed in reinfarction or stroke rates.

52. GISSI-3. Effects of lisinopril and transdermal glyceryl trinitrate singly and together on 6-week mortality and ventricular function after acute MI. *Lancet* 1994;343:1115–1122.

Design: Prospective, randomized, open-label, 2 × 2 factorial, multicenter study. Primary outcomes were 6-week all-cause mortality and combination of death, heart failure at 5 days after MI, and EF of 35% or less or 45% or more myocardial segments with abnormal motion.

Purpose: To evaluate the effect of lisinopril and nitrates, alone and in combination, on all-cause mortality and LV function after AMI.

Population: 18,895 patients seen within 24 hours with 1 mm or more ST elevation or depression in at least one limb lead or 2 mm or more in at least one precordial lead.

Exclusion Criteria: Severe heart failure, SBP <100 mm Hg, serum creatinine more than 177 μM, and severe comorbidity.

Treatment: (a) Lisinopril, 5 mg in the first 24 hours and then 10 mg once daily for 6 weeks or open control; (b) glyceryl nitrate (GTN), 5 μg/min i.v., and increased by 5 to 20 μg/min or until SBP was lowered by 10%. At 24 hours, transdermal GTN was started (10 mg/day, 14 hours each day) for 6 weeks. If not tolerated, isosorbide mononitrate (50 mg once daily) or open control. Overall, 72% of patients received a thrombolytic agent, 31% were taking a β-blocker, and 84% were taking aspirin.

Results: Overall, 6-week mortality rate was only 6.7%. Lisinopril was associated with significant mortality reduction (6.3% vs. 7.1%; OR, 0.88; $p = 0.03$), with survival curves beginning to diverge on the first day. Reduction also was seen in the combined primary outcome (15.6% vs. 17.0%; OR, 0.90; $p = 0.009$). No difference between lisinopril and controls was observed in recurrent infarction, postinfarct angina, cardiogenic shock, and stroke. No difference in mortality was observed between patients with and without GTN (18.4% vs. 18.9%, $p = 0.39$). Of note, 13.3% of controls received nonstudy ACE inhibitors, and 57.1% received nonstudy nitrates.

Comments: At 6 months, the lisinopril group had fewer deaths and LV dysfunction (18.1% vs. 19.3%, $p = 0.03$). A subgroup analysis showed that lisinopril was more beneficial in diabetic patients (6-week mortality, 8.7% vs. 12.4%; OR, 0.68) than in nondiabetic patients ($p < 0.025$).

53. ISIS-4 Collaborative Group. ISIS-4: a randomised factorial assessing early oral captopril, oral mononitrate and intravenous magnesium sulfate in 58,050 patients with suspected acute MI. *Lancet* 1995;345:669–685.

Design: Prospective, randomized, double-blind, partially placebo-controlled (including captopril arm), multicenter study. The primary end point was 5-week mortality rate.

Purpose: To assess the effects of early initiation of captopril, oral nitrate, and intravenously magnesium on mortality and morbidity in AMI patients.

Population: 58,050 patients with suspected AMI (confirmed in 92%) seen within 24 hours (median, 8 hours) of symptom onset.

Exclusion Criteria (Recommended): Cardiogenic shock, persistent severe hypotension, severe fluid depletion, and negligibly low risk of cardiac death.

Treatment: Captopril arm received 6.25 mg, 12.5 mg 2 hours later, 25 mg at 10 to 12 hours, and then 50 mg twice daily for 28 days or placebo. The isosorbide mononitrate (Imdur) arm received 30 mg, 30 mg 10 to 12 hours later, and 60 mg once daily for 28 days; 70% received thrombolytic therapy, and 94% antiplatelet therapy.

Results: Captopril was associated with a 7% reduction in mortality—7.19% versus 7.69% ($p^2 = 0.02$). The benefit doubled in high-risk groups (prior MI, CHF, anterior ST elevation). More hypotension was seen with captopril, but no increased deaths were seen among patients with low BP (90 to 100 mm Hg). Imdur administration did not have a significant effect on mortality (7.34% vs. 7.54%).

54. Dickstein K, et al.; the OPTIMAAL Steering Committee, for the OPTIMAAL Study Group. Effects of losartan and captopril on mortality and morbidity in high-risk patients after acute myocardial infarction: the OPTIMAAL randomised trial. *Lancet* 2002;360:752–760.

Design: Prospective, randomized, double-blind, multicenter study. The primary end point was all-cause mortality. The mean follow-up was 2.7 years.

Purpose: To determine whether losartan is superior or noninferior to captopril at decreasing all-cause mortality in high-risk patients after AMI.

Population: 5,477 patients enrolled within 10 days of presentation and with (a) AMI and signs or symptoms of heart failure (rales, S_3, treatment with diuretics or vasodilators, persistent sinus tachycardia, or radiographic evidence of heart failure); (b) AMI and EF <35%, or LV end-diastolic diameter (LVEDD) >65 mm; (c) new

Q-wave anterior wall MI; or (d) reinfarction with previous pathologic Q waves in the anterior wall.

Exclusion Criteria: Included SBP <100 mm Hg, current ACE inhibitor or ARB therapy, unstable angina, stenotic valvular heart disease, and planned coronary revascularization.

Treatment: Losartan (target dose, 50 mg orally once daily) or captopril (target dose, 50 mg orally three times each day).

Results: At follow-up, no significant difference in all-cause mortality was found between the two groups (losartan, 18.2%; captopril, 16.4%; $p = 0.069$). The CI boundary (<1.10) showed that losartan did not fulfill criteria for noninferiority. No significant increase in mortality was found in either group when stratified by β-blocker use. The losartan group had a significantly lower CV mortality than did the captopril group (15.3% vs. 13.3%, $p = 0.032$). Losartan was better tolerated than captopril, with 17% discontinuing losartan for any reason compared with 23% with captopril ($p < 0.0001$).

Comments: Data from the RENAAL and LIFE trials suggest that higher doses of losartan may be more beneficial.

55. Pfeffer MA, et al.; for the Valsartan in Acute Myocardial Infarction Trail (VALIANT) Investigators. Valsartan, captopril, or both in myocardial infarction complicated by heart failure, left ventricular dysfunction, or both. N Engl J Med 2003;349:1893–1906.

Design: Prospective, randomized, double-blind, multicenter, international trial. The primary end point was death from any cause at median follow-up of 24.7 months.

Purpose: To compare the efficacy of angiotensin II receptor blockade (with valsartan) versus ACE inhibitor (captopril) or both in patients with acute MI.

Population: 14,703 patients aged 18 or older, with recent MI (0.5 to 10 days prior), and evidence of heart failure clinically or LV systolic dysfunction (EF ≤35% on echo or angiography, ≤40% on radionucleotide scan).

Exclusion Criteria: Previous intolerance to ACE inhibitors or ARBs.

Treatment: Valsartan, valsartan plus captopril (combination), or captopril alone.

Results: Overall mortality at follow-up was similar among the three groups (hazard ratio for valsartan compared to captopril 1.00, 97.5% CI, 0.90 to 1.11; $p = 0.98$; hazard ratio for combination group compared to captopril 0.98, 97.5% CI, 0.89 to 1.09; $p = 0.73$). These comparisons met the prespecified test for noninferiority ($p = 0.004$). The highest rate of drug-related adverse events occurred in the combination-therapy group.

THROMBOLYTIC THERAPY

Review Articles and Meta-Analyses

56. Fibrinolytic Therapy Trialists (FTT) Collaborative Group. Indications for fibrinolytic therapy in suspected acute MI: collaborative overview of early mortality and major morbidity results from all randomised trials of >1000 patients. *Lancet* 1994;343:311–322.

This analysis focused on nine studies (GISSI-1, ISAM, AIMS, ISIS-2 and ISIS-3, ASSET, USIM, EMERAS, and LATE) with more than 1,000 patients (58,600 total). During days 0 and 1, the use of thrombolytics was associated with a higher mortality rate, especially in the elderly and those treated more than 12 hours after symptom onset. However, much greater benefit was seen on days 2 to 35. Thrombolytic-treated patients with ST-segment elevation or BBB had a 3% lower mortality rate when treated from 0 to 6 hours versus 2% lower at 7 to 12 hours and only 1% lower ($p = NS$) at 13 to 18 hours.

57. Boersma E, et al. Early thrombolytic therapy in acute MI: reappraisal of the golden hour. *Lancet* 1996;348:771–775.

This analysis focused on 22 randomized trials enrolling 100 or more patients (total, 50,246 patients). Substantial mortality benefit (6.5% absolute reduction) was seen when a thrombolytic was given within 1 hour of onset of symptoms (vs. 2.6% at 1 to 2 hours, 2.6% at 2 to 3 hours, and 2.9% at 3 to 6 hours). Comparing those treated within 2 hours with those treated after 2 hours, the proportional mortality reduction was −44% versus −20% (p = 0.001). These data fit a nonlinear regression equation (i.e., most benefit early). In contrast, a similar prior analysis by the Fibrinolytic Therapy Trialists (FTT) Collaborative Group had generated a linear model (1.6 additional lives per 1,000 treated patients for each hour of delay). However, their analysis included data from 4,250 patients who had unstable angina (USIM trial) and minimal or no ST elevation (ISIS-3).

58. Eagle KA, et al.; Practice variation and missed opportunities for reperfusion in ST-segment-elevation myocardial infarction: findings from the Global Registry of Acute Coronary Events (GRACE). *Lancet* 2002;359:373–377.

This study assessed current treatment practices of STEMI from prospectively collected data in the multinational (14 countries) Global Registry of Acute Coronary Events. Of 9,251 patients enrolled, 1,763 were seen within 12 hours of symptom onset with STEMI; of these, 30% did not receive reperfusion therapy. Patients less likely to receive reperfusion therapy were elderly patients (aged 75 years or older), those seen without chest pain, and those with a history of diabetes, CHF, MI, or coronary bypass surgery. A substantial percentage of eligible patients failed to receive reperfusion treatment. The United States had the highest rate of primary PCI. The rate at sites with a catheterization laboratory was only 19%.

59. de Belder MA. Acute myocardial infarction: failed thrombolysis. *Heart* 2001;85:104–112.

This review highlights the risk of failed thrombolysis in acute MI—the incidence, potential mechanisms, and means of diagnosis. It finishes with a discussion of potential management options.

60. Llevadot J, et al. Bolus fibrinolytic therapy in acute myocardial infarction. *JAMA* 2001;286:442–449.

The authors review studies that evaluated the fibrinolytic agents, reteplase, lanoteplase, and TNK; specifically, they assessed pharmacokinetics and pharmacodynamics, as well as angiographic and clinical outcomes. They found an overall similarity in rates of efficacy and mortality among the four agents (they compared all three to tPA). However, lanoteplase and heparin bolus plus infusion increased the rate of intracranial hemorrhage significantly.

Thrombolytic Comparative Studies
61. TIMI-I, The thrombolysis in MI (TIMI) trial. Phase I findings. *N Engl J Med* 1985;312:932–936.

Design: Prospective, randomized, double-blind, placebo-controlled, multicenter study. The primary end point was IRA patency at 90 minutes.

Purpose: To evaluate the efficacy of intravenously administered thrombolytic therapy and to compare the effects of tPA and SK.

Population: 316 patients younger than 76 years seen 7 hours or less from onset of symptoms with chest pain lasting 30 minutes or longer and ST-segment elevation in at least two ECG leads.

Treatment: SK, 1.5 million U over a 60-minute period and a 3-hour infusion of tPA placebo, or a 3-hour infusion of plasminogen activator [80 mg (40 mg in the 1st hour and then 20 mg for 2 hours)] and a 1-hour infusion of SK placebo.

Results: The 290 patients received treatment; 26 had a <50% reduction in the diameter of the IRA not treated. Among the 214 patients with total baseline occlusion, tPA achieved better reperfusion at 90 minutes: 60% versus 35% (TIMI grade 2 or 3 flow; $p < 0.001$). No significant differences in rates of bleeding events were observed.

62. Gruppo Italiano per lo Studio della Streptochinasi nell'Infarto Miocardico (GISSI-2). GISSI-2: a factorial randomised trial of alteplase vs. streptokinase and heparin vs. no heparin among 12,490 patients with acute MI. *Lancet* 1990;336:65–71.

Design: Prospective, randomized, open, parallel-group, 2×2 factorial, multicenter study. The primary end points were death, clinical heart failure, and EF of 35% or less.

Purpose: To compare the efficacy of i.v. SK and tPA for the treatment of suspected acute STEMI and to study the effects of heparin on the incidence of recurrent ischemia.

Population: 12,490 patients seen within 6 hours of onset of symptoms with chest pain and 1 mm or more ST elevation in any limb lead or 2 mm or more in any precordial lead.

Treatment: (a) SK, 1.5 million U over a 30- to 60-minute period, and heparin, 12,500 U s.c. twice daily (starting 12 hours after initiation of the thrombolytic and continued through hospital discharge); (b) tPA, 10-mg bolus, then 50 mg over 1 hour, and then 40 mg over 2 hours, and heparin, 12,500 U s.c. twice daily; (c) SK, 1.5 million U over 30 to 60 minutes without heparin; or (d) tPA, 10-mg bolus, then 50 mg over 1 hour, and then 40 mg over 2 hours without heparin.

Results: No significant difference was observed in combined end points between SK and tPA [22.5% vs. 23.1% (mortality, 8.6% vs. 9.0%)]. No difference was observed in the rates of recurrent infarction, postinfarction angina, stroke, or bleeding. No differences were observed between heparin and no heparin, except for increased bleeding with heparin (1.0% vs. 0.6%; RR, 1.64; 95% CI, 1.09 to 2.45).

63. ISIS-3 Collaborative Group. A randomised comparison of streptokinase versus tissue plasminogen activator versus anistreplase and of aspirin and heparin versus aspirin alone among 41,299 cases of suspected acute MI. *Lancet* 1992;339:753–770.

Design: Prospective, randomized, double-blind (thrombolytic agents) and open-label (heparin), 3×2 factorial, multicenter study. The primary end point was 35-day mortality rate.

Purpose: To compare the effects on mortality of tPA, SK, and acylated plasminogen–streptokinase activator complex (APSAC) and to compare aspirin alone with aspirin plus s.c. administered heparin.

Population: 41,299 patients with suspected MI seen within 24 hours of onset of symptoms (no ECG criteria).

Exclusion Criteria (Suggested): Recent severe trauma, stroke, GI bleeding or ulcer, and SK allergy.

Treatment: (a) SK, 1.5 million U over 60 minutes; (b) rtPA, 0.6 million U/kg over 4 hours (0.04 million U/kg as a bolus, 0.36 million U/kg over 1 hour, and then 0.067 million U/kg/h for 3 hours); or (c) APSAC 30 U over 3 minutes. All patients received aspirin (162.5 mg daily), and half of the patients also received heparin, 12,500 U twice daily s.c. for 7 days (started 4 hours after initiation of thrombolytic therapy).

Results: No differences in 35-day mortality rate were seen between the three thrombolytic groups—SK, 10.6%; tPA, 10.3%; and APSAC, 10.5%. The SK group did have fewer strokes (1.04% vs. 1.39% for tPA, $p < 0.01$), whereas tPA was associated with fewer reinfarctions [2.9% vs. 3.5% (SK)]. A trend toward a lower mortality difference was seen with heparin while it was being administered [7-day mortality rate, 7.4% vs. 7.9% (aspirin alone), $p = 0.06$], but this disappeared at 35-day and 6-month follow-ups. Heparin was associated with an excess of major noncerebral and cerebral hemorrhages (1.0% vs. 0.8%, $p < 0.01$; 0.56% vs. 0.40%, $p < 0.05$), but no difference was seen in the total stroke rate (1.28% vs. 1.18%).

Comments: No difference in mortality seen with tPA and SK, but questions remained because of the suboptimal heparin regimen (i.e., delayed and subcutaneous).

64. GUSTO I. The Global Utilization of Streptokinase and tPA for Occluded Coronary Arteries Study (GUSTO) Investigators. An international randomized trial comparing four thrombolytic strategies for acute MI. *N Engl J Med* 1993;329:673–682.

Design: Prospective, randomized, open-label, multicenter study. The primary end point was 30-day all-cause mortality rate.

Purpose: To compare the effects of four thrombolytic regimens using SK and/or tPA.

Population: 41,021 patients seen <6 hours from onset of symptoms with chest pain lasting more than 20 minutes and ST elevation 1 mm or more in at least two limb leads or 2 mm or more in at least two precordial leads.

Exclusion Criteria: Prior stroke, active bleeding, prior treatment with SK or anistreplase, and recent trauma or major surgery; relative contraindication was SBP 180 or greater unresponsive to therapy.

Treatment: (a) SK, 1.5 million U over 60 minutes, with s.c. heparin, 12,500 U twice daily; (b) SK, 1.5 million U over 60 minutes and i.v. heparin (5,000-U bolus and then 1,000 U/h); (c) accelerated tPA [15-mg bolus, then 0.75 mg/kg (maximum, 50 mg) over 30 minutes, and then 0.5 mg/kg (maximum, 35 mg) over 60 minutes] with i.v. heparin (5,000-U bolus and then 1,000 U/h); or (d) tPA, 1.0 mg/kg over 60 minutes (10% given as a bolus; maximum dose, 90 mg), and SK, 1 million U over 60 minutes with i.v. heparin (5,000-U bolus and then 1,000 U/h).

Results: Accelerated tPA with i.v. heparin (c) was associated with the lowest 30-day mortality rate—6.3% (vs. 7.2%, 7.4%, and 7.0% for regimens a, b, and c), which corresponds to a 14% reduction compared with the SK-only regimens ($p = 0.001$). Despite an increased intracranial hemorrhage risk seen with tPA (0.72% vs. 0.49%, 0.54%, and 94%), tPA still was associated with a significant reduction in the combined end point of death or disabling stroke (6.9% vs. 7.8% in SK-only groups; $p = 0.006$). tPA appeared to confer a greater benefit in patients with anterior MI (8.6% vs. 10.5% mortality). A mortality benefit similar to that of tPA overall was seen in patients older than 75 years (1.3% vs. 1.1%), although limited numbers prevented the subgroup analysis from having the power to achieve statistical significance.

Comments: The mortality rate was only 4.3% in patients treated within 2 hours versus 5.5% at 2 to 4 hours and 8.9% at 4 to 6 hours. Thus, time to therapy also is an important factor. A secondary analysis showed age to be a powerful mortality predictor: 3% if younger than 65 years old versus 9.5%, 19.6%, and 30.3% if 65 to 74, 75 to 85, and older than 85 years, respectively. One-year follow-up showed a persistent benefit of tPA with an increase in mortality of only 1.4% from 30 days to 1 year. Another secondary analysis showed the optimal PTT range to be 50 to 70 seconds (lowest 30-day mortality, stroke, and bleeding rates) with a clustering of reinfarctions in the first 10 hours after discontinuation of heparin. Finally, a cost-effectiveness analysis showed that tPA costs $32,678 per year of life saved.

65. The GUSTO Angiographic Investigators. The effects of tissue plasminogen activator, streptokinase, or both on coronary artery patency, ventricular function and survival after acute MI. *N Engl J Med* 1993;329:1615–1622.

Design: Prospective, randomized, open-label, multicenter study. The primary end point was TIMI grade 2 or 3 flow at 90 minutes.

Purpose: To compare the patency rates and the effect on LV function of tPA and SK.

Population: 2,431 patients seen <6 hours from onset of symptoms with chest pain lasting more than 20 minutes and ST elevation 1 mm or more in at least two limb leads or 2 mm or more in at least two precordial leads.

Exclusion Criteria: See GUSTO-I trial summary.

Treatment: Four thrombolytic regimens (see GUSTO-I trial summary). Patients were then randomized to cardiac catheterization at 90 minutes, 180 minutes, 24 hours, or 5 to 7 days. The 90-minute group underwent repeated catheterization at 5 to 7 days.

Results: The highest patency (TIMI grade 2 or 3 flow) at 90 minutes was seen with tPA and intravenous heparin—81% versus 54% with SK and s.c. heparin, 60% with SK and i.v. heparin, and 73% with combination therapy ($p < 0.001$ for tPA vs. SK groups). Normal flow (TIMI grade 3) was seen in 54% of the tPA patients versus 29%, 32%, and 38% in the other three groups. Surprisingly, the differences between the tPA and SK groups disappeared at 180 minutes. The reocclusion rate was low and similar in all four groups (4.9% to 6.4%). LV function paralleled patency at 90 minutes, with the tPA group having better regional wall motion. Mortality also was strongly correlated with 90-minute patency: a low 4.4% with TIMI grade 3 flow versus 8.9% with grade 1 flow ($p = 0.009$).

Comments: Results support the open-artery theory asserting that early reperfusion of the IRA results in improved outcome (see accompanying editorial). A subsequent analysis of the 559 patients who underwent catheterization twice (at 90 minutes and 5 to 7 days) showed that early patency results were not predictive of reocclusion. Another analysis showed that the mortality benefit of achieving 90-minute TIMI grade 3 flow was amplified beyond the initial 30 days: unadjusted mortality hazard ratio (TIMI grade 3 vs. 2 or less) from 30 to 688 days was only 0.39 (vs. 0.57 at 30 days).

66. Cannon CP, et al. TIMI-4. Comparison of front-loaded recombinant tissue plasminogen activator, anistreplase and combination thrombolytic therapy for acute MI. J Am Coll Cardiol 1994;24:1602–1610.

This prospective, double-blind, multicenter study randomized 382 patients seen within 6 hours of symptom onset to front-loaded rtPA [15-mg bolus, then 0.75 mg/kg (maximum, 50 mg) over a 30-minute period, and then 0.50 mg/kg (maximum, 35 mg) over a 30-minute period]; anistreplase, 30-U bolus over 2 to 5 minutes; or rtPA [15-mg bolus and then 0.75 mg/kg (maximum, 50 mg) over 30 minutes] and anistreplase, 20-U bolus. All received i.v. heparin and aspirin. The rtPA group had higher patency (TIMI grade 2 or 3 flow) at 60 minutes: 78% versus 59% for two other groups ($p = 0.02$). Similar results were observed at 90 minutes [TIMI grade 3 flow in 60%, 43% (anistreplase only), and 44% (combination)]. No significant differences were seen in the composite primary end point, consisting of in-hospital death, severe CHF or cardiogenic shock, low EF, reinfarction, TIMI grade flow <2 at 90 minutes or 18 to 36 hours, reocclusion (on sestamibi imaging), major spontaneous hemorrhage, and severe anaphylaxis (rtPA, 41.3%; anistreplase, 49%; combination, 53.6%). However, the 6-week mortality rate was the lowest in the rtPA group: 2.2% versus 8.8% with anistreplase ($p = 0.02$) and 7.2% with combination therapy ($p = 0.06$).

67. International Joint Efficacy Comparison of Thrombolytics (INJECT). Randomized, double-blind comparison of reteplase double-bolus administration with streptokinase in acute MI: trial to investigate equivalence. Lancet 1995;346:329–336.

Design: Prospective, randomized, double-blind, double-dummy, multicenter study. The primary end point was 35-day mortality rate.

Purpose: To determine whether the effect of reteplase on 35-day mortality is at least equivalent to that of SK.

Population: 6,010 patients seen within 12 hours of onset of symptoms with chest pain lasting 30 minutes or longer and ST elevation 1 mm or more in at least two of the three inferior leads or leads I and aVL, 2 mm or more in at least two contiguous precordial leads, or new LBBB.

Treatment: SK, 1.5 million U over a 60-minute period, or reteplase, 10 million U bolus, and repeated 30 minutes later. All patients received heparin for 24 hours.

Results: The 35-day mortality rates were similar—9.0% (reteplase) and 9.5% (SK). Results show that reteplase is at least as effective as SK. Reinfarction and bleeding rates also were similar (5.0% vs. 5.4%; 0.7% vs. 1.0%), whereas the reteplase group had less atrial fibrillation (7.2% vs. 8.8%, $p < 0.05$), cardiogenic shock (4.7% vs. 6.0%, $p < 0.05$), heart failure (23.6% vs. 26.3%, $p < 0.05$), and hypotension (15.5% vs. 17.6%, $p < 0.05$).

68. Bode C, et al.; for the RAPID II Investigators. Randomized comparison of coronary thrombolysis achieved with double-bolus reteplase (recombinant plasminogen activator) and front-loaded, accelerated alteplase (recombinant tissue plasminogen activator) in patients with acute MI. *Circulation* 1996;94:891–898.

Design: Prospective, randomized, open-label, parallel-group, multicenter study.

Purpose: To compare the bolus-administered thrombolytic reteplase with an accelerated infusion of alteplase on infarct-related patency and major events.

Population: 324 patients aged 18 to 75 years seen within 12 hours (from onset of symptoms to planned administration of treatment) with chest pain lasting 30 minutes or longer and ST elevation 1 mm or more in at least two of the three inferior leads or lateral leads or 2 mm or more in at least two contiguous leads, or LBBB.

Treatment: Reteplase, 10 million U, over 2 to 3 minutes, and then 10 million U repeated 30 minutes later, or front-loaded alteplase. All patients received aspirin and i.v. heparin.

Results: The reteplase group had better TIMI grade 3 flow at 90 minutes (60% vs. 45%, $p = 0.01$) and 51% fewer coronary interventions (13.6% vs. 26.5%, $p < 0.01$); a >50% statistically nonsignificant mortality reduction (4.1% vs. 8.4%) also was observed, as were similar rates of transfusion, hemorrhage, and stroke.

69. GUSTO III Investigators. A comparison of reteplase with alteplase for acute MI. *N Engl J Med* 1997;337:1118–1123 (editorial, 1159–1161).

Design: Prospective, randomized (2:1), open-label, parallel-group, multicenter study. The primary end point was 30-day mortality rate.

Purpose: To determine whether reteplase is superior to alteplase in reducing mortality in AMI.

Population: 15,059 patients seen with 30 minutes or more of continuous symptoms and within 6 hours of their onset and 1 mm or more ST elevation in at least two limb leads or 2 mm or more in precordial leads, or BBB.

Exclusion Criteria: Active bleeding, history of stroke, recent major surgery, SBP 200 mm Hg or higher or DBP 110 mm Hg or higher, and requirement for oral anticoagulation.

Treatment: Reteplase given as two 10 million U boluses 30 minutes apart or an accelerated infusion of alteplase [15-mg bolus, then 0.75 mg/kg (maximum, 50 mg) over a 30-minute period, and then 0.50 mg/kg (maximum, 35 mg) over 60 minutes].

Results: Reteplase and alteplase groups had similar 30-day mortality rates: 7.47% versus 7.24% ($p = 0.54$; 95% CI for absolute difference in mortality rates was −1.1% to 0.66%). Stroke rate and combined end points of death or nonfatal, disabling stroke were both similar (1.64% vs. 1.79%; 7.89% vs. 7.91%).

Comments: Although this trial was designed as a superiority trial, the accompanying editorial points out that these results do not demonstrate equivalence according to the GUSTO trial margin of benefit. Nonetheless, clinical equivalence of reteplase was observed in this large trial.

70. Cannon CP, et al.; for the TIMI-10B Investigators. TNK-tissue plasminogen activator compared with front-loaded alteplase in acute MI. *Circulation* **1998;98:2805–2814.**

This prospective, randomized, multicenter trial was composed of 886 acute STEMI patients seen within 12 hours of onset of symptoms. Patients received TNK, 30 or 50 mg, or front-loaded tPA. All patients underwent immediate angiography. The 50-mg dose of TNK was discontinued early because of an increased rate of intracranial hemorrhage and was replaced by a 40-mg dose and heparin doses were decreased. TNK, 40 mg, and tPA produced similar rates of TIMI grade 3 flow at 90 minutes (62.8% vs. 62.7%; p = NS; TNK, 30 mg; 54.3%; p = 0.035). TNK doses of 0.5 mg/kg resulted in higher TIMI grade 3 flow and lower median CTFCs (i.e., faster flow) than did lower doses. Lower rates of major bleeding and intracranial hemorrhage were observed after the heparin doses were lowered and titration of heparin was begun at 6 hours.

71. Assessment of the Safety and Efficacy of a New Thrombolytic: TNK-tPA (ASSENT-2). Single-bolus tenecteplase compared with front-loaded alteplase in acute MI: the ASSENT-2 double-blind randomized trial. *Lancet* **1999;354:716–722.**

Design: Prospective, randomized, open-label, multicenter study. The primary end point was all-cause mortality at 30 days.

Purpose: To assess the efficacy and safety of TNK compared with alteplase (tPA).

Population: 16,949 patients seen within 6 hours of symptom onset with ST-segment elevations of 1 mm or more in two or more limb leads or 2 mm or more in two or more contiguous precordial leads or new LBBB.

Treatment: TNK administered over 5 to 10 seconds (30 mg if >60 kg; 35 mg if 60 to 60.9 kg; 40 mg if 70 to 79.9 kg; 45 mg if 80 to 89.9 kg; 50 mg if 90 kg or more) or accelerated infusion of tPA over a 90-minute period (100 mg or less).

Results: All-cause mortality rate at 30 days was nearly identical in the two groups: 6.18% (TNK) and 6.15% (tPA). Intracranial hemorrhage rates also were similar [0.43% (TNK), 0.44% (tPA)], but fewer noncerebral bleeding complications (26.4% vs. 29.0%, p = 0.0003) and less need for blood transfusion (4.3% vs. 5.5%, p = 0.0002) were observed with TNK. Subgroup analysis showed that the mortality rate among patients treated more than 4 hours after the onset of symptoms was significantly lower with TNK (7.1% vs. 9.2%, p = 0.018). This finding may be owing to the increased fibrin specificity of TNK.

72. The Assessment of the Safety and Efficacy of a New Thrombolytic Regimen (ASSENT-3) Investigators. Efficacy and safety of tenecteplase in combination with enoxaparin, abciximab, or unfractionated heparin: the ASSENT-3 randomized trial in acute myocardial infarction. *Lancet* **2001;358:605–613.**

Design: Prospective, randomized, open-label, multicenter trial. Primary composite end point at 30 days: death, in-hospital MI, or in-hospital refractory ischemia.

Purpose: To evaluate whether the combination of TNK plus enoxaparin or abciximab is safe and efficacious compared with TNK and UFH in AMI patients.

Population: 6,095 AMI patients seen within 6 hours of symptom onset.

Treatment: Three groups: (a) full-dose TNK and enoxaparin for a maximum of 7 days, (b) half-dose TNK with weight-adjusted low-dose UFH and a 12-hour infusion of abciximab, or (c) full-dose TNK with weight-adjusted UFH for 48 hours.

Results: The enoxaparin and abciximab groups had a lower incidence of the primary efficacy end point compared with the UFH group (11.4% and 11.1% vs. 15.4%, respectively; RR, 0.74 and 0.72; both p < 0.001). Similarly, the efficacy plus safety end point (in-hospital intracranial hemorrhage or in-hospital major bleeding complications) was significantly lower for the enoxaparin group [13.7% vs. 17.0% (UFH), p = 0.0146] and trended to be lower in the abciximab group (14.2% vs. 17.0%, $p = 0.057$). Among patients older than 75 years, the incidence of efficacy or safety events was *higher* in the abciximab group compared with the UFH group (36.9% vs. 28.0%, $p = 0.001$); a similar finding was seen among diabetic patients (22.3% vs. 16.5%, $p = 0.0007$). Overall, the abciximab group had nearly twice the risk of major hemorrhage compared with the UFH group (4.3% vs. 2.2%; $p = 0.0002$; enoxaparin group, 3.0%; $p = $ NS vs. UFH).

73. GISSI-1. Effectiveness of intravenous thrombolytic treatment in acute MI. *Lancet* 1986;327:397–401.

Design: Prospective, randomized, open, parallel-group, multicenter study. The primary end point was 21-day mortality rate.

Purpose: To evaluate the safety and efficacy of i.v. SK in AMI and to determine whether any effect is dependent on the interval between onset of pain and treatment.

Population: 11,806 patients seen within 12 hours of onset of symptoms with chest pain and ST elevation or depression 1 mm or more in any limb lead or 2 mm or more in any precordial lead.

Treatment: SK, 1.5 million U over a 60-minute period.

Results: SK-treated patients had a 21-day mortality rate that was 18% lower than that of controls (10.7% vs. 13.0%, $p = 0.0002$). The largest mortality advantage [23% ($p = 0.0005$)] was associated with administration to those seen within 3 hours of onset of symptoms (RR, 0.74 vs. 1.19 for 9 to 12 hours). At 1 year, the mortality benefit persisted (17.2% vs. 19.0%, $p = 0.0008$).

Comments: The 10-year follow-up showed that the mortality benefit was still significant, with 19 lives saved/1,000 patients ($p = 0.02$).

74. ISIS-2 Collaborative Group. Randomised trial of intravenous streptokinase, oral, both, or neither among 17,187 cases of suspected acute MI. *Lancet* 1988;332:349–360.

Design: Prospective, randomized, double-blind, placebo-controlled, multicenter study. The primary end point was vascular mortality.

Purpose: To assess the separate and combined effects on mortality of i.v. SK and oral aspirin in patients with suspected AMI.

Population: 17,187 patients with suspected MI seen within 24 hours (median, 5 hours) of onset of symptoms.

Exclusion Criteria: Any history of stroke, GI hemorrhage, or ulcer. Possible contraindications included recent trauma, severe persistent hypertension (not defined), and allergy to SK or aspirin.

Treatment: SK, 1.5 million U over a 60-minute period, and/or aspirin, 162.5 mg daily; or placebo.

Results: SK and aspirin-alone groups had 25% and 23% lower 5-week vascular mortality rates, respectively [9.2% vs. 12.0% (placebo), $p < 0.00001$; 9.4% vs. 11.8%, $p < 0.00001$]. The SK-and-aspirin group had an even larger 42% mortality reduction (8% vs. 13.2%). Combination therapy also was effective in patients with LBBB (mortality, 14% vs. 27.7%). SK was associated with hypotension in 10% and more bleeds requiring transfusion (0.5% vs. 0.2%) but fewer strokes (0.6% vs. 0.8%). Aspirin reduced nonfatal reinfarction and stroke rates (1.0% vs. 2.0%; 0.3% vs. 0.6%).

75. Wilcox RG, et al.; Anglo-Scandinavian Study of Early Thrombolysis (ASSET). Trial of tissue plasminogen activator for mortality reduction in acute MI. *Lancet* 1988;332:525–530.

Design: Prospective, randomized, double-blind, placebo-controlled, multicenter study. The primary end point was mortality at 1 month.

Purpose: To evaluate the effects of tPA on mortality after AMI.

Population: 5,013 patients aged 18 to 75 years with suspected AMI who were treated within 5 hours of onset of symptoms.

Treatment: tPA, 10-mg bolus, followed by 50 mg over a 1-hour period, and then 20 mg/h for 2 hours (100 mg total), or placebo.

Results: The tPA group had a 26% lower 1-month mortality rate—7.2% versus 9.8% [26% hazard ratio (95% CI, 11% to 39%)]. This benefit persisted at 6 months: 10.4% versus 13.1%. Among patients with proven MI, the mortality difference was more impressive: 12.6% versus 17.1%. The tPA group had more bleeding and more frequent bradycardia (27 patients vs. 5 patients).

76. The European MI Project (EMIP) Group. Prehospital thrombolytic therapy in patients with suspected MI. N *Engl J Med* 1993;329:383–389.

Prospective, randomized, double-blind, crossover, multicenter study of 5,469 patients seen within 6 hours with 1 mm or greater ST elevation in two or more limb leads or 2 mm or more in two or more precordial leads. Patients received anistreplase, 30 U, before hospitalization, followed by placebo in hospital or placebo followed by anistreplase. Trial was terminated early because of failure to reach target of 10,000 patients in a 2-year period. Patients in the prehospital group received anistreplase 55 minutes earlier on average than did those in the hospital group. Prehospital anistreplase was associated with a nonsignificant 13% overall mortality reduction (9.7% vs. 11.1%, $p = 0.08$) and a significant 16% cardiac mortality reduction (8.3% vs. 9.8%, $p = 0.049$). More adverse events [VF ($p = 0.02$), shock ($p < 0.001$), symptomatic hypotension ($p < 0.001$), bradycardia ($p = 0.001$)] occurred in the prehospital group before hospitalization, but this was offset by a higher incidence during the hospital period in the hospital group.

77. Late Assessment of Thrombolytic Efficacy (LATE) Study Group. Late assessment of thrombolytic efficacy study with alteplase 6–24 hours after onset of MI. *Lancet* 1993;342:759–766.

Design: Prospective, randomized, double-blind, placebo-controlled, multicenter study. The primary end point was 35-day mortality rate.

Purpose: To compare administration of alteplase with placebo in AMI patients seen at 6 to 24 hours.

Population: 5,711 patients seen 6 to 24 hours after onset of symptoms with 1 mm or more ST elevation in at least two limb leads, 2 mm or more ST elevation in at least two precordial leads, ST depression 2 mm or more in at least two leads, pathologic Q waves, or abnormal T-wave inversion in at least two leads thought to represent a non-Q wave infarct.

Treatment: Alteplase, 100 mg over a 3-hour period (10-mg bolus, 50 mg for 1 hour, 20 mg/h for 2 hours), or placebo.

Results: Intention-to-treat analysis showed a nonsignificant 14% 35-day mortality reduction in the alteplase group (8.9% vs. 10.3%). However, prespecified survival analysis according to treatment within 12 hours showed that the alteplase group had a 25.6% mortality reduction (8.9% vs. 11.9%, $p = 0.023$). Treatment for 12 to 24 hours was associated with a nonsignificant 5% mortality reduction (8.7% vs. 9.2%). Alteplase was not associated with a higher cardiac rupture rate, but rather earlier occurrence of rupture (within 24 hours after thrombolysis).

Prehospital Thrombolysis Studies

78. Weaver WD, et al.; MI Triage and Intervention (MITI). Pre-hospital versus hospital-initiated thrombolytic therapy. JAMA 1993;270:1211–1216.

Design: Prospective, randomized, open, parallel-group study. The primary end point was a composite score that combined death, stroke, major bleeding, and infarct size.

Purpose: To compare prehospital and hospital initiation of thrombolytic therapy in patients with chest pain and ST-segment elevation.

Population: 360 patients aged 75 years or younger seen within 6 hours of onset of symptoms with ST elevation.

Exclusion Criteria: History of stroke, recent bleeding or surgery, and SBP <180 mm Hg or DBP >120 mm Hg.

Treatment: Prehospital or hospital administration of alteplase (100 mg over a 3-hour period) plus aspirin (325 mg).

Results: Despite earlier time to treatment in the prehospital-initiated group (77 minutes vs. 110 minutes), no significant differences were seen in primary composite end point score ($p = 0.64$), mortality rate (5.7% vs. 8.1%, $p = 0.49$), EF, or infarct size. A secondary analysis showed that when treatment was initiated at sooner than 70 minutes, prehospital therapy was associated with a lower mortality rate (1.2% vs. 8.7%) and better EF (53% vs. 49%, $p = 0.03$). However, at 2-year follow-up, the mortality benefit in this subgroup was no longer statistically significant [2% (<70 minutes) vs. 12%, $p = 0.12$].

79. Rawles J, et al.; on behalf of the Grampian Region Early Anistreplase Trial (GREAT) Group. Halving of mortality at one year by domiciliary thrombolysis in the GREAT. *J Am Coll Cardiol* 1994;23:1–5.

Design: Prospective, randomized, double-blind, parallel-group, multicenter study.

Purpose: To evaluate the feasibility, safety, and efficacy of home-administered thrombolysis by general practitioners compared with hospital thrombolysis.

Population: 311 patients with suspected MI seen by their general practitioners within 4 hours of symptom onset (ECG recordings required but not reported).

Treatment: Anistreplase, 30 U, at home or in hospital.

Results: Home-administered anistreplase was given more than 2 hours sooner, at a median 101 minutes versus 240 minutes. The home-treated group had a 52% lower 1-year mortality rate (10.4% vs. 21.6%, $p = 0.007$).

80. Morrow DA, et al. Evaluation of the time saved by prehospital initiation of reteplase for ST-elevation myocardial infarction: results of the Early Retavase-Thrombolysis in Myocardial Infarction (ER-TIMI 19) trial. *J Am Coll Cardiol* 2002;40:71–77.

Design: Prospective, randomized, controlled, open, multicenter trial. Time from EMS arrival to fibrinolytic administration was compared between study patients receiving prehospital rPA and sequential control patients from 6 to 12 months before the study who received a fibrinolytic in the hospital.

Purpose: To test the feasibility of prehospital initiation of the bolus fibrinolytic reteplase and determine the time saved by prehospital rPA in the setting of contemporary emergency cardiac care.

Population: 315 patients with STEMI at 20 North American emergency medical systems; 630 controls were treated in-hospital with fibrinolytic therapy.

Treatment: Prehospital administration of reteplase (10 U over a 2-minute period followed by second bolus 30 minutes later, either in ambulance or in ED). All received aspirin and i.v. UFH [60-U/kg bolus (maximum, 4,000 U) and then 12 U/kg/h (maximum, 800 U/h)].

Results: AMI was verified in 98%. The median time from EMS arrival to initiation of reteplase was 31 minutes. The time from EMS arrival to in-hospital fibrinolytic for 630 control patients was 63 minutes, resulting in a time saved of 32 minutes ($p < 0.0001$).

By 30 minutes after first medical contact, 49% of study patients had received the first bolus of fibrinolytic compared with only 5% of controls ($p < 0.0001$). In-hospital mortality was 4.7%. Intracranial hemorrhage occurred in 1.0%.

PERCUTANEOUS CORONARY INTERVENTION

Reviews

81. Keeley EC, et al. Primary PCI for myocardial infarction with ST-segment elevation. N Engl J Med 2007;356:47–54.

The authors present a case vignette and then review the pathophysiology and treatment effect for primary PCI in STEMI. They discuss the clinical evidence for such a strategy, indications for PCI versus fibrinolysis, as well as potential adverse events. The manuscript concludes with a discussion of still uncertain areas, as well as a review of the current guidelines.

82. Nallamothu BK, et al. Time to treatment in primary percutaneous coronary intervention. N Engl J Med 2007;357:1631–1638.

In light of guidelines to reduce door-to-balloon times, the authors review the pathophysiology of MI, use of fibrinolysis, as well as primary PCI. The evidence and rationale behind expediting reperfusion time is discussed, as well as guidance on selecting the most appropriate reperfusion strategy. Helpful strategies for reducing door-to-balloon times are presented, and the manuscript concludes with future challenges to meeting such goals and improving care.

Meta-Analyses

83. Weaver WD, et al. Comparison of primary coronary angioplasty and intravenous thrombolytic therapy for acute MI: a quantitative review. JAMA 1997;278:2093–2098.

Data analysis from 10 randomized trials with a total of 2,606 patients. Mortality at 30 days or less was significantly lower in patients treated with primary PTCA compared with thrombolysis (4.4% vs. 6.5%; OR, 0.66; 95% CI, 0.46 to 0.94; $p = 0.02$). Primary PTCA also was associated with lower rates of reinfarction [7.2% vs. 11.9% or 0.58% (95% CI, 0.44 to 0.75), $p < 0.001$]. Authors point out that the primary angioplasty results were primarily achieved in specialized, high-volume centers.

84. Keeley EC, et al. Primary angioplasty versus intravenous thrombolytic therapy for acute myocardial infarction: a quantitative review of 23 randomised trials. Lancet 2003;361:13–20.

This analysis identified 23 studies with a total of 7,739 patients. SK was used in 8 trials ($n = 1,837$), and fibrin-specific agents in 15 ($n = 5,902$). Stents were used in 12 trials. Primary PTCA had lower short-term mortality compared with thrombolytic therapy (7% vs. 9%, $p = 0.0002$), nonfatal MI (3% vs. 7%, $p < 0.0001$), and stroke (1% vs. 2%, $p = 0.0004$). Results with primary PTCA remained better during long-term follow-up.

85. Dalby M, et al. Transfer for primary angioplasty versus immediate thrombolysis in acute myocardial infarction: a meta-analysis. Circulation 2003;108:1809–1814.

To further identify the best strategy for patients with acute MI presenting to hospitals without catheterization services, the authors analyzed six trials including 3,750 patients comparing immediate thrombolysis with transfer for primary PCI (within 3 hours). For the combined primary end point of death, reinfarction, or stroke, there was a significant 42% reduction ($p < 0.001$) in the group transferred for primary PCI, compared with immediate thrombolysis. This was primarily driven by significant reductions in reinfarction (68%, $p < 0.001$) and stroke (56%, $p = 0.015$), with a nonsignificant trend for overall mortality favoring PCI (19% reduction, $p = 0.08$).

86. Keeley EC, et al. Comparison of primary and facilitated percutaneous coronary interventions for ST-elevation myocardial infarction: quantitative review of randomised trials. *Lancet* 2006;367:579–588.

The authors identified 17 trials of facilitated versus primary PCI for STEMI, including a total of 4,504 patients. The primary end points were short-term outcomes of death, stroke, reinfarction, urgent TVR, and major bleeding at 6 weeks. While early TIMI grade 3 flow favored the facilitated approach (37% vs. 15%; OR, 3.18; 95% CI, 2.22 to 4.55), final TIMI grade 3 flow rates were similar (89% vs. 88%; OR, 1.19; 95% CI, 0.86 to 1.64). However, worse outcomes in the facilitated PCI group were observed for death (5% vs. 3%; OR, 1.38; 95% CI, 1.01 to 1.87), reinfarction (3% vs. 2%; OR, 1.71; 95% CI, 1.16 to 2.51), and urgent TVR (4% vs. 1%; OR, 2.39; 95% CI, 1.23 to 4.66), as well as major bleeding (7% vs. 5%; OR, 1.51; 95% CI, 1.10 to 2.08). The authors note that the majority of adverse events were observed in the thrombolytic-based facilitated PCI groups.

87. Wijeysundera HC, et al. Rescue angioplasty or repeat fibrinolysis after failed fibrinolytic therapy for ST-segment myocardial infarction: a meta-analysis of randomized trials. *J Am Coll Cardiol* 2007;49:422–430.

The authors compiled results from eight trials of 1,177 patients randomized to rescue PCI or conservative therapy, with follow-up data to 6 months. Though they found no difference in overall mortality with rescue PCI (RR, 0.69; 95% CI, 0.46 to 1.05), there were significant reductions in heart failure (RR, 0.73; 95% CI, 0.54 to 1.00) and reinfarction (0.58; 95% CI, 0.35 to 0.97) when rescue PCI was compared to conservative therapy. However, there were increased rates of stroke (RR, 4.98; 95% CI, 1.10 to 22.5) and minor bleeding (RR, 4.58; 95% CI, 2.46 to 8.55). Repeat thrombolysis yielded only higher bleeding rates when compared to conservative therapy (RR, 1.84; 95% CI, 1.06 to 3.18), without any improvement in overall mortality (RR, 0.68; 95% CI, 0.41 to 1.14) or reinfarction (RR, 1.79; 95% CI, 0.92 to 3.48).

Primary PCI

88. Grines CL, et al. Primary Angioplasty in MI (PAMI). A comparison of immediate angioplasty with thrombolytic therapy for acute MI. *N Engl J Med* 1993;328:673–679.

Design: Prospective, randomized, open, multicenter study. End points included in-hospital death, reinfarction, and intracranial bleeding and EF at 6 weeks.

Purpose: To compare immediate PTCA with thrombolytic therapy in AMI.

Population: 395 patients seen within 12 hours of ischemic pain with 1 mm or more ST elevation in at least two contiguous ECG leads.

Exclusion Criteria: Complete LBBB, cardiogenic shock, and increased bleeding risk.

Treatment: tPA, 100 mg i.v. (or 1.25 mg/kg if patient weighed <65 kg) over a 3-hour period; or immediate PTCA. All patients received i.v. heparin for 3 to 5 days.

Results: A 97% PTCA success rate was observed. The PTCA group had a 60% lower in-hospital mortality rate (2.6% vs. 6.5%, $p = 0.06$) and a significant 58% reduction in in-hospital death or reinfarction (5.1% vs. 12.0%, $p = 0.02$). The PTCA group also had less intracranial bleeding (none vs. 2.0%; $p = 0.05$). No difference was seen between groups in EF at 6 weeks (both at rest and during exercise). The benefits of primary angioplasty were maintained at 2-year follow-up: lower incidence of death or MI (14.9% vs. 23%; $p = 0.034$), less recurrent ischemia (36.4% vs. 48%; $p = 0.026$), lower reintervention rates (27.2% vs. 46.5%, $p < 0.0001$), and lower rehospitalization rates (58.5% vs. 69.0%, $p = 0.035$).

Comments: A short randomization to balloon time was observed (average, 60 minutes vs. 42 minutes for door-to-thrombolysis time). Editorial asserts that high-risk patients are most likely to benefit from immediate PTCA (e.g., older than 75 years, anterior MI, cardiogenic shock).

89. Every NR, et al.; for the MI Triage and Intervention (MITI) Investigators. A comparison of thrombolytic therapy with primary coronary angioplasty for acute MI. N Engl J Med 1996;335:1253–1260.

Design: Retrospective cohort analysis of MITI Registry (19 Seattle area hospitals, 10 with primary angioplasty capability).

Purpose: To compare outcomes in AMI patients receiving thrombolytic therapy and primary angioplasty.

Population: 3,145 MITI patients (thrombolytic group, n = 2,095; PTCA group, n = 1,050) treated between 1988 and 1994.

Exclusion Criteria: Lack of ECG data and angioplasty more than 6 hours after admission.

Treatment: Thrombolysis with alteplase (65%), SK (32%), or urokinase (3%; 8% were treated before hospitalization) or coronary angiography within 6 hours of admission followed by angioplasty if indicated.

Results: No significant differences were observed between thrombolysis and PTCA in the in-hospital [5.6% (thrombolytic) vs. 5.5%] or 3-year mortality rates. At 3-year follow-up, the thrombolysis group had 30% less coronary angiography, 15% fewer coronary angioplasties, and 13% lower costs. Thrombolysis patients were treated faster (1 hour vs. 1.7 hours after arrival) and sooner after chest pain than the PAMI thrombolysis group (198 minutes vs. 230 minutes). Low-volume-PTCA hospitals did provide later treatment (2.3 hours vs. 1.5 hours) and had higher in-hospital mortality rates (8.1% vs. 4.5%).

90. GUSTO IIb Angioplasty Substudy. The global use of strategies to open occluded arteries in acute coronary syndromes: angioplasty Substudy Investigators. N Engl J Med 1997;336:1621–1628.

Design: Prospective, randomized, open, multicenter substudy (57 sites; all performed 200 angioplasties/year, with one operator doing 50 per year). The 30-day primary end points were death, MI, and stroke.

Purpose: To compare thrombolytic therapy with primary angioplasty in patients with acute STEMI.

Population: 1,138 patients seen within 12 hours of STEMI.

Exclusion Criteria: Same as main GUSTO-IIb trial.

Treatment: Accelerated tPA [15-mg i.v. bolus, then 0.75 mg/kg over a 30-minute period (maximum, 50 mg), 0.50 mg/kg over a 60-minute period (maximum, 35 mg)] or primary angioplasty (average door-to-balloon time, 1.9 hours).

Results: PTCA group had one-third lower rate of death, MI, and stroke (OR, 0.67; 9.6% vs. 13.7%; p = 0.033). Most of the observed benefit occurred from days 5 to 10. By 6 months, the difference was no longer significant (14% vs. 16%). Breakdown by end point (at 30 days): death, 5.7% versus 7% (p = 0.37); MI, 4.5% versus 6.5% (p = 0.13); and stroke, 0.2% versus 0.9% (p = 0.11). PTCA was not associated with any extra benefit in high-risk groups. PTCA achieved TIMI grade 3 flow in a surprisingly low 73% of cases (technical success rate, 93%), which was associated with a 1.6% mortality rate (vs. 21.4%, 14.3%, and 19.9% for TIMI flow grades 0 to 2).

91. Grines CL, et al. A randomized trial of transfer for primary angioplasty vs. on-site thrombolysis in patients with high risk myocardial infarction: the Air PAMI Study. J Am Coll Cardiol 2002;39:1713–1719.

Design: Prospective, randomized, open, multicenter study. The primary end point was a 30-day composite of death, recurrent MI, and disabling stroke.

Purpose: To evaluate whether early transfer for primary PTCA of AMI results in better outcomes than on-site thrombolysis.

Population: High-risk MI patients (older than 70 years, anterior MI, Killip class II/III, HR >100 beats/min, or SBP < 100 mm Hg) who were eligible for thrombolytic therapy and seen in hospitals without on-site PCI.

Treatment: On-site thrombolysis or emergency transfer for primary PCI.

Results: Because of slow recruitment, the study was terminated after 138 patients enrolled (32% of the projected sample size). Median door-to-therapy time was 51 minutes in the thrombolytic group and 155 minutes in the transfer group. The long delay in the transfer group was mostly due to initiation of transfer (43 minutes) and transport time (26 minutes), as time from arrival in hospital to catheterization laboratory was 11 minutes, and catheterization laboratory arrival to treatment was only 14 minutes. No deaths occurred during transfer. In the transfer group, all patients underwent catheterization, and 89% had primary PCI. At 30-day follow-up, a nonsignificant 38% reduction in the primary composite end point in the transfer group was found compared with the thrombolytic group (8.4% vs. 13.6%; $p = 0.331$). Multivariate logistic regression analysis identified randomization to transfer as independent predictor of a reduction in the primary end point (OR, 0.159; 95% CI, 0.031 to 0.820; $p = 0.028$). The transfer group had a reduced hospital stay (6.1 days vs. 7.5 days, $p = 0.015$) and less ischemia (12.7% vs. 31.8%, $p = 0.007$).

92. Aversano T, et al.; Atlantic Cardiovascular Patient Outcomes Research Team (C-PORT). Thrombolytic therapy versus primary percutaneous coronary intervention for myocardial infarction in patients presenting to hospitals without on-site cardiac surgery: a randomized controlled trial. JAMA 2002;287:1943–1951.

Design: Prospective, randomized trial conducted from July 1996 to December 1999 at 11 community hospitals without on-site cardiac surgery or existing PCI programs. The primary end point at 6 months was death, recurrent MI, or stroke.

Purpose: To determine whether treatment of acute MI with primary PCI is superior to thrombolytic therapy at hospitals without on-site cardiac surgery.

Population: 451 thrombolytic-eligible patients with acute STEMI seen within 12 hours of symptom onset.

Exclusion Criteria: Included those ineligible for thrombolytic therapy.

Treatment: Primary PCI program was developed at all sites. Patients were randomized to receive primary PCI or accelerated tPA.

Results: The primary PCI group had a significantly lower incidence of the primary composite end point at 6 weeks (10.7% vs. 17.7%, $p = 0.03$) and 6 months (12.4% vs. 19.9%, $p = 0.03$). The benefit was primarily driven by a lower incidence of recurrent MI (at 6 months: 5.3% vs. 10.6%, $p = 0.04$). Mortality rates were similar (6.2% vs. 7.1%, $p = 0.72$), whereas stroke occurred in 2.2% and 4.0%, respectively ($p = 0.28$). The primary PCI group also had a shorter median length of stay (4.5 days vs. 6.0 days, $p = 0.02$).

93. Andersen HR, et al.; for the DANAMI-2 Investigators. A comparison of coronary angioplasty with fibrinolytic therapy in acute myocardial infarction. N Engl J Med 2003;349:733–742.

Design: Prospective, randomized, open, multicenter trial. The primary end point at 30 days was death, clinical reinfarction, or significant disabling stroke.

Purpose: To demonstrate that a primary PCI strategy will be superior in both patients seen at on-site interventional facilities (no transfer of patient required) and without (transfer of patient required).

Population: 1,572 patients seen within 12 hours with a sum of >4-mm ST elevation in all leads.

Exclusion Criteria: Included contraindications to thrombolytic therapy; expected time between randomization and arrival in catheterization laboratory longer than 3 hours for patients randomized in referral hospitals, and more than 2 hours in invasive-equipped hospitals.

Treatment: Primary PCI or front-loaded tPA. PCI patients were transferred to referring center if catheterization laboratory facilities were not available on-site. All received aspirin (300 mg and then 75 to 150 mg daily) and heparin (5,000-U bolus + 1,000 U/h infusion for at least 48 hours in patients randomized to tPA; 10,000-U initial bolus + additional heparin to keep the ACT between 350 and 450 seconds during the procedure in patients randomized to PCI).

Results: The trial was terminated early because of a clear benefit for PCI. The PCI group had 40% reduction in the primary composite end point compared with the fibrinolytic group (8.5% vs. 14.2%, $p = 0.002$), primarily because of a lower incidence of recurrent MI (6.3% vs. 1.6%, $p < 0.001$). The 30-day mortality was 7.8% in the fibrinolysis group versus 6.6% in the PCI group ($p = 0.35$), and disabling stroke occurred in 2.0% and 1.1% ($p = 0.15$), respectively. A similar benefit with PCI was seen in patients who were transferred and those who were not transferred (time difference to balloon inflation between the referred and on-site patients was only 10 minutes).

94. PRAGUE-2; Widimsky P, et al. Long distance transport for primary angioplasty vs immediate thrombolysis in acute myocardial infarction. *Eur Heart J* 2003;24:94–104.

This prospective, randomized trial enrolled 850 patients with acute STEMI seen within 12 hours in a community hospital and compared on-site thrombolysis (SK) with transfer for primary PCI. Exclusion criteria included contraindications to thrombolytic therapy and failure to initiate transfer within 30 minutes. Routine glycoprotein IIb/IIIa receptor antagonists before planned PCI were not used. At 30 days, mortality rates were not significantly different [10.4% (thrombolysis) vs. 6.0% (PCI), $p < 0.05$]. However, among those seen at 3 to 12 hours (vs. < 3 hours), the PCI group had a stronger relative mortality reduction (6% vs. 15.3%, $p < 0.02$). The incidence of death, MI, and stroke also was significantly lower in the PCI group (8.4% vs. 15.2%, $p < 0.003$).

PCI After Thrombolysis

95. Topol EJ, et al.; the Thrombolysis and Angioplasty in MI (TAMI) Study Group. A randomized trial of immediate versus delayed elective angioplasty after intravenous tissue plasminogen activator in acute MI. *N Engl J Med* 1987;317:581–588 (editorial, 624–626).

Design: Prospective, randomized, multicenter study. The primary end points were infarct-related vessel patency and global LV function.

Purpose: To compare immediate with delayed elective angioplasty in patients undergoing thrombolysis for AMI.

Population: 386 patients met initial criteria (75 years or younger, within 6 hours of onset of symptoms, and 1 mm or more ST elevation in at least two contiguous leads); 197 patients had appropriate catheterization findings (i.e., lesions amenable to angioplasty) and were randomized to immediate or delayed angioplasty.

Exclusion Criteria: Contraindications related to angiographic findings included more than 50% left main stenosis, severe/diffuse disease, and infarct-related vessel unidentifiable.

Treatment: Predominantly single-chain tPA, 150 mg i.v. over a 6- to 8-hour period followed by angiography with either immediate angioplasty or deferred angioplasty (latter performed at 7 to 10 days and if indicated). The immediate group also had angiography at 7 to 10 days to assess for reocclusion and LV function.

Results: Immediate PTCA success rate was 86%. Similar reocclusion rates were observed [11% (immediate) vs. 13%]. Neither group had an improvement in global LV function. In the delayed group, 14% did not require angioplasty (residual stenosis < 50%), but a higher crossover rate was found to emergency angioplasty (16% vs. 5%).

Immediate angioplasty had its own risks. Seven of nine patients with abrupt closure required emergency CABG surgery.

96. Rogers WJ, et al.; for the TIMI-IIA Investigators. Comparison of immediate invasive, delayed invasive and conservative strategies after tissue-type plasminogen activator. *Circulation* 1990;81:1457–1476.

Design: Prospective, randomized, open, multicenter study. The primary end point was predischarge LVEF.

Purpose: To compare immediate versus delayed (at 18 to 48 hours) PTCA or CABG versus conservative treatment in AMI patients treated with tPA.

Population: 586 patients 75 years or younger seen within 4 hours of chest pain and with 1 mm or more ST elevation in at least two contiguous ECG leads.

Treatment: All patients received tPA [first 195 patients, 150 mg over a 6-hour period; next 391 patients, 100 mg over a 6-hour period (6-mg bolus, then 54 mg over the 1st hour, 20 mg in the 2nd hour, and 5 mg/h for 4 hours)]; 195 underwent immediate invasive treatment, 194 delayed invasive treatment, and 197 conservative treatment [angiography ± angioplasty allowed with ischemic symptoms (spontaneous or provoked with testing)]. All patients received heparin for 5 days.

Results: All groups had similar predischarge LVEF (average, 49.3%) and IRA patency (TIMI grade 2 or 3 flow; mean, 83.7%). The immediate invasive group had a significantly higher CABG rate [7.7% vs. 2.1% (delayed invasive) vs. 2.5% (conservative), $p < 0.01$], and more transfusions were required among non-CABG patients (13.8% vs. 3.1% vs. 2.0%). Similar 1-year mortality rates were observed despite higher PTCA rates in immediate and delayed invasive groups (76% vs. 64% vs. 24%).

97. Califf RM, et al.; for the TAMI Study Group. Evaluation of combination thrombolytic therapy and timing of cardiac catheterization in acute MI. *Circulation* 1991;83:1543–1556.

Design: Prospective, randomized, open, parallel-group, factorial (3 × 2), multicenter study. The primary end point was global LVEF.

Purpose: To evaluate combination thrombolytic therapy by comparing with monotherapy and to compare an aggressive with a deferred angiography strategy.

Population: 575 patients aged 75 years or younger seen within 6 hours of symptoms and with >1-mm ST elevation in at least two contiguous ECG leads.

Treatment: Urokinase (1.5 million U i.v. bolus and then 1.5 million U over a 60-minute period), rtPA [100 mg over a 3-hour period (6-mg i.v. bolus, 60 mg over a 1-hour period, 20 mg/h for 2 hours)], or combination therapy [urokinase, 1.5 million U over a 1-hour period and rtPA, 1 mg/kg, over a 1-hour period (10% as i.v. bolus; maximum dose, 90 mg)]. Aggressive strategy consisted of immediate angiography, whereas deferred strategy involved angiography before discharge (days 5 to 10).

Results: Global LVEF was well preserved and nearly identical at predischarge angiography (54%), regardless of thrombolytic or catheterization strategy. Combination thrombolysis resulted in higher 90-minute patency: TIMI grade 2 or 3 flow in 76% [tPA, 71% (p = NS); urokinase, 62% (p = 0.049)]. Less reocclusion [2% vs. 12% (p = 0.04) and 7% (p = NS)] and recurrent ischemia (25% vs. 31% vs. 35%) were observed. An aggressive strategy yielded better results with fewer adverse outcomes: death, stroke, reinfarction, heart failure, or recurrent ischemia in 55% versus 67% (p = 0.004), as well as a trend toward a higher predischarge patency rate (94% vs. 90%, p = 0.065).

98. Should We Intervene Following Thrombolysis (SWIFT) Trial Study Group. SWIFT trial of delayed elective intervention vs conservative treatment after thrombolysis with anistreplase in acute MI. *BMJ* 1991;302:555–560.

In this prospective, multicenter ($n = 21$) trial of 800 patients younger than 70 years, patients randomized to early angiography and appropriate intervention (PTCA, 43%; CABG, 15%) or conservative care [PTCA, 2.5%; CABG, 1.7% (initial admission)]. All patients were treated with anistreplase, 30 U over a 5-minute period. No differences in 1-year mortality (5.8% vs. 5%) and reinfarction rates (15% vs. 13%) were observed. Intervention group did have longer stay (11 days vs. 10 days).

99. Madsen JK, et al.; Danish Trial in Acute MI (DANAMI). Danish multicenter randomized study of invasive vs. conservative treatment in patients with inducible ischemia after thrombolysis in acute MI (DANAMI). Circulation 1997;96: 748–755.

Design: Prospective, randomized, open, multicenter study. Median follow-up period was 2.4 years. The primary end points were death, AMI, and admission with unstable angina.

Purpose: To compare an invasive strategy of PTCA or CABG with a conservative strategy in patients with inducible ischemia after thrombolysis for MI.

Population: 1,008 patients younger than 70 years with first MI and inducible ischemia [spontaneous ischemia 36 hours or less after admission or positive bicycle exercise tolerance test result (0.1 mm or more ST depression, 0.2 mm or more ST elevation)].

Exclusion Criteria: Prior MI, PTCA, or CABG; incomplete thrombolysis; BP decrease during exercise; significant noncoronary disease; and ECG abnormalities precluding ST-segment evaluation during exercise (e.g., LBBB).

Treatment: Invasive therapy group received angiography within 2 weeks, PTCA and CABG if significant disease (50% or greater stenosis). In the conservative arm, angiography was allowed if severe angina developed (e.g., Canadian Cardiovascular Society class 3 or 4).

Results: In the invasive group, PTCA was performed in 52.9% and CABG in 29.2% (at 2 to 10 weeks). In the conservative group, at 2 months, only 1.6% had undergone revascularization (at 1 year, 15%). At follow-up, no significant mortality difference was observed [3.6% (invasive) vs. 4.4%], but the invasive group had 47% fewer MIs (5.6% vs. 10.5%, $p = 0.0038$) and fewer unstable angina admissions (17.9% vs. 29.5%, $p < 0.00001$). Overall, the invasive group had 36% fewer primary end points (death, MI, and unstable angina) at 2 years (23.5% vs. 36.6%, $p < 0.0001$).

Comments: Editorial points out that few US cardiologists follow ACC/AHA guidelines that recommend stress testing before invasive testing and propose performing angiography for medium or large MIs and revascularization if evidence of an incomplete infarct is present (e.g., lower than expected CK peak, ECG evolution, preserved wall motion of infarct zone) and stress testing first those with only small MIs (e.g., leads II, III, aVF only).

100. Ross AM, et al. A randomized trial comparing primary angioplasty with a strategy of short-acting thrombolysis and immediate planned rescue angioplasty in acute myocardial infarction: the PACT trial. J Am Coll Cardiol 1999;34:1954–1962.

Design: Prospective, randomized, open, multicenter trial. The primary end point was predischarge EF. Follow-up was 1 year.

Purpose: To evaluate the effectiveness and safety of a "facilitated" PCI approach to AMI management.

Population: 606 patients seen 6 hours or less after symptom onset with ST 0.1 mV or more in two or more limb leads or 0.2 mV or more in two or more contiguous leads.

Treatment: Precatheterization thrombolysis (tPA, 50-mg bolus) or placebo followed by immediate angiography. If TIMI grade 3 flow is present, second bolus of tPA, 50 mg, is administered. If TIMI grade 0 to 2 flow is present, PCI is performed.

Results: Initial angiography demonstrated that the tPA group had higher TIMI grade 3 flow (32.8% vs. 14.8%) and patency (TIMI grade 2 or 3; 61% vs. 34%; $p = 0.001$). After angioplasty, TIMI flow grade was similar between the two groups [TIMI grade 3 flow in 77% (rescue) and 79% (primary)], indicating that tPA administration did not adversely affect procedural outcomes. No significant difference was noted between the groups in predischarge EF (primary end point), but the EF was higher in those with TIMI 3 flow on catheterization laboratory arrival (62.4%). The small group of patients (12%) who had PTCA performed <1 hour after the tPA bolus also had better EFs (62.5% vs. 57.3%). No significant differences were found in bleeding rates, suggesting that immediate angioplasty could be performed safely after reduced-dose tPA.

101. Assessment of the Safety and Efficacy of a New Treatment Strategy with Percutaneous Coronary Intervention (ASSENT-4 PCI) Investigators. Primary versus tenecteplase facilitated percutaneous coronary intervention in patients with ST-segment elevation acute myocardial infarction (ASSENT-4 PCI): randomized trial. *Lancet* 2006;367:569–578.

Design: Prospective, randomized, open, multicenter trial. The primary end point was death, CHF, or shock within 90 days.

Purpose: To evaluate the effectiveness of full-dose TNK to facilitate delayed PCI, in cases of acute STEMI.

Population: 1,667 (4,000 planned) patients with STEMI, symptom duration of <6 hours, and scheduled to undergo primary PCI with an anticipated delay of 1 to 3 hours.

Treatment: Standard primary PCI or PCI preceded by full-dose TNK ("facilitated" PCI). All patients received aspirin and only a bolus of UFH (no infusion).

Results: The trial was stopped early, as recommended by the Data and Safety Monitoring Board, due to higher mortality in the facilitated PCI group (6% vs. 3%; $p = 0.01$). There was a higher rate of the primary end point in the facilitated PCI group (19% vs. 13%; $p = 0.0045$), as well as significantly more strokes (1.8% vs. 0%; $p < 0.0001$). Median time from TNK to balloon inflation was 104 minutes. Major, noncerebral bleeding was similar (6% for facilitated vs. 4% in the standard PCI group; $p = 0.3118$), yet there were higher rates of reinfarction (6% vs. 4%; $p = 0.0279$) and repeat TVR (7% vs. 3%; $p = 0.0041$).

102. Ellis SG, et al.; for the FINESSE Investigators. Facilitated PCI in patients with ST-elevation myocardial infarction. *N Engl J Med* 2008;358:2205–2217.

Design: Prospective, randomized, double-blind, placebo-controlled, international, multicenter trial. The primary end point was a composite of death, VF (>48 hours after randomization), cardiogenic shock, or CHF within 90 days.

Purpose: To evaluate strategy of early abciximab or abciximab plus half-dose reteplase to facilitate primary PCI in patients with STEMI.

Population: 2,452 patients with STEMI who presented within 6 hours of symptoms.

Treatment: Standard primary PCI, abciximab-facilitated PCI, or combination-facilitated PCI (with abciximab and half-dose reteplase). All patients received UFH or enoxaparin prior to PCI, as well as a 12-hour infusion of abciximab after PCI.

Results: The rates of primary events were 9.8%, 10.5%, and 10.7% in the combination-facilitated, abciximab-facilitated, and standard PCI groups, respectively ($p = 0.55$), with 90-day mortality rates of 5.2%, 5.5%, and 4.5%, respectively ($p = 0.49$). However, patients in the combination-facilitated group were significantly more likely to have early ST-segment resolution (43.9%), compared with abciximab-facilitated (33.1%) or standard PCI (31.0%, $p = 0.01$ and 0.003, respectively).

103. Di Mario C, et al.; on behalf of the CARESS-in-AMI Investigators. Immediate angioplasty versus standard therapy with rescue angioplasty after thrombolysis in the Combined Abciximab Reteplase Stent Study in Acute Myocardial Infarction (CARESS-in-AMI): an open, prospective, randomised, multicentre trial. *Lancet* 2008;371:559–568.

Design: Prospective, randomized, open, multicenter trial. The primary end point was a composite of death, reinfarction, or refractory ischemia at 30 days.

Purpose: To identify the best subsequent management of patients with STEMI who received thrombolytic therapy.

Population: 600 patients <76 years old with acute MI with one or more high-risk features (ST-segment elevation, new LBBB, previous MI, Killip class >2, or LVEF ≤35%).

Treatment: All patients received half-dose reteplase, abciximab, heparin, and aspirin and were either managed conservatively locally or transferred to another center for PCI.

Results: Rates of events in the primary end point were significantly lower in the group receiving PCI (4.4% vs. 10.7%, $p = 0.004$), and 30.3% of patients in the conservative therapy arm underwent rescue PCI. Rates of major bleeding were not significantly different (3.4% in the conservative group vs. 2.3% in the PCI group, $p = 0.47$), and neither were rates of strokes (0.7% vs. 1.3%, $p = 0.50$).

104. Bonnefoy E, et al.; on behalf of the Comparison of Angioplasty and prehospital Thrombolysis in Acute Myocardial infarction (CAPTIM) Study Group. Primary angioplasty versus prehospital fibrinolysis. *Lancet* 2002;360:825–829.

Design: Prospective, randomized, open, multicenter trial. The primary end points were death, nonfatal reinfarction, and nonfatal disabling stroke at 30 days.

Purpose: To determine whether primary angioplasty is better than prehospital fibrinolysis followed by transfer to an interventional facility for possible rescue PTCA.

Population: 840 patients seen within 6 hours of symptom onset with 2 mm or more ST elevation in at least two contiguous leads or LBBB.

Treatment: Prehospital fibrinolysis (accelerated alteplase) with angiography only for ongoing chest pain or ECG signs of continuing ischemia OR primary angioplasty. Each ambulance was staffed with a physician.

Results: The median delay between onset of symptoms and treatment was 130 minutes in the fibrinolysis group and 190 minutes (time to first balloon inflation) in the primary PTCA group. Rescue angioplasty was performed in 26% of fibrinolysis patients. No significant differences were seen between the groups in the incidence of the primary composite end point (primary PTCA, 6.2%; fibrinolysis, 8.2%; $p = 0.29$).

Comments: Study was underpowered—planned enrollment was 1,200 patients, which would have allowed a detection of a 40% relative reduction in the incidence of the primary end point.

105. Fernandez-Avilés F, et al.; on behalf of the GRACIA Group. Routine invasive strategy within 24 hours of thrombolysis versus ischaemia-guided conservative approach for acute myocardial infarction with ST-segment elevation (GRACIA-1): a randomised controlled trial. *Lancet* 2004;364:1045–1053.

Design: Prospective, randomized, open, multicenter, international trial. The primary end point was a composite of death, nonfatal reinfarction, or revascularization at 12 months.

Purpose: To determine the role for early postthrombolysis PCI in patients with STEMI in the era of contemporary therapies.

Population: 500 patients with STEMI who received thrombolytics.

Treatment: Early angiography within 24 hours, with intervention if indicated versus conservative, ischemia-guided interventional approach.

Results: At 1 year, the interventional group had a significantly lower incidence of primary end point events (9% vs. 21%, $p = 0.0008$). Rates of death or reinfarction were also nonsignificantly reduced in the early interventional group (7% vs. 12%, $p = 0.07$). Importantly, rates of major bleeding were similar, and length of hospitalization was shorter in the early intervention group.

106. Schweiger MJ, et al.; for the TIMI 10B and TIMI 14 Investigators. Early coronary intervention following pharmacologic therapy for acute myocardial infarction (the combined TIMI 10B-TIMI 14 experience). *Am J Cardiol* 2001;88:831–836.

This study analyzed 1,938 AMI patients from TIMI 10B (tPA vs. TNK) and TIMI 14 (thrombolytic therapy with or without abciximab). All patients underwent angiography at 90 minutes. Patients who underwent PCI were described as having a rescue procedure (TIMI 0 or 1 flow at 90 minutes), an adjunctive procedure (TIMI 2 or 3 flow at 90 minutes), or a delayed procedure [performed > 150 minutes after symptom onset (median, 2.8 days)]. Among patients with TIMI 0 or 1 flow, a trend was found toward lower 30-day mortality with rescue PCI compared with no PCI (6% vs. 17%, $p = 0.01$, adjusted $p = 0.28$). Patients who underwent adjunctive PCI had 30-day mortality and/or reinfarction rates similar to those who underwent delayed PCI. In a multivariate model, adjunctive and delayed PCI patients had lower 30-day mortality and/or reinfarction rates ($p = 0.02$) than did patients with "successful thrombolysis" (i.e., TIMI 3 flow at 90 minutes) who did not undergo revascularization. Thus, early PCI after AMI is associated with favorable outcomes. Randomized trials of an early invasive strategy after thrombolysis are warranted.

107. Cantor WJ, et al.; for the TRANSFER-AMI Trial Investigators. Routine early angioplasty after fibrinolysis for acute myocardial infarction. *N Engl J Med* 2009;360: 2705–2718.

Design: Prospective, randomized, open, multicenter, trial. The primary end point was a composite of death, reinfarction, recurrent ischemia, new or worsening CHF, or cardiogenic shock at 30 days.

Purpose: To identify the optimal timing of routine PCI following thrombolysis for acute STEMI.

Population: 1,059 patients with STEMI who received fibrinolytics at a center without PCI capability.

Treatment: Early angiography within 6 hours requiring transfer to another institution, or routine conservative therapy (including rescue PCI if necessary or delayed angiography).

Results: In the early invasive group, median time to PCI was 2.8 hours; for the standard-therapy group, 88.7% of patients underwent PCI at a median time of 32.5 hours after randomization. Incidence of primary end point events occurred in 11.0% of patients in the early invasive group versus 17.2% in the standard-therapy group ($p = 0.004$). Rates of major bleeding were similar in the two groups.

108. Bohmer E, et al. Efficacy and safety of immediate angioplasty versus ischemia-guided management after thrombolysis in acute myocardial infarction in areas with very long transfer distances, results of the NORDISTEMI. *J Am Coll Cardiol* 2010;55(2):102–110.

Design: Randomized, controlled, multicenter trial. The primary end point was a composite of death, reinfarction, stroke, or new ischemia at 12 months.

Purpose: To compare the effects of 2 different management strategies after thrombolysis in patients presenting with STEMI: (a) transfer all patients immediately for PCI or (b) an ischemia-guided strategy.

Population: 266 patients aged 18 to 75 with symptoms of MI for <6 hours, ECG indicative of STEMI, and expected time delay from first medical contact to PCI >90 min received TNK fibrinolysis.

Exclusion Criteria: Contraindications to thrombolytics, serious renal failure, cardiogenic shock or serious arrhythmias, pregnancy, life expectancy <12 months, and psychiatric or other conditions that could reduce compliance (drug abuse, dementia, etc.).

Treatment: All patients received standard weight-adjusted dose TNK, aspirin 300 mg, enoxaparin 30 mg IV followed by a subcutaneous dose of 1 mg/kg repeated every 12 hours, and 300-mg clopidogrel on the 1st day.

Results: There was no significant difference in the composite primary end points of death, reinfarct, stroke, and new ischemia between the two groups [27.3% in the conservative arm vs. 20.9% in the early invasive arm; HR, 0.72 (95% CI, 0.44 to 1.18); $p = 0.18$]; however, there was a significant decrease in death, reinfarct, and stroke in the early invasive arm [15.9% vs. 6.0%; HR, 0.36 (95% CI, 0.16 to 0.81); $p = 0.01$].

Rescue PCI

109. Ellis SG, et al.; RESCUE. Randomized comparison of rescue angioplasty with conservative management of patients with early failure of thrombolysis for acute anterior MI. *Circulation* 1994;90:2280–2284.

Design: Prospective, randomized, multicenter study. The primary end point was LVEF at 25 to 35 days.

Purpose: To assess the clinical benefit of rescue angioplasty in a relatively high-risk population.

Population: 151 patients aged 21 to 79 years seen with ST elevation 2 mm or more in at least two precordial leads.

Exclusion Criteria: Cardiogenic shock, prior MI, and left main stenosis 50% or more.

Treatment: Thrombolysis followed by PTCA or aspirin, heparin, and vasodilators.

Results: Rescue PTCA was successful in 92%. The rescue PTCA group had less death and severe heart failure (6% vs. 17%, $p = 0.05$) and better exercise (but not rest) EFs (43% vs. 38%, $p = 0.04$).

110. Gershlick AH, et al.; for the REACT Trial Investigators. Rescue angioplasty after failed thrombolytic therapy for acute myocardial infarction. *N Engl J Med* 2005;353:2758–2768.

Design: Prospective, randomized, multicenter study. The primary end point was a composite of death, reinfarction, stroke, or severe CHF at 6 months.

Purpose: To compare emergent PCI with repeated thrombolysis in patients with STEMI who fail to reperfuse following initial thrombolysis.

Population: 427 patients with STEMI had <50% ST-segment resolution 90 minutes after thrombolytic therapy.

Exclusion Criteria: Any contraindication to thrombolysis and cardiogenic shock.

Treatment: Conservative treatment (no intervention or further lysis), repeat thrombolysis, or emergent, rescue PCI.

Results: More patients in the rescue PCI group were event free (84.6%), compared with conservative therapy (70.1%), or repeat thrombolysis (68.7%, overall $p = 0.004$). Overall mortality among the three groups was similar. Revascularization-free survival at 6 months was statistically similar but tended to favor the PCI group (86.2% for the rescue PCI group vs. 77.6% in the conservative therapy arm vs. 74.4% in the repeat thrombolysis group, overall $p = 0.05$).

Comments: The benefits of rescue PCI persisted for at least 1 year, as described in the long-term follow-up analysis of the REACT trial (see *J Am Coll Cardiol* 2009;54:118–126).

Operator and Hospital Volumes

111. Thiemann DR, et al. The association between hospital volume and survival after acute myocardial infarction in elderly patients. *N Engl J Med* 1999;340:1640.

This retrospective cohort analysis focused on 98,898 Medicare patients aged 65 years or older with a principal discharge diagnosis of AMI. Patients admitted to hospitals in the lowest quartile of volume of invasive procedures had a 17% higher in-hospital mortality rate compared with patients at highest-volume-quartile hospitals (hazard ratio, 1.17; 95% CI, 1.09 to 1.26; $p < 0.001$).

112. Magid DJ, et al. Relation between hospital primary angioplasty volume and mortality for patients with acute MI treated with primary angioplasty vs thrombolytic therapy. *JAMA* 2000;284:3131–3138.

This retrospective cohort study analyzed 62,299 AMI patients at 446 acute care hospitals treated with primary angioplasty or thrombolytic therapy from June 1994 to July 1999. At hospitals with intermediate volume (17 to 48 procedures/year) and high volume (>49 procedures), mortality was significantly lower among patients undergoing angioplasty compared with thrombolysis (4.5% vs. 5.9%, $p < 0.001$; 3.4% vs. 5.4%, $p < 0.001$). At low-volume hospitals, no significant difference in mortality was found between the two treatment modalities (6.2% vs. 5.9%, $p = 0.58$).

113. Srinivas VS, et al. Effect of physician volume on the relationship between hospital volume and mortality during primary angioplasty. *J Am Coll Cardiol* 2009;53:574–579.

This, the most contemporary analysis of the New York State PCI registry, looked at 7,321 patients receiving primary PCI for acute MI. It compared risk-adjusted in-hospital mortality between high-volume hospitals (>50 cases/year) and high-volume operators (>10 cases/year) versus lower volume centers and physicians. ORs for in-hospital mortality in high-volume hospitals (0.58; 95% CI, 0.38 to 0.88) and high-volume operators (OR, 0.66; 95% CI, 0.48 to 0.92) were significantly lower than those for their lower volume counterparts. Furthermore, physician volume modified hospital outcome as well—low-volume physicians had higher mortality outcomes in both low- and high-volume hospitals. The absolute difference was highest in low-volume hospitals (8.4% in-hospital mortality for low-volume physicians vs. 4.8% for high-volume physicians; OR, 1.44; 95% CI, 0.68 to 3.03). The difference was significant in high-volume hospitals (3.8% for high-volume physicians vs. 6.5% for low-volume physicians; OR, 0.58; 95% CI, 0.39 to 0.86).

Stenting in STEMI

114. Antoniucci D, et al.; Florence Randomized Elective Stenting in Acute Coronary Occlusions (FRESCO). A clinical trial comparing primary stenting of the infarct-related artery with optimal primary angioplasty for acute MI. *J Am Coll Cardiol* 1998;31:1234–1239.

This prospective, randomized, multicenter study enrolled 150 patients seen within 6 hours of onset of symptoms with STEMI and who underwent successful primary PTCA. Patients were randomized to primary PTCA or primary PTCA followed by stenting. No PTCA was attempted if stenosis was <70% or the IRA could not be identified. No randomization to PTCA alone or stenting was performed if the reference diameter was <2.5 mm. Stenting success rate was 100%. At 6 months, the incidence of death, reinfarction, and repeated TVR due to recurrent ischemia at 6 months (primary end point) was only 9% in the stent group versus 28% in the PTCA group ($p = 0.003$). Repeated angiography was performed at 6 months, and the incidence of restenosis or reocclusion was 17% in the stent group and 43% in the PTCA group ($p = 0.001$).

115. Suryapranata H, et al. Randomized comparison of coronary stenting with balloon angioplasty in selected patients with acute MI. *Circulation* 1998;97:2502–2505.

This prospective, single-center study randomized 227 AMI patients seen within 6 hours of symptom onset (or after 6 to 24 hours if ongoing ischemia) to primary stenting (Palmaz–Schatz) or angioplasty (with bailout stenting only if prolonged inflation unsuccessful). Initial patients received warfarin for 3 months, but patients enrolled after January 1996 received ticlopidine, 250 mg/day for 2 weeks. Exclusion criteria were cardiogenic shock, prior bypass surgery or angioplasty, and prior MI. Angiographic exclusion criteria included unprotected left main, significant side branch jeopardy, excessive tortuosity, extensive thrombus, or inability to cross lesion with guide wire. Overall 6-month mortality rate was 2%. The stent group had fewer reinfarctions (1% vs. 7%, $p = 0.036$) and less need for subsequent TVR (4% vs. 17%, $p = 0.0016$). The stent group also had better cardiac event-free survival rate (95% vs. 80%, $p = 0.012$). The stent group had a larger reference vessel.

116. Grines CL, et al.; for the Stent PAMI Study Group. Coronary angioplasty with or without stent implantation for acute myocardial infarction. *N Engl J Med* 1999;341:1949–1956.

Design: Prospective, randomized, open, multicenter trial. The primary end point was the 6-month incidence of death, reinfarction, and disabling stroke or ischemia-driven TVR.

Purpose: To compare stent implantation with primary angioplasty alone in AMI.

Population: 900 patients within 12 hours of symptom onset with ST elevation 1 mm or more in at least two contiguous leads or a nondiagnostic ECG with evidence of AMI in the catheterization laboratory and with lesions amenable to stenting.

Exclusion Criteria: Included prior administration of thrombolytic agents for index infarction, current use of warfarin, stroke in prior month, and cardiogenic shock.

Treatment: Angioplasty alone or stenting (heparin-coated Palmaz–Schatz).

Results: Acute procedural success rates were >99% in both groups. The postprocedural TIMI grade 3 flow rates were 89.4% in the angioplasty group and 92.7% in the stent group ($p = 0.10$). At 6 months, the stent group had a larger mean luminal diameter (2.56 mm vs. 2.12 mm, $p < 0.001$) and lower restenosis rate (20.3% vs. 33.5%, $p < 0.001$). Stenting was associated with a significant reduction in the 6-month composite primary end point (12.6% vs. 20.1%, $p < 0.01$). This difference was driven entirely by a decreased need for TVR because of ischemia (7.7% vs. 17%, $p < 0.001$). The 6-month mortality rate was 4.2% in the stent group and 2.7% in the angioplasty group ($p = 0.27$). Bleeding rates were similar.

Comments: The use of glycoprotein IIb/IIIa inhibitors was infrequent (5%), rigid early generation stents were used (increased thrombus embolization), and high-pressure deployment and oversizing of the stent were common. Many of these practice patterns have now changed, and this finding should be re-evaluated in future studies.

117. Le May MR, et al. Stenting versus thrombolysis in acute myocardial infarction trial (STAT). *J Am Coll Cardiol* 2001;37:985–991.

A total of 123 patients with STEMI were randomized to primary stenting or accelerated tPA. Patients with cardiogenic shock, active bleeding, history of stroke, major surgery, severe hypertension, prolonged CPR, inadequate vascular access, PTCA within 6 months, prior stenting of culprit artery, and prior CABG were excluded. The primary end point was a 6-month composite of TVR. At 6-month follow-up, the primary end point (death, reinfarction, stroke, or repeated TVR) had occurred in 24.2% of stent patients and 55.7% of TPA patients ($p < 0.001$); this difference was due to a significant reduction in TVR in the stent group (14.5% vs. 49.2%, $p < 0.001$).

118. Kastrati A, et al.; for the Stent versus Thrombolysis for Occluded Coronary Arteries in Patients with Acute Myocardial Infarction (STOPAMI-2) Study. Myocardial salvage after coronary stenting plus abciximab versus fibrinolysis plus abciximab in patients with acute myocardial infarction: a randomised trial. *Lancet* 2002;359:920–925.

Design: Prospective, randomized, open, multicenter trial. The primary end point was the salvage index (the ratio of the degree of myocardial salvage to the initial perfusion defect).

Purpose: To determine whether AMI patients benefit from the addition of glycoprotein IIb/IIIa inhibitors to fibrinolytic or mechanical reperfusion strategies.

Population: 162 patients with AMI seen within 12 hours of onset of symptoms.

Treatment: Stenting or alteplase. All received abciximab. Technetium-99m sestamibi scintigraphy was done at admission and at a median of 11 days in 141 (87%) patients.

Results: Stenting was associated with greater myocardial salvage than was alteplase (median, 13.6% vs. 8.0% of the left ventricle; p = 0.007). The salvage index was greater in the stent group than in the alteplase group [median, 0.60 (0.37 to 0.82) vs. 0.41 (0.13 to 0.58); p = 0.001]. Six-month mortality rate was 5% in the stent group and 9% in the alteplase group [RR, 0.56 (95% CI, 0.17 to 1.88); p = 0.35].

119. Stone GW, et al.; for the Controlled Abciximab and Device Investigation to Lower Late Angioplasty Complications (CADILLAC) Investigators. Comparison of angioplasty with stenting, with or without abciximab, in acute myocardial infarction. *N Engl J Med* 2002;346:957–966 (see Ref. 152, full summary).

This 2,082-patient trial found a significantly lower incidence of major events with stenting compared with angioplasty, regardless of abciximab use (see Ref. 54 for full summary).

120. Valgimigli M, et al.; for the Multicentre Evaluation of Single High-dose Bolus Tirofiban vs Abciximab With Sirolimus-eluting Stent or Bare Metal Stent in Acute Myocardial Infarction Study (MULTISTRATEGY) Investigators. Comparison of angioplasty with infusion of tirofiban or abciximab and with implantation of sirolimus-eluting or uncoated stents for acute myocardial infarction: the multistrategy randomized trial. *JAMA* 2008;299(15):1788–1799.

Design: Prospective, randomized, open-label, 2 × 2 factorial design, multicenter, international trial. The primary end point for the stent comparison was a composite of death, reinfarction, or clinically driven TVR at 8 months. The primary end point for the drug comparison was at least 50% ST-segment resolution at 90 minutes, with a prespecified noninferiority margin.

Purpose: To evaluate alternative glycoprotein IIb/IIIa inhibitor strategies (using tirofiban), as well as the use of DES, in patients with STEMI.

Population: 745 patients with STEMI or new LBBB.

Treatment: Patients were first randomized to either high-dose bolus tirofiban or abciximab infusion; they were also randomized to receive a sirolimus-eluting stent (SES) or an uncoated BMS.

Results: For the drug comparison, 83.6% of patients had ST-segment resolution in the abciximab group versus 85.3% in the tirofiban group (p < 0.001 for noninferiority). Each group had a similar rate of ischemic and bleeding adverse events. The primary end point in the stenting comparison was met in 14.5% of patients in the BMS group compared with 7.8% in the SES group (p = 0.004), which was significantly driven by a reduction in repeat revascularization (10.2% vs. 3.2%). They reported a similar incidence of stent thromboses in the two groups.

121. De Luca G, et al. Efficacy and safety of drug-eluting stents in ST-segment elevation myocardial infarction: a meta-analysis of randomized trials. *Int J Cardiol* 2009;133:213–222.

The reviewers compiled results from 11 trials, including 3,605 patients, comparing SES, paclitaxel-eluting stents (PES), and BMS in patients undergoing primary PCI for STEMI. End points for SES and PES were combined into the DES group. At follow-up of 12 months, there were no differences in overall mortality (4.1% vs. 4.4%, $p = 0.59$), reinfarction (3.1% vs. 3.4%, $p = 0.38$), or stent thrombosis (1.6% vs. 2.2%, $p = 0.22$). However, the DES groups had lower rates of TVR (5.0% vs. 12.6%, $p < 0.0001$). In four trials of 1,178 patients, data at 18 and 24 months were similar.

122. De Luca G, et al. Short and long-term benefits of sirolimus-eluting stent in ST-segment elevation myocardial infarction: a meta-analysis of randomized trials. *J Thromb Thrombolysis* 2009;28:200–210. doi: 10.1007/s11239-009-0305-7.

The authors repeated the previous meta-analysis, now limited to SES only and including more contemporary trials. They combined data on 2,769 patients from nine randomized trials comparing BMS and SES in patients receiving primary PCI for STEMI. Follow-up at 12 months yielded significantly fewer incidents of TVR (4.9% vs. 13.6%, $p < 0.0001$) in the SES group, with a nonsignificant trend toward decreased mortality (2.9% vs. 4.2%, $p = 0.08$) and reinfarction (3.0% vs. 4.3%, $p = 0.06$). Rates of stent thrombosis appeared similar between the two groups (1.9% vs. 2.5%, $p = 0.36$). They report that long-term data at 2 to 3 years of follow-up from four of the trials (encompassing 569 patients) were similar.

123. Chechi T, et al. ST-segment elevation myocardial infarction due to early and late stent thrombosis: a new group of high-risk patients. *J Am Coll Cardiol* 2008;51:2396–2402.

The investigators explored a retrospective sample of patients with stent thrombosis who presented with STEMI (92 or 80% of thromboses), as compared with 98 patients with de novo STEMI. All received primary PCI therapy; however, those who presented with stent thrombosis were significantly less likely to achieve successful reperfusion ($p < 0.0001$) and had higher rates of distal embolization ($p = 0.01$). Patients with stent thrombosis had higher rates of major adverse cardiovascular and cerebrovascular events ($p = 0.03$), yet among hospital survivors, mortality was similar ($p = 0.7$).

124. Steg PG, et al.; for the Global Registry of Acute Coronary Events (GRACE) Investigators. Mortality following placement of drug-eluting and bare-metal stents for ST-segment elevation acute myocardial infarction in the Global Registry of Acute Coronary Events. *Eur Heart J* 2009;30:321–329.

In this multinational, observational registry of acute coronary syndromes, the investigators reviewed outcomes in 5,093 patients with STEMI receiving DES ($n = 1,313$) compared with those receiving BMS ($n = 3,780$). Baseline characteristics did differ significantly (with patients receiving BMS having higher risk characteristics); however, in risk-adjusted and propensity analyses, postdischarge mortality was not different at 6 months ($p = 0.21$) or 1 year ($p = 0.34$). Mortality from 6 months to 2 years and from 1 to 2 years was significantly higher in the DES group (hazard ratio 4.90, $p = 0.01$, and hazard ratio 7.06, $p = 0.02$, respectively).

125. Di Lorenzo E, et al.; The PASEO (PaclitAxel or Sirolimus-Eluting Stent Versus Bare Metal Stent in Primary Angioplasty) randomized trial. *J Am Coll Cardiol Intvervent* 2009;2:515–523.

Design: Prospective, randomized, open-label, trial. The primary end point was TLR at 1 year.

Purpose: To compare the two most common DES with each other and with BMS for acute STEMI.

Population: 270 patients with STEMI within 12 hours of symptom onset.

Treatment: Primary angioplasty with implantation of either BMS, SES, or PES.

Results: After 1 year, rates of TLR significantly favored the DES—BMS (14.4%), PES (4.4%, p = 0.023), and SES (3.3%, p = 0.016). There were no differences in the rates of death and/or reinfarction at 2 years.

126. Brar SS, et al. Use of drug-eluting stents in acute myocardial infarction a systematic review and meta-analysis. *J Am Coll Cardiol* 2009;53:1677–1689.

The authors combined results from 13 randomized trials encompassing 7,352 patients comparing BMS and DES in STEMI. Rates of TVR favored DES over BMS (RR, 0.44; 95% CI, 0.35 to 0.55), with no effect on death (RR, 0.89; 95% CI, 0.70 to 1.14), reinfarction (RR, 0.82; 95% CI, 0.64 to 1.05), or stent thrombosis (RR, 0.97; 95% CI, 0.73 to 1.28). These results remained consistent over 2 years of follow-up. They also reviewed results form 18 registry studies including 26,521 patients; similarly, DES significantly reduced TVR (RR, 0.54; 95% CI, 0.40 to 0.74). While mortality was significantly lower at 1 year, rates were similar between DES and BMS at 2 years.

ANTITHROMBOTIC REGIMENS
Antithrombins

127. Ross AM, et al. Randomized comparison of enoxaparin, a low-molecular-weight heparin with unfractionated heparin adjunctive to recombinant tissue plasminogen activator thrombolysis and aspirin: second trial of Heparin and Aspirin Reperfusion Therapy (HART II). *Circulation* 2001;104:648–652.

Design: Prospective, randomized, open-label, parallel-group, international trial. The primary end point was IRA patency (TIMI grade 2 or 3 flow) at 90 minutes.

Purpose: To demonstrate noninferiority of enoxaparin compared with UFH as an adjunctive therapy during thrombolytic treatment for acute MI.

Population: 400 patients seen within 12 hours and with ST elevation 0.1 mV or more in two or more limb leads or ST elevation of 0.2 mV or more in two or more contiguous precordial leads.

Exclusion Criteria: Contraindications to thrombolysis and serum creatinine more than 2 mg/dL.

Treatment: Enoxaparin or UFH for at least 3 days. All received accelerated tPA regimen and aspirin.

Results: Patency rates at 90 minutes were 80.1% and 75.1% in the enoxaparin and UFH groups, respectively. TIMI grade 3 flow was observed in 52.9% and 47.6%, respectively. Reocclusion at 5 to 7 days from TIMI grade 2 or 3 to TIMI 0 or 1 flow and TIMI grade 3 to TIMI 0 or 1 flow, respectively, occurred in 5.9% and 3.1% of the enoxaparin group versus 9.8% and 9.1% in the UFH group. Bleeding and 30-day mortality rates were similar in both groups.

Comments: The results of this study complement the findings of the larger ASSENT-3 trial (98).

128. Antman EM, et al. Enoxaparin as adjunctive antithrombin therapy for ST-elevation myocardial infarction: results of the ENTIRE-Thrombolysis in Myocardial Infarction (TIMI) 23 trial. *Circulation* 2002;105:1642–1649.

Design: Prospective, randomized, open, 2 × 2 factorial, multicenter trial. The primary end point was TIMI grade 3 flow at 60 minutes.

Purpose: To evaluate enoxaparin with full-dose TNK and half-dose TNK plus abciximab.

Population: 483 patients with STEMI seen <6 hours from symptom onset.

Exclusion Criteria: Included contraindications to thrombolysis; abciximab within the prior 7 days or eptifibatide or tirofiban within the prior 24 hours; treatment with any LMWH or UFH within 24 hours.

Treatment: Full-dose TNK and either UFH (60-U/kg bolus and then 12 U/kg/h) or enoxaparin (1.0 mg/kg s.c. every 12 hours ± initial 30-mg i.v. bolus) or half-dose TNK plus abciximab and either UFH (40-U/kg bolus and then 7 U/kg/h) or enoxaparin (0.3 to 0.75 mg/kg s.c. every 12 hours ± initial i.v. bolus of 30 mg).

Results: With full-dose TNK and UFH, TIMI grade 3 flow at 60 minutes was 52% and was 48% to 51% with enoxaparin. With combination therapy, the TIMI 3 flow was achieved in 48% with UFH and 47% to 58% with enoxaparin. The rate of TIMI 3 flow among all UFH patients was 50% compared with 51% among enoxaparin patients. At 30 days, death or recurrent MI occurred with the full-dose TNK group in 15.9% of patients with UFH compared with only 4.4% with enoxaparin ($p = 0.005$). With combination therapy, the rates were 6.5% with UFH and 5.5% with enoxaparin. Major hemorrhage with full-dose TNK occurred in 2.4% with UFH and 1.9% with enoxaparin; with combination therapy, 5.2% with UFH and 8.5% with enoxaparin.

Comments: Major finding is that in patients receiving full-dose TNK, enoxaparin was associated with similar TIMI 3 flow rates but fewer ischemic events at 30 days compared with UFH.

129. Antman EM, et al.; for the ExTRACT-TIMI 25 Investigators. Enoxaparin versus unfractionated heparin with fibrinolysis for ST-elevation myocardial infarction. N Engl J Med 2006;354:1477–1488.

Design: Prospective, randomized, double-blind, international, multicenter trial. The primary end point was death or nonfatal recurrent MI at 30 days.

Purpose: To compare efficacy and safety of enoxaparin versus UFH in patients with STEMI receiving fibrinolytic therapy.

Population: 20,056 patients with STEMI seen <6 hours from symptom onset and eligible for fibrinolysis.

Exclusion Criteria: Included cardiogenic shock, pericarditis, symptoms of aortic dissection, contraindications to fibrinolysis, receipt of a low-molecular-weight heparin within the prior 8 hours, known renal insufficiency (serum creatinine > 2.5 mg/dL for men, 2.0 mg/dL for women), or life expectancy <12 months.

Treatment: UFH for at least 48 hours versus enoxaparin throughout hospitalization (or 8 days, whichever was shorter). Enoxaparin dosing was reduced in patients 75 years of age or older. All patients received aspirin and fibrinolysis (the agent at the physician's discretion), and clopidogrel was given at the physician's discretion.

Results: Enoxaparin significantly reduced the primary end point (9.9% vs. 12.0%, $p < 0.001$), with the majority of the benefit in reduction of reinfarction. Major bleeding was significantly higher in the enoxaparin group (2.1% vs. 1.4%, $p < 0.001$). When ischemic and bleeding events were combined (death, reinfarction, intracranial hemorrhage), this net clinical effect favored enoxaparin (10.1% vs. 12.2%, $p < 0.001$).

Comments: The superiority of enoxaparin over UFH was subsequently verified in multiple prespecified, post hoc analyses of different subgroups of the trial, including age stratification (*Eur Heart J* 2007;28:1066–1071), patients with impaired renal function (*J Am Coll Cardiol* 2007;49:2249–2255), patients who did and did **not** receive clopidogrel (*J Am Coll Cardiol* 2007;49:2256–2263), each type of fibrinolytic agent (*Eur Heart J* 2007;28:1566–1573), and also those patients in the ExTRACT-TIMI 25 trial who subsequently underwent PCI as a "rescue" strategy or for recurrent symptoms (*J Am Coll Cardiol* 2007;49:2238–2246).

130. Murphy SA, et al. Efficacy and safety of the low-molecular weight heparin enoxaparin compared with unfractionated heparin across the acute coronary syndrome spectrum: a meta-analysis. *Eur Heart J* 2007;28:2077–2086.

The investigators combined patient-level data from 12 randomized studies (6 each of both STEMI and UA/NSTEMI), including 49,088 patients. The net clinical events end point was a composite of death, MI, or major bleeding at 30 days. Across the spectrum of ACS, enoxaparin proved superior to UFH for ischemic events (9.8% vs. 11.4% for death or MI, $p < 0.001$) and reduced the net clinical event rate nonsignificantly (12.5% vs. 13.5%, $p = 0.051$). Major bleeding remained higher in the enoxaparin group (4.3% vs. 3.4%, $p = 0.019$). When isolated to STEMI patients only, the net clinical events end point significantly favored enoxaparin (OR, 0.94; $p = 0.015$).

131. Yusuf S, et al.; for the CREATE Trial Group Investigators. Effects of reviparin, a low-molecular weight heparin, on mortality, reinfarction, and strokes in patients with acute myocardial infarction presenting with ST-segment elevation. *JAMA* 2005;293:427–435.

Design: Prospective, randomized, double-blind, placebo-controlled, multicenter, international trial. The primary end point was a composite of death, reinfarction, or stoke at 7 and 30 days.

Purpose: To compare the effects of reviparin versus placebo, in addition to standard therapy, for patients with STEMI.

Population: 15,570 patients with STEMI presenting within 12 hours of symptoms.

Treatment: Reviparin twice daily or placebo for 7 days.

Results: Reviparin significantly reduced the primary outcome at 7 days (9.6% vs. 11%, $p = 0.005$), and the effect persisted at 30 days (11.8% vs. 13.6%, $p = 0.001$). Overall mortality at 30 days was also significantly reduced in the reviparin group (9.8% vs. 11.3%, $p = 0.005$), as well as reinfarction (2.0% vs. 2.6%, $p = 0.01$) without a change in stroke rate (1.0% vs. 0.8%, $p = 0.19$). There was a significant time-to-benefit effect with reviparin ($p = 0.04$ for trend to increased benefit for every 2 hours the sooner it was given). Life-threatening bleeding occurred at a higher, albeit nonsignificant, rate in the reviparin group at 7 days (0.2% vs. 0.1%, $p = 0.07$).

132. Montalescot G, et al. Intravenous enoxaparin or unfractionated heparin in primary percutaneous coronary intervention for ST-elevation myocardial infarction: the international randomized open-label ATOLL trial. *Lancet* 2011;378:693–703.

Design: Randomized, open-label, international, multicenter trial. The primary end point was a composite end point of death, complication of MI, procedural failure, or major bleeding.

Purpose: Comparison of traditional IV UFH with IV enoxaparin in primary PCI.

Population: 910 patients with STEMI or new LBBB, age ≥ 18, presentation within 12 hours or if 12 to 24 hours with persistent symptoms or persistent/recurrent ST elevations, cardiogenic shock from STEMI, or cardiac arrest (<10 min) from STEMI.

Exclusion Criteria: Anticoagulation use prior to randomization, use of thrombolytics, short life expectancy, and childbearing potential.

Treatment: IV bolus of enoxaparin 0.5 mg/kg versus IV bolus of UFH 70 to 100 IU/kg (if no concurrent GP IIb/IIIa) or 50 to 70 IU/kg (if concurrent GP IIb/IIIa).

Results: There was no statistically significant difference in the primary composite end point of death/MI complications/procedural failure/major bleeding between the two groups [34% in the UFH group vs. 28% in the enoxaparin group; RR, 0.83 (95% CI, 0.68 to 1.01); $p = 0.06$].

133. The OASIS-6 Trial Group. Effects of fondaparinux on mortality and reinfarction in patients with acute ST-segment elevation myocardial infarction: the OASIS-6 randomized trial. **JAMA 2006;295:1519–1530.**

Design: Prospective, randomized, double-blind, multicenter, international trial. The primary end point was a composite of death or reinfarction at 30 days. Additional secondary analyses at 9 days, 3 months, and 6 months.

Purpose: To compare efficacy and safety of fondaparinux versus control (either placebo or UFH) for treatment in patients with STEMI in whom UFH is indicated and in patients in whom it is not indicated.

Population: 12,092 patients with STEMI, presenting within 12 to 24 hours of symptom onset; enrollment was stratified by whether the clinician–investigator felt UFH was indicated.

Treatment: Patients in whom UFH was not indicated (stratum 1) were randomized to either fondaparinux or placebo (control group); patients in whom UFH was indicated (stratum 2) were randomized to either fondaparinux or UFH. If patients went for PCI, blinded study drug was maintained, with dosing adjusted depending on whether they received UFH and/or glycoprotein IIb/IIIa inhibitors prior to randomization. Both strata were combined [comparing fondaparinux vs. control (placebo or UFH)] for reporting of the primary outcome.

Results: The primary end point was significantly decreased in the fondaparinux group, compared to control (9.7% vs. 11.2%, $p = 0.008$). This benefit was significant at 9 days ($p = 0.003$). In patients in stratum 2 not undergoing PCI, fondaparinux nonsignificantly reduced rates of death and reinfarction at 30 days, compared with UFH (hazard ratio, 0.82; $p = 0.08$). For patients undergoing primary PCI, there was no difference in outcomes between fondaparinux and either control. With respect to the primary outcome, fondaparinux proved superior to control in patients receiving thrombolytic therapy (hazard ratio, 0.79; $p = 0.003$) and among those receiving no reperfusion therapy (hazard ratio, 0.80; $p = 0.03$).

Direct Thrombin Inhibitors

134. Antman EM, et al.; for the TIMI-9B Investigators. Hirudin in AMI. *Circulation* 1996;94:911–921.

Design: Prospective, randomized, double-blind, parallel-group, multicenter study. The primary end point was 30-day incidence of death, nonfatal MI, severe CHF, and cardiogenic shock.

Purpose: To compare the safety and effectiveness of hirudin with heparin in patients undergoing thrombolysis for acute MI.

Population: 3,002 patients within 12 hours of onset of symptoms and with >1-mm ST elevation in at least two contiguous ECG leads; mean age of 60 ± 12 years.

Exclusion Criteria: Contraindications to thrombolytic therapy, creatinine more than 2.0 mg/dL, cardiogenic shock, and therapeutic anticoagulation (PT, 14 seconds; aPTT, 60 seconds).

Treatment: Heparin, 5,000-U i.v. bolus and then 1,000 U/h, or hirudin, 0.1-mg/kg i.v. bolus and then 0.1 mg/kg/h (maximum, 15 mg/h) for 96 hours. Infusions were started before or immediately after thrombolysis (front-loaded tPA or SK) and adjusted to keep aPTT at 55 to 85 seconds. All patients were given thrombolysis.

Results: No significant difference in primary end points was observed—12.9% (hirudin) versus 11.9%—nor were any differences observed in hemorrhage and intracranial hemorrhage rates (4.6% vs. 5.3; 0.4% vs. 0.9%). Target aPTT was achieved more frequently with hirudin.

135. White HD, et al.; on behalf of the Hirulog Early Perfusion/Occlusion (HERO) Trial Investigators. Randomized, double-blind comparison of hirulog versus heparin in patients receiving streptokinase and aspirin for acute MI (HERO). *Circulation* 1997;96:2155–2161 (editorial, 2118–2120).

Design: Prospective, randomized, double-blind, multicenter study. The primary outcome was TIMI grade flow at 90 to 120 minutes.

Purpose: To evaluate and compare the safety and efficacy of two hirulog regimens with heparin in acute MI patients receiving SK.

Population: 412 patients seen within 12 hours of symptom onset and with 1-mm ST elevation or greater in at least two contiguous limb leads and/or V_4 to V_6 or 2 mm or more in V_1 to V_3.

Exclusion Criteria: Prior SK, cardiogenic shock, and contraindications to thrombolysis.

Treatment: Heparin (5,000-U i.v. bolus and then 1,000 to 1,200 U/h), low-dose hirulog (0.125 mg/kg i.v. bolus, 0.25 mg/kg/h for 12 hours, and then 0.125 mg/kg/h), or high-dose hirulog (0.25-mg/kg intravenously bolus, 0.5 mg/kg/h for 12 hours, and then 0.25 mg/kg/h).

Results: Hirulog groups had better TIMI grade 3 flow at 90 to 120 minutes (primary outcome)—46% and 48% versus 35% (heparin vs. hirulog, p = 0.023; heparin vs. high-dose hirulog, p = 0.03). However, no significant difference in rates of reocclusion was observed at 48 hours (5% and 1% vs. 7%) or death, shock, and reinfarction at 35 days (14% and 12.5% vs. 17.9%). Hirulog also was associated with less major bleeding: 14% and 19% versus 28% (low-dose hirulog vs. heparin, p < 0.01).

136. Behar S, et al. Argatroban versus heparin as adjuvant therapy for thrombolysis for acute myocardial infarction: safety considerations ARGAMI-2 study [abstract]. *Circulation* 1998;98(1 Suppl):I453–I454.

This prospective, randomized, placebo-controlled study was composed of 1,200 patients seen within 6 hours and with ST elevation in two or more leads. Exclusion criteria included CNS events, elevated creatinine, and increased bleeding risk(s). Patients were randomized to argatroban (60 μg + 2 μg/kg/min or 120 μg + 4 μg/kg/min for 72 hours) or heparin (5,000 IU + 1,000 IU/h for 72 hours) with dose adjustment(s) to achieve aPTT of 55 to 85 seconds. All received aspirin and tPA or SK. Low-dose argatroban arm was closed after interim analysis of first 609 patients. At 30 days, no difference was found between the high-dose argatroban and heparin groups in total cardiovascular events, mortality, recurrent MI, heart failure/cardiogenic shock, need for revascularization, or stroke. The argatroban group had a lower incidence of major bleeding, intracranial hemorrhage, and stroke. Maintaining aPTT was easier with argatroban, with only 35% of having an aPTT value <55 seconds at 24 hours compared with 68% in the heparin group.

137. The Hirulog and Early Reperfusion or Occlusion (HERO)-2 Trial Investigators. Thrombin-specific anticoagulation with bivalirudin versus heparin in patients receiving fibrinolytic therapy for acute myocardial infarction: the HERO-2 randomized trial. *Lancet* 2001;358:1855–1863.

Design: Prospective, randomized, open, multicenter study. The primary end point was 30-day mortality.

Purpose: To evaluate the effect on 30-day mortality of bivalirudin versus UFH in acute MI patients treated with SK.

Population: 17,073 patients with acute STEMI seen within 6 hours of symptom onset and with 1 mm or more of ST elevation in two limb leads or 2 mm or more in two contiguous precordial leads or presumed new LBBB.

Exclusion Criteria: Included contraindications to thrombolysis, LMWH therapy within 12 hours, and previous SK therapy.

Treatment: Bivalirudin (0.25-mg/kg bolus, then 0.5 mg/kg/h for 12 hours, and then 0.25 mg/kg/h for 36 hours) or UFH. All received SK, 1.5 MU over a 30- to 60-minute period, and aspirin, 150 to 325 mg once daily.

Results: At 30 days, no significant difference appeared between the two groups in unadjusted mortality (bivalirudin, 10.8%; heparin, 10.9%) and adjusted mortality (10.5% vs. 10.9%). At 96 hours, the bivalirudin group had a 30% reduction in reinfarction compared with the heparin group (1.6% vs. 2.3%, $p = 0.001$). Nonsignificant trends were seen toward increased severe bleeding and intracerebral bleeding with bivalirudin (0.7% vs. 0.5%, $p = 0.07$; 0.6% vs. 0.4%, $p = 0.09$), whereas significant increased risks of both moderate and mild bleeding were noted (1.4% vs. 1.1%, $p = 0.05$; 12.8% vs. 9.0%, $p < 0.001$).

138. The Direct Thrombin Inhibitor Trialists' Collaborative Group. Direct thrombin inhibitors in acute coronary syndromes: principal results of a meta-analysis based on individual patients' data. *Lancet* 2002;359:294–302.

This meta-analysis examined 11 randomized trials (35,970 total patients) comparing a direct thrombin inhibitor (DTI; hirudin, bivalirudin, argatroban, efegatran, or inogatran) with heparin. Compared with heparin, DTIs were associated with a lower risk of death or MI at the end of treatment [4.3% vs. 5.1%; OR, 0.85 (95% CI, 0.77 to 0.94); $p = 0.001$] and at 30 days [7.4% vs. 8.2%; OR, 0.91 (95% CI, 0.84 to 0.99); $p = 0.02$]. This was due primarily to a reduction in MI [2.8% vs. 3.5%; OR, 0.80 (95% CI, 0.71 to 0.90); $p < 0.001$] with no significant effect on mortality [1.9% vs. 2.0%; OR, 0.97 (95% CI, 0.83 to 1.13); $p = 0.69$]. Subgroup analyses suggested a benefit of DTIs on death or MI in trials of both acute coronary syndromes and PCIs. Compared with heparin, an increased risk of major bleeding with hirudin was seen, but a reduction with bivalirudin. No increased incidence of intracranial hemorrhage was found with DTIs.

139. Stone GW, et al.; for the HORIZONS-AMI Trial Investigators. Bivalirudin during primary PCI in acute myocardial infarction. *N Engl J Med* 2008;358:2218–2230.

Design: Prospective, randomized, open-label, multicenter study. Two coprimary end points: (a) major bleeding and (b) combined adverse clinical events (major bleeding, death, reinfarction, TVR for ischemia, or stroke), both at 30 days.

Purpose: To evaluate the strategy of bivalirudin as anticoagulation for patients undergoing primary PCI for STEMI, as compared with a combination of UFH and glycoprotein IIb/IIIa inhibitor.

Population: 3,602 patients with STEMI, presenting within 12 hours of symptom onset, undergoing primary PCI.

Treatment: Bivalirudin alone versus UFH plus a glycoprotein IIb/IIIa inhibitor.

Results: Treatment with bivalirudin resulted in decreased rates of clinical adverse events (9.2% vs. 12.1%, $p = 0.005$), mainly driven by reduced rates of major bleeding (4.9% vs. 8.3%, $p < 0.001$). However, there was a significant increase in acute stent thrombosis in the bivalirudin group at 24 hours (1.3% vs. 0.3%, $p < 0.001$). Despite this, 30-day rates of stent thrombosis (1.7% vs. 1.2%, $p = 0.28$) were similar, and cardiac mortality (1.8% vs. 2.9%, $p = -0.03$) and overall mortality (2.1% vs. 3.1%, $p = 0.047$) were both reduced at 30 days.

140. Steg PG, et al. Bivalirudin started during emergency transport for primary PCI (the European Ambulance Acute Coronary Syndrome Angiography [EUROMAX] trial). *N Engl J Med* 2013;369(23):2207–2217.

Design: International, randomized, multicenter, open-label trial. The primary outcome was a composite of death from any cause or major bleeding not related to CABG at 30 days.

Purpose: To evaluate bivalirudin (with GP IIb/IIIa inhibitor use allowed for giant thrombus or no reflow) versus UFH or enoxaparin (with GP IIb/IIIa inhibitor use at the discretion of the individual physicians) in STEMI patients.

Population: 2,218 patients ≥18 years old with STEMI undergoing primary PCI.

Exclusion Criteria: The main exclusion criteria were treatment with any injectable anticoagulant before randomization, oral anticoagulation, recent surgery, and a history of bleeding.

Treatment: Bivalirudin 0.75 mg/kg followed by an infusion of 1.75 mg/kg/h versus heparin 100 IU/kg without a GP IIb/IIIa inhibitor or 60 IU/kg with a GP IIb/IIIa inhibitor or enoxaparin bolus 0.5 mg/kg (the heparin group was considered the "control" arm).

Results: The primary outcome occurred in 5.1% of the bivalirudin group and 8.5% of the heparin (control) group [RR, 0.60 (95% CI, 0.43 to 0.82); $p = 0.001$]. Non-CABG major bleeding occurred more in the control arm [6.0% vs. 2.6%; RR, 0.43 (95% CI, 0.28 to 0.66); $p < 0.001$].

141. Shahzad A, et al. Unfractionated heparin versus bivalirudin in primary percutaneous coronary intervention (HEAT-PPCI): an open-label, single centre, randomised controlled trial. *Lancet* 2014;384:1849–1858. doi: 10.1016/S0140-6736(14)60924-7.

Design: Prospective, randomized, single center, parallel assignment, open-label trial. The primary outcome was MACE: incidence of all-cause mortality, CVA, reinfarction, and additional unplanned TLR at 28 days.

Purpose: To compare UFH to bivalirudin (with provisional GP IIb/IIIa inhibitor bailout) in STEMI patients undergoing primary PCI.

Population: 1,829 patients with suspected acute MI.

Treatment: UFH (70 U/Kg) versus bivalirudin (0.75 mg/kg followed by an infusion of 1.75 mg/kg/h). GP IIb/IIIa inhibitor bailout was used in 13.5% of the bivalirudin group and 15.5% of the heparin group.

Results: MACE occurred at a rate of 8.7% in the bivalirudin arm and 5.7% in the heparin arm [RR, 1.52 (95% CI, 1.1 to 2.1); $p = 0.01$]. Definite or probable stent thrombosis occurred more frequently in the bivalirudin arm [RR, 3.91 (95% CI, 1.6 to 9.5); $p = 0.001$]. Major bleeding was not significantly different between the two arms (3.5% in the bivalirudin arm vs. 3.1% in the heparin arm).

Oral Anticoagulants

142. Smith P, et al.; Warfarin Reinfarction Study (WARIS). The effect of warfarin on mortality and reinfarction after MI. *N Engl J Med* 1990;323:147–152.

Design: Prospective, randomized, double-blind, placebo-controlled, multicenter study. The mean follow-up period was 37 months. The primary end points were all-cause mortality and reinfarction.

Purpose: To evaluate the effects of warfarin on mortality, reinfarction, and cerebrovascular events in post-MI patients.

Population: 1,214 patients aged 75 years or younger; mean time since index MI, 27 days.

Exclusion Criteria: Required anticoagulant use and significant bleeding risk.

Treatment: Warfarin dose adjusted to achieve target INR of 2.8 to 4.8 or placebo.

Results: Warfarin group had 24% lower all-cause mortality (15.5% vs. 20.3%, $p = 0.03$), 34% fewer reinfarctions (13.5% vs. 20.4%, $p < 0.001$), and 55% fewer cerebrovascular accidents (CVAs; 3.3% vs. 7.2%; $p = 0.0015$). Serious bleeding rate in the warfarin group was 0.6% per year (intracranial hemorrhage rate, 0.2% per year).

143. Anticoagulants in Secondary Prevention of Events in Coronary Thrombosis (ASPECT) Research Group. Effect of long-term anticoagulant treatment on mortality and cardiovascular morbidity after MI. *Lancet* 1994;343:499–503.

Design: Prospective, randomized, double-blind, placebo-controlled, multicenter study. The mean follow-up period was 37 months. The primary end point was all-cause mortality.

Purpose: To evaluate the impact of long-term anticoagulation in the secondary prevention of morbidity and mortality after acute MI.

Population: 3,404 patients with cardiac serum marker evidence of acute MI (2× or more than the upper limit of normal).

Exclusion Criteria: Need for long-term anticoagulation, anticoagulation therapy in the prior 6 months, increased bleeding tendency, and anticipated coronary revascularization procedure.

Treatment: Phenprocoumon or nicoumalone started within 6 weeks of hospital discharge to achieve an INR of 2.8 to 4.8, or placebo.

Results: No significant mortality difference was observed between groups [10% (anticoagulation) vs. 11.1%]. Anticoagulation was associated with a reduction in two secondary end points: more than 50% fewer recurrent MIs (6.7% vs. 14.2%) and approximately 40% fewer cerebrovascular events (2.2% vs. 3.6%). The anticoagulation group had more major bleeding complications (4.3% vs. 1.1%).

Comments: A post hoc analysis showed that the optimal INR was 3 to 4. The rate of major bleeding plus thromboembolic complications was 3.2 per 100 patient-years (INR, <2, 8.0; 2 to 3, 3.9; 4 to 5, 6.6; >5, 7.7).

144. Julian DG, et al.; for the Aspirin/Anticoagulants Following Thrombolysis with Eminase in Recurrent infarction (AFTER) Study Group. A comparison of aspirin and anticoagulation following thrombolysis for MI (the AFTER study): a multicentre unblinded randomised clinical trial. *BMJ* 1996;313:1429–1431.

Design: Prospective, randomized, unblinded, multicenter study. Follow-up period was 1 year. The primary end points were cardiac death and nonfatal MI at 30 days.

Purpose: To compare aspirin with heparin followed by oral anticoagulation therapy in MI patients undergoing thrombolysis with anistreplase.

Population: 1,036 patients treated with anistreplase within 6 hours of onset of symptoms (ECG criteria, 2 mm or more ST elevation in at least two adjacent precordial leads or 1 mm or more in at least two limb leads).

Treatment: Aspirin, 150 mg/day, or heparin, 1,000 U/h for 24 hours (started 6 hours after anistreplase, 30 U) followed by oral anticoagulation to achieve a target INR of 2.0 to 2.5. Therapy was discontinued after 3 months.

Results: Similar 30-day incidences of cardiac death and reinfarction were observed [11.2% (aspirin) vs. 11%]. The anticoagulation group had more severe bleeding and strokes: at 3 months, 3.9% versus 1.7% (*p* = 0.04).

145. Coumadin Aspirin Reinfarction Study (CARS) Investigators. Randomised double-blind trial of fixed low-dose warfarin with aspirin after MI. *Lancet* 1997;350:389–396.

Design: Prospective, randomized, double-blind, multicenter study. Median follow-up period was 14 months. The primary end points were MI, stroke, and cardiovascular death.

Purpose: To compare long-term administration of aspirin alone with lower dose aspirin in combination with fixed low-dose regimens of oral anticoagulation in acute MI patients.

Population: 8,803 patients aged 21 to 85 years with documented MI 3 to 21 days before enrollment.

Treatment: Aspirin, 160 mg/day; aspirin, 80 mg/day; and warfarin, 1 mg/day, or aspirin, 80 mg/day, and warfarin, 3 mg/day.

Results: Average measured INRs at week 4 were 1.02 (aspirin alone), 1.05 (aspirin and warfarin, 1 mg/day), and 1.27 (aspirin and warfarin, 3 mg/day). No significant difference in primary end point (MI, stroke, or cardiovascular death) was observed [1-year rates, 8.6% (aspirin), 8.8% (aspirin and warfarin, 1 mg/day), 8.4% (aspirin and warfarin, 3 mg/day)]. However, the warfarin, 3 mg/day, group had a higher rate of spontaneous major hemorrhage versus aspirin alone: 0.74% per year versus 1.4% per year ($p = 0.014$).

146. Fiore LD, et al.; for the Combination Hemotherapy and Mortality Prevention (CHAMP) Study. Department of Veterans Affairs Cooperative Studies Program clinical trial comparing combined warfarin and aspirin with aspirin alone in survivors of acute myocardial infarction: primary results of the CHAMP study. *Circulation* 2002;105:557–563.

Design: Prospective, randomized, open-label, multicenter. The primary end point was all-cause mortality. Median follow-up was 2.7 years.

Purpose: To determine if the combination of aspirin and warfarin is more effective than aspirin monotherapy in the secondary prevention of vascular events and death after AMI.

Population: 5,059 patients with AMI within 14 days. Diagnosis of AMI as defined by the presence of two of the following: (a) chest discomfort typical of AMI, (b) ECG changes typical of AMI, and (c) blood enzyme changes typical of AMI.

Exclusion Criteria: Included more than 14 days after MI, ongoing bleeding or bleeding risk, alternative indication for anticoagulant therapy, treatment with high-dose aspirin or NSAID, and hypersensitivity to aspirin or warfarin.

Treatment: Warfarin (target INR, 1.5 to 2.5) plus aspirin (81 mg once daily) or aspirin alone (162 mg once daily).

Results: At follow-up, all-cause mortality was similar in the two groups [17.6% (combination group) vs. 17.3% (aspirin only)]. No significant difference was seen between the groups in recurrent MI (13.3% vs. 13.1%, respectively; log-rank $p = 0.78$) or stroke (3.1% vs. 3.5%, respectively; log-rank $p = 0.52$). Major bleeding, primarily GI, occurred more often in the combination-therapy group than in the aspirin group (1.28 events per 100 patient-years vs. 0.72 events per 100 patient-years, respectively; $p < 0.001$).

147. van Es RF, et al.; for the Antithrombotics in the Secondary Prevention of Events in Coronary Thrombosis-2 (ASPECT-2) Research Group. Aspirin and coumadin after acute coronary syndromes (the ASPECT-2 study): a randomised controlled trial. *Lancet* 2002;360:109–113.

Design: Prospective, randomized, open-label, multicenter trial. The primary composite end point was MI, stroke, or death.

Purpose: To determine whether the combination of aspirin and oral anticoagulants provides a greater benefit than either of these agents alone, without excessive risk of bleeding.

Population: 999 patients with AMI or unstable in previous 8 weeks.

Exclusion Criteria: Included established indication(s) for oral anticoagulation or platelet inhibitors, planned revascularization, increased risk of bleeding, bleeding diathesis, history of stroke, and pregnancy.

Treatment: Low-dose aspirin (80 mg), high-intensity oral anticoagulation (target INR, 3.0 to 4.0), or combined low-dose aspirin and moderate-intensity oral anticoagulation (target INR, 2.0 to 2.5).

Results: The anticoagulant and combination-therapy groups had a significantly lower incidence of the primary composite end point compared with the aspirin group [hazard ratio, 0.55 (95% CI, 0.30 to 1.00); $p = 0.0479$; hazard ratio, 0.50 (0.27 to 0.92); $p = 0.03$], respectively. Major bleeding was similar in the three groups (1% to 2%). Frequency of minor bleeding was 5%, 8% [1.68 (0.92 to 3.07), $p = 0.20$], and 15% [3.13 (1.82 to 5.37); $p \leq 0.0001$], in the aspirin, anticoagulant, and combination groups, respectively.

148. Hureln M, et al. Warfarin, aspirin, or both after myocardial infarction: WARIS-II (Warfarin–Aspirin Reinfarction Study). N Engl J Med 2002;347:969–974.

Design: Prospective, randomized, open-label, multicenter trial. The primary end points were death, nonfatal MI, and stroke. The mean follow-up was 4 years.

Purpose: To compare the efficacy and safety of long-term treatment with warfarin alone, aspirin alone, or the two combined in survivors of AMI.

Population: 3,630 patients aged 20 to 74 years with two or more of following—ischemic chest pain, ECG changes typical of AMI, CK >250 U/L, and/or aspartate aminotransferase >50 U/L of probable cardiac origin.

Exclusion Criteria: Included history of serious bleeding or bleeding diathesis, spontaneous bleeding with aspirin or warfarin, and any contraindication to or indication for aspirin or warfarin.

Treatment: Randomized on hospital discharge to warfarin (target INR, 2.8 to 4.2) or aspirin (160 mg/day) or warfarin (target INR, 2.0 to 2.5) and aspirin (75 mg/day). The average INR was 2.8 in the warfarin-alone group and 2.2 in the warfarin + aspirin group; however, measured INRs were below target one-third of the time.

Results: The incidence of death, nonfatal MI, and stroke was 20.0% in the aspirin-alone group compared with 16.7% in the warfarin-alone group [relative risk ratio compared with aspirin, 0.81 (95% CI, 0.67 to 0.98); $p = 0.028$] and 15.0% in the aspirin + warfarin group [relative risk ratio compared with aspirin, 0.71 (95% CI, 0.58 to 0.86); $p = 0.0005$]. The aspirin + warfarin group had a significantly higher cumulative probability of survival compared with the aspirin-alone group ($p = 0.0033$), whereas no significant difference was seen between the warfarin-alone and the warfarin + aspirin groups. However, major bleeding rates (bleeding requiring transfusion or surgical intervention) were higher in the warfarin groups (0.58/100 patient-years with warfarin alone and 0.52/100 patient-years in the warfarin + aspirin group) compared with aspirin alone (0.15/100 patient-years in the aspirin group). Minor bleeding rates were 0.81, 2.16, and 2.75/100 patient-years, respectively.

Comments: The exclusion of patients 75 years or older likely attenuated the excess warfarin-associated bleeding risk. Only 35% of patients underwent revascularization (PCI or CABG). The efficacy of warfarin as part of an early revascularization strategy and in conjunction with thienopyridine therapy is unknown.

149. Brouwer MA, et al. Aspirin plus coumarin versus aspirin alone in the prevention of reocclusion after fibrinolysis for acute myocardial infarction: results of the Antithrombotics in the Prevention of Reocclusion in Coronary Thrombolysis (APRICOT)-2 trial. Circulation 2002;106:659–665.

Design: Prospective, randomized, open, multicenter trial. The primary end point was angiographic reocclusion at 3 months.

Purpose: To evaluate a prolonged anticoagulation regimen as an adjunct to aspirin in the prevention of reocclusion and recurrent ischemic events after fibrinolysis for STEMI.

Population: 308 STEMI patients receiving aspirin and IVH and angiography within 48 hours showing TIMI grade 3 flow in IRA.

Treatment: Standard in-hospital heparinization and aspirin or aspirin and coumarin for 3 months (target INR, 2.0 to 3.0; median achieved INR, 2.6).

Results: The incidence of reocclusion (TIMI grade 2 flow or less) at 3 months was significantly lower in aspirin and coumarin compared with aspirin alone (15% vs. 28%; RR, 0.55; 95% CI, 0.33 to 0.90; $p < 0.02$). TIMI grade 0 to 1 flow rates were 9% and 20%, respectively (RR, 0.46; 95% CI, 0.24 to 0.89; $p < 0.02$). Aspirin and coumarin were also associated with lower rate of death, reinfarction, and revascularization (14% vs. 34%, $p < 0.01$). Bleeding rates (TIMI major and minor) were similar (5% vs. 3%, $p = $ NS).

Glycoprotein IIb/IIIa Inhibitors

150. Brener SJ, et al.; on behalf of the Reopro and Primary PTCA Organization and Randomized Trial (RAPPORT) Investigators. Randomized, placebo-controlled trial of primary glycoprotein IIb/IIIa blockade with primary angioplasty for acute MI. *Circulation* 1998;98:734–741.

Design: Prospective, randomized, double-blind, placebo-controlled, multicenter study. The primary end points (at 6 months) were death, MI, and any TVR.

Purpose: To evaluate whether platelet IIb/IIIa receptor blockade with abciximab reduces ischemic events in AMI patients undergoing primary angioplasty.

Population: 483 patients seen within 12 hours of onset of symptoms with ischemic chest pain lasting more than 20 minutes accompanied by significant ST elevation in at least two contiguous leads or new LBBB.

Exclusion Criteria: Included severe thrombocytopenia, baseline PTT >1.2× control, previous stroke, severe uncontrolled hypertension, PTCA of IRA in prior 3 months, cardiogenic shock, and prior abciximab or thrombolytic therapy.

Treatment: Abciximab, 0.25-mg/kg bolus and then 0.125 μg/kg/min (maximum, 10 μg/min) for 12 hours. All patients received aspirin and heparin, 100-U/kg bolus before PTCA [with further boluses as needed to keep activated clotting time (ACT) longer than 300 seconds]. Stenting was discouraged but was allowed for residual dissection with more than 50% restenosis and for abrupt or threatened closure.

Results: No difference was observed between the two groups in the incidence of 6-month primary end points (28.1% vs. 28.2%). However, the abciximab group had lower rates of death, MI, and urgent TVR at 7 days (3.3% vs. 9.9%, $p = 0.003$), 30 days (5.8% vs. 11.2%, $p = 0.03$), and 6 months (11.6% vs. 17.8%, $p = 0.05$). The abciximab group had 42% less bailout stenting (11.9% vs. 20.4%, $p = 0.008$). Abciximab was associated with increased major bleeding (defined as hematocrit decrease of >5; 16.6% vs. 9.5%; $p = 0.02$), mostly at the arterial access site. On-treatment analysis showed that abciximab was associated with decreased death and MI at 7 days (1.4% vs. 4.7%, $p = 0.047$) with a trend at 6 months (6.9% vs. 12%, $p = 0.07$).

Comments: Increased bleeding with abciximab was likely due to double-blind design, as the investigators were unwilling to discontinue heparin immediately after procedure(s) for early sheath removal.

151. Montalescot G, et al.; for the ADMIRAL Investigators. Platelet glycoprotein IIb/IIIa inhibition with coronary stenting for acute myocardial infarction. *N Engl J Med* 2001;344:1895–1903.

Design: Prospective, randomized, multicenter, double-blind, placebo-controlled trial. Primary composite end point at 30 days: death, reinfarction, or urgent TVR.

Purpose: To compare the combination of primary stenting and platelet glycoprotein IIb/IIIa receptor inhibition with primary stenting alone in AMI.

Population: 300 patients seen within 12 hours of onset of symptoms with 1 mm or more ST elevation in two or more contiguous leads.

Exclusion Criteria: Included bleeding diathesis, thrombolytic administration for current episode, recent stroke, uncontrolled hypertension, recent surgery, oral anticoagulant therapy, and known contraindications to aspirin, ticlopidine, or heparin.

Treatment: Abciximab (0.25-mg/kg bolus and then 0.125 μg/kg/min for 12 hours) plus stent implantation or primary stenting alone. Therapy was initiated before sheath insertion and coronary angiography. Follow-up angiography at 24 hours and 6 months.

Results: Abciximab group had a significantly higher initial TIMI grade 3 flow compared with placebo (16.8% vs. 5.4%, $p = 0.01$; grade 2 or 3, 25.8% vs. 10.8%, $p = 0.006$). TIMI grade 3 flow after procedure and at 6 months also was higher in the abciximab group (95.1% vs. 86.7%, $p = 0.04$; 94.3% vs. 82.8%, $p = 0.04$). At 30 days, the abciximab group had a nearly 60% lower incidence of the primary end point (6.0% vs. 14.6%, $p = 0.01$; at 6 months, 7.4% vs. 15.9%). Much of this benefit was from a lower rate of urgent TVR with abciximab (at 30 days, 1.3% vs. 6.6%, $p = 0.02$), although mortality also trended lower (at 30 days, 3.4% vs. 6.6%, $p = 0.19$). The abciximab group had a significantly higher LVEF at 24 hours (57.0% vs. 53.9%, $p < 0.05$) and at 6 months (61.1% vs. 57.0%, $p = 0.05$).

152. Stone GW, et al.; for the Controlled Abciximab and Device Investigation to Lower Late Angioplasty Complications (CADILLAC) Investigators. Comparison of angioplasty with stenting, with or without abciximab, in acute myocardial infarction. N *Engl J Med* 2002;346:957–966.

Design: Prospective, randomized, open, 2 × 2 factorial, multicenter trial. The primary end points at 6 months were death, reinfarction, disabling stroke, and ischemia-driven TVR.

Purpose: To determine whether the addition of coronary stenting and/or glycoprotein IIb/IIIA inhibitors to PTCA alone can further improve outcomes in AMI patients.

Population: 2,082 patients seen within 6 hours who underwent urgent cardiac catheterization and were eligible for stent placement.

Exclusion Criteria: Included cardiogenic shock, bleeding diathesis, CVA in previous 2 years, history of leukopenia, thrombocytopenia, or hepatic or renal dysfunction.

Treatment: PTCA alone, PTCA plus abciximab, stenting alone (Multilink stent), or stenting plus abciximab.

Results: TIMI grade 3 flow rates were similar in the four groups (95% to 97%). At 6 months, the primary composite end point occurred in 20.0% of the PTCA-alone group, 16.5% with PTCA plus abciximab, 11.5% with stenting, and 10.2% with stenting plus abciximab ($p < 0.001$). No significant differences were found in 6-month mortality between the four groups (PTCA alone, 4.5%; PTCA + abciximab, 2.5%; stenting, 3.0%; stenting + abciximab, 4.2%). Stroke and reinfarction rates also were similar. The difference in the incidence of the primary end point was owing to differences in the rates of TVR (15.7% with PTCA alone, 13.8% with PTCA + abciximab, 8.3% with stenting, and only 5.2% with stenting + abciximab; $p < 0.001$). Follow-up angiography demonstrated a lower restenosis rate with stenting compared with PTCA (22.2% vs. 40.8%, $p < 0.001$). Reocclusion rates of the IRA were 11.3% and 5.7% ($p = 0.01$), respectively, and both were independent of abciximab use.

Comments: Inclusion criteria were "soft" because patients with infarct suspicion and angiographic evidence were enrolled; as a result, fewer than 90% had ST elevation or new LBBB.

153. Montalescot G, et al. Abciximab in primary coronary stenting of ST-elevation myocardial infarction: a European meta-analysis on individual patients' data with long-term follow-up. *Eur Heart J* 2007;28:443–449.

The authors combined patient-level data from the ISAR-2, ACE, and ADMIRAL trials, comparing clinical outcomes in patients receiving primary PCI for STEMI between those who received abciximab adjunctive therapy with stenting and those who received standard heparin only. The primary end point was a composite of death or reinfarction at 3 years of follow-up. The total population summed to 1,101, and patients in the abciximab group had significantly fewer primary events (hazard ratio, 12.9% vs. 19.0%; $p = 0.008$), as well as a nonsignificant trend toward lower overall mortality (10.9% vs. 14.3%, $p = 0.052$). Major bleeding episodes were similar (2.5% for the abciximab group vs. 2.0% without abciximab, $p = $ NS).

154. De Lusa G, et al. Benefits from small molecule administration as compared with abciximab among patients with ST-segment elevation myocardial infarction treated with primary angioplasty: a meta analysis. *J Am Coll Cardiol* 2009;53:1668–1673.

The authors combined six randomized trials comparing abciximab to small-molecule glycoprotein IIb/IIIa inhibitors (high-dose tirofiban in five trials, eptifibatide in one) in primary PCI, including a total of 2,197 patients. For all outcomes, abciximab was *not* superior to small-molecule inhibitors; this included postprocedural TIMI flow grade 3 (89.8% vs. 89.1%, $p = 0.72$), ST-segment resolution (67.8% vs. 68.2%, $p = 0.66$), 30-day mortality (2.2% vs. 2.0%, $p = 0.66$), and reinfarction (1.2% vs. 1.2%, $p = 0.88$).

155. Van't Hof AW, et al. Prehospital initiation of tirofiban in patients with ST-elevation myocardial infarction undergoing primary angioplasty (On-TIME 2): a multicentre, double-blind, randomised controlled trial. *Lancet* 2008;372:537–546.

Design: Double-blind, randomized, placebo-controlled, multicenter, international trial. The primary end point was residual ST-segment elevation 1 hour after PCI.

Purpose: To identify the benefit, if any, of early, high-dose tirofiban (compared with placebo), in addition to aspirin, heparin, and clopidogrel in patients with STEMI undergoing PCI.

Population: 984 patients with STEMI undergoing PCI.

Treatment: High-dose, bolus tirofiban or placebo, randomized in the ambulance.

Results: Patients who received tirofiban had significantly lower residual ST-segment elevation at 1 hour ($p = 0.003$), without higher bleeding rates.

156. Mehilli J, et al.; for the Bavarian Reperfusion Alternatives Evaluation-3 (BRAVE-3) Study Investigators. Abciximab in patients with acute ST-segment-elevation myocardial infarction undergoing primary percutaneous coronary intervention after clopidogrel loading: a randomized double-blind trial. *Circulation.* 2009;119:1933–1940.

Design: Randomized, double-blind, placebo-controlled trial. The primary end point was infarct size, as measured by sestamibi, at discharge.

Purpose: To identify the benefit, if any, of abciximab added to clopidogrel in patients with STEMI undergoing primary PCI.

Population: 800 patients with STEMI undergoing primary PCI.

Treatment: Abciximab or placebo prior to transfer to the catheterization laboratory.

Results: There was no significant difference in infarct size between the two groups (15.7% for abciximab vs. 16.6% for placebo, $p = 0.47$). Bleeding complications occurred at equal rates between the two groups. At 30 days, rates of the composite of death, recurrent MI, stroke, or urgent TVR were similar (5.0% for abciximab vs. 3.8% for placebo, $p = 0.40$).

Glycoprotein IIb/IIIa Inhibitors and Reduced-Dose Thrombolysis

157. Antman EM, et al. for the TIMI-14 Investigators. Abciximab facilitates the rate and extent of thrombolysis. *Circulation* 1999;99:2720–2732 (editorial, 2714–2716).

Design: Prospective, randomized, dose-ranging, multicenter study. The primary end point was IRA TIMI grade 3 flow at 90 minutes (also see ASSENT-3, Ref. 97).

Purpose: To determine whether abciximab is an effective and safe addition to reduced-dose thrombolytic regimens for STEMI.

Population: 888 patients aged 18 to 75 years seen within 12 hours of symptom onset with 1 mm or greater ST elevation in at least two contiguous ECG leads.

Exclusion Criteria: LBBB, 6,000-U heparin in the hour before randomization, prior CABG surgery, PCI or thrombolytic therapy in prior 7 days, and history of stroke or TIA.

Treatment: (a) 100 mg of accelerated-dose alteplase (control); (b) abciximab (0.25-mg/kg bolus and then 0.125 μg/kg/min for 12 hours) plus reduced-dose SK (500,000 to 1.5 million U); (c) abciximab plus reduced-dose alteplase (20 to 65 mg); or (d) abciximab alone. All patients received aspirin. Control patients received standard weight-based heparin (70-U/kg bolus; initial infusion, 15 U/kg/h), whereas the abciximab groups received low-dose heparin (60-U/kg bolus and then 7 U/kg/h). Very low-dose heparin also was tested in the dose-confirmation phase (30-U/kg bolus and then 4 U/kg/h).

Results: Abciximab alone achieved TIMI grade 3 flow at 90 minutes in only 32% and abciximab plus SK, 500,000 to 1.25 million U in only 34% to 46%. Higher rates of TIMI grade 3 flow at 60 and 90 minutes were seen with increasing duration of alteplase infusion, progressing from bolus alone to bolus and 30- or 60-minute infusion ($p <$ 0.02). The best regimen was abciximab and alteplase, 50 mg (15-mg bolus, 35 mg over 60 minutes), which produced TIMI 3 flow in 77% at 90 minutes (vs. 62% with alteplase alone, $p = 0.02$). TIMI 3 flow at 60 minutes also was significantly better with this regimen [72% vs. 43% (alteplase alone), $p = 0.0009$]. Major hemorrhage occurred in 3% receiving abciximab alone, 6% with alteplase alone, 10% with SK plus abciximab, 7% with 50-mg alteplase plus abciximab plus low-dose heparin, and 1% with 50-mg alteplase plus abciximab plus very low-dose heparin.

158. Strategies for Patency Enhancement in the Emergency Department (SPEED) Group. Trial of abciximab with and without low-dose reteplase for acute myocardial infarction. *Circulation* 2000;101:2788–2794.

This prospective, randomized, open-label, multicenter, phase II study enrolled 528 patients with STEMI within 6 hours of chest pain onset. Patients were randomized in a 4:1 fashion to abciximab alone ($n = 63$) or with 5, 7.5, 10, 5 + 2.5, or 5 + 5 U of reteplase ($n = 241$). Phase B tested the best phase A strategy (abciximab plus 5 + 5 U of reteplase, $n = 115$) against 10 + 10 U of reteplase alone ($n = 109$). Initial angiography was performed at a median of 63 minutes from the beginning of reperfusion therapy. In phase A, 62% of the abciximab–reteplase 5 + 5-U group had TIMI grade 3 flow (primary end point) versus 27% of the abciximab-only patients ($p = 0.001$). In phase B, 54% of the abciximab–reteplase 5 + 5-U group had grade 3 flow versus 47% of the reteplase-only patients ($p = 0.32$). TIMI grade 3 flow rates were 61% for a 60-U/kg heparin bolus and abciximab–reteplase 5 + 5 U, 51% for a 40-U/kg heparin bolus and abciximab–reteplase 5 + 5 U ($p = 0.22$), and 47% for reteplase alone ($p = 0.05$ vs. the 60-U/kg heparin group). Major bleeding rates in phase A were 3.3% for abciximab alone and 5.3% for abciximab–reteplase 5 + 5 U; rates in phase B were 9.8% for abciximab–reteplase 5 + 5 U and 3.7% for reteplase alone. Major bleeding rates were not significantly different with standard- or low-dose heparin (6.3% vs. 10.5%, $p = 0.30$). An analysis of the 323 (61%) patients who underwent early PCI found that it was used more frequently in patients with initial TIMI flow grade 0 or 1 versus flow grade 2 or 3 (83% vs. 60%, $p < 0.0001$) (see *J Am Coll Cardiol* 2000;36:1489). The early PCI group had a significantly lower incidence of reinfarction [1.2% vs. 4.9% (no early PCI), $p = 0.03$], urgent revascularization (1.6% vs. 9.3%, $p = 0.001$), transfusion requirement (9.0% vs. 16%, $p = 0.02$), and a significantly higher freedom from death, reinfarction, urgent revascularization, major bleeding, or transfusion at 30 days (85.4% vs. 70.4%, $p < 0.001$).

159. Topol EJ.; The GUSTO-V Investigators. Reperfusion therapy for acute myocardial infarction with fibrinolytic therapy or combination reduced fibrinolytic therapy and platelet glycoprotein IIb/IIIa inhibition: the GUSTO-V randomised trial. *Lancet* 2001;357:1905–1914.

Design: Prospective, randomized, open, multicenter trial. The primary end point was 30-day mortality, and secondary end points included various complications of MI.

Purpose: To compare the effect of reteplase alone with reteplase plus abciximab in patients with AMI.

Population: 16,588 patients seen within 6 hours of symptom onset with ST elevation.

Exclusion Criteria: Included planned PCI and contraindications to thrombolysis.

Treatment: Standard-dose reteplase (two 10-U boluses, 30 minutes apart) or half-dose reteplase (two 5-U boluses) and full-dose abciximab.

Results: No significant differences were seen between the two groups in 30-day mortality [5.9% (reteplase) vs. 5.6% (OR, 0.95), $p = 0.43$]; the 0.3% absolute decrease with combination therapy fulfilled the criteria of noninferiority. At 1 year, mortality rates were identical (8.38% in both groups) (*JAMA* 2002;288:2130). The combination-therapy group had significantly lower rates of death and reinfarction (7.4% vs. 8.8%, $p = 0.0011$) and reinfarction (at 7 days: 2.3% vs. 3.5%). Reinfarction was associated with much higher 1-year mortality (22.6% vs. 8.0%). However, more nonintracranial bleeding complications were seen in the combination group (4.6% vs. 2.3%). The rates of intracranial hemorrhage and nonfatal disabling stroke were similar.

160. Brenner SJ, et al.; for the INTRO AMI Investigators. Eptifibatide and low-dose tissue plasminogen activator in acute myocardial infarction: the integrelin and low-dose thrombolysis in acute MI (INTRO AMI) trial. *J Am Coll Cardiol* 2002;39: 277–286.

This prospective, randomized, open-label, multicenter trial enrolled 649 patients with acute STEMI seen within 6 hours of symptom onset. In phase A, patients were randomized to eptifibatide, single or double bolus (30 minutes apart) of 180, 180/90, or 180/180 μg/kg, followed by infusion of 1.33 or 2.0 μg/kg/min (sequentially added to 25 or 50 mg of tPA). In phase B, patients were randomized to (a) double-bolus eptifibatide, 180/90 (30 minutes apart) and 1.33 μg/kg/min infusion with 50-mg tPA (group I); (b) 180/90 (10 minutes apart) and 2.0 g/kg/min with 50-mg tPA (group II); or (c) full-dose, weight-adjusted tPA (group III). In phase A, the highest rate of TIMI flow grade 3 (primary end point) was seen with eptifibatide 180/90/1.33 and 50-mg tPA (65% and 78% at 60 and 90 minutes, respectively). In phase B, the incidence of TIMI grade 3 flow at 60 minutes was 42%, 56%, and 40%, for groups I through III, respectively ($p = 0.04$, group II vs. group III). The median CTFCs were 38, 33, and 50, respectively ($p = 0.02$). No differences were found between the three groups in TIMI major bleeding or intracranial hemorrhage. Mortality, reinfarction, and revascularization rates at 30 days also were similar.

161. Giugliano RP, et al.; on behalf of the INTEGRETI Investigators. Combination reperfusion therapy with eptifibatide and reduced-dose tenecteplase for ST-elevation myocardial infarction: results of the integrelin and tenecteplase in acute myocardial infarction (INTEGRETI) Phase II Angiographic trial. *J Am Coll Cardiol* 2003;41: 1251–1260.

This prospective, randomized, open-label, multicenter trial enrolled 438 STEMI patients seen within 6 hours. In the dose-finding phase, 189 patients were randomized to different combinations of double-bolus eptifibatide and reduced-dose TNK. In dose confirmation, 249 patients were randomized to eptifibatide, 180-μg/kg boluses, 2-μg/kg/min infusion, and a second bolus 10 minutes later (180/2/180) plus half-dose TNK (0.37 mg/kg), or standard-dose (0.53 mg/kg) TNK monotherapy. All received aspirin and UFH [60-U/kg bolus and then 7 U/kg/h (combination therapy) or 12 U/kg/h (monotherapy)].

In dose finding, TIMI grade 3 flow rates at 60 minutes (primary end point) were similar across groups (64% to 68%). Arterial patency (TIMI grade 2 or 3 flow) was highest for eptifibatide, 180/2/180, plus TNK (96%, $p = 0.02$) versus eptifibatide, 180/2/90, plus half-dose TNK. In dose confirmation, this combination, compared with TNK monotherapy, tended to achieve better TIMI 3 flow (59% vs. 49%, $p = 0.15$), arterial patency (85% vs. 77%, $p = 0.17$), and ST resolution (71% vs. 61%, $p = 0.08$). However, it was associated with increased rates of noncerebral major bleeding (7.6% vs. 2.5%, $p = 0.14$) and transfusion (13.4% vs. 4.2%, $p = 0.02$).

162. De Luca G, et al. Benefits from small molecule administration as compared with abciximab among patients with ST-segment elevation myocardial infarction treated with primary angioplasty: a meta-analysis. *J Am Coll Cardiol* 2009;53: 1668–1673.

Six trials comparing abciximab with small-molecule IIb/IIIa inhibitors in a total of 2,197 patients undergoing primary PCI for STEMI were combined in this analysis. Angiographic and clinical outcomes were available: there was no difference in rates of postprocedural TIMI 3 flow (89.8% for abciximab vs. 89.1% for small molecules, $p = 0.72$) or ST-segment resolution ($p = 0.66$). Mortality at 30 days was not different (2.2% vs. 2.0%, $p = 0.66$) nor were reinfarction rates (1.2% vs. 1.2%, $p = 0.88$) or bleeding rates (1.3% vs. 1.9%, $p = 0.27$).

OTHER THERAPIES

Nitrates

163. Yusuf S, et al. Effect of intravenous nitrates on mortality in acute MI: an overview of the randomized trials. *Lancet* 1988;1:1088–1092.

Analysis of data from seven small i.v. NTG trials enrolling 851 patients found that use of i.v. NTG was associated with a significant 41% mortality reduction (12.0% vs. 20.5%, $p < 0.001$). Analysis of three trials studying i.v. nitroprusside found that its use was associated with a nonsignificant mortality reduction (14.3% vs. 17.8%).

164. ISIS-4 Collaborative Group. ISIS-4: a randomised factorial assessing early oral captopril, oral mononitrate and intravenous magnesium sulfate in 58,050 patients with suspected acute MI. *Lancet* 1995;345:669–685.

This megatrial that enrolled 58,050 patients with suspected AMI admitted within 24 hours of symptom onset included a randomization to oral mononitrate (30 mg, 30 mg 10 to 12 hours later, and then 60 mg/day for 28 days), or placebo. In the nitrate arm, a nonsignificant reduction was seen in 35-day mortality (7.34% vs. 7.54%). Nearly half the placebo group received i.v. nitrate therapy, which could have diluted the results. See Ref. (171) for a full summary.

Calcium Channel Blockers

165. Wilcox RG, et al.; Trial of early nifedipine in acute MI (TRENT) study. *BMJ* 1986;293:1204–1208.

Design: Prospective, randomized, double-blind, placebo-controlled, multicenter study. The primary end point was all-cause mortality rate.

Purpose: To evaluate the effects of early nifedipine on mortality in acute MI patients.

Population: 4,491 patients aged 70 years or younger seen within 24 hours of onset of chest pain.

Exclusion Criteria: SBP <100 mm Hg or DBP <50 mm Hg; HR, more than 120 beats/min; and current treatment with calcium channel blocker.

Treatment: Nifedipine, 10 mg four times daily, or placebo.

Results: Of the patients, 64% had confirmed MI. Nifedipine was associated with a nonsignificant 7% increase in mortality at 1 month (6.7% vs. 6.3%).

166. The Multicenter Diltiazem Post-Infarction Trial (MDPIT) Research Group. The effect of diltiazem on mortality and reinfarction after MI. *N Engl J Med* 1988;319:385–392.

Design: Prospective, randomized, double-blind, placebo-controlled, multicenter study. The mean follow-up period was 25 months. The primary end points were total mortality, cardiac death, and nonfatal MI.

Purpose: To evaluate the effects of long-term diltiazem on mortality or reinfarction rates after documented MI.

Population: 2,466 patients aged 25 to 75 years with a documented MI (enzyme confirmation required).

Exclusion Criteria: Included cardiogenic shock; second- or third-degree heart block; HR <50 beats/min; and requirement for calcium antagonist.

Treatment: Diltiazem, 60 mg twice or four times daily, or placebo.

Results: No difference was observed in total mortality between the diltiazem and placebo groups (166 and 167 patients, respectively). However, among patients without pulmonary congestion (1,909 patients), diltiazem was associated with fewer cardiac events (hazard ratio, 0.77; 95% CI, 0.61 to 0.98), whereas diltiazem-treated patients with pulmonary congestion had more cardiac events (hazard ratio, 1.41; 95% CI, 1.01 to 1.96).

167. The Danish Study Group on Verapamil in MI (DAVIT II). Effect of verapamil on mortality and major events after acute MI (DAVIT II). *Am J Cardiol* 1990;66:779–785.

Design: Prospective, randomized, double-blind, placebo-controlled, multicenter study. Average follow-up period was 16 months. The primary end points were death and reinfarction.

Purpose: To evaluate the effect on total mortality and major cardiac events of verapamil started in the 2nd week after MI.

Population: 1,975 patients younger than 75 years enrolled 7 to 15 days after proven MI.

Exclusion Criteria: Included BP <90 mm Hg and second- or third-degree heart block at 3 days.

Treatment: Verapamil, 120 mg three times daily (once- or twice-daily dosing allowed in cases of adverse drug reactions), or placebo.

Results: Verapamil group had 17% fewer major events (18.0% vs. 21.6%, $p = 0.03$) and 20% lower mortality (11.1% vs. 13.8%, $p = 0.11$). A significant mortality reduction was seen in patients with CHF (7.7% vs. 11.8%, $p = 0.02$), whereas no benefit was seen in those without CHF (17.9% vs. 17.5%).

168. Goldbourt U, et al.; Secondary Prevention Reinfarction Israel Nifedipine Trial (SPRINT 2). Early administration of nifedipine in suspected acute MI. *Arch Intern Med* 1993;153:345–353.

Design: Prospective, randomized, double-blind, placebo-controlled study. The primary end point was 6-month all-cause mortality rate.

Purpose: To evaluate the effect on mortality of nifedipine started early after AMI in high-risk patients.

Population: 1,006 patients aged 50 to 79 years meeting at least one of the following criteria—prior MI, angina in preceding month, hypertension, NYHA class II or higher, anterior MI, and lactate dehydrogenase three times the upper limit of normal.

Treatment: Nifedipine, 20 mg three times daily (6-day titration period), or placebo.

Results: Trial was terminated early. The nifedipine group had a 20% higher 6-month mortality rate (18.7% vs. 15.6%; 95% CI, 0.94 to 1.84). The majority of the mortality difference was owing to excessive mortality during the first 6 days (7.8% vs. 5.5%; CI, 0.86 to 3.0). No differences were observed in reinfarction rates (5.1% vs. 4.2%) or in outcomes based on CHF status.

169. Rengo F, et al.; Calcium antagonist reinfarction Italian study (CRIS). A controlled trial of verapamil in patients after acute MI: results of the CRIS. *Am J Cardiol* 1996;77:365–369 (editorial, 421–422).

Design: Prospective, randomized, double-blind, placebo-controlled study. Mean follow-up period was 2 years. The primary end point was all-cause mortality rate.

Purpose: To evaluate the effects of verapamil on mortality and major cardiac end points in AMI patients.

Population: 1,073 patients aged 30 to 75 years who survived 5 days after an AMI.

Exclusion Criteria: NYHA class III/IV heart failure; HR <50 beats/min; SBP <90 mm Hg or >190 mm Hg; DBP >110 mm Hg; long-term therapy with calcium antagonists or β-blockers.

Treatment: Verapamil, 120 mg orally every 8 hours, or placebo started 7 to 21 days (mean, 13.8 days) after admission.

Results: No differences were observed between the verapamil and placebo groups in all-cause mortality (30 and 29 deaths, respectively). The verapamil group had 20% fewer reinfarctions and 20% less angina.

Comments: Editorial reports that pooled data from nine trials show that verapamil is associated with a favorable effect on reinfarction (OR, 0.81; 95% CI, 0.67 to 0.98) but no overall mortality benefit (OR, 0.93; 95% CI, 0.78 to 1.10).

170. Boden WE, et al.; for the Incomplete Infarction Trial of European Research Collaborators Evaluating Prognosis Post-thrombolysis (INTERCEPT). Diltiazem in acute myocardial infarction treated with thrombolytic agents: a randomised placebo-controlled trial. *Lancet* 2000;355:1751–1756.

Design: Prospective, randomized, double-blind, multicenter, international, placebo-controlled study. The primary end point was a composite of cardiac death, reinfarction, or refractory ischemia.

Purpose: To evaluate the effects of diltiazem on clinical outcomes in patients with acute MI who receive thrombolytic agents.

Population: 874 patients with acute MI, without CHF, who received thrombolytic agents.

Treatment: Diltiazem 300 mg daily or placebo, started within 36 to 96 hours of symptom onset, for a duration of up to 6 months.

Results: At 6 months, the diltiazem group had a nonsignificant 21% hazard reduction in death, MI, and refractory ischemia (hazard ratio, 0.79; 95% CI, 0.61 to 1.02; $p = 0.07$). The diltiazem group had a significant reduction in the incidence of nonfatal reinfarction or refractory ischemia (hazard ratio, 0.76; 95% CI, 0.58 to 1.00). There was a significant reduction in the need for repeat revascularization in the diltiazem group (hazard ratio, 0.61; 95% CI, 0.39 to 0.96).

Antiarrhythmics

171. Burkart F, et al.; Basel Antiarrhythmic Study of Infarct Survival (BASIS). Effect of antiarrhythmic therapy on mortality in survivors of MI with asymptomatic complex ventricular arrhythmias: BASIS. *J Am Coll Cardiol* 1990;16:1711–1718.

Design: Prospective, randomized, three-center study. Follow-up period was 1 year.

Purpose: To compare individualized antiarrhythmic therapy with low-dose amiodarone and no therapy.

Population: 312 of 1,220 consecutively screened MI survivors younger than 71 years with asymptomatic, complex ventricular arrhythmias (Lown class 3 or 4b) on 24-hour ECG before hospital discharge.

Treatment: (a) Individualized, initially quinidine or mexiletine (if both failed, others tried: ajmaline, disopyramide, flecainide, propafenone, sotalol); (b) amiodarone, 1 g/d for 5 days and then 200 mg/day for 1 year; or (c) no therapy, drugs are allowed if arrhythmias developed.

Results: Amiodarone group had a lower overall 1-year mortality rate compared with controls—5.1% versus 13.2% ($p < 0.05$); mortality for individually treated patients was 10% (p = NS vs. amiodarone).

Comments: Post hoc analysis showed that the benefit of amiodarone was restricted to those with an EF of 40% (1.5% vs. 8.9% 1-year mortality, $p < 0.03$). Late follow-up showed persistent benefit of amiodarone (after discontinuation at 1 year) compared with placebo: at 7 years, 30% versus 45% mortality (p = 0.03).

172. The Cardiac Arrhythmia Suppression Trial (CAST) Investigators. Preliminary report: effect of encainide and flecainide on mortality in a randomized trial of arrhythmia suppression after myocardial infarction. N Engl J Med 1989;321:406–412.

Design: Prospective, randomized, open-label (initial phase), double-blind (main phase), placebo-controlled, multicenter study. Follow-up period was 10 months.

Purpose: To evaluate whether suppression of asymptomatic or mildly asymptomatic ventricular arrhythmias after MI reduces death due to arrhythmia.

Population: 1,727 patients with MI in prior 6 days to 2 years, at least six ventricular premature contractions per hour on 24-hour Holter monitoring, EF of 0.55 or less if 90 days or less after MI or 0.40 or less if more than 90 days after MI (if EF is30%, patients are not eligible to receive flecainide), and suppressibility during open-label phase (at 4 to 10 days, 80% reduction of ventricular premature contractions and 90% reduction of unsustained runs of VT).

Exclusion Criteria: Ventricular arrhythmias associated with severe symptoms; unsustained VT with 15 beats at 120 beats/min; contraindications to drugs; and ECG abnormalities making rhythm interpretation difficult.

Treatment: Encainide, 35 or 50 mg orally three times daily; flecainide, 100 or 150 mg twice daily; or moricizine, 200 or 250 mg three times daily.

Results: Encainide and flecainide arms were discontinued early. Encainide and flecainide patients had more arrhythmic deaths [4.5% vs. 1.2% (placebo); RR, 3.6; 95% CI, 1.7 to 8.5], as well as higher overall mortality (7.7% vs. 3.0%; RR, 2.5; 95% CI, 1.6 to 4.5).

Comments: The moricizine arm of the trial continued. Later analysis showed that those patients with easily suppressible arrhythmias (n = 1,778) had fewer arrhythmic deaths than the 1,173 patients with difficult-to-suppress arrhythmias (RR, 0.59; p = 0.003). This likely explains the low placebo mortality rate (1.2%).

173. Waldo AL, et al.; for the Survival with Oral d-sotalol (SWORD) Investigators. Effect of D-sotalol on mortality in patients with left ventricular dysfunction after recent and remote MI. Lancet 1996;348:7–12.

Design: Prospective, randomized, double-blind, placebo-controlled, multicenter study. Mean follow-up period was 148 days. The primary end point was all-cause mortality rate.

Purpose: To determine if the NYHA class III antiarrhythmic agent D-sotalol can decrease all-cause mortality in high-risk MI survivors.

Population: 3,121 patients with an EF of 40% or less and recent MI (6 to 42 days) or symptomatic heart failure (class II or III) with remote (longer than 42 days) MI.

Exclusion Criteria: Unstable angina, class IV heart failure, history of life-threatening arrhythmia, PTCA, or CABG in previous 14 days, and creatinine clearance 50 mL/min or less.

Treatment: D-sotalol, 200 mg orally twice daily, or placebo.

Results: The trial was terminated early because of 65% higher overall mortality in the sotalol group: 5.0% versus 3.1% ($p = 0.006$). Increased arrhythmic deaths (RR, 1.77; $p = 0.008$) accounted for the excess mortality. The effect was greatest in those with an EF of 30% or less (RR, 4.0 vs. 1.2; EF, 31% to 40%; $p = 0.007$).

174. Julian DG, et al.; for the European MI Amiodarone Trial (EMIAT) Investigators. Randomised trial of effect of amiodarone on mortality in patients with left-ventricular dysfunction after recent MI: EMIAT. *Lancet* 1997;349:667–674.

Design: Prospective, randomized, double-blind, placebo-controlled, multicenter study. Mean follow-up period was 21 months. The primary end point was all-cause mortality rate.

Purpose: To evaluate the effect of amiodarone on mortality in post-MI patients with LV dysfunction.

Population: 1,486 patients aged 18 to 75 years with MI in the prior 5 to 21 days and EF of 40% or less by multiple-gated nuclear angiography (approximately 45% with an EF of 30% or less).

Exclusion Criteria: Amiodarone in the previous 6 months; HR <50 beats/min; second- or third-degree AV block; significant hepatic or thyroid dysfunction; and need for antiarrhythmic(s) other than β-blockers or digoxin.

Treatment: Amiodarone (800 mg/day for 14 days, 400 mg/day for 14 weeks, and then 200 mg/day) or placebo.

Results: Among all patients, total mortality was 13.4%, with no difference between amiodarone and placebo (RR, 0.99). No difference was observed in cardiac mortality (RR, 0.94; $p = 0.67$). The amiodarone group had fewer arrhythmic deaths (RR, 0.35; $p = 0.04$).

175. Cairns JA, et al.; for the Canadian Amiodarone MI Arrhythmia Trial (CAMIAT) Investigators. Randomised trial of outcome after MI in patients with frequent or repetitive ventricular premature depolarisations: CAMIAT. *Lancet* 1997;349:675–682.

Design: Prospective, randomized, double-blind, placebo-controlled, multicenter study. Median follow-up period was 1.8 years. The primary end point was resuscitated VF or arrhythmic death.

Purpose: To determine the effect of amiodarone on overall mortality in post-MI patients with frequent or repetitive ventricular premature depolarizations.

Population: 1,202 patients with MI in the prior 6 to 45 days, EF of 40% or less, and 24-hour ECG monitoring showing 10 ventricular premature depolarizations per hour or one run of three beats of VT at 100 to 120 beats/min.

Exclusion Criteria: Contraindications to amiodarone (prior intolerance), HR < 50 beats/min, heart block (any degree), QT interval >480 msec, and VT at more than 120 beats/min.

Treatment: Amiodarone, 10 mg/kg/d for 2 weeks, 300 to 400 mg/day for 3 to 5 months, 200 to 300 mg/day for 4 months, and 200 mg for 5 to 7 days/week for 16 months, or placebo.

Results: Amiodarone group with nearly 50% fewer arrhythmic deaths plus resuscitated VF [3.3% vs. 6.0%, $p = 0.016$ (intention-to-treat analysis, $p = 0.029$)]. Total mortality was not different.

Comments: Primary analysis was not based on intention-to-treat analysis. The trial also had many dropouts (221 amiodarone and 152 placebo patients; >70% and >50%, respectively, stopped because of adverse effects).

176. Teo KK, et al. Effects of prophylactic antiarrhythmic drug therapy in acute MI. *JAMA* 1993;270:1589–1595.

This analysis focused on 138 randomized trials with approximately 98,000 enrolled patients. Lower mortality was seen with β-blockers (26,973 patients; OR, 0.81; p = 0.00001) and amiodarone (778 patients; OR, 0.71; p = 0.03). Higher mortality was seen with class I agents (11,712 patients; OR, 1.14; p = 0.03). A statistically nonsignificant impact of calcium channel blockers was observed (10,154 patients; OR, 1.04; p = 0.41).

177. Sadowski ZP, et al. Multicenter randomized trial and a systematic overview of lidocaine in acute myocardial infarction. *Am Heart J* 1999;137:792–798.

A total of 903 patients seen within 6 hours of symptom onset with ST elevation were randomized to lidocaine (four boluses of 50 mg each every 2 minutes, then 3 mg/min for 12 hours, and then 2 mg/min for 36 hours) or no lidocaine. The lidocaine group had significantly less VF (2.0% vs. 5.7%, p = 0.004) but tended toward increased mortality (9.7% vs. 7.0%, p = 0.145). A meta-analysis of these results and those from 20 other randomized studies with more than 11,000 patients revealed nonsignificant trends toward reduced VF (OR, 0.71; 95% CI, 0.47 to 1.09) and increased mortality rates (OR, 1.12; 95% CI, 0.91 to 1.36) with lidocaine.

178. Amiodarone Trials Meta-Analysis Investigators. Effect of prophylactic amiodarone on mortality after acute myocardial infarction and in congestive heart failure: meta-analysis of individual data from 6500 patients in randomised trials. *Lancet* 1997;350:1417–1424.

The investigators pooled data from 13 trials, 8 in post-MI patients and 5 in CHF, 9 of which were double blind and placebo controlled. The resulting cohort of 6,553 patients demonstrated a significant reduction in mortality by 13% (OR, 0.87; p = 0.03) for those taking amiodarone, with a particular reduction in sudden death (OR, 0.71; p = 0.0003). These results did not differ between the post-MI and CHF populations; however, the risk of sudden death was higher for those in the CHF group. They calculated an excess risk of pulmonary toxicity to be 1% per year.

Magnesium

179. Woods KL, et al.; Second Leicester Intravenous Magnesium Intervention Trial (LIMIT-2). Intravenous magnesium sulfate in suspected acute MI: results of LIMIT-2. *Lancet* 1992;339:1553–1558.

This prospective, randomized, double-blind, placebo-controlled, single-center study randomized 2,316 patients with suspected AMI (no ECG criteria specified) seen within 24 hours. Patients received magnesium sulfate, 8 mmol over a 5-minute period, followed by 65 mmol over a 24-hour period, or saline. AMI was confirmed in 65%. The magnesium group had a 24% lower 28-day mortality rate (7.8% vs. 10.3%, p = 0.04). Long-term follow-up (mean, 2.7 years) showed persistent significant mortality benefit (16%) associated with magnesium.

180. ISIS-4 Collaborative Group. ISIS-4: a randomised factorial assessing early oral captopril, oral mononitrate and intravenous magnesium sulfate in 58,050 patients with suspected acute MI. *Lancet* 1995;345:669–685.

This megatrial of 58,050 patients with suspected AMI included a randomization to magnesium (8-mmol bolus over a 15-minute period and then 72 mmol over a 24-hour period) or no magnesium. The magnesium group had a nonsignificant 6% increase in mortality (7.64% vs. 7.24%) and a higher incidence of CHF (+12/1,000), hypotension

(+11/1,000), and cardiogenic shock (+5/1,000). No benefit of magnesium was seen in any subgroup.

181. The Magnesium in Coronaries (MAGIC) Trial Investigators. Early administration of intravenous magnesium to high-risk patients with acute myocardial infarction in the Magnesium in Coronaries (MAGIC) trial: a randomized controlled trial. *Lancet* 2002;360:1189–1196.

This prospective, randomized, placebo-controlled, multicenter trial enrolled 6,213 high-risk AMI patients aged 65 years or older seen within 6 hours of symptom onset who were ineligible for reperfusion or eligible for reperfusion. Exclusion criteria included high-grade AV block, cardiogenic shock, and renal failure. Patients received i.v. magnesium (2-g i.v. bolus over a 15-minute period and then 17 g over a 24-hour period) or placebo. Of patients who underwent reperfusion (primarily thrombolysis), 96% received the magnesium at the time of reperfusion. At 30 days, no difference was found between the two groups in all-cause mortality (15% in both groups). No differences occurred when the patients were stratified by sex, geography, EF, concomitant medications, and other variables.

Glucose–Insulin–Potassium

182. Malmberg K, et al. Diabetic insulin–glucose infusion in acute MI (DIGAMI). Randomized trial of insulin–glucose infusion followed by subcutaneous insulin treatment in diabetic patients with acute MI: effects on mortality at 1 year. *J Am Coll Cardiol* 1995;26:57–65.

Design: Prospective, randomized, open, multicenter study. The primary end point was all-cause mortality.

Purpose: To evaluate whether rapid improvement of metabolic control in diabetic patients with an insulin/glucose infusion decreases early mortality and subsequent morbidity.

Population: 620 patients with suspected MI and blood glucose 11 mM on admission (with or without prior diagnosis of diabetes).

Treatment: Continuous i.v. insulin infusion for 24 hours (started at 5 U/h) or until normoglycemia was achieved (goal of 7 to 10 mM) and then s.c. insulin for 3 months or conventional therapy.

Results: At 24 hours, the insulin-/glucose-treated patients had lower glucose (9.6 mM vs. 11.7 mM) and 29% lower mortality at 1 year (18.6% vs. 26.1%, $p = 0.027$). Mortality reduction was most marked (52%) in patients with a low cardiovascular risk profile or no previous insulin therapy. Only 10% stopped insulin because of hypoglycemia with no associated morbidity.

Comments: Intense insulin may restore impaired platelet function, decrease plasminogen activator inhibitor (PAI)-1 activity, and possibly improve metabolism of noninfarcted areas. Long-term follow-up showed that lower mortality was maintained at a mean 3.4 years: 33% versus 44% (RR, 0.72; $p = 0.011$), with the largest benefit seen in patients with no prior insulin therapy (RR, 0.49).

183. Fath-Ordoubadi F, et al. Glucose–insulin–potassium therapy for treatment of acute MI. *Circulation* 1997;96:1152–1156.

This analysis focused on nine well-designed randomized, placebo-controlled trials with 1,932 patients (all prethrombolytic era). GIK was associated with lower hospital mortality (16.1% vs. 21%; OR, 0.72; $p = 0.004$). A 48% reduction was seen in the four trials using high-dose GIK (to suppress free fatty acid levels maximally).

184. Diaz R, et al.; on behalf of the Estudios Cardiologicos Latinoamerica (ECLA) Glucose–Insulin–Potassium Pilot Trial Collaborative Group. Metabolic modulation of acute MI. *Circulation* 1998;98:2227–2234.

Design: Prospective, randomized, open, multicenter study.

Purpose: To evaluate the feasibility of GIK administration in contemporary practice and to assess its effect on clinical end points in patients with AMI.

Population: 407 patients with suspected AMI seen within 24 hours of symptom onset.

Exclusion Criteria: Severe renal impairment or hyperkalemia.

Treatment: High-dose GIK (25% glucose, 50 IU insulin/L, and 80 mM KCl at 1.5 mL/kg/h for 24 hours), low-dose GIK (10% glucose, 20 IU insulin/L, and 40 mM KCl at 1.0 mL/kg/h for 24 hours), or control. GIK was started an average 10 to 11 hours after onset of symptoms.

Results: GIK-treated patients had nonsignificant reductions in several in-hospital events, including severe heart failure, cardiogenic shock, VF, and reinfarction. Among the 252 (61.9%) patients treated with reperfusion strategies (thrombolysis, 95%; PTCA, 5%), GIK-treated patients had a significant 66% reduction in in-hospital mortality (5.2% vs. 15.2%; RR, 0.34; $p = 0.008$). At 1-year follow-up, only the high-dose GIK patients undergoing reperfusion had a significant mortality benefit (RR, 0.37; log-rank test, 0.046). The GIK group had a higher frequency of phlebitis (severe in only 2%) and serum changes in plasma concentration of glucose or potassium.

Comments: High-dose regimen achieves maximal suppression of free fatty acid levels. A meta-analysis of 1,932 patients showed no interaction between GIK and reperfusion.

185. The CREATE-ECLA Trial Group Investigators. Effect of glucose–insulin–potassium infusion on mortality in patients with acute ST-segment elevation myocardial infarction: the CREATE-ECLA randomized controlled trial. *JAMA* 2005;293:437–446.

Design: Prospective, randomized, multicenter, international trial. The primary end points were death, cardiac arrest, cardiogenic shock, and reinfarction at 30 days.

Purpose: To evaluate the benefit, if any, of GIK infusion in patients with STEMI.

Population: 20,201 patients presenting with STEMI within 12 hours of symptom onset.

Treatment: High-dose GIK infusion for 24 hours or standard care.

Results: GIK infusion resulted in no significant changes in the rates of 30-day mortality (hazard ratio, 1.03; $p = 0.45$), cardiac arrest (hazard ratio, 0.93; $p = 0.51$), cardiogenic shock (hazard ratio, 1.05; $p = 0.38$), or reinfarction (hazard ratio, 0.98; $p = 0.81$). Rates of heart failure were similar at 7 days (hazard ratio, 1.01; $p = 0.72$).

Comments: The subsequent OASIS 6-GIK trial of GIK infusion in STEMI was stopped early on publication of these results (see also *JAMA* 2007;298:2399–2405).

INFARCT TYPES
Left Ventricular Infarctions
186. Stone PH, et al. Prognostic significance of location and type of MI: independent adverse outcome associated with anterior location. *J Am Coll Cardiol* 1988;11:453–463.

This retrospective analysis focused on 471 Multicenter Investigation of the Limitation of Infarct Size (MILIS) patients with first MI showing an anterior location associated with poor outcome. Anterior versus inferior patients: larger infarcts (higher CK-MB fraction, $p < 0.001$), approximately three times more heart failure (40.7% vs. 14.7%), more than four times more in-hospital deaths (11.9% vs. 2.8%, $p < 0.001$), and higher cumulative cardiac mortality (27% vs. 11%, $p < 0.001$). Q wave versus non-Q wave: worse in-hospital course [higher CK-MB, lower EF, and more heart failure and deaths (9.3% vs. 4.1%, $p < 0.05$)], but no significant difference in long-term cardiac mortality (21% vs. 16%). After adjustment for infarct size, anterior patients still had higher mortality rates. If location and type were considered, anterior patients still had worse outcomes (whether Q wave or non-Q wave).

187. Patel MR, et al. Intra-aortic balloon counterpulsation and infarct size in patients with acute anterior myocardial infarction without shock: the CRISP AMI randomized trial. JAMA 2011;306:1329–1337.

Design: Randomized, prospective, open, multicenter trial. The primary end point was 30-day all-cause mortality. The primary outcome was infarct size, as a percentage of LV mass by cardiac MRI, 3 to 5 days postinfarct.

Purpose: To evaluate the benefit of IABP support in patients with acute anterior MI without cardiogenic shock undergoing early revascularization.

Population: 337 patients with acute anterior STEMI without cardiogenic shock and with planned early revascularization.

Treatment: IABP before PCI for at least 12 hours versus no IABP (PCI alone).

Results: Time to first intracoronary device was slightly longer in the IBAP group (median time 77 minutes vs. 68, p = 0.04). The mean infarct size was not different between the groups (42% vs. 38%, p = 0.06). While there were no significant differences in the rates of bleeding or vascular complications, the numbers were very low.

188. Berger PB, et al. Incidence and prognostic implications of heart block complicating inferior MI treated with thrombolytic therapy: results from TIMI II. *J Am Coll Cardiol* 1992;20:533–540.

This retrospective analysis focused on 1,786 patients. Complete heart block occurred in 12% (6.3% at presentation). The complete heart block group had a higher unadjusted 21-day mortality rate (7.1% vs. 2.7%, p = 0.007), but adjusted RR was not statistically significant. Mortality was nearly five times higher in those with complete heart block after thrombolysis (9.9% vs. 2.2%, p < 0.001). Increased deaths were attributable to more severe cardiac dysfunction.

189. Behar S, et al. Complete atrioventricular block complicating inferior acute wall MI: short and long-term prognosis. *Am Heart J* 1993;125:1622–1627.

This analysis focused on 2,273 SPRINT Registry patients with inferior Q-wave MIs. An 11% incidence of complete heart block was observed (women, 14%; age 70 years, 15%). The complete heart block group had more than a threefold higher in-hospital mortality rate (37% vs. 11%; p < 0.0001; adjusted OR, 2.0; 95% CI, 1.12 to 3.57). However, no difference in 5-year mortality was observed among hospital survivors (28% vs. 23%).

190. Peterson ED, et al. Prognostic significance of precordial ST segment depression during inferior MI in the thrombolytic era: results in 16,521 patients. *J Am Coll Cardiol* 1996;28:305–312.

This post hoc GUSTO-I analysis focused on 6,422 patients without any precordial depression. The ST depression group had a 47% higher 30-day mortality rate (4.7% vs. 3.2%; at 1 year, 5% vs. 3.4%; p < 0.001). Magnitude of depression (sum of V_1 through V_6) added significant prognostic information after risk factor adjustment: 36% higher mortality per 0.5 mm.

191. Matetzky S, et al. Significance of ST segment elevations in posterior chest leads (V_7 to V_9) in patients with acute inferior MI: application for thrombolytic therapy. *J Am Coll Cardiol* 1998;31:506–511.

This analysis showed that ST elevation in V_7 to V_9 correlates with posterolateral involvement, and such patients benefit more from thrombolysis. Eighty-seven patients who had a first inferior MI and were treated with rtPA were stratified according to the presence (46 patients) or absence (41 patients) of ST elevation in V_7 to V_9. The ST elevation group had a higher incidence of posterolateral wall motion abnormalities (p < 0.001) on radionuclide ventriculography, a larger infarct area (higher peak CK, p < 0.02), lower predischarge EF (p < 0.008), and higher incidence of death, reinfarction, or heart failure

($p < 0.05$). Patency of the IRA in the V_7 to V_9 elevation group resulted in an improved EF at discharge ($p < 0.012$), whereas EF in the nonelevation patients was unchanged, regardless of IRA patency.

Right Ventricular Infarction

192. Zehender M, et al. Right ventricular infarction as an independent predictor of prognosis after acute MI. N Engl J Med 1993;328:981–988.

This analysis of 200 consecutive patients showed that ST elevation in lead V_4R was highly predictive of RVI: sensitivity, 88%, and specificity, 78%. ST elevation in V_4R also was associated with higher mortality (31% vs. 19% overall) and more in-hospital complications (64% vs. 28%).

193. Kinch JW, et al. Right ventricular infarction. N Engl J Med 1994;330:1211–1217.

This excellent overview discusses the pathophysiology, diagnosis, complications, treatment, and prognosis of patients with RVI.

194. Zehender M, et al. Eligibility for and benefit of thrombolytic therapy in inferior MI: focus on the prognostic importance of right ventricular infarction. J Am Coll Cardiol 1994;24:362–369.

This prospective analysis focused on 200 patients with an inferior MI. Thrombolytic therapy (accelerated tPA regimen) was received by 36%; this group of patients had a lower mortality than did patients ineligible for tPA (8% vs. 25%, $p < 0.001$). However, benefit of tPA was restricted to patients with RVI complicating acute inferior MI: 76% lower mortality (10% vs. 42%, $p < 0.005$) and fewer overall complications (34% vs. 54%, $p < 0.05$). In the absence of RVI, no difference was observed in mortality (7% vs. 6%), whether or not patients received tPA.

195. Bowers TR, et al. Effect of reperfusion on biventricular function and survival after right ventricular infarction. N Engl J Med 1998;338:933–940.

This prospective study was composed of 53 inferior MI patients with echocardiographic evidence of RVI (RV free wall dysfunction, dilatation, and depressed global performance). Complete reperfusion was achieved by balloon angioplasty in 77% of patients (i.e., normal flow in the right coronary artery and its major RV branches) and led to recovery of RV function [mean score for free wall motion, 1.4 (at 3 days) vs. 3.0 (baseline), $p < 0.001$]. In contrast, unsuccessful reperfusion (no RV branch flow) was associated with a lack of RV recovery, as well as persistent hypotension and low cardiac output (83% vs. 12%, $p = 0.002$) and markedly higher mortality (58% vs. 2%, $p = 0.001$).

196. Zeymer U, et al. Effects of thrombolytic therapy in acute inferior MI with or without right ventricular involvement. J Am Coll Cardiol 1998;32:876–881.

This analysis of 522 inferior MI patients from the HIT-4 trial showed that RV involvement is not an independent predictor of survival. RV involvement was associated with higher 30-day cardiac mortality rates (5.9% vs. 2.5%), but this was related to larger infarct size rather than to RVI. Among large inferior MI patients (sum ST elevation >0.8 mV or precordial depression), a proximal right coronary artery lesion was seen in 52% with and 23% without RVI. Among small-MI patients, lesions were mostly distal in location, and cardiac mortality was <1% irrespective of the presence of RVI.

TREATMENT OF CARDIOGENIC SHOCK

197. Berger PB, et al. Impact of an aggressive invasive catheterization and revascularization strategy on mortality in patients with cardiogenic shock in the GUSTO I trial. Circulation 1997;96:122–127.

This analysis focused on 2,200 patients with SBP <90 mm Hg for 1 hour who survived 1 hour after onset of shock. The early angiography (24 hours or less) group had a lower 30-day mortality rate (38% vs. 62%, p = 0.0001). After multiple logistic regression analysis, the early angiography group was found to be younger (63 years vs. 68 years), to have had fewer prior MIs (19% vs. 27%), and to have been given thrombolysis earlier (2.9 hours vs. 3.2 hours). An aggressive strategy is still associated with a lower 30-day mortality rate (OR, 0.43; p = 0.0001). A subsequent GUSTO-I analysis showed that most patients (88%) with cardiogenic shock who were alive at 30 days survived at least 1 year and that those who underwent revascularization within 30 days had better 1-year survival than did patients not revascularized.

198. Hochman JS, et al. Should We Emergently Revascularize Occluded Coronaries for Cardiogenic Shock (SHOCK) Investigators. **Early revascularization in acute MI complicated by cardiogenic shock.** *N Engl J Med* 1999;341:625–634 (editorial, 686–688).

This prospective, randomized, multicenter trial was composed of 302 patients with STEMI (or new LBBB); pulmonary capillary wedge pressure, 15 mm Hg or more; cardiac index, 2.2 or less; SBP more than 90 mm Hg for 30 minutes before inotropes/vasopressors or IABP initiated; and HR, 60 beats/min. Patients underwent ERV within 6 hours (PTCA or CABG) or medical management [thrombolysis recommended (given in 64%), delayed revascularization allowed at 54 hours]. The ERV group had a 97% angiography rate and 87% revascularization rate [PTCA, 49% (at average 0.9 hours); CABG, 38% (average 2.7 hours)]. Among initial medical stabilization (IMS) patients, 4% had revascularization performed before 54 hours, and 22% underwent late revascularization. No significant difference was found in 30-day all-cause mortality (primary end point) between the two groups (ERV, 46.7%, vs. IMS, 56.0%; p = 0.11); however, at 6 months, a significant mortality benefit was associated with early revascularization strategy (50.3% vs. 63.1%, p = 0.027). In the subgroup of patients aged 75 years or younger, ERV was significantly better than IMS (at 30 days, 41% vs. 57%, p < 0.01; 6 months, 48% vs. 69%, p < 0.01). The PTCA success rate was 76%, and the mortality rate was 100% if PTCA did not achieve TIMI grade 2 or 3 flow.

Percutaneous Assist Devices

199. Ohman EM, et al.; IABP trial. Use of aortic counterpulsation to improve sustained coronary artery patency during acute MI. *Circulation* 1994;90:792–799.

Design: Prospective, randomized, multicenter study. The primary end point was angiographically detected reocclusion of IRA during initial hospitalization.

Purpose: To determine whether 48 hours of aortic counterpulsation therapy after reperfusion established during emergency catheterization would reduce the rate of reocclusion of the IRA.

Population: 182 AMI patients who underwent catheterization within 24 hours with successful restoration of IRA patency.

Exclusion Criteria: Included cardiogenic shock, pulmonary edema requiring aortic counterpulsation, severe PVD, more than 75% restenosis in one or two major epicardial arteries and TIMI grade 2 or 3 flow achieved in IRA with thrombolytic therapy, and contraindication(s) to heparin.

Treatment: IABP for 48 hours or standard care.

Results: Primary angioplasty was performed in 106 patients, rescue angioplasty in 51 patients, and other methods (e.g., intracoronary thrombolysis) in the remaining 25 patients. Both groups had a similar incidence of severe bleeding complications and transfusions. Catheterization performed at a median of 5 days demonstrated that the aortic counterpulsation group had a lower IRA reocclusion rate (8% vs. 21%) and nearly 50% fewer clinical events (death, stroke, reinfarction, ERV, and recurrent ischemia; 13% vs. 24%; p < 0.04).

200. Stone GW, et al. A prospective, randomized evaluation of prophylactic intraaortic balloon pump (IABP) counterpulsation in high risk patients with acute MI treated with primary angioplasty. *J Am Coll Cardiol* 1997;29:1459–1467.

Design: Prospective, randomized, multicenter study. The primary end points were death, MI, IRA occlusion, stroke, new heart failure, and sustained hypotension.

Purpose: To determine whether AMI patients stratified as high-risk benefit from a routine IABP strategy after PTCA.

Population: 437 PAMI II patients classified as high risk (meeting at least one of the following criteria: age older than 70 years, three-vessel disease, EF of 45% or less, saphenous vein graft occlusion, persistent malignant ventricular arrhythmia, or suboptimal angioplasty result).

Exclusion Criteria: Cardiogenic shock, bleeding diathesis, and thrombolytic therapy before catheterization.

Treatment: IABP for 36 to 48 hours or standard care.

Results: The two groups had similar outcomes [composite end point incidence 28.9% (IABP) vs. 29.2%]. The IABP group had fewer unscheduled repeated catheterizations (7.6% vs. 13.3%, $p = 0.05$) but had more strokes (2.4% vs. 0%, $p = 0.03$). The authors suggest that the IABP effect may not have been detected because of low control group mortality (3.1%) and IRA occlusion rate (5.5%).

201. Anderson RD, et al. Use of intraaortic balloon bump counterpulsation in patients presenting with cardiogenic shock: observations from the GUSTO-I study. *J Am Coll Cardiol* 1997;30:708–715.

This analysis focused on 68 GUSTO-I patients with cardiogenic shock who had an IABP placed (91% within 1 day). Early IABP use was associated with increased bleeding (moderate, 47% vs. 12%, $p = 0.0001$; severe, 10% vs. 5%, $p = 0.16$). IABP use also was associated with increased arrhythmias, procedures, and bypass surgery. However, these increases were owing longer time to death (2.8 days vs. 7.2 hours). However, in part, a trend toward lower 30-day mortality was seen with IABP use [57% vs. 67%, adjusted $p = 0.11$ (if revascularization patients were excluded; 47% vs. 64%, $p = 0.07$)].

202. Thiele H, et al. Percutaneous left ventricular assist devices in acute myocardial infarction complicated by cardiogenic shock. *Eur Heart J* 2007;28:2057–2063.

The authors introduce novel percutaneous left ventricular assist devices (LVADs) and their design, implantation, advantages, and disadvantage. These include percutaneous cardiopulmonary bypass, axial flow pumps, and left atrial-to-femoral arterial LVADs. The authors compare these devices to the current standard, the IABP. Limitations of these therapies, as well as future directions of research, are also discussed.

203. Seyfarth M, et al. A randomized clinical trial to evaluate the safety and efficacy of a percutaneous left ventricular assist device versus intra-aortic balloon pumping for treatment of cardiogenic shock caused by myocardial infarction (Efficacy study of LV assist device to treat patients with cardiogenic shock [ISAR-SHOCK]). *J Am Coll Cardiol* 2008;52:1584–1588.

Design: Prospective, randomized, open trial. The primary end point was change in cardiac index at 30 minutes. Secondary end points were lactic acidosis, hemolysis, and mortality at 30 days.

Purpose: To determine the benefit, if any, of the newer Impella LP2.5 LVAD over standard IABP for hemodynamic support in cardiogenic shock secondary to acute MI.

Population: 26 patients with acute MI complicated by cardiogenic shock (a device was implanted in 25; 1 died prior to implant).

Treatment: Implantation of the Impella LP2.5 percutaneous LVAD versus implantation of a standard IABP.

Results: Cardiac index was significantly higher in the LVAD group at 30 minutes (change in cardiac index 0.49 for LVAD vs. 0.11 for IABP, p = 0.02). Overall mortality was similar in both groups (46%).

204. Sjauw KD, et al. **A systematic review and meta-analysis of intra-aortic balloon pump therapy in ST-elevation myocardial infarction: should we change the guidelines?** *Eur Heart J* 2009;30:459–468.

The authors reviewed data from trials and observational cohorts of patients with STEMI complicated by cardiogenic shock. Their first analysis included seven randomized trials of 1,009 patients, demonstrating no change in 30-day survival between patients who did and did not receive an IABP, despite significantly higher bleeding and stroke rates in the IABP groups. In their second analysis of nine cohorts of 10,529 patients, use of IABP in patients receiving thrombolysis was associated with an 18% lower mortality at 30 days (p < 0.0001), at the expense of higher revascularization rates in this group. However, in those undergoing primary PCI, IABP was associated with a 6% higher 30-day mortality (p < 0.0008). While there were important methodological caveats to the results of the cohort meta-analysis, these results challenge the current guideline recommendations.

205. Thiele H et al. **Intraaortic Balloon Support for Myocardial Infarction with Cardiogenic Shock (IABP-SHOCK II).** **N Engl J Med 2012;367:1287–1296.**

Design: Randomized, prospective, open-label, multicenter trial. The primary end point was 30-day all-cause mortality.

Purpose: To evaluate the benefit of IABP support in patients with acute MI and cardiogenic shock undergoing early revascularization.

Population: 600 patients with acute MI (approximately 70% STEMI) and cardiogenic shock with planned early revascularization. Cardiogenic shock was defined as systolic BP <90 mm Hg for >30 min or use of catecholamines to maintain a systolic pressure above 90 mm Hg, clinical signs of pulmonary congestion, and impaired end-organ perfusion.

Treatment: IABP before or immediately after PCI versus no IABP. Crossover from control to IABP was allowed only if mechanical complications (acute mitral regurgitation, ventricular septal rupture) occurred after randomization.

Results: 30-day all-cause mortality occurred in 39.7% of the IABP group and in 41.3% of the control group [RR, 0.96 (95% CI, 0.79 to 1.17); p = 0.69]. Of note, there were no significant differences between the groups for any of the secondary or safety end points.

Assessment and Prognosis

REVIEWS AND META-ANALYSES

206. Shaw LJ, et al. **A meta-analysis of pre-discharge risk stratification after acute MI with stress electrocardiography myocardial perfusion and ventricular function imaging.** **Am J Cardiol 1996;78:1327–1337.**

This analysis of 54 studies (76% retrospective) with 19,874 patients shows the low positive predictive value of predischarge noninvasive testing.

207. Morrow DA, et al. **TIMI risk score for ST-elevation myocardial infarction: a convenient, bedside, clinical score for risk assessment at presentation: an intravenous nPA for treatment of infarcting myocardium early II trial substudy.** *Circulation* 2000;102:2031–2037.

The TIMI risk score for STEMI was created as the arithmetic sum of independent mortality predictors based on a logistic regression analysis of the 14,114-patient intravenous nPA for treatment of infarcting myocardium early II (InTIME II) trial. The 10 baseline variables constituting the TIMI risk score accounted for 97% of the predictive capacity of the multivariate model. These included age 65 to 74 years (2 points); age older than 75 years (3 points); diabetes, hypertension, or angina (1 point); SBP <100 mm Hg (3 points); HR more than 100 beats/min (2 points); Killip class II to IV (2 points); weight <67 kg (1 point); anterior STEMI or LBBB (1 point); and time to treatment more than 4 hours (1 point). The risk score showed a more than 40-fold graded increase in mortality (<1% with a score of 0 vs. 35.9% for a score >8). The prognostic capacity of the TIMI risk score was similar to the full multivariable model (c statistic, 0.779 vs. 0.784). External validation in the TIMI 9 trial showed similar prognostic capacity (c statistic, 0.746).

208. Morrow DA, et al. Application of the TIMI risk score for ST-elevation MI in the National Registry of Myocardial Infarction 3. JAMA 2001;286:1356–1359.

The TIMI risk score was evaluated in 84,029 STEMI patients treated from 1998 to 2000 and data recorded in the NRMI 3 registry. Only 48% received reperfusion therapy. NRMI 3 patients were older and more often female and with a history of CAD than were those in the derivation set. A significant graded increase in mortality was found with increasing TIMI risk score (range of 1.1% to 30.0%, $p < 0.001$ for trend). The risk score showed strong prognostic capacity overall ($c = 0.74$ vs. 0.78 in derivation set). It was equally predictive in those treated with fibrinolysis ($c = 0.79$) and primary PCI ($c = 0.80$). Among patients not receiving fibrinolytic therapy, absolute mortality rates were much higher for a given risk score, but the same pattern (higher score, higher risk) was seen, although with lower discriminatory capacity ($c = 0.65$).

209. Eagle KA, et al. for the GRACE Investigators. A validated prediction model for all forms of acute coronary syndrome: estimating the risk of 6-month postdischarge death in an international registry. JAMA 2004;291:2727–2733.

The researchers used data from the GRACE multinational registry of patients with ACS, including 17,142 presentations, to develop a risk prediction model for 6-month outcomes. A separate cohort of 7,638 was subsequently used to validate the model. In multivariable analyses, they identified significant predictors of 6-month mortality: older age, history of MI, history of CHF, increased pulse at presentation, lower SBP at presentation, elevated initial creatinine, elevated initial cardiac biomarkers, ST-segment depression on initial ECG, and not having PCI in-hospital (see also Arch Int Med 2003;163:2345–2353; BMJ 2006;333:1091 for additional risk prediction analyses from GRACE).

ELECTROCARDIOGRAPHY, ARRHYTHMIAS, AND CONDUCTION DISEASE

210. Volpi A, et al. In-hospital prognosis of patients with acute MI complicated by primary ventricular fibrillation. N Engl J Med 1987;317:257–261.

This analysis focused on 11,112 GISSI patients. Primary VF (defined as not due to shock or MI) occurred in 2.8% and was associated with a nearly twofold higher in-hospital mortality rate (10.8% vs. 5.9%; RR, 1.94; 95% CI, 1.35 to 2.78).

211. Multicenter Investigation of the Limitation of Infarct Size (MILIS). Prognosis after cardiac arrest due to ventricular tachycardia or ventricular fibrillation associated with acute MI. Am J Cardiol 1987;60:755–761.

This analysis focused on 849 MILIS study patients aged 75 years or younger with a confirmed MI. Mean follow-up period was 32 months. VT and VF patients had a fourfold higher in-hospital mortality rate (27% vs. 7%, $p < 0.001$). This difference was attributable to a sevenfold higher risk in patients with secondary causes of VT and VF (e.g., presence of heart failure, hypotension). A worse outcome was attained if the episode occurred after

72 hours (57% vs. 20%, $p < 0.05$). No cases of primary VT and VF occurred after 72 hours. No difference in mortality at follow-up was seen among hospital survivors.

212. Berger PB, et al. Incidence and significance of ventricular tachycardia and fibrillation in the absence of hypotension or heart failure in acute MI treated with recombinant tissue-type plasminogen activator: results from the Thrombolysis in Myocardial Infarction (TIMI) phase II trial. *J Am Coll Cardiol* 1993;22:1773–1779.

This analysis focused on 2,456 TIMI II patients without CHF or hypotension during the first 24 hours after study entry. Sustained VT or VF developed in 1.9% within 24 hours. Among patients undergoing angiography at 18 to 48 hours (per protocol), the VT and VF group had lower IRA patency (68% vs. 87%, $p = 0.01$). Mortality at 21 days was more than 10 times higher in the VT and VF patients (20.4% vs. 1.6%, $p < 0.001$). Survival from 21 days to 1 year was similar in both groups.

213. Schroder R, et al. Extent of early ST segment elevation resolution: a strong predictor of outcome in patients with acute MI and a sensitive measure to compare thrombolytic regimens. *J Am Coll Cardiol* 1995;26:1657–1664.

This prospective study was composed of 1,398 INJECT patients seen within 6 hours of symptom onset. ST resolution at 3 hours was classified into three groups: complete (>70%), partial (30% to 70%), and no (<30%) resolution. The 35-day mortality rates in these groups were 2.5%, 4.3%, and 17.5% ($p < 0.0001$). Even after baseline characteristics were included, ST resolution was the most powerful predictor of 35-day mortality.

214. Mont L, et al. Predisposing factors and prognostic value of sustained monomorphic ventricular tachycardia in early phase of acute MI. *J Am Coll Cardiol* 1996;28:1670–1676.

This retrospective analysis focused on 1,120 consecutive cardiac care unit patients. The incidence of monomorphic VT was 1.9%. This group had larger infarcts (peak CK-MB, 435 IU/L vs. 168 IU/L) and four times higher mortality (43% vs. 11%, $p < 0.001$). VT was an independent mortality predictor, whereas independent predictors of VT were CK-MB (OR, 11.8), Killip class (OR, 4.0), and bifascicular block (OR, 3.1).

215. Hathaway WR, et al. Prognostic significance of the initial electrocardiogram in patients with acute MI. *JAMA* 1998;279:387–391.

This retrospective analysis focused on 34,166 GUSTO-I patients without paced or ventricular rhythms or LBBB. In multivariate analysis, 30-day mortality predictors were found to be the sum of ST deviation (depression and elevation; OR, 1.53), hazard ratio (OR, 1.49), and QRS duration.

216. Volpi A, et al. Incidence and prognosis of early primary ventricular fibrillation in acute MI: results of the GISSI-2 database. *Am J Cardiol* 1998;82:265–271.

This retrospective analysis focused on 9,720 patients with first MI. Early (4 hours or less) and late (>4 to 48 hours) primary VF occurred in 3.1% and 0.6%, respectively. Recurrence rates were 11% and 15%. Early primary VF occurred more frequently if SBP was <120 mm Hg and in the presence of hypokalemia. In-hospital mortality was higher in patients with both early and late primary VF [ORs, 2.47 (95% CI, 1.48 to 4.13) and 3.97 (95% CI, 1.51 to 10.48)]. Mortality from hospital discharge to 6 months was similar for both primary VF subgroups and controls.

217. Go AS, et al. Bundle-branch block and in-hospital mortality in acute MI. *Ann Intern Med* 1998;129:690–697.

This large retrospective cohort study of 297,832 patients from 1,571 hospitals showed that the prevalences of RBBB and LBBB are similar (6.2% and 6.7%, respectively) and that RBBB is a stronger independent predictor of in-hospital death [adjusted OR, 1.64 vs. 1.34 (LBBB)].

218. Cheema AN, et al. Nonsustained ventricular tachycardia in the setting of acute MI. *Circulation* 1998;98:2030–2036.

This prospective database analysis showed that contrary to prevailing opinion, NSVT that occurs beyond several hours after AMI is associated with adverse outcomes. NSVT was identified in 118 patients within 72 hours of AMI. The control group was matched for age, sex, type of MI, and thrombolytic therapy. The NSVT group had more frequent in-hospital VF (9% vs. none, $p < 0.001$), but in-hospital mortality (10% vs. 4%) and follow-up mortality (10% vs. 17%) were not significantly different. However, a multivariate analysis showed that time from presentation to NSVT was the strongest mortality predictor (risk became significant at 13 hours and peaked at 24 hours; RR, 7.5).

219. Savonitto S, et al. Prognostic value of the admission electrocardiogram in acute coronary syndromes. *JAMA* 1999;281:707–713.

This retrospective analysis focused on 12,142 GUSTO-IIb patients. Presenting ECG characteristics included T-wave inversion in 22%, ST elevation in 28%, ST depression in 35%, and 15% with a combination of ST elevation and depression. The 30-day incidence of death or MI was 5.5% in patients with T-wave inversion, 9.4% in those with ST elevation, 10.5% in those with ST depression, and 12.4% in those with both ST elevation and depression. After adjusting the factors associated with increased death or MI at 30 days, compared with those with T-wave inversion only, patients with ST-segment changes were at significantly increased risk (ORs, 1.68, 1.62, and 2.27 for ST elevation, ST depression, and both, respectively). Admission CK levels were associated with increased risk of death (OR, 2.36) and death or MI (OR, 1.56). In a multivariate analysis, ECG category and CK levels at admission remained highly predictive of death and MI.

EXERCISE TESTING

220. Hamm LF, et al. Safety and efficacy of exercise testing early after acute MI. *Am J Cardiol* 1989;63:1193–1197.

This analysis focused on 151,949 tests performed at 570 institutions; 42% were symptom-limited tests. Overall, only 41 fatal (0.03%) and 141 major cardiac complications (0.09%) were noted. Symptom-limited testing was associated with a similar mortality rate but with 1.9 times more major cardiac complications.

221. Chaitman BR, et al. Impact of treatment strategy on predischarge exercise test in TIMIII. *Am J Cardiol* 1993;71:131–138.

This analysis focused on 3,339 patients showing a fourfold higher 1-year mortality rate if no predischarge exercise test was done (7.7% vs. 1.8%, $p < 0.001$). No predictive value of ST depression or chest pain was observed: conservative RR, 0.6 (95% CI, 0.1 to 2.9), and invasive RR, 2.1 (95% CI, 0.5 to 9.4). However, catheterization and revascularization are recommended if ETT is positive.

222. Jain A, et al. Comparison of symptom-limited and low level exercise tolerance tests early after MI. *J Am Coll Cardiol* 1993;22:1816–1820.

This analysis focused on 150 consecutive patients [44 others were excluded (death, ischemia at rest or with minimal ambulation, complications, physician/patient preference)]. Bruce protocol was performed at 6.4 ± 3.1 days. Low-level test results were positive in only 23% versus 40% with symptom-limited tests ($p < 0.001$). At follow-up (15 ± 5 months), only 5 patients with a negative maximal test result versus 14 patients with a nondiagnostic symptom-limited test had cardiac events.

223. Zaret BL, et al. Value of radionuclide rest and exercise left ventricular ejection fraction in assessing survival of patients after thrombolytic therapy for acute MI: results of TIMI II Study. *J Am Coll Cardiol* 1995;26:73–79.

The 2,567 patients were studied at average of 9 hours after onset of symptoms. Rest EF was strongly associated with 1-year mortality (overall, 9.9%). The RR for EF of 30% to 39% was 3.1; 40% to 49%, 2.2; and 50% to 59%, 1.2. The differential between rest and exercise EF was not helpful.

224. Villella A, et al. Prognostic significance of maximal exercise testing after MI treated with thrombolytic agents: the GISSI-2 data base. *Lancet* 1995;346:523–529.

This post hoc analysis focused on 6,295 GISSI-2 patients who were tested an average of 28 days after AMI. The same mortality rate (7.1%) was observed among those with a positive ETT result as in those who did not undergo testing; lower rates were associated with nondiagnostic and negative tests (1.3% and 0.9%, respectively). Independent predictors of mortality were symptomatic ischemia and low work capacity (RRs, 2.1 and 1.8).

ECHOCARDIOGRAPHY AND OTHER NONINVASIVE TESTS

225. Sutton MSJ, et al. Quantitative two-dimensional echocardiography measurements are major predictors of adverse cardiovascular events after acute MI. *Circulation* 1994;89:68–75.

A total of 521 SAVE trial patients had echocardiograms at 11.1 ± 3.2 days. At 1 year, LVED and LV end-systolic areas were smaller in the captopril group (p = 0.038, 0.015). The captopril group had 35% fewer cardiovascular events. In these patients with cardiovascular events, a more than threefold increase in LV cavity areas was observed.

226. Picano E, et al. Stress echocardiography results predict risk of reinfarction early after uncomplicated acute MI: large-scale multicenter study. *J Am Coll Cardiol* 1995;26:908–913.

The 1,080 patients underwent a dipyridamole echocardiography study at 10 ± 5 days. Follow-up period was 14 months. A positive test result (44%) was associated with a higher reinfarction rate (6.3% vs. 3.3%, p < 0.01).

227. Sicari R, et al.; ECHO Dobutamine International Cooperative (EDIC) Study. Prognostic value of dobutamine-atropine stress echocardiography early after acute MI. *J Am Coll Cardiol* 1997;29:254–260.

In this prospective, observational, multicenter trial, 778 patients with first MI were tested at an average of 12 days, with follow-up testing at 9 ± 7 months. Positive test results were attained in 56%. No difference in event rates (death, MI, unstable angina, angioplasty, bypass surgery) was observed regardless of positive or negative test results: 14% versus 12% (p = 0.3). However, when only spontaneously occurring events were considered, myocardial viability was the best predictor (hazard ratio, 2.0; p < 0.002). Wall motion stroke index is a very strong predictor of cardiac deaths only (hazard ratio, 9.2; p < 0.0001).

228. Migrino RQ, et al. End-systolic volume index at 90 to 180 minutes into reperfusion therapy for acute MI is a strong predictor of early and late mortality. *Circulation* 1997;96:116–121.

The 1,300 patients underwent left ventriculography. End-systolic volume index of 40 mL/m² or less was independently associated with increased 30-day and 1-year mortality rates [adjusted ORs, 3.4 (95% CI, 2.0 to 5.9) and 4.1 (95% CI, 2.6 to 6.2); p < 0.001]. Independent predictors of high end-systolic volume index of 40 or less were SBP <110 mm Hg, anterior MI, male, prior angina or MI, weight <70 kg, and HR 80 beats/min or less.

FLOW, VESSEL PATENCY, AND ANGIOGRAPHY

229. Dewood MA, et al. Prevalence of total coronary occlusion during the early hours of transmural MI. *N Engl J Med* 1980;303:897–902.

This classic angiography study demonstrated the central role of thrombotic occlusion in the pathogenesis of transmural MI. A total of 322 patients underwent catheterization at <24 hours. Total occlusion of the IRA was seen in 87% at <4 hours versus 65% at 12 to 24 hours.

230. Gibson CM, et al. Angiographic predictors of reocclusion after thrombolysis: results from TIMI-4. J Am Coll Cardiol 1995;25:582–589.

The 278 patients were randomized to APSAC, rtPA, or combination therapy. Higher reocclusion (at 18 to 36 hours) was associated with TIMI grade 2 versus 3 flow (10% vs. 2%, $p = 0.003$), ulcerated lesions (10% vs. 3%, $p = 0.009$), and positive collateral vessels (18% vs. 5.6%, $p = 0.03$). Similar trends were seen for eccentric (7% vs. 2%, $p = 0.06$) and thrombotic lesions (8% vs. 3%, $p = 0.06$). Reocclusion also was associated with more severe mean stenosis at 90 minutes (78% vs. 74%, $p = 0.04$).

231. Simes RJ, et al. Link between the angiographic substudy and mortality outcomes in a large randomized trial of myocardial reperfusion: importance of early and complete infarct artery reperfusion. Circulation 1995;91:1923–1928.

This GUSTO-I substudy of 1,210 patients showed that TIMI grade 3 flow at 90 minutes was associated with decreased mortality. A model was developed that assumed any difference in treatment effects on 30-day mortality were mediated through differences in 90-minute IRA patency. The model showed a strong correlation ($r = 0.97$) between actual and predicted mortality rates. These data provide support for the idea that improved survival is due to achievement of early and complete reperfusion.

232. Lenderink T, et al. Benefit of thrombolytic therapy is sustained throughout 5 years and is related to TIMI perfusion grade 3 but not grade 2 flow at discharge. Circulation 1995;92:1110–1116.

This study showed the benefits of achieving TIMI grade 3 flow. Five-year follow-up data were analyzed on 923 hospital survivors enrolled in the ECSG studies. Patients with TIMI grade 3 flow had a 91% 5-year survival rate compared with 84% for the TIMI grade 0 to 1 and TIMI grade 2 groups ($p^2 = 0.01$).

233. Anderson JL, et al. Meta-analysis of five reported studies on the relation of early coronary patency grades with mortality and outcomes after acute MI. Am J Cardiol 1996;78:1–8.

This meta-analysis focused on five studies with 3,969 patients. The mortality rate was 8.8% for TIMI grade 0/1, 7% for grade 2, and only 3.7% for grade 2 patients (grade 3 vs. grade 2, $p = 0.001$). TIMI grade 3 flow also was associated with better EFs and less time to CK peak.

234. Reiner JS, et al. Evolution of early TIMI 2 flow after thrombolysis for acute MI. Circulation 1996;94:2441–2446.

This analysis of the GUSTO Angiography Study showed the benefit of progressing from early TIMI grade 2 flow to grade 3 at follow-up. Of 914 patients with TIMI grade 2 flow, 278 underwent angiography at both 90 minutes and 5 to 7 days. In the group that improved to grade 3 flow by the second catheterization (67%), a higher mean EF (57.5% vs. 52.8%, $p = 0.02$), better infarct zone wall motion ($p = 0.01$), and less visible thrombus (26% vs. 38%, $p = 0.04$) were found. However, TIMI grade 3 flow at 90 minutes remained the best, with less thrombus (42% vs. 58%, $p < 0.0001$) and the highest 5- to 7-day EF (61.7% vs. 57.5%, $p = 0.002$).

235. Pilote L, et al. Determinants of the use of angiography and revascularization after thrombolysis for acute MI. N Engl J Med 1996;335:1198–1205.

This post hoc analysis focused on 21,772 GUSTO-I patients; 71% had predischarge angiography, of whom 58% underwent revascularization (PTCA, 73%). Overall, the best predictor of angiography use was age [if younger than 73 years, 76% (vs. 53%)]. Among young patients, PTCA availability was the most important predictor [83% vs. 67% (no PTCA)]. The number two predictor was recurrent ischemia. Reassuringly, coronary anatomy was the top predictor of the use and type of revascularization. However, the study yielded several unexpected findings: (a) similar revascularization rate in those with three-vessel disease and LV dysfunction and those with an EF <50% and one- or two-vessel disease and LAD stenosis of 50% or less, (b) many without symptoms had revascularization for one- or two-vessel disease, and (c) patients younger than 80 years with CHF or cardiogenic shock had similar angiography rates to those without these findings.

236. Barbagelata NA, et al. TIMI grade 3 flow and reocclusion after intravenous thrombolytic therapy: a pooled analysis. *Am Heart J* 1997;133:273–282.

Analysis of 15 TIMI flow studies with 5,475 angiograms and 27 reocclusion studies with 3,147 angiograms. TIMI grade 3 flow rates at 60 and 90 minutes were as follows: with accelerated tPA, 57.1/63.2%; standard tPA, 39.5/50.2%; APSAC, 40.2/50.1%; and SK, 31.5% (90 minutes). Reocclusion rates were as follows: with accelerated tPA, 6.0%; standard tPA, 11.8%; APSAC, 3.0%; and SK, 4.2%.

237. Gibson CM, et al. Relationship between TIMI frame count and clinical outcomes after thrombolytic administration. *Circulation* 1999;99:1945–1950.

CTFC was measured in 1,248 patients in TIMI 4, TIMI 10A, and TIMI 10B trials. Patients who died in the hospital and by 30 to 42 days had higher CTFCs (69.6 vs. 49.5, $p = 0.0003$; 66.2 vs. 49.9, $p = 0.006$). In a multivariate model, CTFC was an independent predictor of in-hospital mortality (OR, 1.21 per 10-frame increase). The risk of in-hospital mortality increased in a graded fashion from none in patients with the fastest flow (0 to 13 frames, hyperemia, TIMI grade 4 flow) to 2.7% in patients with CTFC of 14 to 40 (CTFC 40 is the cutoff for TIMI grade 3 flow) and to 6.4% in patients with CTFC >40 ($p = 0.003$).

238. Gibson CM, et al.; for the TIMI Study Group. Relationship of TIMI myocardial perfusion grade to mortality after administration of thrombolytic drugs. *Circulation* 2000;101:125–130.

The TMP grade system was developed to assess the filling and clearance of contrast in the myocardium. TMPG 0 was defined as no apparent tissue-level perfusion (no ground glass appearance of blush or opacification of the myocardium) in culprit artery distribution; TMPG 1 indicates presence of myocardial blush but no clearance from the microvasculature (blush or a stain was present on the next injection); TMPG 2 blush clears slowly (blush is strongly persistent and diminishes minimally or not at all during three cardiac cycles of the washout phase); and TMPG 3 indicates that blush begins to clear during washout (blush is minimally persistent after three cardiac cycles of washout). Among 762 patients enrolled in the TIMI 10B trial, a significant mortality gradient was found across TMPGs, with mortality lowest in those patients with TMPG 3 (2.0%), intermediate in TMPG 2 (4.4%), and highest in TMPGs 0 and 1 (6.0%, three-way $p = 0.05$). Even among patients with TIMI grade 3 flow in the epicardial artery, the TMPGs allowed further risk stratification of 30-day mortality: 0.73% for TMPG 3; 2.9% for TMPG 2; 5.0% for TMPG 0 or 1 ($p = 0.03$ for TMPG 3 vs. grades 0, 1, and 2; three-way $p = 0.066$). TMPG 3 flow was a multivariate correlate of 30-day mortality (OR, 0.35; 95% CI, 0.12 to 1.02; $p = 0.054$) in a multivariate model that was adjusted for the presence of TIMI 3 flow ($p = NS$), CTFC (OR, 1.02; $p = 0.06$), presence of an anterior MI (OR, 2.3; $p = 0.03$), admission hazard ratio ($p = NS$), female sex ($p = NS$), and age (OR, 1.1; $p < 0.001$).

239. Gibson CM, et al. Relationship of the TIMI myocardial perfusion grades, flow grades, frame count, and percutaneous coronary intervention to long-term outcomes after thrombolytic administration in acute myocardial infarction. *Circulation* 2002;105:1909–1913.

This analysis examined 848 patients from the TIMI 10B trial (compared tPA with TNK) who had 2-year follow-up. Improved survival was associated with TIMI grade 2/3 flow (Cox hazard ratio, 0.41; $p = 0.001$), reduced CTFCs ($p = 0.02$), and an open microvasculature (TMPG, 2/3; hazard ratio, 0.51; $p = 0.038$). Rescue PCI of closed arteries (TFG, 0/1) at 90 minutes was associated with lower mortality ($p = 0.03$), and mortality trended lower with adjunctive PCI of open (TFG, 2/3) arteries ($p = 0.11$). In a multivariate model correcting for previously identified correlates of mortality (age, sex, pulse, LAD as culprit vessel, and any PCI during initial hospitalization), patency (TFG, 2/3; hazard ratio, 0.32; $p < 0.001$), CTFC ($p = 0.01$), and TMPG 2/3 remained associated with reduced mortality (hazard ratio, 0.46; $p = 0.02$).

240. Gibson CM, et al.; for the TIMI Study Group. Association of duration of symptoms at presentation with angiographic and clinical outcomes after fibrinolytic therapy in patients with ST-segment elevation myocardial infarction. *J Am Coll Cardiol* 2004;44:980–987.

This analysis of 3,845 patients in various TIMI trials examined the relationship between TMPG and symptom duration in patients receiving thrombolysis for acute STEMI. Patients with impaired myocardial perfusion had longer median times from symptom onset to treatment (3 hours for TMPG 0/1 vs. 2.7 hours for TMPG 2/3, $p = 0.001$). This relationship remained robust in a multivariable model ($p = 0.007$). Furthermore, delayed time from onset of symptoms was also associated with increased 30-day mortality (6.6% for time >4 hours vs. 3.3%, $p < 0.001$). These findings highlight the potential pathophysiologic background for poorer clinical outcomes linked to delayed presentation.

OTHER PROGNOSTIC FACTORS

241. Grines CL, et al. Effect of cigarette smoking on outcome after thrombolytic therapy for MI. *Circulation* 1995;91:298–303.

This study showed that better outcomes in smokers with MI may be due to a low-risk profile. Analysis of 1,619 patients treated with tPA, urokinase, or both in six MI trials showed that smokers had similar 90-minute patency (but higher grade 3 flow: 41.1% vs. 34.6%, $p = 0.03$) but lower in-hospital mortality rates (4% vs. 8.9%, $p = 0.0001$). However, after adjustments [lower age (54 years vs. 60 years), more inferior MIs (60% vs. 53%), less three-vessel disease (16% vs. 22%), and higher baseline EF (53% vs. 50%)], no independent prognostic significance was associated with smoking.

242. Lee KL, et al. Predictors of 30-day mortality in the era of reperfusion for acute MI: results from an international trial of 41,021 patients. *Circulation* 1995;91:1659–1668.

Multivariate analysis showed the strong influence of age on mortality rate (only 1.1% if younger than 45 years, 20.5% if older than 75 years). Other factors associated with mortality included lower SBP, higher Killip class, elevated HR, and anterior infarct. These five factors contribute approximately 90% of prognostic information.

243. Woodfield SL, et al. Gender and acute MI: is there a different response to thrombolysis? *J Am Coll Cardiol* 1997;29:35–42.

This GUSTO angiography substudy analysis showed female gender to be an independent risk factor for mortality. The women had some high-risk features (e.g., older, more hypertension, diabetes, and heart failure) and some low-risk features (e.g., fewer prior MIs and bypass surgery, less smoking). The unadjusted 30-day mortality rate was nearly three times higher (13.1% vs. 4.8%, $p < 0.001$), and after multivariate analysis, female gender remained an independent mortality predictor.

244. Case RB, et al. Living alone after MI. *JAMA* 1992;267:515–519.

This analysis of 1,234 MI patients with an average follow-up of 2.1 years showed that living alone was associated with 54% more end points (nonfatal MI plus cardiac death).

245. Frasure-Smith N, et al. Depression following MI. JAMA 1993;270:1819–1825.

This small study was composed of 222 MI patients who survived to hospital discharge. Patients were interviewed at average 7 days (major depression, 2 weeks). Depression was associated with a 4.3-fold higher mortality rate ($p = 0.013$). The impact was at least equivalent to that of LV dysfunction (Killip class) and prior MI. Editorial points out that typically 15% to 20% of post-MI patients have major depression.

246. Kuhl EA, et al. Relation of anxiety and adherence to risk-reducing recommendations following myocardial infarction. Am J Cardiol 2009;103:1629–1634.

Among 278 patients with acute MI, in multivariable analysis, anxiety predicted poorer adherence to many risk-reducing therapies (pharmacologic and nonpharmacologic). It was the only predictor of poor adherence to smoking cessation.

247. Jollis JG, et al. Outcome of acute MI according to the specialty of the admitting physician. N Engl J Med 1996;335:1880–1887.

This retrospective analysis of 8,241 Medicare patients showed that cardiologists provide optimal care for MI patients. All-cause 1-year mortality HRs (based on admitting physician) were as follows: cardiologists, 0.88; family medicine, 0.98; general practitioner, 1.06; and other, 1.16. Cardiologist-treated patients were younger and healthier and had less diabetes, more Killip class I, lower predicted 30-day mortality rates (GUSTO-I model; 18% vs. 20%), and longer hospital stay (9.3 days vs. 7.3 to 8.6 days). Cardiologists used thrombolysis about twice as often; used angiography, revascularization, treadmill tests, nuclear imaging, Holter monitoring, and echocardiography more frequently; and gave more patients aspirin, β-blockers, and heparin. In an analysis of all 1992 Medicare claims (approximately 220,000 patients), the same mortality pattern emerged: with cardiologists, 30%; internists, 37%; family medicine, 39%; and general practitioners, 40%. Although 82% of the attending physicians were the same as the admitting physician, the roles of consultants and transfers were not assessed.

248. Bradley EH, et al. Hospital quality for acute myocardial infarction correlation among process measures and relationship with short-term mortality. JAMA 2006;296:72–78.

The investigators sought to correlate quality-of-care measures, as determined by Centers for Medicare & Medicaid Services (CMS) and the Joint Commission on Accreditation of Healthcare Organizations (JCAHO), with 30-day clinical outcomes for acute MI in the NRMI. Core measures, such as β-blocker use at admission/discharge, aspirin at admission/discharge, and ACE use, were significantly correlated with 30-day mortality rates of hospitals (correlation coefficients ≥ 0.40, $p < 0.001$ for pairwise comparisons). However, these measures captured only explained a small fraction of variability in hospitals' mortality rates (approximately 6%).

249. Williams SC, et al. Performance of top-ranked heart care hospitals on evidence-based process measures. Circulation 2006;114:558–564.

Hospitals at the top of U.S. News & World Report's "America's Best Hospitals" were assessed for compliance with measures from the American College of Cardiology and AHA's clinical treatment guidelines for heart failure and acute MI. They aggregated 10 rate-based performance measures into a cardiovascular composite score. While on the whole, hospitals at the top of the list did better than the rest (86% of measures met vs. 83%, $p < 0.05$), only 23 of "America's Best Hospitals" met such standards more frequently than the overall average.

Complications of Myocardial Infarction

ARRHYTHMIAS, BUNDLE BRANCH BLOCK

250. Solomon SD, et al. Ventricular arrhythmias in trials of thrombolytic therapy for acute MI: a meta-analysis. *Circulation* 1993;88:2575–2581.

This analysis focused on 15 randomized trials with 39,606 patients. Thrombolytic administration was associated with lower risk of VF during the entire hospitalization (OR, 0.83; 95% CI, 0.76 to 0.90; $p < 0.0001$) but not in the first 6 or 24 hours after thrombolysis (ORs, 0.98 and 1.00). Thrombolytic use also was associated with a higher incidence of VT during hospitalization (OR, 1.34; 95% CI, 1.15 to 1.55; $p < 0.0001$).

251. Newby KH, et al. Incidence and clinical relevance of the occurrence of bundle branch block in patients treated with thrombolytic therapy. *Circulation* 1996;94:2424–2428.

This study was composed of 681 TAMI-9 and GUSTO-I patients who underwent continuous 12-lead ECG monitoring for 36 to 72 hours. BBB occurred in 23.6% (RBBB, 13%; LBBB, 7%; alternating, 3.5%). Mortality was 2.5 times higher in BBB patients compared with those without BBB (8.7% vs. 3.5%, $p = 0.007$). The highest mortality rate was observed in those with persistent BBB [19.4% vs. 5.6 (transient) and 3.5% (none); $p < 0.001$]. BBB patients also had decreased EF, increased peak CK, and more diseased vessels.

252. Crenshaw BS, et al. Atrial fibrillation in the setting of acute MI: the GUSTO I experience. *J Am Coll Cardiol* 1997;30:406–413.

Atrial fibrillation was present on admission ECG in 2.5%, and increased to 7.9% after study enrollment. The group with early and late AF had more three-vessel disease, less TIMI grade 3 flow, more in-hospital strokes (3.1% vs. 1.3%, $p = 0.0001$), and more than twofold higher unadjusted 30-day and 1-year mortality rates (14.3% vs. 6.2%, $p = 0.0001$; 21.5% vs. 8.6%, $p < 0.0001$). In multivariate analysis, late AF predictors were age, peak CK, Killip class, and HR. Adjusted ORs of mortality were 1.1 for baseline AF (85% CI, 0.88 to 1.3) and 1.4 for late AF (95% CI, 1.3 to 1.5).

CARDIAC RUPTURE

253. Becker RC, et al. Cardiac rupture associated with thrombolytic therapy: impact of time to treatment in the LATE (Late Assessment of Thrombolytic Efficacy) study. *J Am Coll Cardiol* 1995;25:1063–1068.

This analysis of 5,711 LATE patients found that cardiac rupture was the listed cause of death in 53 (9.7%) of 547 patients who died in the first 35 days. No increased risk of rupture was found in the group receiving rtPA at 6 to 24 hours compared with the placebo group. However, rupture events did occur earlier in the thrombolytic group (treatment × time to death interaction, $p = 0.03$).

254. Becker RC, et al. A composite view of cardiac rupture in the U.S. National Registry of MI. *J Am Coll Cardiol* 1996;27:1321–1326.

In this analysis of 350,755 patients, thrombolytic administration (approximately 12,000 patients) was associated with 5.9% mortality (no thrombolytic therapy, 12.9%). Cardiac rupture was reported as the cause of death in 12% of patients who received thrombolysis [vs. 6% (no thrombolysis)] and occurred more frequently within the first 24 hours.

255. Becker RC, et al. Fatal cardiac rupture among patients treated with thrombolytic agents and adjunctive thrombin antagonists. *J Am Coll Cardiol* 1999;33:479–487.

This analysis of 3,759 patients enrolled in the TIMI 9A and TIMI 9B trials showed a 1.7% incidence of cardiac rupture. By multivariate analysis, independent predictors of rupture were age older than 70 years (OR, 3.77; 95% CI, 2.06 to 6.91), female gender

(OR, 2.87; 95% CI, 1.44 to 5.73), and prior angina (OR, 1.82; 95% CI, 1.05 to 3.16). No association was found between the intensity of anticoagulation or type of thrombin inhibition (e.g., heparin or hirudin) and cardiac rupture.

256. Moreno R, et al. Primary angioplasty reduces the risk of left ventricular free wall rupture compared with thrombolysis in patients with acute myocardial infarction. *J Am Coll Cardiol* 2002;39:598–603.

This analysis consisted of 1,375 patients with AMI seen within 12 hours of symptom onset; 55.4% underwent primary angioplasty, and 44.6% were treated with thrombolytic therapy. FWR was diagnosed when sudden death occurred because of PEA with large pericardial effusion on an echocardiogram or when demonstrated postmortem or at surgery. The overall incidence of FWR was 2.5% (angioplasty, 1.8%; thrombolysis, 3.3%; $p = 0.69$). In the univariate analysis, the following were risk factors for FWR: age older than 70 years (5.2% vs. 1.2%, $p < 0.001$), female gender (5.1% vs. 1.8%, $p = 0.006$), anterior location (3.3% vs. 1.4%, $p = 0.02$), and treatment more than 2 hours after symptom onset (3.6% vs. 1.7%, $p = 0.043$). In the multivariate analysis, independent risk factors were age older than 70 (OR, 4.12; 95% CI, 2.04 to 8.62; $p < 0.001$) and anterior location (OR, 2.91; 95% CI, 1.36 to 6.63; $p = 0.008$), whereas treatment with primary angioplasty was an independent protective factor (OR, 0.46; 95% CI, 0.22 to 0.96; $p = 0.037$).

INTRACRANIAL HEMORRHAGE IN THROMBOLYSIS

257. Maggioni AP, et al. Risk of stroke in patients with acute MI after thrombolytic and antithrombotic therapy. *N Engl J Med* 1992;327:1–6.

This analysis focused on GISSI-2 and International Study patients; complete data were available on 20,768 patients. The in-hospital stroke rate was 1.14% (hemorrhagic, 0.36%; ischemic, 0.48%; undefined cause, 0.30%). Patients treated with tPA had a small but significant excess of stroke versus SK-treated patients (1.33% vs. 0.94%; adjusted OR, 1.42; 95% CI, 1.09 to 1.84). Factors associated with increased risk of stroke were older age, higher Killip class, and anterior infarction.

258. Simoons ML, et al. Individual risk assessment for intracranial hemorrhage during thrombolytic therapy. *Lancet* 1993;342:1523–1528.

This analysis focused on data from the Netherlands registry, ECSG, GISSI-2 and International Study Group trials, TIMI II trials, TAMI trials, and ISAM study. By multivariate analysis, independent predictors of intracranial hemorrhage were age older than 65 years (OR, 2.2; 95% CI, 1.4 to 3.5), body weight <70 kg (OR, 2.1; 95% CI, 1.3 to 3.2), hypertension on hospital admission (OR, 2.0; 95% CI, 1.2 to 3.2), and administration of alteplase (OR, 1.6; 95% CI, 1.0 to 2.5).

259. Gurwitz JH, et al. Risk for intracranial hemorrhage after tissue plasminogen activator for acute MI. *Ann Intern Med* 1998;129:597–604.

This analysis focused on 71,073 patients from the NRMI 2 treated with tPA between June 1994 and September 1996. The in-hospitalization intracranial hemorrhage rate was 0.95% [0.88% confirmed (CT or MRI)]. In multivariate models, the following were intracranial hemorrhage predictors: older age, female sex, black ethnicity, SBP more than 140 mm Hg, DBP >100 mm Hg, history of stroke, tPA dose more than 1.5 mg/kg, and lower body weight.

REOCCLUSION, RECURRENT ISCHEMIA, AND REINFARCTION

260. Benhorin J, et al. Prognostic significance of nonfatal myocardial reinfarction. *J Am Coll Cardiol* 1990;15:253–258.

This analysis focused on 1,234 placebo patients in the multicenter diltiazem trial. At follow-up (1 to 4 years), nonfatal MI had occurred in 9.4%, with a higher frequency in women and those with prior cardiac symptoms. Nonfatal MI was associated with a three-fold higher risk of subsequent cardiac mortality (5.4 times higher if the index event was a first MI).

261. Ohman EM, et al. Consequences of reocclusion after successful reperfusion therapy in acute MI. *Circulation* 1990;82:781–791.

This analysis focused on 810 TAMI patients with repeated angiography at average 7 days that showed a reoccluded IRA in 12.4% (58% with symptoms). At follow-up, occluded patients had a similar EF but worse infarct zone function and increased in-hospital mortality (11% vs. 4.5%, $p = 0.01$).

262. Kornowski R, et al. Predictors and long-term prognostic significance of recurrent infarction in the year after a first MI. *Am J Cardiol* 1993;72:883–888.

This retrospective analysis focused on 3,695 SPRINT patients, with a 1-year reinfarction rate of 6% (associated in-hospital mortality, 30%). Reinfarction predictors were peripheral vascular disease (adjusted RR, 2.12), anterior MI (RR, 1.62), angina before MI (RR, 1.53), CHF on admission (RR, 1.34), diabetes (RR, 1.33), hypertension (RR, 1.28), and age increment (RR, 1.13). Reinfarction rates were as follows: zero or one risk factor, 4.0%, and five or six risk factors, 23.3%. Recurrent MI is the strongest long-term mortality predictor (adjusted RR, 4.76).

263. Mueller HS, et al. Prognostic significance of nonfatal reinfarction during 3 year follow-up of the TIMI II clinical trial. *J Am Coll Cardiol* 1995;26:900–907.

The incidence of reinfarction was 10.1% (43 of 339 died). Relative risks of death were 1.9 if reinfarction occurred at <42 days, 6.2 at 43 to 365 days, and 2.9 at 1 to 3 years.

264. Verheught FWA, et al. Reocclusion: the flip of coronary thrombolysis. *J Am Coll Cardiol* 1996;27:766–773.

This analysis focused on 61 studies with 6,061 patients undergoing angiography twice. Reocclusion usually occurs within weeks. Overall, an 11% reocclusion rate was observed, but a 16% incidence was seen in true occlusion studies; thus, initial occlusion is a risk factor. Aspirin and heparin were not associated with benefit in prevention (APRICOT, HART trials). Hirudin and hirulog appear beneficial. Half of reocclusions are clinically silent. Revascularization is helpful, especially if symptoms are present.

265. Bauters C, et al. Angiographically documented late reocclusion after successful coronary angioplasty of an infarct-related lesion is a powerful predictor of long-term mortality. *Circulation* 1999;99:2243–2250.

Retrospective analysis of 528 patients who had a patent IRA after balloon angioplasty procedure 10 ± 6 days after MI. At 6-month follow-up angiography, IRA reocclusion occurred in 17% (TIMI flow grade 0 or 1). At long-term follow-up (median, 6.4 years), the reocclusion group had a 2.5-fold higher mortality rate (20% vs. 8%, $p = 0.002$). The actuarial 8-year total mortality rates were 28% and 10% ($p = 0.0003$), and the CV mortality rates were 25% and 7% ($p < 0.0001$). The mortality differences between reoccluded and patent IRA patients were greater in patients with an anterior MI.

266. Ernst NM, et al.; on behalf of the Zwolle Myocardial Infarction Study Group. Impact of failed mechanical reperfusion in patients with acute myocardial infarction treated with primary angioplasty. *Am J Cardiol* 2005;96:332–334.

Among 1,683 patients undergoing primary PCI for acute MI at a single center, nearly 7% in this cohort did not achieve mechanical reperfusion—roughly half had failed primary angioplasty and the other half had late reocclusion. Predictors of failed PCI in univariate analysis were Killip class >1, LAD IRA, and TIMI flow grade 0/1 prior to PCI. In-hospital, 30-day, and 1-year mortality rates were all higher in the patients with failed reperfusion ($p < 0.001$ for each).

LEFT VENTRICULAR THROMBI

267. Gueret P, et al. Effects of full-dose heparin anticoagulation on the development of left ventricular thrombosis in acute transmural MI. *J Am Coll Cardiol* 1986;8: 419–426.

This small prospective study showed that thrombi occur frequently in anterior MIs. Ninety patients (46 anterior, 44 inferior) seen an average of 5.2 hours after onset of symptoms were randomized to heparin or no heparin. No thrombi were detected on first echocardiograms (done at 10.3 ± 8 hours). In the anterior MI group, 46% had thrombi at 4.3 ± 3.0 days [38% (heparin) vs. 52% (no heparin), $p = 0.76$]. No thrombi formed in the inferior group.

268. Vecchio C, et al. Left ventricular thrombus in anterior acute MI after thrombolysis. *Circulation* 1991;84:512–519.

This GISSI-2 ancillary echocardiography study was composed of 180 consecutive patients with first MI. Echocardiography was performed within 48 hours and before discharge. LV thrombi were found in 28% (no difference between the four treatment groups). Mural shape was more common, especially in heparinized patients. Only one in-hospital embolic event was documented.

269. Vaitkus PT, et al. Embolic potential, prevention and management of mural thrombus complicating anterior MI: a meta-analysis. *J Am Coll Cardiol* 1993;22: 1004–1009.

This analysis focused on 11 studies with 856 patients. Thrombus by echocardiography was associated with an OR of embolization of 5.45 (11% vs. 2%). In anterior MI patients, the OR was 8.0. Anticoagulation was associated with 86% less embolization. Primary anticoagulation led to 68% less embolization, whereas thrombolytic therapy was associated with 52% less embolization (16% vs. 32%).

270. Greaves SC, et al. Incidence and natural history of left ventricular thrombus following anterior wall acute MI. *Am J Cardiol* 1997;80:442–448.

This analysis focused on 309 Healing and Early Afterload Reducing Treatment (HEART) substudy patients, 78% with Q-wave anterior MIs. Echocardiography was performed on days 1, 14, and 90. LV thrombus rates were low: day 1, 0.6%; day 14, 3.7%; and day 90, 2.5%. Only one thrombus was detected on two echocardiograms. Thrombus patients had a greater LV size increase and wall-motion abnormalities.

271. Weinsaft JW, et al. Detection of left ventricular thrombus by delayed-enhancement cardiovascular magnetic resonance: prevalence and markers in patients with systolic dysfunction. *J Am Coll Cardiol* 2008;52:148–157.

In 784 patients with impaired systolic function (EF < 50%), LV thrombus was detected in 7% (both intracavitary and mural thrombi). In multivariable analyses, risk factors for thrombus included low EF, ischemic cardiomyopathy, and increased myocardial scarring on magnetic resonance.

VALVULAR DAMAGE AND SEPTAL DEFECTS

272. Lehmann KG, et al. Mitral regurgitation in early MI: incidence, clinical detection and prognostic implications. *Ann Intern Med* 1992;117:10–17.

This analysis focused on 206 TIMI I patients with contrast left ventriculography within 7 hours of symptom onset. Mitral regurgitation was present in 27 (13%) patients and associated with a markedly increased 1-year mortality rate (RRs, 12.2 and 7.5 by univariate and multivariate analyses, respectively).

273. Lamas GA, et al. Clinical significance of mitral regurgitation after acute MI. *Circulation* 1997;96:827–833.

This study was composed of 727 SAVE patients with catheterization and left ventriculography data (done within 16 days of MI). Mitral regurgitation (19.4%) patients were more likely to have a persistently occluded IRA (27.2% vs. 15.2%, $p = 0.001$). At follow-up (median, 3.5 years), mitral regurgitation patients had a more than twofold higher CV mortality rate (29% vs. 12%, $p < 0.001$), more severe CHF (24% vs. 16%, $p = 0.015$), and a higher rate of CV mortality, severe CHF, and reinfarction (47% vs. 29%, $p < 0.001$). In multivariate analysis, mitral regurgitation was an independent CV mortality predictor [RR, 2.0; 95% CI, 1.28 to 3.04].

274. Crenshaw BS, et al.; for the GUSTO-I (Global Utilization of Streptokinase and TPA for Occluded Coronary Arteries) Trial Investigators. Risk factors, angiographic patterns, and outcomes in patients with ventricular septal defect complicating acute myocardial infarction. *Circulation* 2000;101:27–32.

VSD complicated 0.2% of STEMIs in the GUSTO-I trial (84 of 41,021). Predisposing factors included older age, anterior infarct, females, and no previous smoking; additionally, VSD is more common when the IRA was the LAD and when it was totally occluded. Mortality was significantly higher at 30 days in patients with VSD (73.8% vs. 6.8%, $p < 0.001$), and surgical therapy showed mortality benefit over medical management (30-day mortality, 47% vs. 94%, $p < 0.001$).

275. Birnbaum Y, et al. Ventricular septal rupture after acute myocardial infarction. *N Engl J Med* 2002;347:1426–1432.

This review article discusses numerous topics, including the incidence, risk factors, pathogenesis, hemodynamics, time course, clinical manifestations, angiographic findings, medical and surgical therapy, and prognosis of ventricular septal rupture after acute MI.

chapter 5

Heart Failure

Benjamin A. Steinberg and Christopher P. Cannon

EPIDEMIOLOGY

Congestive heart failure (HF) is responsible for more than 1 million hospital admissions each year in the United States, and one-quarter of those hospitalized will return within 1 month. Total annual costs for HF care in the United States are estimated at $30 billion (1).

The aging of the population and improved survival after myocardial infarction (MI) (*Circulation* 2008;118(20):2057–2062) has resulted in an increasing prevalence of HF, which is projected to continue. Data from the Framingham Heart Study suggest that the incidence of HF over the past 50-year period has declined among women but not among men, whereas survival has continued to improve in both sexes (by 12% per decade), which accounts for the increasing prevalence (12). However, a large population-based study of Olmsted County, MN, residents showed no significant decline in incidence in either sex, and survival improved in both sexes but much more so in younger men than in women and older patients (10). Furthermore, hospitalizations for HF with *preserved* left ventricular ejection fraction (HFpEF) have dramatically increased over the last decade (11).

Most studies show women surviving longer than men (8,12; see also *J Am Coll Cardiol* 1992;20:301–306 and *Circulation* 1999;99:1816–1821), whereas the Studies of Left Ventricular Dysfunction (SOLVD) trial found the opposite. The explanation for this discrepancy may be that the SOLVD trial enrolled a higher percentage of women with coronary artery disease (CAD), and HF due to an ischemic etiology is associated with increased mortality. But analysis of the Candesartan in Heart Failure: Assessment of Reduction in Mortality and Morbidity (CHARM) trial data suggests that the gender difference cannot be fully explained by a difference in the prevalence of CAD between sexes (13).

Factors associated with an increased risk of HF are advanced age, male gender, black race, diabetes, obesity, smoking, CAD/previous MI, and hypertension

(7–9). The Olmsted County data suggest the highest population attributable risk stems from CAD and hypertension (see *Am J Med* 2009;122:1023–1028). Among women, those with hypertension and diabetes are more likely than men to develop HF. Echocardiographic findings associated with increased risk include low left and/or right ventricular ejection fraction (EF), left ventricular (LV) dilatation, and valvular disease (28).

The American Heart Association (AHA)/American College of Cardiology (ACC) guidelines for HF developed a revised classification system for HF, involving four stages in its development, A through D. These were not intended to replace the New York Heart Association (NYHA) classification system, discussed below, but rather to complement it with a staging system that does not change with response to therapy. It also recognizes that there are established risk factors and structural prerequisites for the development of HF, which may provide the opportunity for therapeutic intervention before the manifestation of LV systolic dysfunction or symptoms.

- Stage A: at high risk for HF but without structural heart disease or symptoms of HF
- Stage B: structural heart disease but without signs or symptoms of HF
- Stage C: structural heart disease with prior or current symptoms of HF
- Stage D: refractory HF requiring specialized interventions

Among those diagnosed with HF, severity of signs and symptoms is predicted by functional class. Most of the NYHA classes are contained within Stage C (see above). The NYHA classification is as follows:

- Class I: no limitation
- Class II: slight HF; comfortable at rest but ordinary activity causes fatigue, dyspnea, or angina
- Class III: marked failure; less than ordinary activity causes symptoms
- Class IV: severe failure; symptoms of HF at rest

The mortality rate in NYHA class III patients with peak oxygen consumption of 10 to 15 mL/kg/min is 15% to 20% per year, and it increases to 50% per year or more in class IV patients with oxygen consumption of <10 mL/kg/min.

Also noteworthy is the Killip classification system, first developed in 1967. It stratifies post-MI patients based on their level of HF signs and symptoms. Patients with a lower Killip class have a lower 30-day mortality post-MI than do patients with a higher Killip class:

- Killip class I: no clinical signs of HF
- Killip class II: rales or crackles in the lungs, an S_3 gallop, and elevated jugular venous pressure (JVP)
- Killip class III: frank acute pulmonary edema
- Killip class IV: cardiogenic shock or hypotension (measured as systolic blood pressure [SBP] lower than 90 mm Hg) and evidence of peripheral vasoconstriction (oliguria, cyanosis, or sweating)

Lastly, the Interagency Registry for Mechanically Assisted Circulatory Support (INTERMACS) has developed a separate list of profiles for patients with severe HF who might be considered for cardiac transplant (1). The profiles range from 7 (the patient with advanced NYHA III HF) to profile 1 (those with acute, life-threatening cardiac insufficiency requiring immediate hemodynamic support) and may assist clinicians in identifying patients in need of advanced HF care.

The acute HF syndrome is the presentation of symptomatic, decompensated HF (6). This is frequently triggered in the setting of other acute medical or surgical illness (commonly infectious), dietary or medication nonadherence, or acute coronary syndrome events. Such hospitalizations account for a significant morbidity in such patients, in addition to enormous health care resource expenditures. Rehospitalization rates within 30 days are high, as are rates of postdischarge events. While outpatient management strategies have accumulated a significant evidence base, inpatient management has remained focused predominantly on fluid removal and symptomatic treatment with relatively few supporting data (as discussed herein).

HISTORY AND PHYSICAL EXAMINATION

Symptoms include dyspnea, fatigue, paroxysmal nocturnal dyspnea, orthopnea, and nocturia. Orthopnea appears to be the most sensitive symptom for predicting elevated pulmonary capillary wedge pressure (PCWP) (14). Impaired concentration may occur in individuals with decreased cardiac output at rest.

The physical examination may be notable for rales (often not present if chronic or gradual in onset), elevated JVP, presence of third heart sound, peripheral edema, cool extremities, narrowed pulse pressure, and tachycardia (**Table 5.1**). Hepatomegaly and ascites are often seen with right HF. Most of these signs have limited sensitivity at predicting elevated PCWP. In one study, jugular venous distention, at rest or inducible by a hepatojugular test, had a sensitivity of 80% for predicting elevated PCWP (15). JVD and third heart sound have been shown to have prognostic significance (18). In another study, low

Table 5.1	Findings of Physical Examination	
	Systolic Dysfunction	**Diastolic Dysfunction**
Third heart sound	Frequent	Rare
Fourth heart sound	Rare	Frequent
Rales	Occasional	Occasional
Peripheral edema	Frequent	Rare
Jugular venous distention	Frequent	Rare
Cardiomegaly	Usual	Rare

Modified from **Braunwald E.** *Heart disease*. Philadelphia, PA: W.B. Saunders; 1997.

pulse pressure was an excellent predictor of poor cardiac output, with a pulse pressure of <25% having a 91% sensitivity and 83% specificity for a cardiac index of 2.2 L/min/m^2 or less (14).

ETIOLOGY

Systolic dysfunction is due to pump failure, typically from ischemic cardiomy-opathy, nonischemic dilated cardiomyopathy, hypertensive heart disease, or valvular disease. Alcohol and viral illnesses are responsible for some cases of nonischemic dilated cardiomyopathy, but many are idiopathic. High-output causes of HF are less common and include anemia, hyperthyroidism, and pregnancy. Rare causes include Paget disease, arteriovenous fistula, pheochromocytoma, and beriberi.

Diastolic dysfunction is a component in approximately one-half of HF cases (11). Most of these are classified as HFpEF, though it should be noted that diastolic function is often abnormal in HF with reduced EF (HFrEF). HFpEF is most commonly associated with hypertension but also hypertrophic cardiomyopathy and infiltrative disease. It is most prevalent among elderly women, most of whom have hypertension, diabetes, or both. Unlike systolic HF, there is a dearth of large clinical trials to guide the management of these patients. Current recommendations are to control hypertension, control ventricular rate to allow diastolic filling, treat symptoms with diuretics, and address the underlying etiology if possible (e.g., coronary revascularization for CAD) (1).

An important precipitating factor of HF is noncompliance with a prescribed drug regimen and poor diet (e.g., high salt intake). In one study of patients hospitalized for HF, more than 60% were found to be noncompliant with drugs and/or diet (see *Arch Intern Med* 1988;148:2013). Abrupt/acute precipitating causes of HF include acute MI, acute pulmonary embolism, acute mitral regurgitation and aortic insufficiency, acute ventricular septal defect, and infection. More chronic precipitating causes of HF include drugs [nonsteroidal anti-inflammatory drugs (vasoconstriction), potentially even aspirin in nonischemic HF (107, WATCH trial); verapamil, diltiazem, and procainamide (due to negative inotropy, though amlodipine and felodipine appear to be safe in HF); estrogens, androgens, minoxidil, and thiazolidinediones (see the RECORD trial, *Lancet* 2009;373:2125–3215) (water retention); doxorubicin (adriamycin)], depression, and sleep apnea.

DIAGNOSTIC TESTING

1. Laboratory tests. The use of B-type natriuretic peptide (BNP) and NT-proBNP have been found to be beneficial in the evaluation and triage of patients with acute dyspnea in the emergency department (ED; also see *J Am Coll Cardiol* 2011;58:1881 and *Eur Heart J* 2006;27:839). One of the largest such studies, the *BNP* multinational study, demonstrated the statistically significant

impact of adding BNP levels to other clinical criteria, to make the diagnosis of HF as an explanation for patients presenting with dyspnea (21,22). Moreover, BNP level was more predictive than any other single clinical criterion for making the diagnosis of acute HF. Data on BNP have expanded to include support for BNP-guided outpatient management, as demonstrated by the STARS-BNP study (24); however, these results could not be replicated in the TIME-HF study (25). Nevertheless, additional studies of goal-directed care with BNP are ongoing. Small studies of using BNP to aid in discharge planning and decrease length of stay have yielded mixed results (23,26).

Low serum sodium is common (neurohormonal activation) and linearly predictive of poor outcome (19); elevated creatinine and liver function tests also are predictors of poor outcome. Finally, inflammatory markers (e.g., C-reactive protein, TNF-alpha, IL-6) appear to be elevated in HF patients (see *Circulation* 2003;107:1486). Their prognostic role requires further study.

2. Chest radiograph. Findings of increased pulmonary capillary pressure are seen in approximately 50% of patients; bilateral pleural effusions and cardiomegaly also may be present.

3. Electrocardiography (ECG). Q waves and left bundle branch block are good predictors of systolic dysfunction. A wide QRS (more than 220 milliseconds) is predictive of increased mortality. Longer QRS duration is also a predictor of response to resynchronization therapy (see below).

4. Echocardiogram. A simple and useful tool, echocardiography can help determine systolic versus diastolic dysfunction and left and/or right ventricular impairment.

5. Six-minute walk test. Short distance correlates with higher mortality and increased HF-related hospitalizations (28).

6. Metabolic stress testing. Used to measure oxygen consumption; a peak oxygen consumption of <12 to 14 mL/kg/min portends a poor prognosis (27). The test is also used in the evaluation of candidates for cardiac transplantation.

7. Endomyocardial biopsy (EMB). Biopsy may be useful in selected cases, such as suspected amyloidosis, sarcoidosis, and giant cell myocarditis (1,20). However, it is not recommended in the routine workup of HF patients.

TREATMENT

Treatment of Acute Heart Failure

1. Diuretics. Furosemide is administered intravenously to alleviate lung edema due to volume overload, again by reducing preload. (Initial dose should be based on prior diuretic history.) Addition of a thiazide (e.g., metolazone or chlorothiazide) may help potentiate diuresis. In cases of massive fluid overload that respond poorly to diuretics, ultrafiltration may be effective (102). Data from the DOSE trial failed to demonstrate the superiority of continuous-infusion diuresis (compared to bolus dosing) but did advocate for higher

intensity dosing of bolus intravenous diuretics (up to 2.5 × the outpatient oral dose).

   a. Nitrates. Nitroglycerin is given sublingually or intravenously in cases in which preload reduction is necessary to more rapidly reduce pulmonary congestion. IV nitroglycerin is ideal for patients with HF and hypertension, coronary ischemia, or significant mitral regurgitation. In the case of severe HF, nitroprusside administration should be considered if both PCWP and systemic vascular resistance (SVR) are elevated. Nitroprusside has a balanced arteriodilating/venodilating effect and also dilates the pulmonary vasculature.

2. Nesiritide. This form of human BNP causes vasodilation and appeared to result in rapid symptomatic and hemodynamic improvement in patients with acutely decompensated HF (76). It was an attractive alternative to inotropes because it caused rapid symptom relief without the risk of arrhythmias. However, subsequent studies suggested that nesiritide may be associated with worsening renal function (see *Circulation* 2005;111:1487–1491) and possibly even an increased risk of mortality (78). Following this, two major clinical trials of nesiritide failed to demonstrate a significant clinical benefit with the drug (79,80), and it maintains a IIb recommendation for the treatment of dyspnea symptoms (1).

3. Inotropic agents. No single agent has been found to be clinically superior, but adrenergic agents (such as dobutamine and dopamine and the phosphodiesterase inhibitor, milrinone) each may have a role in certain hemodynamic states such as relative hypotension with poor response to vasodilators and diuretics. Dopamine may be preferable in those with low blood pressure because dobutamine reduces SVR to a greater extent, but the gain in cardiac output added to the decrease in SVR with dobutamine typically leads to a slight *increase* in blood pressure. Milrinone has greater vasodilating–unloading properties and works on both the systemic and pulmonary systems. This agent was evaluated for short-term use in acute exacerbations of HF in the OPTIME-HF trial and was not shown to be beneficial (87).

4. Vasopressin antagonists: Not only is the presence of hyponatremia a poor prognostic sign, but severe hyponatremia can have serious neurologic sequelae. Thus, the vasopressin antagonists conivaptan and tolvaptan are approved and recommended (class IIb) for the treatment of hypervolemic hyponatremia in patients with or at risk for cognitive impairment (1,88,90).

Data from small clinical trials and anecdotal case experience suggest that inotropic agents reduce hospitalization, lead to hemodynamic and clinical improvement, and may serve as a bridge to transplantation. Some reports have suggested that intermittent infusion therapy in outpatients also may be effective in attenuating HF symptoms in the long term (see *J Heart Lung Transplant* 2000;19:S49), but the safety of prolonged outpatient use of these agents has been questioned. Data from more than 1,000 patients with chronic HF randomized to milrinone or placebo showed an increase in mortality (30% vs. 24%) with more adverse reactions, including syncope and hypotension [Prospective Randomized Milrinone Survival Evaluation (PROMISE); (84)]. The increase in mortality has led some to suggest that inotropic drugs used in this fashion may exacerbate arrhythmias with subsequent sudden cardiac death. Intermittent outpatient infusion of either vasoactive drugs such as nesiritide or positive inotropic drugs has not been shown to improve symptoms or survival in patients with advanced HF.

Treatment of Chronic Heart Failure

ANGIOTENSIN-CONVERTING ENZYME INHIBITORS

Clearly indicated if LV dysfunction is present (**Table 5.2**), angiotensin-converting enzyme (ACE) inhibitors should be initiated before aggressively performing diuresis in HF patients. They are first-line therapy in patients with systolic HF. The Cooperative North Scandinavian Enalapril Survival Study (CONSENSUS I) showed that enalapril reduced 1-year mortality by 31% in NYHA class IV patients (32), whereas the larger SOLVD trial enrolled NYHA class II and III patients and showed that enalapril reduced mortality by 16% (average follow-up, 41 months) (33). Subsequent trials have shown similar benefits with other ACE inhibitors [e.g., Veterans Administration Cooperative Vasodilator-Heart Failure Trial II (V-HEFT II), Acute Infarction Ramipril Efficacy Study (AIRE) (35)] (**Table 5.3**). A meta-analysis of 32 studies found ACE inhibitor therapy to be associated with significant reductions in total mortality and mortality or hospitalization for HF ($p < 0.001$ for both) (30).

The beneficial effect of administering larger versus lower doses of ACE inhibition has been demonstrated, though the benefit seems limited to reducing the risk of hospitalization. Effects on symptoms and mortality did not appear to differ (ATLAS; 37). The ATLAS trial randomized 3,164 patients with NYHA class II to IV HF and EF $\leq$30% to low-dose (2.5 to 5 mg/day) versus high-dose (32.5 to 35 mg/day) lisinopril. This trial demonstrated a nonsignificant 8% lower mortality and significant 24% fewer hospitalizations in patients treated with high-dose lisinopril.

Table 5.2	Differential Diagnosis		
	Acute Heart Failure	**Decompensated Chronic Heart Failure**	**Chronic Heart Failure**
Severity of symptoms	Severe	Severe	Mild to moderate
Pulmonary edema	Rare	Common	Rare
Peripheral edema	Rare	Common	Common
Weight gain	None to minimal	Moderate to severe	Mild to moderate

Modified from **Braunwald E.** *Heart disease.* Philadelphia, PA: W.B. Saunders; 1997.

Table 5.3 Major ACE inhibitor Trials

	Number of Patients	Patient Characteristics	Placebo Mortality	Hazard Ratio
V-HeFT II (57)	804	NYHA I-III	25% at 2 y[a]	0.72
CONSENSUS I (36)	253	NYHA IV	52% at 1 y	0.69
SOLVD (37)	2,569	NYHA II, III	40% at 3.4 y	0.84
SOLVD Prevention (38)	4,228	NYHA I	16% at 3.1 y	0.91
AIRE (39)	2,006	Post-MI, clinical HF	23% at 1.3 y	0.73
SAVE (Chapter 4)	2,231	Post-MI, EF ≤40%	25% at 3.5 y	0.81
ISIS-4 (Chapter 4)	58,050	24-h post-MI[b]	7.7% at 5 wk	0.93

This table demonstrates that studies that enrolled higher-risk patients showed a strong benefit (15%–30% lower mortality) from ACE inhibitor therapy, whereas a modest benefit was seen in the lower-risk populations (SOLVD Prevention, ISIS-4).

[a]Hydralazine and isosorbide.

[b]No HF required for enrollment.

EF, ejection fraction; HF, heart failure; NYHA, New York Heart Association; MI, myocardial infarction; ACE, angiotensin-converting enzyme.

The use of ACE inhibition in HFpEF has not shown a proven benefit, however. The Perindopril in Elderly People with Chronic Heart Failure (PEP-HF) trial randomized 850 HF patients who were at least 70 years of age and had a left ventricular ejection fraction (LVEF) of ≥45% and echocardiographic features suggesting possible diastolic dysfunction to receive perindopril at 4 mg/day or placebo. The primary end point was a composite of all-cause mortality and unplanned HF–related hospitalization with a minimum follow-up of 1 year. Though there was a trend toward benefit, the study was underpowered to make any treatment recommendations. However, data from the CHARM-Preserved trial demonstrated a reduction in hospitalizations associated with candesartan among 3,023 patients randomized and followed out to 3 years (41; see also *Lancet.* 2003;362:777–781).

ANGIOTENSIN II RECEPTOR ANTAGONISTS

Recent trial data comparing angiotensin II receptor antagonists (ARBs) with ACE inhibitors have found similar outcomes with the two classes of drugs, with somewhat better tolerability of ARBs. The ELITE II study compared captopril with losartan in 3,152 patients. After a median follow-up of 1.5 years, losartan was not superior to captopril in reducing mortality but was better tolerated (38). In the Val-HEFT trial, valsartan was compared with placebo in more than 5,000 HF patients with NYHA class II to IV symptoms (39). Whereas no difference in mortality was noted, patients had improved quality of life (QOL) and fewer hospitalizations with valsartan. In addition, subgroup analysis showed a trend toward increased mortality in patients receiving valsartan, ACE inhibition, and β-blockers. In the Valsartan in Acute Myocardial Infarction (VALIANT) trial, 14,703 patients were recruited up to 10 days post-MI and randomized to one of the three treatment arms: captopril in a target dose of 50 mg t.i.d., valsartan target dose 160 mg b.i.d., or the combination of captopril 50 mg t.i.d. and valsartan 80 mg b.i.d. Valsartan was demonstrated to be as effective as a proven dose of captopril in reducing mortality as well as cardiovascular events including MI, but it was noninferior and did not show superiority over captopril alone (40).

The CHARM trial evaluated the use of candesartan in various groups of patients in NYHA class II to IV (41). The trial compared candesartan to placebo and evaluated three groups of patients with (a) LVEF ≤40% treated with an ACE inhibitor (CHARM-added, n = 2,300); (b) LVEF of 40% or less, ACE inhibitor intolerant (CHARM-alternative, n = 1,700); and (c) LVEF >40%, not treated with ACE inhibitors (CHARM-preserved, n = 2,500; see below). In CHARM-added, 2548 patients with LV dysfunction and HF were randomized to candesartan versus placebo, in addition to ACE inhibition. Over median follow-up of 41 months, the primary outcome of cardiovascular death or HF admission was significantly lower in the candesartan group (38% vs. 42%, unadjusted hazard ratio 0.85 [95% CI, 0.75–0.96], p = 0.011). In the CHARM-alternative trial, 2029 patients with LV dysfunction and HF who were previously intolerant to ACE inhibitor were randomly assigned to *either* candesartan or placebo. The results demonstrated tolerance of valsartan in these patients intolerant of

ACE inhibition, and the patients assigned to candesartan had a lower risk of the primary outcome of cardiovascular death or hospitalization at follow-up of 33.7 months (33% vs. 40%, unadjusted hazard ratio 0.77 [95% CI, 0.67–0.89], $p = 0.0004$). The CHARM program was also analyzed overall, and the results showed that candesartan reduced the composite outcomes, cardiovascular mortality, hospital admissions for HF, and all-cause mortality, particularly among patients with reduced LV systolic function (41).

A trial of high-dose versus low-dose losartan on clinical outcomes in patients with HF (HEAAL study) suggested that a higher dose of losartan provides mortality benefit over lower doses in patients with systolic HF intolerant of ACE inhibitors (43). This trial suggests that incremental inhibition of the RAS system is beneficial, and it does not necessarily require two different types of agents. Notably, losartan is not currently approved for HF in the United States, only for hypertension.

ARB therapy in HFpEF initially showed some promise with the results of the CHARM-preserved arm of the CHARM trial. In that arm of the trial, the addition of candesartan to the treatment regimen for patients with symptomatic HF and relatively preserved EF significantly reduced morbidity but did not reach the primary end point of CV death. However, the Irbesartan in Patients with Heart Failure and Preserved Ejection Fraction (I-PRESERVE) trial again did not show any difference in outcomes when irbesartan was compared to placebo in HFpEF patients (42).

DUAL RAS BLOCKADE (ACE/ARB)

The Randomized Evaluation of Strategies for Left Ventricular Dysfunction (RESOLVD) trial evaluated the effects of candesartan alone, enalapril alone, and their combination on exercise tolerance, ventricular function, QOL, neurohormone levels, and tolerability in HF (44). There were no differences among groups with regard to 6-minute walk distance (6MWD), NYHA functional class, or QOL. However, there was a trend toward benefit on LV remodeling with the combination therapy.

The bulk of the data on dual RAS blockade, however, come from CHARM-added, VALIANT, ONTARGET, and Val-HeFT trials (39–41; see also *N Engl J Med* 2008;358:1547). CHARM added was the only trial that showed a reduction in cardiovascular deaths with dual therapy, and it also showed a lower rate of hospitalization for HF. However, all-cause mortality did not differ between groups. In post hoc analysis, Val-HeFT actually showed that dual therapy increased morbidity and mortality. Two recent meta-analyses suggest that dual RAS therapy is not beneficial (*Arch Intern Med* 2007;167:1930–1936; *J Card Fail* 2008;14(3):181–188), and there is a higher risk of discontinuation of therapy because of adverse effects such as hyperkalemia, renal dysfunction, and hypotension. Though there may be a subset of patients that benefit from dual RAS therapy, such as young patients with good renal function, the available data do not support the routine addition of an ARB to ACE-I therapy in HF patients.

β-BLOCKERS

β-Blockers are safe when given carefully in controlled fashion in patients with HFrEF, but only three β-blockers—bisoprolol, metoprolol succinate (XL), and carvedilol—have been shown to be effective in reducing the risk of death in patients with chronic HF. Recommendations advocate the use of these three β-blockers in patients with Stage C HF. However, they should not be used in those with severe, decompensated HF. All β-blocker trials of more than 1-month duration have shown improved LV function, and a meta-analysis of 17 randomized trials with approximately 3,000 patients showed an approximately 30% mortality reduction, mostly due to fewer sudden deaths.

The Cardiac Insufficiency Bisoprolol Study (CIBIS II) enrolled more than 2,600 NYHA class III or IV patients with an EF of <35% and found that bisoprolol-treated patients had a mortality rate approximately one-third lower than that of placebo-treated patients, whereas the Metoprolol CR/XL Randomized Intervention Trial in HF (MERIT-HF) trial enrolled nearly 4,000 patients with an EF of <40% and found that metoprolol succinate reduced mortality by 35% compared with placebo (54).

The largest published experience to date of the nonselective β-blocker and α_1-antagonist carvedilol pooled data from different small studies (46,47) and found an impressive 65% mortality reduction at 6 months in carvedilol-treated patients (48). Carvedilol also was shown to be beneficial in improving EF and NYHA functional class and reducing LV volumes (see *J Am Coll Cardiol* 2001;37:407). The Carvedilol Prospective Randomized Cumulative Survival (COPERNICUS) trial extended these results to a more advanced patient population with NYHA class IV symptoms (50). Patients with far advanced HF symptoms and those who could not reach compensation were not enrolled, nor were significant numbers of black patients. The Carvedilol or Metoprolol European Trial (COMET) directly compared these two agents in 3,029 patients. At a mean follow-up of more than 3 years, carvedilol was associated with a significantly lower mortality than metoprolol therapy (51). It should be noted, however, that this trial (and all others comparing the two agents head-to-head) used the shorter-acting metoprolol tartrate, not the extended-release metoprolol succinate.

Some trials suggest a benefit of β-blockers in asymptomatic HF patients, that is, those with Stage B HF. A post hoc analysis of the SOLVD-Prevention trial, looking at asymptomatic patients with an LVEF ≤35%, suggests a synergistic effect of β-blockers and ACE-I leading to significantly lower rates of mortality due to HF compared to ACE-I alone (56). The Carvedilol Post-infarct Survival Control in Left Ventricular Dysfunction (CAPRICORN) study evaluated the addition of carvedilol versus placebo in post-MI patients with LVEF ≤40% (57). Carvedilol reduced mortality risk by 23% and was equally effective in patients with or without HF symptoms. The Carvedilol ACE Inhibitor Remodeling Mild HF Evaluation (CARMEN) trial and Reversal of Ventricular Remodeling with Toprol-XL (REVERT) trial suggest the importance of high-dose β-blocker therapy in reducing cardiac remodeling in asymptomatic HF patients (58,59).

Not all trials of β-adrenergic blockade have shown positive results. The β-blocker Evaluation of Survival Trial (BEST) compared bucindolol with placebo in 2,708 patients with NYHA class III or IV symptoms and found no difference in overall mortality rates (52). However, bucindolol did significantly reduce cardiovascular mortality by 14% versus placebo ($p = 0.04$). Additionally, several subgroup analyses have yielded important genetically based differences in treatment effect, which have led to further study of this drug in patients with specific genetic polymorphisms.

It is also important to note that β-blockers should be continued in all HF patients unless they show signs of poor perfusion in the setting of decompensation.

DIURETICS

Optimal use of diuretics is the cornerstone of any successful approach to the *symptomatic* treatment of HF. Diuretics are used to control and reduce fluid retention. In most cases, they should be used in conjunction with an ACE inhibitor with or without a β-blocker. Smaller, older studies have demonstrated a reduction in JVP, pulmonary congestion, peripheral edema, and body weight with diuretics. Some longer studies have shown improvement in cardiac function, symptoms, and exercise tolerance. However, there have been no long-term studies of diuretic therapy, and thus, their effects on morbidity and mortality are not known.

ALDOSTERONE BLOCKERS

Blockage of aldosterone provides not just diuresis but has been shown to have potent neurohormonal effects that lead to significantly improved clinical outcomes (in contrast to non–aldosterone-based diuretics). The landmark Randomized Aldactone Evaluation Study (RALES) evaluated the potassium-sparing diuretic spironolactone in patients receiving optimal therapy (including a loop diuretic) and showed a significantly lower mortality rate among spironolactone-treated patients compared with those treated with a loop diuretic alone (62). However, when spironolactone therapy is initiated, hyperkalemia occurs frequently, so careful monitoring of serum potassium levels is necessary (see *N Engl J Med* 2004;351:543–551).

Eplerenone is a later-generation, selective aldosterone blocker that has a favorable side effect profile compared to aldosterone, specifically a lower incidence of gynecomastia. The Eplerenone Post-acute MI Heart Failure Efficacy and Survival Study (EPHESUS) compared eplerenone with placebo in 6,632 MI patients with an EF $\leq 40\%$. The eplerenone group had a significant reduction in all-cause mortality compared to placebo (relative risk 0.85, $p = 0.008$). It was later also studied in the Eplerenone in Mild Patients Hospitalization and Survival Study in Heart Failure (EMPHASIS-HF) trial of 2737 patients with more mild HF (NYHA II) (64). After 21 months, patients treated with up to 50 mg of eplerenone had significantly lower rates of the primary end point, cardiovascular death or HF hospitalization compared with placebo (18.3% vs. 25.9%, $p < 0.001$).

Data regarding the use of aldosterone antagonists in HFpEF had been hopeful based on early-phase trials. The Aldo-DHF randomized trial demonstrated improved measures of diastolic function in patients assigned to spironolactone versus placebo; however, the power to assess clinical outcomes was limited (65). The larger and much-anticipated Trial of Aldosterone Antagonist Therapy in Adults With Preserved Ejection Fraction Congestive Heart Failure (TOPCAT) yielded mixed clinical results in patients with HFpEF assigned to spironolactone versus placebo (66). The primary end point, a composite of cardiovascular death, aborted cardiac arrest, or HF hospitalization, was not reached, but a reduction in HF hospitalization was seen. However, there have been questions regarding the heterogeneity of patients in this trial, including regional differences, since the diagnosis of HFpEF can be challenging and often highly subjective.

DIGOXIN

Although the large Digoxin Investigation Group (DIG) mortality trial (70) found that digoxin had no significant effect on total mortality (positive or negative), it also found that digoxin-treated patients with HF and EF <45% had fewer hospitalizations than did placebo patients. Physicians may consider adding digoxin in patients with persistent symptoms of HF despite therapy with diuretics, an ACE-I (or ARB), and a β-blocker (*Circulation* 2004;109:2942–2946, 2959–2964).

Toxicity is a concern with digoxin, especially in patients over age 70, with impaired renal function, or with a low lean body mass. The DIG trial suggests that risk-adjusted mortality increased as the plasma concentrations exceeded 1.0 ng/mL, though overt toxicity is not often seen until levels are >2 ng/mL. Toxicity at lower levels can be seen if hypokalemia, hypomagnesemia, or hypothyroidism coexist. One analysis suggests that women may not benefit from digoxin therapy and may be at increased risk for death (*N Engl J Med* 2002;347:1403–1411). Given the narrow therapeutic index and lack of mortality benefit of digoxin, the latest AHA/ACC guidelines make it a IIa recommendation in patients with HFrEF to reduce hospitalizations (1).

VASODILATORS

Hydralazine and Isosorbide Dinitrate

This combination was associated with a higher mortality rate than was enalapril in the Veterans Administration Cooperative Vasodilator-Heart Failure Trial (V-HeFT II; 25% vs. 18% at 2 years) (72) but yielded better results than did placebo in V-HeFT I (71). Post hoc analysis of the V-HeFT trials suggested a significant benefit specifically in African Americans. This prompted the design of the African-American Heart Failure Trial (A-HeFT), which only enrolled self-identified black patients (73). The trial was stopped early due to the significant mortality benefit of the study drug combo (in addition to ACE-I and β-blocker). This trial led to the first FDA approval of a drug for a specific race (BiDil), a significant medical milestone. It is untested as to whether there would be added benefit of this combination in nonblack patients when added to a background of ACE-I and/or β-blocker. Despite a lack of studies in ACE-I–intolerant patients, this combination may be considered as a therapeutic alternative in such patients.

Calcium Channel Blockers

Negative inotropic effects are not desirable in systolic dysfunction, and most calcium channel blockers should generally be avoided in HF. However, in the Prospective Randomized Amlodipine Survival Evaluation (PRAISE) trial (74), amlodipine showed a trend toward lower mortality (-16%; $p = 0.07$), with a 46% lower mortality rate among patients with nonischemic cardiomyopathy. PRAISE-2 compared amlodipine with placebo in a group of patients without ischemic heart disease (75). Patients with HF with LVEF <30% were randomized to receive placebo or amlodipine. No significant difference was found in this cohort with regard to all-cause or cardiac mortality. Thus, calcium channel blockers are generally discouraged in the HFrEF population but are not contraindicated.

AMIODARONE

The use of amiodarone to prevent sudden cardiac death is discussed in Chapters 4 and 6. However, it has also been tested in the treatment of chronic HF. One South American study of the Grupo de Estudio de la Sobrevida en la Insuficiencia Cardiaca en Argentina (GESICA) (81) showed a mortality benefit of amiodarone, whereas the better-designed Survival Trial of Antiarrhythmic Therapy in HF (HF-STAT) (82) found no mortality advantage in the amiodarone group. In the HF-STAT, a trend was seen toward a lower mortality rate with amiodarone in the subgroup of patients with nonischemic cardiomyopathy. Analysis of the VALIANT study has shown that amiodarone should not be considered as part of the routine treatment of patients with HF. However, it is one of only two antiarrhythmic drugs recommended for arrhythmia suppression in patients with HF (for either recurrent atrial fibrillation or symptomatic ventricular arrhythmias). Nevertheless, chronic exposure to amiodarone should be minimized if at all possible, given its numerous, significant toxicities (pulmonary, hepatic, ocular, thyroid).

EMERGING MEDICAL THERAPIES

1. Myosin activators—These investigational drugs use a novel mechanism within the myocyte to directly activate myosin without increasing intracellular calcium. The effect is lengthening of systole without the unwanted increase in oxygen demand. Omecantiv mecarbil is one myosin activator demonstrating hopeful results in early, clinical studies (see *Lancet* 2011;378:676–683 and *Lancet* 2011;378:667–675).
2. Relaxin, serelaxin—The naturally occurring peptide (relaxin) is responsible for favorable cardiovascular and neurohormonal changes during pregnancy and has shown early promise in the treatment of acute heart failure. Serelaxin represents and recombinant version (see *Lancet* 2009;373:1429–1439 and *Lancet* 2013;381:29–39).

3. Ivabradine [I$_f$ current inhibitor (SA node)]—Through this agent's novel mechanism, it can decrease heart rate in sinus rhythm, without affected inotropy. It has been shown to reduce the composite of cardiovascular death or HF hospitalization and is now approved in the US (see *Lancet* 2010;376:875–885).

4. Bromocriptine (dopamine 2D agonist)—Though not a new drug, bromocriptine has shown promise as a novel treatment for peripartum cardiomyopathy. However, the pivotal study was small, and bromocriptine has not yet made it into the guidelines (see *Circulation* 121(13):1465–1473).

5. LCZ696 (angiotensin receptor–neprilysin inhibitor)—Neprilysin breaks down endogenous vasoactive peptides and its inhibition improves hemodynamic profiles. Based on earlier work demonstrating compound effect of neprilysin and renin angiotensin system inhibition, this agent was formulated as a combination of valsartan and neprilysin inhibitor sacubitril (combination with ACE inhibition was associated with significant risk of angioedema). In recent trials, LCZ696 has demonstrated promising clinical outcomes: it lowered cardiovascular death or hospitalization in the PARDIGM-HF trial of HFrEF, and it lowered NT-proBNP in the PARAMOUNT trial of patients with HFpEF (see also *N Engl J Med* 2014;371:993 and *Lancet* 2012;380:1387).

BIVENTRICULAR PACING

Among those with chronic HF due to systolic dysfunction, 30% or more have electrical conduction defects (bundle branch block or intraventricular conduction delay) that cause delayed activation of portions of the ventricular myocardium. This dyssynchrony decreases efficiency of ventricular contraction and worsens systolic function and symptoms. Please see Chapter 6 for a discussion of biventricular (BiV) pacing, also known as cardiac resynchronization therapy (CRT).

SURGICAL THERAPIES
Left Ventricular Assist Device

Many variations of an "artificial heart" have been developed, each with various advantages and limitations. However, the most contemporary, widely used incarnation of fully implantable cardiac support is the left ventricular assist device (LVAD). The first-generation HeartMate was the first device to reach late-stage clinical development and use; initially, it was shown to be effective as a short-term solution to "bridge" patients to cardiac transplant, significantly improving peak oxygen consumption (92). It was subsequently tested as destination therapy (i.e., long-term cardiac support) in the REMATCH trial. A significant survival advantage was noted in patients with end-stage HF who received the HeartMate, but this device was limited by device malfunction, the high incidence of infection, and the fact that only 25% of patients receiving LVAD were alive at 2 years (94).

The next-generation of LVAD represented a significant advance in the development of the technology—the HeartMate II is a continuous-flow pump, which lead better durability. It was compared to the older pulsatile-flow HeartMate XVE in 200 transplant-ineligible patients (as destination therapy) (95). Patients with continuous-flow devices had improved survival rates at 2 years (58% vs. 24%; $p = 0.008$). As compared with patients with a pulsatile-flow LV device, there were significant reductions in the rates of major adverse events among patients with a continuous-flow LVAD—including hardware-related or non–hardware-related infection, arrhythmia, RV failure, respiratory failure, and renal failure. The incidence of stroke did not differ significantly between the continuous-flow group and the pulsatile-flow group. There was a 38% relative reduction in the rate of rehospitalization among patients with a continuous-flow LVAD as compared with those with a pulsatile-flow device. The HeartMate II has since been approved for use both as a bridge to heart transplant and as a destination therapy.

Additional devices have also been developed, and the latest to be approved is the HeartWare LVAD system. Continuing the trend of minimizing device size and wear and tear, this pump sits within the pericardium and uses centrifugal flow technology to minimize any metal-on-metal contact and improve durability. The pivotal trial was the ADVANCE study, which enrolled 180 patients receiving the HeartWare and compared them to 499 patients receiving other, commercially available LVADs (96). They demonstrated similar device success rates (roughly 90%) and improvements in 6-minute walk and other quality of live metrics. Currently, the HeartWare is indicated only as a bridge to transplantation.

There remain significant knowledge gaps regarding the management of patients receiving these devices. Most require anticoagulation to prevent pump thrombosis; however, major bleeding can become a significant, limiting factor (see N Engl J Med 2014;370:33–40). A phenomenon of acquired von Willebrand disease in these patients has been well described (see J Am Coll Cardiol 2010;56:1207–1213) and is thought to contribute to the high incidence of bleeding rates. Further study is needed, and hopefully future advances in pump technology will help reduce this risk.

Coronary Artery Bypass Graft Surgery

In HF patients with CAD and moderate-to-severe LV dysfunction (EF <40%), coronary artery bypass graft (CABG) improves 3-year survival by 30% to 50%. However, it is not clear that this benefit extends to patients with more severe LV dysfunction (LVEF <35%) and significant CAD. Prior observational studies found that revascularization of hibernating myocardium in patients with ischemic cardiomyopathy improves both survival and LV function compared to medical therapy [see J Am Coll Cardiol 2005;46(4):567–574]. The Surgical Treatment for Ischemic Heart Failure (STICH) trial was a multicenter, international, randomized trial from the NHLBI to determine whether there was a benefit to surgical revascularization in patients with CAD and LVEF <35% (97). Among 1,212 patients randomized to CABG versus medical therapy, the primary outcome of death from any cause at median follow-up of 55 months was not significantly different between the two groups (36% for CABG vs. 41%

for medical therapy; HR, 0.86; p = 0.12). However, the CABG group experienced significant reductions in cardiovascular death (HR, 0.81; p = 0.05) and the composite of all-cause mortality or cardiovascular hospitalization (HR, 0.74; p < 0.001). Additional analyses from this trial, specifically investigating the utility of myocardial viability testing, have provided a wealth of information (see *N Engl J Med.* 2011;364:1617–1625). See below for results of the STICH ventricular restoration surgery arm.

Cardiac Transplantation

Heart transplantation should be considered if peak oxygen consumption is below 10 to 15 mL/kg/min on chronic, optimal medical therapy. Other eligibility criteria also must be met (typically, age 65 years or younger, no active infection, and no malignancy). While the use of cardiac transplantation is largely limited by the available donor pool, refinement in patient selection and expanded donor criteria have helped to maximize the availability of this therapy.

Other Surgical Treatments

1. Surgical ventricular restoration: Dor procedure—This procedure was evaluated in a separate arm of the STICH trial, as is an attempt to restore the LV's elliptical geometry at the time of CABG in ischemic cardiomyopathy patients (98). The procedure entails an anterior left ventriculotomy centered in the zone of anterior asynergy, a suture encircling the scar, and then a cinching of the suture to bring the healthy portions of the ventricular walls in contact with one another. In STICH, surgical ventricular reconstruction reduced the end-systolic volume (ESV) index by 19%, as compared with a reduction of 6% with CABG alone. Cardiac symptoms and exercise tolerance improved from baseline to a similar degree in the two study groups. However, no significant difference was observed in the primary outcome of death or cardiac rehospitalization at 48 months (59% in the CABG-alone group vs. 58% for CABG plus SVR; p = 0.90).

2. Mitral valve repair—This option has been used in patients with HF due to DCM, which is complicated by severe, refractory mitral regurgitation ("functional" MR). In one study, mitral valve reconstruction resulted in significant NYHA class improvement and a 2-year survival rate of more than 70% (see *J Thorac Cardiovasc Surg* 1998;115:381–386). However, a more recent study evaluating MV repair at the time of CABG for ischemic MR showed no improvement in survival and no significant difference in NYHA functional class versus CABG alone [see *Ann Thorac Surg* 2004;78(3):794–799]. The most recent major trial compared mitral valve repair with chordal-sparing mitral valve replacement in patients with severe, ischemic MR, with or without concomitant CABG (100). Prior data suggested improved perioperative outcomes with repair and longer durability with replacement, and there appeared to be more durable correction in MR in this trial. However, there was no difference in the primary end point of LV ESV index (including deaths), or other clinical outcomes, at 12 months.

Additional Therapeutic Considerations

HEMODYNAMIC MONITORING

Routine invasive hemodynamic monitoring with pulmonary artery catheters is *not* considered standard of care for most hospitalized patients with symptoms of worsening HF. This trend stems primarily from the Evaluation Study of Congestive Heart Failure and Pulmonary Artery Catheterization Effectiveness (ESCAPE) trial, a large randomized multicenter trial of tailored therapy with PA catheters versus clinical assessments in patients hospitalized with severe HF refractory to standard of care therapy (101). A meta-analysis of 13 randomized trials published at the time of the ESCAPE trial found similar results (see JAMA 2005;294:1664–1670).

The latest AHA/ACC guidelines recommend that invasive hemodynamic monitoring should be performed in patients with (1) poor perfusion and/or respiratory distress in whom intracardiac pressures cannot be determined by clinical assessment (class I) or (2) those with persistent, severe symptoms or end-organ damage despite optimized medical therapy (including those who are candidates for or receiving intravenous inotropes or mechanical circulatory support; class IIa). Additional data on remote, device-based hemodynamic monitoring have demonstrated promising results for the management of chronic, outpatient HF and reduction of hospitalizations; however, they have yet become broadly available (104).

EXERCISE TRAINING AND REHABILITATION

Numerous studies have shown tolerability and benefits of exercise in most patients, and it is now recommended for most stable outpatients with chronic HF. Regular exercise typically results in increased peak oxygen uptake and increased peak workload; however, few randomized data were available. Thus, the Heart Failure: A Controlled Trial Investigating Outcomes of Exercise Training (HF ACTION) study was conducted (111). The investigators randomized 2,331 patients with chronic, stable HFrEF to 36 sessions of supervised, aerobic exercise or usual care, for a primary end point of all-cause mortality or hospitalization at median follow-up of 30 months. In the prespecified analysis, the primary outcome was no significantly different between the groups (65% vs. 68%;, HR, 0.93; $p = 0.13$). However, after adjustment for high-risk features, the investigators identified a modest, significant benefit to the exercise intervention for death or hospitalization (HR, 0.89; $p = 0.03$). In the latest US guidelines, regular, exercise activity in capable patients with chronic HF is a class I recommendation.

PREVENTION OF SUDDEN CARDIAC DEATH

CAD is the major substrate of sudden cardiac death, and cardiomyopathies, valvular heart disease, and abnormalities of the conduction system also are implicated; the baseline EF is a significant predictor of sudden cardiac risk. Sudden cardiac death is responsible for 30% to 70% of deaths among those with HF. The incidence is 2% to 3% per year in those with asymptomatic LV dysfunction and up to 20% per year in those with severe HF. Patients with advanced HF who have a syncopal episode have a high incidence of subsequent sudden death [in one study, 45% at 1 year (100)]. The incidence of sudden cardiac death appears lower in patients receiving ACE inhibitors.

Whereas predictors of sudden cardiac death have been established in patients with prior MI and reduced EF (see Chapter 6, MADIT, MADIT II, and MUSTT), risk stratification is difficult because few clinical predictors are specific for sudden cardiac death in those with nonischemic HF. However, the Sudden Cardiac Death in Heart Failure Trial (SCD-HeFT) showed a significant decrease in mortality in patients with NYHA class II and III HF and EF <35% (see Chapter 6 for trial details), and ICD implantation is now recommended for these patients with ischemic or nonischemic cardiomyopathy.

REFERENCES

Guidelines and Reviews

1. Yancy CW, et al. 2013 ACCF/AHA guideline for the management of heart failure: a report of the American College of Cardiology Foundation/American Heart Association Task Force on practice guidelines. *Circulation* 2013;128:e240–e327.

This most recent update to the US guidelines expanded HF definitions to include HFpEF, encouraged consideration of heritable causes of HF, and highlighted the proven motility benefits of evidence-based care. They specifically discouraged oral anticoagulation in HF patients without additional risk factors for stroke (e.g., AF) and emphasized dietary and exercise therapies, as well as the benefits of a multidisciplinary team (including palliative care).

2. Costanzo MR, et al. The International Society of Heart and Lung Transplantation Guidelines for the care of heart transplant recipients. *J Heart Lung Transplant* 2010;29:914–956.

These represent some of the first, structured guidelines for the care of heart transplantation recipients and are the result of three different tasks forces charged with identifying best practices at each stage of transplantation (perioperative care, treatment of rejection, and long-term care). However, it should be noted that the majority of recommendations therein are supported only by level of evidence "C," due to the limited numbers of patients available to generate robust, clinical outcomes data and lack of randomized, clinical trials.

3. Feenstra J, et al. Drug-induced heart failure. *J Am Coll Cardiol* 1999;33:1152–1162.

This review discusses anthracyclines, cyclophosphamide, paclitaxel, mitoxantrone, other chemotherapeutic agents, nonsteroidal anti-inflammatory drugs, immunomodulating agents (e.g., interferons, interleukin-2), and antidepressants. The contributory roles of three major cardiac drug classes in causing HF also are reviewed: antiarrhythmics, β-blockers, and calcium channel blockers.

4. Jessup M, et al. Heart failure. *N Engl J Med* 2003;348:2007–2018.

This article reviews the epidemiology, pathophysiology, and etiologies of HF. Treatment modalities are then discussed for patients in various stages (A to D) of HF. Two final sections briefly review nonpharmacologic therapies.

5. Maeder MT, et al. Heart failure with normal left ventricular ejection fraction. *J Am Coll Cardiol* 2009;53:905–918.

In this "State-of-the-Art" paper, the authors describe the population of patients with "heart failure with normal ejection fraction" (HFNEF), as well as pathophysiologic mechanisms. They detail a diagnostic criteria algorithm, echocardiographic measures, and biomarkers in support of future therapeutic options.

6. Pang PS, et al. The current and future management of acute heart failure syndromes. *Eur Heart J* 2010;31:784–793.

This review focuses on the enormous problem of acute, symptomatic, decompensated HF, termed "acute heart failure syndromes." The authors highlight the significance of the problem, its triggers, and outcomes. They also call to attention the disparity in evidence base in therapies for inpatient, versus outpatient, management of HF. Future therapeutic approaches are discussed, in an effort to emphasize the need for improved outcomes in these patients.

Epidemiology

7. Levy D, et al. The progression from hypertension to congestive heart failure. *JAMA* 1996;275:1557–1562.

This analysis focused on 5,143 Framingham Study subjects with a mean follow-up period of 14.1 years. Hypertension antedated 91% of new HF cases. After risk factor adjustment, hypertension was associated with relative risks of developing HF of approximately 2.0 (men) and 3.0 (women). Poor 5-year survival was observed among hypertensive HF subjects: 24% in men and 31% in women.

8. Adams KF Jr, et al. Relation between gender, etiology and survival in patients with symptomatic heart failure. *J Am Coll Cardiol* 1996;28:1781–1788.

This prospective, observational study was composed of 557 patients (177 women; nonischemic etiology in 68%). At a mean follow-up of 2.4 years, the all-cause mortality rate was 36%. Women had better survival ($p < 0.001$), primarily due to the lower mortality associated with a nonischemic etiology (men vs. women, relative risk 2.36; $p < 0.001$).

9. Bibbins-Domingo K, et al. Racial differences in incident heart failure among young adults. *N Engl J Med* 2009;360:1179–1190.

In a prospective, 20-year cohort study, the investigators assessed the incidence of HF during follow-up among 5,115 blacks and whites aged 18 to 30 (at baseline). All but 1 of the 27 participants who developed HF was black ($p = 0.001$ for black vs. white), and preexisting hypertension, obesity, or systolic dysfunction were high-risk features for earlier development of HF.

10. Roger VL, et al. Trends in heart failure incidence and survival in a community-based population. *JAMA* 2004;292:344–350.

To assess survival rates in patients with HF among various demographics, the investigators enrolled 4,537 patients with HF of Olmsted County, Minnesota, between 1979 and 2000. They found that men had a higher incidence of HF (378 per 100,000 for men vs. 289 per 100,000 for women), and survival was worse among men at mean follow-up of 4.2 years (RR, 1.33; 95% CI, 1.24 to 1.43). Five-year survival rates did improve from 1979–1984 to 1996–2000 (age-adjusted survival, 43% for 1979 to 1984 vs. 52% for 1996 to 2000; $p < 0.001$); however, these gains were predominantly limited to men and younger patients at the expense of little to no improvement among women and the elderly. The incidence of HF has not declined over two decades; however, overall survival has improved, at least in this community-based cohort.

11. Steinberg BA, et al. Trends in patients hospitalized with heart failure and preserved left ventricular ejection fraction: prevalence, therapies, and outcomes. *Circulation* 2012;126:65–75.

Using data from the AHA's national Get With The Guidelines registry, this study assessed the prevalence and trends in prevalence of HFpEF, relative to HFrEF, among 110,621 inpatient admissions for HF. The analysis demonstrated a near even split between HFrEF and HFpEF, with increasing proportion of HFpEF overall. While in-hospital mortality was lower for the HFpEF patients, there remains opportunities for improved evidence-based care in this group.

12. Levy D, et al. Long-term trends in the incidence of and survival with heart failure. *N Engl J Med* 2002;347:1397–1402 (editorial, 1442–1444).

This analysis consisted of 1,075 Framingham Heart Study participants who developed HF from 1950 to 1999. As compared with the period from 1950 to 1969, the incidence of HF remained virtually unchanged among men in the three subsequent periods (1970 to 1979, 1980 to 1989, 1990 to 1999) but declined by 31% to 40% among women (rate ratio for 1990 to 1999, 0.69; 95% CI, 0.51 to 0.93). Survival after onset of HF improved in both sexes. The 30-day, 1-year, and 5-year age-adjusted mortality rates among men declined from 12%, 30%, and 70% in the period from 1950 to 1969 to 11%, 28%, and 59% from 1990 to 1999. Corresponding rates among women were 18%, 28%, and 57% (1950 to 1969) and 10%, 24%, and 45% (1990 to 1999). Overall, the survival after HF onset improved by 12% per decade ($p = 0.01$ for men, $p = 0.02$ for women).

13. O'Meara E, et al. Sex differences in clinical characteristics and prognosis in a broad spectrum of patients with heart failure: results of the Candesartan in Heart Failure: Assessment of Reduction in Mortality and Morbidity (CHARM) program. *Circulation* 2007;115:3111–3120.

The CHARM trial consisted of three independent but related trials in which patients with NYHA class II to IV HF were randomized to placebo or candesartan based on EF and prior ACE experience—CHARM-Alternative (EF ≤40%, intolerant of ACE-I) with 2,028 patients, CHARM-Added (EF ≤40%, already taking an ACE-I) with 2,548 patients, and CHARM-Preserved (EF >40%) with 3,023 patients. The primary outcome for each of the trials was the composite of cardiovascular death or unplanned admission for HF; there was a primary end point for the overall program, as well: all-cause mortality.

O'Meara et al. used the results of the CHARM trial to assess differences in outcome based on gender alone. They found that women had lower all-cause mortality (21.5% vs. 25.3% in men; adjusted HR, 0.77; $p < 0.001$), as well as cardiovascular death or HF admission (30.4% vs. 33.3% for men; adjusted HR, 0.83; $p < 0.001$). Risk of death in women was unrelated to cause of HF or EF (see below for additional description of the CHARM program).

Diagnosis and Prognosis

PHYSICAL EXAMINATION

14. Stevenson LW, et al. The limited reliability of physical signs for estimating hemodynamics in chronic heart failure. *JAMA* 1989;261:884–888.

This prospective study was composed of 50 patients with known chronic HF. Orthopnea within the preceding week was the most sensitive (91%) symptom for predicting elevated PCWP (22 mm Hg or more). Physical signs were not sensitive at predicting elevated PCWP because rales, edema, and elevated mean JVP were absent in 18 (41.9%) of 43 patients. A measured pulse pressure of <25% had a 91% sensitivity and 83% specificity for a cardiac index <2.2 L/min/m^2.

15. Butman SM, et al. Bedside cardiovascular exam with severe chronic heart failure: importance of rest or inducible jugular venous distention. *J Am Coll Cardiol* 1993;22:968–974.

This prospective study was composed of 52 patients with chronic HF who underwent right heart catheterization. The presence of jugular venous distention had a 57% sensitivity and 93% specificity for a PCWP of 18 mm Hg. The combination of jugular venous distension at rest or inducible by an hepatojugular test had a sensitivity of 81%, specificity of 80%, and 81% predictive accuracy.

16. Badgett RG, et al. Can the clinical examination diagnose left-sided heart failure in adults? *JAMA* 1997;277:1712–1719.

This review of the literature asserts that the best findings for detecting increased filling pressure are jugular venous distention and radiographic redistribution. The best findings for detecting systolic dysfunction are abnormal apical impulse, cardiomegaly (by radiograph), and Q waves or left bundle branch block on ECG.

17. Nohria A, et al. Clinical assessment identifies hemodynamic profiles that predict outcomes in patients admitted with heart failure. *J Am Coll Cardiol* 2003;41:1797–1798.

In this seminal paper, the investigators identify clinical findings in inpatients with HF that help to categorize them into four different hemodynamic profiles: cold–wet, cold–dry, warm–wet, and warm–dry. The primary conclusion found that such a categorization could help predict outcomes in patients with HF (with the cold–wet patients fairing the worst). However, these profiles also provide a foundation on which to base decisions for clinical therapies and aggressiveness of interventions.

18. Drazner MH, et al. Prognostic importance of elevated jugular venous pressure and a third heart sound in patients with heart failure. *N Engl J Med* 2001;345:574–581.

This is a retrospective analysis of the SOLVD treatment trial, in which 2,569 patients with a history of symptomatic HF were randomly assigned to receive enalapril or placebo and followed for a mean of 32 months. Elevated JVP or a third heart sound was identified on physical examination at trial enrollment and used to predict outcomes of hospitalization for HF and/or progression of HF. In multivariable analyses, the risk of all end points was increased in patients with an elevated JVP and/or third heart sound ($p < 0.05$ for hospitalization for HF, death or hospitalization for HF, and death from pump failure).

DIAGNOSTIC TESTING

19. Gheorghiade M, et al. Relationship between admission serum sodium concentration and clinical outcomes in patients hospitalized for heart failure: an analysis from the OPTIMIZE-HF registry. *Eur Heart J* 2007;28:980–988.

The investigators used the OPTIMIZE-HF registry, a cohort of patients hospitalized with HF, to measure 60- to 90-day outcomes based on serum sodium concentration at admission. In multivariable analyses of 48,612 patients from 259 hospitals, the risk of in-hospital death, follow-up mortality, and death or rehospitalization increased by 19.5%, 10%, and 8%, respectively, for each 3 mmol/L decrease in admission serum sodium below 140 mmol/L.

20. Cooper LT, et al. The role of endomyocardial biopsy in the management of cardiovascular disease: a scientific statement from the American Heart Association, American College of Cardiology, and the European Society of Cardiology. *Circulation* 2007;116:2216–2233.

This writing group provides 14 clinical scenarios in which EMB may be considered, with the strength of evidence supporting biopsy for each group. The writers intended to more specifically describe the evidence for and against EMB, balancing the procedural risk of potential clinical benefit, for each scenario.

21. Maisel AS, et al.; for the Breathing Not Properly (BNP) Multinational Study Investigators. Rapid measurement of B-type natriuretic peptide in the emergency diagnosis of heart failure. *N Engl J Med* 2002;347:161–167.

Design: Prospective, blinded, multicenter study. The primary end point was diagnostic accuracy at the optimum cutoff of BNP and at 80% or more ED physician estimate of clinical probability of HF.

Purpose: To assess the correlation of serum BNP levels with the clinical diagnosis of HF.

Population: 1,538 patients with clinical suspicion for HF determined by the ED attending physician.

Exclusion Criteria: Advanced renal failure (creatinine clearance, <15 mL/min), acute MI, and overt cause of dyspnea (e.g., chest wall trauma).

Treatment: Standard evaluation and management for HF.

Results: The final diagnosis, as determined by two blinded independent cardiologists, was HF in 47% (744), with no findings of HF in 49% (770). BNP level, alone, was more diagnostic of HF than was any other clinical marker. At a level of 100 pg/mL, diagnostic accuracy was 83.4%, with a negative predictive value of 96% at a cutoff of 50 pg/mL. In multivariable analyses, BNP added significantly to diagnostic certainty of HF.

22. McCullough PA, et al. B-type natriuretic peptide and clinical judgment in emergency diagnosis of heart failure: analysis from Breathing Not Properly (BNP) Multinational Study. *Circulation* 2002;106:416–422.

In this additional analysis of the BNP study, the investigators sought to quantify the additional diagnostic certainty provided by BNP in assessment of patients in the ED with possible HF (see above for further details of the BNP study). At an 80% cutoff level of certainty of HF, clinical judgment had a sensitivity of 49% and specificity of 96%. At 100 pg/mL, BNP had a sensitivity of 90% and specificity of 73%. In determining the correct diagnosis (HF vs. no HF), adding BNP to clinical judgment would have enhanced diagnostic accuracy from 74% to 81%. In those participants with an intermediate (21% to 79%) probability of HF, BNP at a cutoff of 100 pg/mL accurately classified 74% of the cases. The areas under the receiver operating characteristic curve were 0.86 (95% CI, 0.84 to 0.88), 0.90 (95% CI, 0.88 to 0.91), and 0.93 (95% CI, 0.92 to 0.94) for clinical judgment, for BNP at a cutoff of 100 pg/mL, and for the two in combination, respectively ($p < 0.0001$ for all pairwise comparisons).

23. Mueller C, et al. Use of B-type natriuretic peptide in the evaluation and management of acute dyspnea. *N Engl J Med* 2004;350:647–654.

To assess the impact of BNP-diagnosed HF on length of stay and cost of hospitalization, the investigators randomly assigned 452 patients with dyspnea to a diagnostic strategy involving BNP levels, or standard care. In those who had BNP levels measured, fewer required hospitalization and intensive care ($p = 0.008$ and $p = 0.01$, respectively), compared with the standard care group. Length of stay was lower in the BNP group (8 days vs. 11 days; $p = 0.001$), as was total cost of treatment ($p = 0.006$). Mortality at 30 days was similar ($p = 0.45$). The authors offer that improved, early diagnosis of HF in the ED, as aided by BNP measurement, can lead to more efficient treatment and hospitalization course. However, large-scale validation is required.

24. Jourdain P, et al. Plasma brain natriuretic peptide-guided therapy to improve outcome in heart failure: the STARS-BNP Multicenter Study. *J Am Coll Cardiol* 2007;49:1733–1739.

The investigators sought to assess the utility of BNP-guided therapy in the management of outpatient HF. They enrolled 220 patients with NYHA II or III symptoms and randomized them to conventional HF therapy, or therapy targeting a reduction in BNP to <100 pg/mL. The primary outcome was HF death or hospitalization for HF, and all patients were managed by a HF specialist. Overall, medication changes were more frequent in the BNP group (for all types of medications). This led to significantly higher mean doses of

β-blockers and ACE-Is in the BNP group ($p < 0.05$). Subsequently, fewer patients experienced a primary end point event in the BNP group (24% vs. 52%; $p < 0.001$).

25. Pfisterer M, et al. BNP-guided vs. symptom-guided heart failure therapy: the Trial of Intensified vs Standard Medical Therapy in Elderly Patients With Congestive Heart Failure (TIME-HF) randomized trial. *JAMA* 2009;301:383–392.

In patients 60 years or older, with systolic HF, these investigators sought to demonstrate the superiority of BNP-guided management of outpatient HF, for the improvement of QOL and all-cause hospitalization rate. In all, 499 patients were randomized and stratified by age (60 to 74, 75 and older), and the patients, but not investigators, were blinded to their assignments. At 18 months of follow-up, there was no difference in the rates of rehospitalization (41% for BNP-guided vs. 40% for standard care; $p = 0.39$), and improvement in QOL was similar in the two groups. However, there was a significant interaction between outcome and age group—BNP-guided therapy appeared to improve outcomes only for younger patients (those aged 60 to 74 years).

26. Singer AJ, et al. Rapid Emergency Department Heart Failure Outpatients Trial (REDHOT II): a randomized controlled trial of the effect of serial B-type natriuretic peptide testing on patient management. *Circ Heart Fail* 2009;2:287–293.

To determine the utility of BNP in discharging patients with HF, the investigators randomized 447 patients with acute HF exacerbations to care guided by serial BNP measurements or to usual care. Notably, physicians were not given standardized management instructions in response to BNP measurements; they were only provided with the laboratory result. There were no differences in the primary end points of length of stay (6.5 days for each group), readmission within 30 days, or all-cause mortality. The small sample size and short follow-up, however, limit the conclusions from this study.

NONINVASIVE TESTING

27. Mancini DM, et al. Value of peak exercise oxygen consumption for optimal timing of cardiac transplantation in ambulatory patients with heart failure. *Circulation* 1991;83:778–786.

This study of 114 patients found a peak oxygen consumption of 14 mL/kg/min or less in 62 patients (35 were transplantation candidates and 27 had noncardiac issues) and more than 14 mL/kg/min in 52 patients. All three groups had similar NYHA functional class, LVEF, and cardiac index. Patients with an oxygen consumption of more than 14 mL/kg/min had a lower PCWP and significantly better 1-year survival [94% vs. 70% (transplant candidates) and 47%]. A multivariate analysis found peak oxygen consumption to be the best survival predictor, whereas PCWP added further prognostic information.

28. Bitner V, et al. Prediction of mortality and morbidity with a 6-minute walk test in patients with left ventricular dysfunction. *JAMA* 1993;270:1702–1707.

This analysis focused on 898 SOLVD patients with radiologic evidence of HF and/or EF <45%; mean follow-up period was 8 months. No significant test-related complications were found. Highest versus lowest performance level (distance walked, 450 m or more vs. <300 m): 71% lower mortality (3% vs. 10.2%), 51% fewer hospitalizations (19.9% vs. 40.9%), and 91% fewer HF hospitalizations (2% vs. 22.2%). Logistic regression analysis showed that EF and walk time were equally strong and independent predictors of mortality and hospitalization due to acute HF.

29. Balady GJ, et al. Clinician's Guide to cardiopulmonary exercise testing in adults: a scientific statement from the American Heart Association. *Circulation* 2010;122:191–225.

The AHA released this statement on cardiopulmonary exercise testing (CPX) in order to guide clinicians in the appropriate, standardized implementation of such testing.

The authors also review the appropriate indications and applications of such testing, including supporting evidence and outcomes.

Treatment

ANGIOTENSIN-CONVERTING ENZYME INHIBITORS AND ANGIOTENSIN-II RECEPTOR BLOCKERS

Meta-analyses

30. Garg R, et al. Overview of randomized trials of angiotensin-converting enzyme inhibitors on mortality and morbidity in patients with heart failure. JAMA 1995;273:1450–1456.

This analysis focused on 32 studies with 7,105 patients. All studies were placebo controlled, were 8 weeks in duration, and assessed all-cause mortality by intention to treat. ACE inhibitor therapy was associated with significant reductions in total mortality (odds ratio, 0.77; 95% CI, 0.67 to 0.88; $p < 0.001$) and mortality or hospitalization for HF (odds ratio, 0.65; 95% CI, 0.57 to 0.74; $p < 0.001$). Patients with the lowest EF had the greatest benefit. The mortality reduction was mainly due to fewer deaths from progressive HF (odds ratio, 0.69; 95% CI, 0.58 to 0.83). Nonsignificant reductions were noted in the incidence of arrhythmic deaths (odds ratio, 0.91; 95% CI, 0.73 to 1.12) and fatal MI (odds ratio, 0.82; 95% CI, 0.60 to 1.12). No significant differences were found between several different agents (see **Tables 5.1 and 5.2**).

31. Flather MD, et al. Long-term ACE-inhibitor therapy in patients with heart failure or left-ventricular dysfunction: a systematic overview of data from individual patients. ACE-Inhibitor Myocardial Infarction Collaborative Group. Lancet 2000;355:1575–1581.

The investigators combined data on 12,763 patients with HF randomly assigned to ACE inhibitors or placebo in 4 trials (SAVE, AIRE, TRACE, SOLVD), who were followed for out to 35 months. Compared with placebo, patients in the ACE inhibitor group had lower rates of all-cause mortality (23.0% vs. 26.8%; OR 0.80; 95% CI, 0.74 to 0.87), reinfarction (89.% vs. 11.0%; OR 0.79, 95% CI, 0.70 to 0.89), and HF hospitalization (13.7% vs. 18.9%; OR, 0.67; 95% CI, 0.61 to 0.74). Notably, the treatment effect was early and persistent and did not vary significantly across major subgroups.

Studies

32. The Cooperative North Scandinavian Enalapril Survival Study (CONSENSUS) Group. Effects of enalapril on mortality in severe HF. N Engl J Med 1987;316:1429–1435.

Design: Prospective, randomized, double-blind, placebo-controlled, multicenter study. Average follow-up period was 6 months. The primary end point was all-cause mortality rate.

Purpose: To evaluate the effect of enalapril, in addition to conventional therapy, on mortality in patients with severe HF.

Population: 253 NYHA class IV patients with heart size larger than 600 mL/m² body surface area in men and more than 550 mL/m² in women.

Exclusion Criteria: Acute pulmonary edema, MI in prior 2 months, unstable angina, planned cardiac surgery, and serum creatinine more than 300 μM.

Treatment: Enalapril, 2.5 mg/day orally, up to 20 mg twice daily. All patients were taking diuretics, 94% taking digoxin, and 50% taking vasodilators (mostly isosorbide dinitrate).

Results: Trial was terminated early because of significant mortality benefit in the enalapril group—40% relative risk reduction (RRR) in mortality at 6 months (26% vs. 44%;

$p = 0.0002$), 31% RRR at 1 year (36% vs. 52%; $p = 0.001$), and 27% RRR at end of the study (39% vs. 54%; $p = 0.003$). The entire mortality reduction was seen in patients with progressive HF (approximately 50% lower mortality). No difference in sudden death rates was observed. A significant mortality benefit was maintained at 2-year follow-up.

33. The Studies of Left Ventricular Dysfunction (SOLVD) Investigators. Effect of enalapril on survival in patients with reduced ventricular ejection fraction and congestive heart failure. N Engl J Med 1991;325:293–302.

Design: Prospective, randomized, double-blind, placebo-controlled, multicenter study. Average follow-up period was 41 months. The primary end point was all-cause mortality rate.

Purpose: To evaluate the effect of enalapril on mortality in patients with LV dysfunction and HF symptoms.

Population: 2,569 NYHA class II and III patients aged 21 to 80 years with an EF of 35% or less.

Exclusion Criteria: Active angina requiring surgery, unstable angina, or MI within the preceding month; renal failure; pulmonary disease; and current ACE inhibitor therapy.

Treatment: Enalapril, 2.5 to 5 mg twice daily initially, and then increased at 2 weeks to 5 to 10 mg twice daily; or placebo. Other drugs were not restricted (e.g., diuretics, digoxin, vasodilators).

Results: Enalapril group had 16% lower mortality (35.2% vs. 39.7%, 16% risk reduction; $p = 0.0036$). The majority of this effect was owing to fewer deaths from progressive HF (16.3% vs. 19.5%; $p = 0.0045$). The enalapril group also had a lower rate of death and rehospitalization due to worsening HF (47.7% vs. 57.3%, 26% risk reduction; $p < 0.0001$). Sudden death rates were similar.

34. The SOLVD Investigators. Effect of enalapril on mortality and the development of heart failure in asymptomatic patients with reduced left ventricular ejection fractions. N Engl J Med 1992;327:685–691.

Design: Prospective, randomized, double-blind, placebo-controlled, multicenter study. Follow-up period was 37 months. The primary end point was all-cause mortality rate.

Purpose: To evaluate effect of enalapril on mortality in patients with LV dysfunction without overt HF.

Population: 4,228 patients aged 21 to 80 years with an EF of 35% or less and taking no medications for HF (diuretics allowed for hypertension and digoxin for atrial fibrillation).

Exclusion Criteria: See SOLVD trial earlier.

Treatment: Enalapril, 2.5 to 20 mg orally per day, or placebo.

Results: Total mortality rates were 14.8% and 15.8% in the enalapril and placebo groups, respectively ($p = 0.30$). Most of this nonsignificant difference was due to 12% fewer cardiovascular deaths in the enalapril group (12.5% vs. 14.1%; $p = 0.12$). Fewer enalapril patients developed HF (20.7% vs. 30.2%; $p < 0.001$), and fewer required hospitalization due to HF (8.7% vs. 12.9%; $p < 0.001$).

35. The Acute Infarction Ramipril Efficacy Study (AIRE) Investigators. Effect of ramipril on mortality and morbidity of survivors of acute MI with clinical evidence of heart failure. Lancet 1993;342:821–828.

Design: Prospective, randomized, double-blind, placebo-controlled, multicenter study. Mean follow-up period was 15 months. The primary end point was all-cause mortality.

Purpose: To compare the effects of ramipril with placebo on overall mortality in acute MI survivors with early evidence of HF.

Population: 2,006 patients with an MI 2 to 9 days before study enrollment and clinical evidence of HF at any time since acute MI.

Exclusion Criteria: Severe HF (usually NYHA class IV), unstable angina, and HF of primary valvular or congenital etiology.

Treatment: Ramipril, 2.5 mg orally twice daily for 2 days, and then 5 mg twice daily; or placebo.

Results: Ramipril group had a 27% risk reduction in mortality (17% vs. 23%; p = 0.002). This benefit was already apparent at 30 days. Sudden cardiac deaths were reduced by 30% (p = 0.011).

Comments: AIREX follow-up study analyzed 603 patients at a mean 59 months, and the ramipril group still had a significantly lower mortality rate (RR, 0.64; 27.5% vs. 38.9%; p = 0.002).

36. Pitt B, et al. Evaluation of Losartan in the Elderly (ELITE). Randomized trial of losartan vs. captopril in patients over 65 with heart failure. *Lancet* **1997;349:747–752.**

Design: Prospective, randomized, double-blind, placebo-controlled, multicenter study. The primary end point was increase in creatinine clearance of 0.3 mg/dL.

Purpose: To compare the effects of angiotensin II–receptor inhibitor losartan with captopril on creatinine clearance and major cardiac events in elderly HF patients.

Population: 722 ACE inhibitor–naive patients in NYHA class II to IV and with EF of 40% or less.

Exclusion Criteria: Included SBP <90 mm Hg, acute MI, or coronary angioplasty in the prior 72 hours, bypass surgery in the prior 2 weeks, unstable angina in the prior 3 months, and stroke or transient ischemic attack (TIA) in the prior 3 months.

Treatment: Losartan, 12.5 to 50 mg daily, or captopril, 6.25 to 50 mg three times daily for 48 weeks.

Results: Similar incidence of increased creatinine was observed in both groups (10.5%). Fewer losartan patients discontinued therapy: 12.2% versus 20.8%; p = 0.002 (cough, 0 patient vs. 14 patients). The losartan group showed a trend toward lower rates of death and hospitalization (9.4% vs. 13.2%; p = 0.075) and a significant 45% lower overall mortality rate (4.8% vs. 8.7%; p = 0.035; sudden cardiac death: 5 patients vs. 14 patients). This mortality benefit was seen in all subgroups except women (240 patients, 7.6% vs. 6.6%).

Comments: The study was not designed to examine mortality.

37. Packer M, et al. Comparative effects of low and high doses of the angiotensin-converting enzyme inhibitor, lisinopril, on morbidity and mortality in chronic heart failure (ATLAS). *Circulation* **1999;100:2312–2318.**

Design: Prospective, randomized, double-blind, placebo-controlled, multicenter study. The primary end point was all-cause mortality. Follow-up period was 4 years.

Purpose: To evaluate the comparative efficacy of lisinopril on mortality in patients with LV dysfunction and HF symptoms.

Population: 3,164 patients with NYHA class II to IV HF and an EF of 30% or less.

Exclusion Criteria: Included acute coronary ischemic event or revascularization procedure in the prior 2 months, history of sustained or symptomatic ventricular tachycardia (VT), intolerance to ACE inhibitors, and serum creatinine >2.5 mg/dL.

Treatment: Low-dose lisinopril (2.5 to 5.0 mg daily) or high-dose lisinopril (32.5 to 35 mg daily). Before randomization, all patients received lisinopril for 4 weeks to assess their ability to tolerate the drug. Digitalis, ACE inhibitors, or vasodilators were allowed but not mandated.

Results: Patients in the high-dose group had a nonsignificant 8% lower risk of death (p = 0.13) but a significant 12% lower risk of death or hospitalization for any reason (p = 0.002) and 24% fewer hospitalizations for HF (p = 0.002). Dizziness and renal insufficiency were observed more frequently in the high-dose group, but the two groups were similar in the number of patients requiring cessation of the study medication.

38. Pitt B, et al. Effect of losartan compared with captopril on mortality in patients with symptomatic heart failure: randomised trial—the Losartan Heart Failure Survival Study (ELITE II). *Lancet* 2000;355:1582–1587.

Design: Prospective, randomized, double-blind, placebo-controlled, multicenter study. The primary end point was all-cause mortality.

Purpose: To compare the mortality benefit of the angiotensin II receptor inhibitor losartan with captopril in elderly HF patients.

Population: 3,152 ACE inhibitor–naive patients in NYHA class II through IV and with EF 40% or less.

Exclusion Criteria: Included ACE inhibitor or angiotensin II receptor antagonist intolerance, SBP <90 mm Hg, diastolic blood pressure (DBP) >95 mm Hg, hemodynamically important stenotic valvular heart disease, active myocarditis or pericarditis, ICD implantation, serum creatinine more than 220 mM, PTCA in previous week, and cerebrovascular accident (CVA), or TIA in previous 6 weeks; CABG surgery, acute MI, or unstable angina in previous 2 weeks.

Treatment: Losartan, 12.5 to 50 mg daily, or captopril, 6.25 to 50 mg three times daily.

Results: No significant differences were found between the two groups in all-cause mortality (11.7% vs. 10.4% average annual mortality rate) or sudden death or resuscitated arrests (9.0% vs. 7.3%; p = 0.08). Fewer losartan patients had adverse effects (9.7% vs. 14.7%; p < 0.001), especially cough (0.3% vs. 2.7%).

Comments: These results demonstrate the problem of drawing conclusions from trials enrolling small numbers of patients (i.e., ELITE I). The trial was not designed to address equivalence between the two treatments, so these findings do not provide evidence regarding the efficacy of losartan compared with placebo.

39. Cohn JN, et al. A randomized trial of the angiotensin-receptor blocker valsartan in chronic heart failure (Val-HeFT). *N Engl J Med* 2001;345:1667–1675.

Design: Prospective, randomized, double-blind, placebo-controlled, multicenter study. The primary end point was all-cause mortality.

Purpose: To determine the mortality benefit of adding valsartan to usual therapy for HF in patients with HF.

Population: 5,010 patients with NYHA class II to IV symptoms with EF 40% or less. Patients required to be on stable medical regimens, which could include diuretics, digoxin, ACE inhibition, and β-blockers.

Treatment: Valsartan, 40 to 50 mg daily, or captopril, 6.25 to 50 mg three times daily.

Results: No significant difference in overall mortality was found between the valsartan and captopril groups (19.7% vs. 19.4%). The incidence of the secondary combined end point of death or cardiac arrest with resuscitation, hospitalized for HF, or intravenous inotropic or vasodilator for 4 hours or more was significantly lower with valsartan (RR, 0.87; p = 0.009). This benefit was mainly owing to a lower incidence of hospitalization for HF (13.8% vs. 18.2%; p < 0.001). Treatment with valsartan also was associated with improvements in NYHA class, EF, signs and symptoms of HF, and QOL.

40. Pfeffer MA, et al. Valsartan, captopril, or both in myocardial infarction complicated by heart failure, left ventricular dysfunction, or both (VALIANT). *N Engl J Med* 2003;349(20):1893–1906.

Design: Prospective, randomized, double-blind, multicenter (931 centers, 24 countries) noninferiority study.

Purpose: To compare valsartan, captopril, or both in a population of post-MI patients complicated by LV systolic dysfunction, HF, or both.

Population: 14,808 patients up to 10 days post-MI complicated by clinical or radiologic signs of HF, evidence of LV systolic dysfunction (an EF ≤0.35 on echocardiography or contrast angiography and ≤0.40 on radionuclide ventriculography), or both.

Treatment: Therapy was begun with either 20 mg of valsartan, 20 mg of valsartan plus 6.25 mg of captopril, or 6.25 mg of captopril alone. Doses were gradually increased in four steps, with the goal of reaching step 3 (80 mg of valsartan twice daily, 40 mg of valsartan twice daily, and 25 mg of captopril three times daily, or 25 mg of captopril three times daily) during the initial hospitalization and step 4 (160 mg of valsartan twice daily, 80 mg of valsartan twice daily, and 50 mg of captopril three times daily, or 50 mg of captopril three times daily), if clinically possible, by the 3-month visit.

Results: Mortality from any cause and cause-specific mortality were similar in the three treatment groups. The rate of the secondary end point of death from cardiovascular causes, recurrent MI, or hospitalization for HF was similar in the three groups.

41. Pfeffer MA, et al. Effects of candesartan on mortality and morbidity in patients with chronic heart failure: the CHARM-overall programme. Lancet 2003;362:759–766.

Design: Three parallel, randomized, double-blind, placebo-controlled clinical trials.

Purpose: To evaluate the effect of candesartan versus placebo on all-cause mortality in three different populations of HF patients.

Population: Overall, 7,601 patients (7,599 with data) were randomly assigned candesartan (*n* = 3,803, titrated to 32 mg once daily) or matching placebo (*n* = 3,796) and followed up for at least 2 years.

Treatment: Candesartan titrated to 32 mg daily versus placebo.

Results: Over median follow-up of 37.7 months, all-cause mortality trended to favor the candesartan group (23% vs. 25% in the placebo group, unadjusted HR 0.91, $p = 0.055$; adjusted HR 0.90, $p = 0.032$) and significantly favored cardiovascular death (18% vs. 20%, unadjusted HR 0.88, $p = 0.012$) and HF hospitalization (20% vs. 24%; $p < 0.0001$). Heterogeneity analyses were not significant across the component trials.

Comments: See individual results from the CHARM-added (*Lancet* 2003;362(9386): 767–771), CHARM-alternative (*Lancet* 2003;362(9386):772–776), and CHARM-preserved (*Lancet* 2003;362:777–781) studies.

42. Massie BM, et al. Irbesartan in Patients with Heart Failure and Preserved Ejection Fraction (I-PRESERVE). N Engl J Med 2008;359:2456–2467.

Design: Prospective, randomized, placebo-controlled trial. Primary composite outcome was all-cause mortality or cardiovascular hospitalization (HF, MI, UA, arrhythmia, or stroke).

Purpose: To assess utility of irbesartan in HFpEF.

Population: 4,128 patients at least 60 years of age, with NYHA class II, III, or IV HF and an EF ≥45%.

Treatment: Irbesartan 300 mg daily or placebo.

Results: Irbesartan did not significantly reduce incidence of the primary end point (HR, 0.95; $p = 0.35$), all-cause mortality (HR, 1.00; $p = 0.98$), or rates of cardiovascular hospitalization (HR, 0.95; $p = 0.44$).

Comments: This trial added to the evidence that HFpEF is a unique clinical entity, not responsive (in terms of clinical end points) to classical HF therapies.

43. Konstam MA, et al. Effects of high-dose versus low-dose losartan on clinical outcomes in patients with heart failure (HEAAL study): a randomised, double-blind trial. *Lancet* 2009;374:1840–1848.

Design: Prospective, randomized, double-blind, multicenter (255, 30 countries) trial. The primary end point was all-cause mortality or admission for HF over median 4.7 years of follow-up.

Purpose: To compare high-dose versus low-dose losartan in patients with HF.

Population: 3,846 patients with HF of NYHA class II, III, or IV, EF ≤40%, and intolerance to ACE inhibitors.

Treatment: Losartan 150 mg or losartan 50 mg daily.

Results: Incidence of a primary end point event was significantly lower in the high-dose losartan group (43% vs. 46%; *p* = 0.027); this was predominantly driven by significantly lower rates of HF admissions (HR, 0.87; *p* = 0.025). While expected adverse events were higher in the high-dose group (renal impairment, hypotension, and hyperkalemia), this did not yield significantly higher treatment cessation rates in this group.

44. McKelvie RS, et al.; The RESOLVD Pilot Study Investigators. Comparison of candesartan, enalapril, and their combination in congestive heart failure: randomized evaluation of strategies for left ventricular dysfunction (RESOLVD) pilot study. *Circulation* 1999;100:1056–1064.

Design: Multicenter, double-blind, randomized, placebo-controlled trial.

Purpose: To compare candesartan alone, enalapril alone, and their combination for the end points of exercise tolerance, ventricular function, QOL, neurohormone levels, and tolerability over 43 weeks.

Population: 768 patients with NYHA class II, III, or IV HF, EF <0.40, and a 6MWD <500 m.

Treatment: Candesartan (4, 8, or 16 mg), candesartan (4 or 8 mg) plus 20 mg of enalapril, or 20 mg of enalapril.

Results: Over the 43-week study period, the groups did not differ with regard to 6MWD, NYHA class, or QOL (*p* = NS). End-diastolic volume (EDV) and ESV increased less with combination (candesartan–enalapril) therapy than with candesartan or enalapril alone. The authors conclude that, while candesartan is as safe and effective as enalapril, the combination may have incremental benefit on ventricular remodeling.

β-BLOCKERS
Review Articles and Meta-analyses
45. Lechat P, et al. Clinical effects of β-adrenergic blockade in chronic heart failure. *Circulation* 1998;98:1184–1191.

This meta-analysis focused on 18 double-blind, placebo-controlled, parallel-group studies with a total of 3,023 patients. β-Blocker use was associated with a 29% increase in EF (*p* < 0.0001) and 37% reduction in the risk of death or hospitalization for HF (*p* < 0.001). All-cause mortality was decreased by 32% (*p* = 0.003). A greater reduction for nonselective β-blockers compared with $β_1$-selective agents was seen (49% vs. 18%; *p* = 0.049). The effect of β-blocker use on NYHA functional class was of only borderline significance (*p* = 0.04).

Carvedilol Studies
46. Packer M, et al. Prospective Randomized Evaluation of Carvedilol on Symptoms and Exercise (PRECISE). Double-blind, placebo-controlled study of the effects of carvedilol in patients with moderate to severe heart failure. *Circulation* 1996;94:2793–2799.

Design: Prospective, randomized, double-blind, placebo-controlled, multicenter study. The primary end point was exercise tolerance.

Purpose: To evaluate the clinical effects of carvedilol in patients with moderate-to-severe HF.

Population: 278 patients with moderate-to-severe HF (dyspnea or fatigue at rest or on exertion for 3 months), an EF 35% or less, and receiving digoxin, diuretics, and an ACE inhibitor.

Exclusion Criteria: MI, unstable angina, CABG surgery, or stroke in the prior 3 months; uncorrected primary valvular disease; SBP <85 mm Hg or more than 160 mm Hg or DBP more than 100 mm Hg; heart rate, <68 beats/min; and use of calcium channel blockers or antiarrhythmic drugs.

Treatment: During the open-label run-in period, carvedilol, 6.25 mg twice daily for 2 weeks. If tolerated, the patient was randomized to carvedilol, 12.5 mg twice daily initially, with titration over a 2- to 6-week period to 25 to 50 mg twice daily for 6 months, or placebo.

Results: Carvedilol patients had more frequent improvement in symptoms, as evaluated by changes in NYHA functional class ($p = 0.014$) and global assessments by the patient ($p = 0.002$) and the physician ($p < 0.001$). Carvedilol patients also had a significant increase in EF (+8% vs. +3%; $p < 0.001$) and a significant decrease in morbidity and mortality (19.6% vs. 31.0%; $p = 0.029$). However, no significant effect was seen on exercise tolerance or QOL scores.

47. Bristow MR, et al. **Multicenter Oral Carvedilol Heart Failure Assessment (MOCHA). Carvedilol produces dose-related improvements in left ventricular function and survival in subjects with chronic heart failure.** *Circulation* 1996;94:2807–2816.

Design: Prospective, randomized, double-blind, placebo-controlled, multicenter study. Follow-up period was 6 months. The primary end point was change in walk test distances (6-minute corridor test and 9-minute self-powered treadmill test).

Purpose: To evaluate the effects of carvedilol in addition to standard therapy on clinical events and QOL in chronic HF patients.

Population: 345 patients aged 18 to 85 years with symptomatic, stable HF capable of walking 150 to 450 m in 6 minutes.

Exclusion Criteria: MI or stroke in the prior 3 months, uncorrected primary valvular disease, planned bypass surgery or balloon angioplasty, SBP <85 or more than 160 mm Hg, and use of calcium channel blockers or antiarrhythmic drugs.

Treatment: Carvedilol, 6.25 to 25 mg/day, or placebo. Concomitant therapy included diuretics, digoxin, and ACE inhibitors.

Results: No differences were seen in submaximal exercise performance (as assessed by two walk tests) or HF symptoms. Carvedilol was associated with dose-dependent improvements in LV function (+5%, +6%, and +8% in low-, medium-, and high-dose groups vs. + 2% with placebo; $p < 0.001$) and mortality (6.0%, 6.7%, and 1.1% vs. 15.5%; $p < 0.001$). When the three carvedilol groups were combined, the all-cause actuarial mortality risk was 73% lower ($p < 0.001$). Carvedilol patients also were hospitalized less frequently (by 58% to 64%; $p = 0.01$).

48. Packer M, et al.; U.S. Carvedilol Heart Failure Study Group. **The effect of carvedilol on morbidity and mortality in patients with chronic heart failure.** *N Engl J Med* 1996;334:1349–1355 (editorial, 1396–1397).

Design: Prospective, randomized, double-blind, placebo-controlled, multicenter study. The primary end point was mortality.

Purpose: To evaluate the safety and efficacy of carvedilol in patients with chronic HF.

Population: 1,094 chronic HF patients with an EF 35% or less and taking digoxin, diuretics, and an ACE inhibitor.

Exclusion Criteria: SBP <90 mm Hg, acute MI or coronary angioplasty in the prior 72 hours, bypass surgery in the prior 2 weeks, unstable angina in the prior 3 months, and stroke or TIA in the prior 3 months.

Treatment: After the 2-week open-label phase (5.6% failed to complete this period because of adverse events), patients were assigned to one of the four treatment groups based on exercise capacity [6-minute walk: mild, 426 to 550 m; moderate, 150 to 425 m; severe, <150 m (fourth group, dose-ranging protocol)] and randomized to carvedilol, 6.25 to 50 mg twice daily (titrated over a 2- to 10-week period), or placebo.

Results: At 6 months, carvedilol-treated patients had 65% lower mortality (3.2% vs. 7.8%; $p < 0.001$), 27% fewer CV-related hospitalizations (14.1% vs. 19.6%; $p = 0.036$), and a 38% reduction in death and hospitalization (15.8% vs. 24.6%; $p < 0.001$). Patients with an initial HR of more than 82 beats/min had the most benefit. More placebo patients had worsening HF.

Comments: Analysis combined patients from three different studies [PRECISE, MOCHA, Colucci WS, et al.]. This study had limited follow-up and only 53 total deaths; 7 carvedilol deaths occurred in the run-in period, and 17 (1.4%) patients were excluded because of worsening HF [more problematic in severe HF patients (only 3% of this study population)].

49. Heart Failure Research Collaborative Group, ANZ (Australia/New Zealand). Randomized, placebo-controlled trial of carvedilol in patients with congestive heart failure due to ischaemic heart disease. *Lancet* 1997;349:375–380.

Design: Prospective, randomized, double-blind, placebo-controlled, multicenter study. Average follow-up period was 19 months. The primary end point was changes in LVEF and treadmill exercise duration.

Purpose: To evaluate the longer-term effects on death and other serious clinical events of carvedilol in patients with chronic stable HF.

Population: 415 NYHA class II or III patients with chronic stable HF.

Exclusion Criteria: Current NYHA class IV; primary valvular disease; SBP <90 mm Hg or more than 160 mm Hg or DBP more than 100 mm Hg; and MI, unstable angina, bypass surgery, or coronary angioplasty in the prior 4 weeks.

Treatment: Twenty-seven patients were withdrawn during the 2- to 3-week open-label phase of carvedilol therapy (3.125 mg daily to 6.25 mg twice daily). Carvedilol was then given at 6.25 to 25 mg twice daily or placebo.

Results: At 1 year, the carvedilol group had an increased EF (+5.3%; $p < 0.0001$) and decreased end-diastolic and end-systolic dimensions [−1.7 mm ($p = 0.06$) and −3.2 mm ($p = 0.001$)]. However, no differences were noted in exercise treadmill time, 6MWD, NYHA class, or specific activity score. At 19 months, no difference was seen in the number of HF episodes, but the carvedilol group had a lower incidence of death and hospitalization (50% vs. 63%; RR, 0.74; 95% CI, 0.57 to 0.95).

Comments: ANZ echocardiographic substudy of 123 patients (echocardiograms at baseline and 6 and 12 months) showed that the carvedilol group had a LV end-diastolic volume index (LVEDVI) 14 mL/m^2 lower than placebo ($p = 0.0015$), LV end-systolic volume index (LVESVI) 15.3 mL/m^2 lower than placebo ($p = 0.0001$), and EF 5.8% higher ($p = 0.0015$).

50. Packer M, et al.; for the Carvedilol Prospective Randomized Cumulative Survival Study (COPERNICUS) Group. Effect of carvedilol on survival in severe chronic heart failure. *N Engl J Med* 2001;344:1651–1658.

Design: Prospective, randomized, double-blind, placebo-controlled, multicenter study. The primary end point was changed in LVEF and treadmill exercise duration. Average follow-up period was 10 months.

Purpose: To evaluate the longer-term effects on death and other serious clinical events of carvedilol in patients with chronic stable HF.

Population: 2,289 NYHA class III or IV patients with chronic stable HF.

Exclusion Criteria: Included HF due to uncorrected primary valvular disease or a reversible cardiomyopathy; eligibility for cardiac transplantation; contraindication to β-blocker therapy or use in the previous 2 months; coronary revascularization, acute myocardial or cerebral ischemic event in the previous 2 months; use of α-adrenergic blocker, calcium channel blocker, or class I antiarrhythmic drug in the previous 4 weeks; SBP <85 mm Hg; creatinine more than 2.8 mg/dL.

Treatment: Patients received an initial dose of 3.125 mg of carvedilol or placebo twice daily for 2 weeks, which was then increased at 2-week intervals (if tolerated), first to 6.25 mg, and then to 12.5 mg, and finally to a target dose of 25 mg twice daily.

Results: A 35% decrease was seen in the risk of death with carvedilol (95% CI, 19% to 48%; p = 0.0014). A 24% decrease in the combined risk of death or hospitalization with carvedilol was found (p < 0.001). Fewer patients in the carvedilol group than in the placebo group withdrew because of adverse effects or for other reasons (p = 0.02). A subsequent report showed that more patients felt improved, and fewer patients felt worse in the carvedilol group than in the placebo group after 6 months of maintenance therapy (p = 0.0009; see *Circulation* 2002;106:2194).

Comments: Patients not included were those with far-advanced HF symptoms and those who could not reach compensation. A small proportion of black patients was included.

51. Poole-Wilson PA, et al. Comparison of carvedilol and metoprolol on clinical outcomes in patients with chronic heart failure in the Carvedilol Or Metoprolol European Trial (COMET): randomised controlled trial. *Lancet* 2003;362:7–13.

Design: Prospective, randomized, double-blind, multicenter trial. The primary end points were all-cause mortality and the composite of all-cause mortality or all-cause hospital admission over a mean of 58 months.

Purpose: To compare carvedilol to metoprolol (both twice daily) in chronic HF.

Population: 3,029 patients with chronic HF (NYHA class II, III, or IV), previous cardiovascular hospitalization, EF <35%, and already on ACE inhibitors (as tolerated).

Treatment: Carvedilol (target dose 25 mg twice daily) or metoprolol (metoprolol tartrate, target dose 50 mg twice daily).

Results: The outcome of all-cause mortality heavily favored carvedilol (34% vs. 40%; p = 0.0017) and was consistent across predefined subgroups. However, the composite end point of mortality or all-cause admission was not significantly different between the two groups (74% for carvedilol vs. 76% for metoprolol; p = 0.122), perhaps owing to the high rates of incidence overall.

52. Eichhorn E, et al. A trial of the β-blocker bucindolol in patients with advanced chronic heart failure (BEST). *N Engl J Med* 2001;344:1659–1667.

Design: Prospective, randomized, double-blind, placebo-controlled, multicenter trial. The primary end point was all-cause mortality. Average follow-up, 2.0 years.

Purpose: To evaluate the effect on survival of the β-blocker bucindolol in patients with advanced HF.

Population: 2,708 patients with NYHA III (92%) or IV (8%) HF and LVEF 35% or lower.

Exclusion Criteria: Included decompensated HF, eligibility for heart transplantation, reversible causes of HF, uncorrected primary valvular disease, hypertrophic cardiomyopathy, MI within the previous 6 months, PCI or CABG within 60 days, calcium channel blocking or β-agonists within 1 week, β-blocking agents within 30 days, and amiodarone within 8 weeks.

Treatment: Bucindolol, 3 to 100 mg orally, or placebo.

Results: Trial terminated after seventh interim analysis. Mortality rates were similar between the two groups [411 deaths (bucindolol) vs. 449 deaths; unadjusted $p = 0.16$]. The bucindolol group had a significantly lower incidence of CV death and heart transplantation or death.

Comments: The neutral results of this study are surprising and challenge the concept of a beneficial class effect with β-adrenergic blockade. However, several subsequent, post hoc analyses suggested a genetic-based mechanism that may potentially explain heterogeneity of response to bucindolol and development is ongoing.

Other Studies

53. Waagstein F, et al. Metoprolol in Dilated Cardiomyopathy (MDC). Beneficial effects of metoprolol in idiopathic dilated cardiomyopathy (DCM). *Lancet* 1993;342: 1441–1446.

Design: Prospective, randomized, double-blind, placebo-controlled, parallel-group, multicenter study. Follow-up period was 12 to 18 months. The primary end point was death and need for cardiac transplantation.

Purpose: To evaluate the effects of metoprolol versus placebo in patients with HF due to idiopathic DCM.

Population: 383 patients aged 16 to 75 years with LVEF <0.40; 94% were in NYHA functional class II or III.

Exclusion Criteria: Use of β-blockers or calcium channel blockers, CAD (more than 50% stenosis), SBP <90 mm Hg, heart rate <45 beats/min, obstructive lung disease requiring β-agonists, and insulin-dependent diabetes.

Treatment: If the test dose was tolerated (metoprolol, 5 mg twice daily for 2 to 7 days), then patients were randomized to metoprolol [10 mg/day titrated up to 100 to 150 mg/day (mean, 108 mg/day)] or placebo.

Results: Metoprolol group had 34% risk reduction in death or need for heart transplantation (22.5% vs. 36.5%; $p = 0.058$). At follow-up, the metoprolol group had a significantly better improvement in LVEF (+0.12 vs. +0.06 at 12 months; $p < 0.0001$), increased exercise duration (+76 seconds vs. + 15 seconds at 12 months; $p = 0.046$), and showed a trend toward lower PCWP (−5 mm Hg vs. −2 mm Hg; $p = 0.06$). The metoprolol group had better QOL (based on patient assessment at 12 and 18 months; $p = 0.01$), and a significant correlation was found between the NYHA classification made by the physician and the QOL assessment. A subsequent report showed that the metoprolol group had a significantly improved exercise oxygen consumption index ($p = 0.045$).

54. Cardiac Insufficiency Bisoprolol Study II (CIBIS-II) Investigators. The Cardiac Insufficiency Bisoprolol Study II (CIBIS II): a randomized trial. *Lancet* 1999;353: 9–12.

Design: Prospective, randomized, double-blind, placebo-controlled, multicenter study. Mean follow-up period was 1.3 years. The primary end point was all-cause mortality rate.

Purpose: To evaluate the efficacy of bisoprolol in decreasing all-cause mortality in patients with symptomatic chronic HF.

Population: 2,647 NYHA class III or IV patients with LVEF <35%.

Exclusion Criteria: Uncontrolled hypertension, MI, or unstable angina in the prior 3 months, PTCA or CABG in the prior 6 months, heart rate <60 beats/min, or preexisting or planned therapy with β-blockers.

Treatment: Bisoprolol, 1.25 to 10.0 mg/day, or placebo. All patients were taking diuretics and ACE inhibitors.

Results: Study was terminated because bisoprolol showed a significant mortality benefit—11.8% versus 17.3% (hazard ratio, 0.66; *p* < 0.0001). The bisoprolol group also had a lower incidence of sudden death (3.6% vs. 6.3%; hazard ratio, 0.56; *p* = 0.0011) and 20% fewer hospital admissions; treatment effects were independent of severity or cause of HF.

Comments: No run-in period provided a better estimate of clinical effectiveness of bisoprolol. The low mortality rates suggest that not all patients were NYHA class III and IV patients.

55. MERIT-HF Study Group. Effect of metoprolol CR/XL in chronic heart failure: metoprolol CR/XL randomized intervention trial in congestive heart failure (MERIT-HF). *Lancet* 1999;353:2001–2007.

Design: Prospective, randomized, double-blind, placebo-controlled multicenter study. Mean follow-up period was 1 year. The primary end point was all-cause mortality.

Purpose: To evaluate whether metoprolol CR/XL, once daily, in addition to standard therapy, could lower mortality in symptomatic HF patients with impaired EF.

Population: 3,991 NYHA class II to IV (II, 41%; III, 55%) patients with an EF of 40% or less. Two-thirds of patients had an ischemic etiology of HF; 89% were taking an ACE inhibitor; 90% were taking a diuretic; and 63% were receiving digoxin.

Treatment: Metoprolol CR/XL, 12.5 mg (NYHA III or IV) or 25 mg (NYHA II) once daily; or placebo. Target dose was 200 mg/day with up-titration over an 8-week period. Randomization was preceded by a 2-week single-blind placebo run-in period.

Results: All-cause mortality was significantly lower in the metoprolol group (7.2% vs. 11.0%; RR, 0.66; *p* < 0.001). The metoprolol group also had a 38% reduction in CV mortality (*p* < 0.001), a 41% reduction in sudden death (*p* < 0.001), and a 49% reduction in death due to progressive HF (*p* = 0.002). The incidence of side effects was similar in both groups.

56. Exner DV, et al. Beta-adrenergic blocking agent use and mortality in patients with asymptomatic and symptomatic left ventricular systolic dysfunction: a post hoc analysis of the studies of left ventricular dysfunction. *J Am Coll Cardiol* 1999;33: 916–923.

Design: Retrospective analysis of patients in the SOLVD trial, based on baseline β-blocker use.

Purpose: To determine if β-blocker use was associated with lower morality and if the effect interacts with ACE inhibitor use.

Population: 6,790 patients with HF (4,223 mostly asymptomatic, 2,567 symptomatic).

Results: In all, only 1,015 (24%) asymptomatic and 197 (8%) symptomatic patients were receiving β-blockers at baseline. However, these groups did have fewer symptoms and higher EFs than did those not receiving β-blockers (in univariate analysis). β-Blocker use was associated with significantly lower mortality in both cohorts, an effect that persisted in multivariable analysis for asymptomatic patients. Moreover, this effect was synergistic in patients who added enalapril to their β-blocker.

57. Dargie HG. Effect of carvedilol on outcome after myocardial infarction in patients with left-ventricular dysfunction: the CAPRICORN randomized trial. *Lancet* 2001;357:1385–1390.

Design: Multicenter (163 centers, 17 countries), randomized, double-blind, placebo-controlled trial. The primary end point was all-cause mortality or cardiovascular hospitalization over a mean of 1.3 years.

Purpose: To assess the utility of adding carvedilol to standard medical therapy in post-MI patients with LV dysfunction.

Population: 1,959 post-MI patients with EF ≤40%.

Treatment: Carvedilol 6.25 mg (titrated to 25 mg twice daily, as tolerated) or placebo.

Results: The two groups did not differ significantly in their incidence of primary end point events (35% for carvedilol vs. 37% for placebo). However, all-cause mortality alone was significantly reduced in carvedilol (12% vs. 15%; HR, 0.77; p = 0.03). Additionally, cardiovascular death and nonfatal MI were also lower in carvedilol.

58. Remme WJ, et al. The benefits of early combination treatment of carvedilol and an ACE-inhibitor in mild heart failure and left ventricular systolic dysfunction: the carvedilol and ACE-inhibitor remodeling mild heart failure evaluation trial (CARMEN). *Cardiovasc Drugs Ther* 2004;18:57–66.

Design: Multicenter (63 centers, 13 countries), double-blind, randomized trial. Primary outcome was change in LVESVI at 18 months.

Purpose: To identify the benefit, if any, of combination ACE inhibitor plus β-blocker therapy, on ventricular remodeling in HF.

Population: 572 patients with mild, stable HF (NYHA class I, II, or III) with EF <40%.

Treatment: Carvedilol (n = 191), enalapril (n = 190), or their combination (n = 191). In the latter, carvedilol was up-titrated before enalapril.

Results: LVESVI was significantly reduced by 5.4 mL/m² (p = 0.0015) in the combination therapy group, compared to enalapril alone. However, there was no significant difference between carvedilol alone and enalapril alone. Furthermore, carvedilol significantly reduced LVESVI by 2.8 mL/m² (p = 0.018) compared to baseline, whereas enalapril did not. LVESVI was reduced by 6.3 mL/m² (p = 0.0001) with combination therapy.

59. Colucci WS, et al. Metoprolol reverses left ventricular remodeling in patients with asymptomatic systolic dysfunction: the Reversal of Ventricular Remodeling with Toprol-XL (REVERT) trial. *Circulation* 2007;116:49–56.

Design: Randomized, double-blind, placebo-controlled trial. The primary end point was change in LVESVI from baseline to 12 months.

Purpose: To determine if β-blockers can attenuate LV remodeling in asymptomatic patients with LV systolic dysfunction.

Population: 149 patients with LVEF <40% and mild LV dilatation (LVEDVI >75 mL/m²) due to idiopathic, ischemic, or hypertensive cardiomyopathy (without HF symptoms for at least 2 months).

Treatment: Extended-release metoprolol succinate 200 mg (n = 48) or 50 mg (n = 48) or placebo (n = 53).

Results: At 12 months, there was a 14 mL/m² decrease in LVESVI and a 6 ± 1% increase in EF in the 200-mg group (p < 0.05 vs. baseline and placebo for both). In the 50-mg group, LVESVI and LVEDVI decreased relative to baseline, but not significantly more than was seen with placebo.

DIURETICS AND ALDOSTERONE ANTAGONISTS

60. Dormans TPJ, et al. Diuretic efficacy of high dose furosemide in severe heart failure: bolus injection vs. continuous infusion. *J Am Coll Cardiol* 1996;28:376–382.

In this crossover study, 20 patients were randomized to an equal dosage by intravenous bolus or an 8-hour continuous infusion after a loading dose (20% total). Doses used ranged from 250 to 2,000 mg/24 h. The continuous-infusion group had an increased urinary volume (2.9 vs. 2.3 L; $p < 0.001$) and better sodium excretion. Reversible hearing loss was seen in five intravenous bolus patients (maximal plasma concentration, 95 μg/mL vs. 24 μg/mL; only nine patients, and the bolus plus 48-hour infusion yielded better results than did intravenous boluses three times daily).

61. Felker GM, et al. Diuretic strategies in patients with acute decompensated heart failure. N Engl J Med 2011;364:797–805.

Design: Prospective, double-blind, randomized trial. The coprimary end points were global assessment of symptoms and change in creatinine form baseline at 72 hours.

Purpose: To assess the differences, if any, between bolus-dosed and continuous infusion loop diuretics for the treatment of acute, decompensated, congestive HF.

Population: 308 patients with decompensated HF, including at least 1 symptom and 1 sign of congestion. There was no LVEF inclusion criterion.

Key Exclusion Criteria: Patients in shock, on inotropes and/or intravenous vasodilators, and those with relative hypotension or baseline creatinine >3 mg/dL were excluded.

Treatment: Furosemide administered by intravenous bolus dosing every 12 hours or furosemide administered by continuous, intravenous infusion at either low (equivalent to patient's prior oral dosing) or high dosing (2.5 times the prior oral dosing).

Results: There were no significant differences in either coprimary end point among the dosing strategies ($p = 0.47$ for symptoms, $p = 0.45$ for change in creatinine).

62. Pitt B, et al.; Randomized Aldactone Evaluation Study (RALES) Investigators. The effect of spironolactone on morbidity and mortality in patients with severe heart failure. N Engl J Med 1999;341:709–719 (editorial, 753–755).

Design: Prospective, randomized, double-blind, placebo-controlled, multicenter study. Mean follow-up was 24 months. The primary end point was all-cause mortality.

Purpose: To evaluate whether spironolactone would significantly reduce mortality in patients with severe HF.

Population: 1,663 NYHA class III (69%) or IV (31%) patients with an EF of 35% or less. Ischemic etiology of HF in 54%.

Exclusion Criteria: Included valvular heart disease; unstable angina; hepatic failure; potassium, 5 mM or greater; creatinine, >2.5 mg/dL.

Treatment: Spironolactone, 25 mg, or placebo once daily. Dose could be increased to 50 mg if worsening HF with normal potassium. All patients were taking loop diuretics, 95% were taking ACE inhibitors, and 74% were receiving digoxin.

Results: Spironolactone group had a significant (30%) reduction in mortality compared with placebo (35% vs. 46%; $p < 0.001$). This benefit was attributable to a lower risk of sudden death from cardiac causes (29% RRR) and death from progressive HF (36% RRR). Spironolactone was associated with a higher incidence of gynecomastia (10% vs. 1%; $p < 0.001$), whereas the incidence of serious hyperkalemia was similar (2% vs. 1%).

63. Pitt B, et al.; for the EPHESUS (Eplerenone Post-acute MI Heart Failure Efficacy and Survival Study) Investigators. Eplerenone, a selective aldosterone blocker in patients with left ventricular dysfunction after myocardial infarction. N Engl J Med 2003;348:1309–1321 (editorial, 1380–1382).

Design: Prospective, randomized, placebo-controlled, double-blind, multicenter study. The primary end points were all-cause mortality and cardiovascular death or hospitalization for cardiovascular causes. Mean follow-up was 16 months.

Purpose: To evaluate the effect of eplerenone on morbidity and mortality among patients with acute MI complicated by LV dysfunction.

Population: 6,632 patients with an acute MI 3 to 14 days prior to randomization and LVEF = 40% by echocardiography.

Exclusion Criteria: Included use of potassium-sparing diuretics, creatinine >2.5 mg/dL, and potassium >5.0 mmol/L.

Treatment: Eplerenone, 25 to 50 mg twice daily, or placebo. Nearly all were on ACE inhibitors (94%) and 75% were on β-blockers.

Results: Eplerenone group had a significant reduction in all-cause mortality compared to placebo (14.4% vs. 16.7%; relative risk, 0.85; p = 0.008). It was also associated with a lower rate of cardiovascular death or CV-related hospitalization (RR, 0.87; p = 0.002). Eplerenone also had a 21% relative reduction in sudden cardiac death (p = 0.03). Serious hyperkalemia occurred more frequently with eplerenone (5.5% vs. 3.9%; p = 0.002), while hypokalemia was less common (8.4% vs. 13.1%; p < 0.001).

64. Zannad F, et al.; The EMPHASIS-HF Trial. Eplerenone in patients with systolic heart failure and mild symptoms. N Engl J Med 2011;364:11–21.

Design: Prospective, double-blinded, placebo-controlled, randomized trial. The primary end point was a composite of cardiovascular death or HF hospitalization at a median follow-up of 21 months.

Purpose: To assess the utility of aldosterone antagonism with eplerenone in patients with more mild HF.

Population: 2,737 patients with NYHA II HF and LVEF ≤35%, already treated with beta-blockers and ACE inhibitors (and/or ARBs).

Key Exclusion Criteria: Recent MI, hyperkalemia or severe renal dysfunction at baseline, or NYHA III/IV.

Treatment: Eplerenone titrated to a maximum dose of 50 mg daily or placebo.

Results: The trial was terminated early due to a significant benefit of eplerenone versus placebo for the primary end point (18.3% vs. 25.9%; p < 0.001). There was also a significant reduction in all-cause mortality alone (12.5% vs. 15.5%; p = 0.008). As expected, hyperkalemia was significantly more common in the eplerenone group (11.8% vs. 7.2%; p < 0.001).

65. Edelmann F, et al. Effect of spironolactone on diastolic function and exercise capacity in patients with heart failure with preserved ejection fraction: the Aldo-DHF randomized controlled trial. JAMA 2013;309:781–791.

Design: Prospective, multicenter, double-blinded, placebo-controlled, randomized trial. The coprimary end points were changes in diastolic dysfunction (E/e') on echocardiography and changes in CPX capacity (peak Vo$_2$), both at 12 months.

Purpose: To assess the utility of spironolactone for treatment of HFpEF.

Population: 422 patients with chronic, NYHA II-III HF symptoms, and LVEF ≥50% with evidence of diastolic dysfunction.

Key Exclusion Criteria: History of reduced LVEF, significant active CAD, or hyperkalemia or significant renal dysfunction at baseline.

Treatment: Spironolactone 25 mg daily or placebo.

Results: Diastolic dysfunction decreased significantly in patients assigned to spironolactone (adjusted mean difference in change −1.5, p < 0.001); however, change in peak did not differ significantly between the two groups (adjusted mean difference of change 0.1 mL/min/kg, p = 0.81). Over time, spironolactone did appear to improve neurohormonal markers of HF, however did not have a significant effect on symptom scores and slightly decreased 6MWDs (−15 m, p = 0.03).

Comments: Though disappointing, these data could not definitively measure the effect of spironolactone on clinical outcomes in patients with HFpEF.

66. Pitt B, et al. **Spironolactone for heart failure with preserved ejection fraction. N Engl J Med 2014;370:1383–1392.**

Design: Prospective, international, multicenter, double-blind, placebo-controlled, randomized trial. The primary end point was a composite of cardiovascular death, aborted cardiac arrest, or HF hospitalization at a mean follow-up of 3.3 years.

Purpose: To assess the safety and efficacy of spironolactone for chronic treatment of HFpEF to improve clinical outcomes.

Population: 3,445 patients with symptomatic HF and LVEF ≥45%.

Key Exclusion Criteria: Severe renal dysfunction.

Treatment: Spironolactone (15 to 45 mg daily) or placebo.

Results: There was a nonsignificant reduction in the primary end point in the spironolactone group (18.6% vs. 20.4%; p = 0.14). Among the components, only HF hospitalization was significant reduced in the spironolactone group (12.0% vs. 14.2%; p = 0.04). Rate of hyperkalemia was doubled in the spironolactone group (18.7% vs. 9.1%), but serious adverse events were not.

Comments: The results of TOPCAT were disappointing given the lack of medical therapies available to improve clinical outcomes in HFpEF patients. There has been much speculation on the cause of these results, with focus on possible significant heterogeneity of patients enrolled (HFpEF can be more challenging to define clinically, particularly internationally). Nevertheless, spironolactone cannot be recommended broadly in the treatment of patients with HFpEF.

DIGOXIN

67. Hauptman PJ, et al. Digitalis. *Circulation* 1999;99:1265–1270.

This review discusses the molecular and clinical pharmacology of cardiac glycosides, describes the clinical manifestations and treatment of digitalis toxicity, and examines recent trial data, with a focus on the DIG trial results.

68. Packer M, et al.; Randomized Assessment of Effect of Digoxin on Inhibitors of ACE (RADIANCE) study. Withdrawal of digoxin from patients with chronic HF treated with ACE inhibitor. N Engl J Med 1993;329:1–7.

Design: Prospective, randomized, double-blind, placebo-controlled, multicenter study. The primary end point was study withdrawal due to worsening HF, time to withdrawal, and changes in exercise tolerance.

Purpose: To evaluate the effect of the withdrawal of digoxin from patients with chronic HF who were clinically stable while receiving digoxin, diuretics, and an ACE inhibitor.

Population: 178 NYHA class II or III patients taking digoxin, diuretics, and ACE inhibitors (captopril or enalapril).

Exclusion Criteria: SBP, 160 mm Hg or more or <90 mm Hg; DBP, >95 mm Hg; history of supraventricular arrhythmias or sustained ventricular arrhythmias; MI in the prior 3 months; and stroke in the prior 12 months.

Treatment: Patients were randomized to continue digoxin or to placebo for 12 weeks.

Results: Cessation/placebo group had a markedly higher rate of worsening HF requiring withdrawal from the study (24.7% vs. 4.7; RR, 5.9; p < 0.001), lower EF (p < 0.001), decreased functional capacity (maximal exercise tolerance, p = 0.033; submaximal exercise endurance, p = 0.01; NYHA class, p = 0.019), and poorer QOL scores (p = 0.04).

69. Uretsky BF, et al.; Prospective Randomized Study of Ventricular Failure and Efficacy of Digoxin (PROVED). Randomized study assessing effect of digoxin withdrawal in patients with mild–moderate chronic HF. *J Am Coll Cardiol* 1993;22:955–962.

Design: Prospective, randomized, double-blind, placebo-controlled, multicenter study. The primary end point was incidence of treatment failure, time to treatment failure, treadmill time, and 6MWD.

Purpose: To evaluate the effects of digoxin withdrawal in patients with mild-to-moderate HF.

Population: 88 NYHA class II or III patients in normal sinus rhythm and taking digoxin and diuretics.

Exclusion Criteria: SBP <90 mm Hg, acute MI or coronary angioplasty in the prior 72 hours, bypass surgery in the prior 2 weeks, unstable angina in the prior 3 months, and stroke or TIA in the prior 3 months.

Treatment: Patients were randomized to continue digoxin or to placebo for 12 weeks.

Results: Cessation/placebo group had lower exercise tolerance (−96 seconds vs. −4.5 seconds; p = 0.003), twice as many treatment failures (39% vs. 19%; p = 0.039), decreased time to treatment failure (p = 0.037), lower EF (p = 0.016), and higher heart rate (p = 0.003).

70. Digoxin Investigation Group (DIG). The effect of digoxin on mortality and morbidity in patients with heart failure. *N Engl J Med* 1997;336:525–533.

Design: Prospective, randomized, double-blind, placebo-controlled, multicenter study. Follow-up period was 37 months. The primary end point was all-cause mortality rate.

Purpose: To evaluate the effects of digoxin on mortality from any cause in HF patients.

Population: 6,800 patients with an EF of 45% or less and in normal sinus rhythm. Most patients were taking ACE inhibitors (94%) and diuretics (82%).

Treatment: Digoxin (average dose, 0.25 mg/day) or placebo.

Results: No significant difference in mortality rates (34.8% vs. 35.1%) was observed. The digoxin group had fewer HF hospitalizations (26.8% vs. 34.7%; RR, 0.72; p < 0. 001) and showed a trend toward fewer HF deaths (RR, 0.88; p = 0.06), but this was offset by increased mortality due to other cardiac causes (not a prespecified outcome; 15% vs. 13%; p = 0.04). Subgroup analysis showed that greater reductions in death and hospitalization were due to worsening HF if EF <25% (−23% vs. −16%) or NYHA class III/IV (−22% vs. −18%). An overall decrease in hospital stays of only 9 per 1,000 patient-years was observed. An ancillary trial of 988 patients with EF >45% also showed no difference in mortality (both 23.4%).

Comments: Subsequent post hoc subgroup analysis (see *N Engl J Med* 2002;347:1403) showed that among women, a significantly higher mortality was seen in those assigned to digoxin therapy [33.1% vs. 28.9% (no digoxin)]; in contrast, mortality rates were similar in men. This finding among women persisted after a multivariate analysis was performed. Another post hoc analysis of 3,782 men with LVEF ≤45% found that the optimal serum digoxin concentration was 0.5 to 0.8 mg/mL (higher mortality if ≥0.9 mg/mL; see *JAMA* 2003;289:871).

VASODILATORS

71. Cohn JN, et al.; VA Cooperative Heart Failure Trial (V-HeFT I). Effect of vasodilator therapy on mortality in chronic congestive heart failure. *N Engl J Med* 1986;314:1547–1552.

Design: Prospective, randomized, double-blind, placebo-controlled, multicenter study. Mean follow-up period was 2.3 years. The primary end point was all-cause mortality rate.

Purpose: To determine whether two widely used vasodilator regimens could alter life expectancy in men with stable chronic HF.

Population: 642 men aged 18 to 75 years with chronic HF (defined as cardiac dilatation by chest radiography or echocardiography) or EF <45% in association with reduced exercise tolerance.

Exclusion Criteria: Exercise tolerance limited by chest pain, MI in prior 3 months, and requirement for long-acting nitrates, calcium channel antagonists, and/or β-blockers.

Treatment: Prazosin, 20 mg once daily; hydralazine, 300 mg/day; and isosorbide dinitrate, 160 mg/day; or placebo. Digoxin and diuretics were permitted.

Results: Hydralazine–isosorbide dinitrate group had 38% lower mortality at 1 year [12.1% vs. 19.5% (placebo)], 25% reduction at 2 years [25.6% vs. 34.3% (placebo); $p < 0.028$], and 23% reduction at 3 years (36.2% vs. 46.9%). LVEF increased significantly at 8 weeks and at 1 year in the hydralazine–isosorbide dinitrate group (+2.9%, +4.2%; both $p < 0.001$). No significant benefits were seen with prazosin.

72. Cohn JN, et al.; V-HeFT II. A comparison of enalapril with hydralazine–isosorbide dinitrate in the treatment of chronic HF. N Engl J Med 1991;325:303–310.

Design: Prospective, randomized, double-blind, placebo-controlled, multicenter study. Average follow-up period was 2.5 years. The primary end point was 2-year all-cause mortality rate.

Purpose: To compare the efficacy of enalapril with hydralazine plus isosorbide dinitrate in HF patients.

Population: 804 men aged 18 to 75 years in mostly NYHA class II/III and taking digoxin and diuretics.

Exclusion Criteria: MI or cardiac surgery in the prior 3 months and angina limiting exercise or requiring long-term medical therapy.

Treatment: Enalapril, 20 mg/day, or hydralazine, 300 mg/day, plus isosorbide dinitrate, 160 mg/day.

Results: Enalapril group had a 28% lower 2-year mortality rate (18% vs. 25%; $p = 0.016$) and a 14% lower overall mortality rate (32.8% vs. 38.2%; $p = 0.08$). This mortality difference was owing to fewer sudden cardiac deaths (57 patients vs. 92 patients), mostly in NYHA class I or II patients. At 13 weeks, the enalapril group had a greater reduction in BP, whereas the hydralazine–isosorbide dinitrate group had a greater increase in EF and exercise tolerance.

73. Taylor AL, et al. Combination of isosorbide dinitrate and hydralazine in blacks with heart failure (A-HeFT). N Engl J Med 2004;351:2049–2057.

Design: Prospective, randomized, double-blind, placebo-controlled multicenter trial. The primary end point was a weighted score composed of all-cause mortality, HF hospitalization, and QOL.

Purpose: To determine whether fixed-dose combination isosorbide dinitrate and hydralazine provides additional benefit in blacks with advanced HF.

Population: 1,050 black patients with NYHA class III or IV, dilated HF.

Treatment: Fixed-dose combination isosorbide dinitrate plus hydralazine or placebo.

Results: The study was terminated early due to significantly increased all-cause mortality in the placebo arm (10.2% vs. 6.2%; $p = 0.02$), which also had a lower mean primary composite score (−0.5 vs. −0.1; p = 0.01). All components of the composite score also significantly favored the isosorbide dinitrate plus hydralazine arm.

Comments: This trial led to the first FDA approval of a drug for *a specific racial group.*

74. Packer M, et al.; Prospective Randomized Amlodipine Survival Evaluation (PRAISE). Effect of amlodipine on morbidity and mortality in severe chronic heart failure. N *Engl J Med* 1996;335:1107–1114.

Design: Prospective, randomized, double-blind, placebo-controlled, multicenter study. Average follow-up period was 14 months. The primary end point was mortality and CV morbidity [hospitalization for 24 hours for MI, pulmonary edema, severe hypoperfusion, VT, or ventricular fibrillation (VF)].

Purpose: To assess the safety and efficacy of the calcium channel antagonist amlodipine in patients with severe chronic HF.

Population: 1,153 patients with an EF <30%. HF was associated with ischemic disease in 732 (63.5%) patients.

Exclusion Criteria: Unstable angina or MI in the prior month, cardiac arrest or sustained VT or VF in the prior year, stroke or cardiac revascularization in the prior 3 months, SBP <85 or 160 mm Hg or more, active myocarditis, constrictive pericarditis, and primary valvular disease.

Treatment: Amlodipine, 10 mg/day (5 mg/day for first 2 weeks), or placebo.

Results: Amlodipine group had a nonsignificant 9% lower incidence in the primary end point (39% vs. 42%; p = 0.31). It also had a nonsignificant 16% mortality reduction (33% vs. 38%; p = 0.07). Among nonischemic patients, amlodipine was associated with a 46% lower mortality rate (p < 0.001) and 31% fewer overall events (p = 0.04).

Comments: An interesting ancillary study of cytokines showed that high interleukin-6 levels correlated with increased HF and death (p = 0.048) and were reduced by amlodipine (p = 0.006) but to values still more than five times normal.

75. Packer M, et al. Effect of amlodipine on the survival of patients with severe chronic heart failure due to a nonischemic cardiomyopathy: results of the PRAISE-2 study (prospective randomized amlodipine survival evaluation 2). *JACC Heart Failure* 2013;1:308–314. PRAISE-2 (preliminary results originally presented at the 49th Annual American College of Cardiology Scientific Sessions, Anaheim, CA, November 2000).

Design: Prospective, randomized, double-blind, placebo-controlled, multicenter study. The primary end point was all-cause mortality and CV morbidity (hospitalization for 24 hours for MI, pulmonary edema, severe hypoperfusion, VT, or VF). Median follow-up was 33 months.

Purpose: To assess the safety and efficacy of the calcium channel antagonist amlodipine in patients with severe nonischemic chronic HF.

Population: 1,654 patients with an EF <30% and NYHA class IIIb or IV symptoms despite therapy with diuretics, ACE inhibitors, and digoxin.

Key Exclusion Criteria: Included therapy with calcium channel blockers, β-blockers, or cardiodepressant antiarrhythmic drugs; unstable angina or MI in the prior month; cardiac arrest or sustained VT or VF in the prior year; stroke or cardiac revascularization in the prior 3 months; SBP <85 or 160 mm Hg or greater; primary valvular disease.

Treatment: Amlodipine, 10 mg/day (5 mg/day for first 2 weeks), or placebo.

Results: No significant difference was found between the groups in all-cause mortality [262 (placebo), 278 (amlodipine); hazard ratio for amlodipine, 1.09; 95% CI, 0.92 to 1.29; p = 0.33]. No subgroup was found to receive a mortality benefit with amlodipine.

Comments: Further analysis using the combined population of PRAISE-1 and PRAISE-2 showed no significant differences in all-cause mortality.

76. Colucci WS, et al.; for Nesiritide Study Group. Intravenous nesiritide, a natriuretic peptide, in the treatment of decompensated congestive heart failure. N *Engl J Med* 2000;343:246–253.

Design: Prospective, randomized, partially blinded, partially open, multicenter trial. The primary end point: change in pulmonary capillary pressure from baseline to 6 hours (efficacy trial); global clinical status and clinical symptoms (comparative trial).

Purpose: To evaluate an intravenous infusion of nesiritide, a BNP, in patients with decompensated HF.

Population: Efficacy study—127 patients with a PCWP of 18 mm Hg or more and cardiac index of 2.7 L/min/m^2; comparative trial, 305 patients.

Exclusion Criteria: Included dopamine, dobutamine, or intravenous vasodilator infusion for more than 4 hours; MI or unstable angina in the previous 48 hours; clinically significant valvular stenosis; hypertrophic or restrictive cardiomyopathy; constrictive pericarditis; or active myocarditis.

Treatment: Efficacy trial—Swan–Ganz catheter placed and randomization to double-blind treatment with intravenous placebo or nesiritide (0.015 or 0.030 µg/kg/min) for 6 hours. Comparative trial: hemodynamic monitoring not required and open-label therapy with standard agents or nesiritide for up to 7 days.

Results: In the efficacy trial, at 6 hours, nesiritide was associated with significant reductions in PCWP (6.0 and 9.6 mm Hg for 0.015 and 0.030 µg/kg/min, respectively, versus +2.0 mm Hg with placebo; $p < 0.001$). It was also associated with improved global clinical status in 60% and 67% of patients (vs. 14% in placebo group; $p < 0.001$), less dyspnea [57% and 53% vs. 12% (placebo); $p < 0.001$], and less fatigue [32% and 38% vs. 5% (placebo); $p < 0.001$]. In the comparative trial, the improvements in global clinical status, dyspnea, and fatigue were sustained with nesiritide therapy for up to 7 days and were similar to those seen with standard intravenous therapy for HF. The most common side effect was dose-related hypotension [symptomatic: 11% and 17% vs. 4%, $p = 0.008$ (comparative); 2% and 5% vs. none, $p = 0.55$ (efficacy)].

77. Publication Committee for the VMAC Investigators (Vasodilatation in the Management of Acute HF). Intravenous nesiritide vs nitroglycerin for treatment of decompensated congestive heart failure: a randomized controlled trial. JAMA 2002;287:1531–1540.

Design: Prospective, randomized, double-blind trial. The primary end points were change in PCWP in catheterized patients and self-evaluation of dyspnea at 3 hours after initiation of study drug.

Population: 489 inpatients with dyspnea at rest from decompensated HF, including 246 who received pulmonary artery catheterization (PAC).

Treatment: Intravenous nesiritide, intravenous nitroglycerin, or placebo added to standard medications for 3 hours, followed by nesiritide or nitroglycerin added to standard medication for 24 hours.

Results: At 3 hours, the mean decrease in PCWP from baseline was greater with nesiritide compared with placebo ($p < 0.001$) and nitroglycerin ($p = 0.03$). At 3 hours, nesiritide resulted in improvement in dyspnea compared with placebo ($p = 0.03$), but no significant difference was found between nesiritide and nitroglycerin in dyspnea or global clinical status. At 24 hours, the reduction in PCWP was greater in the nesiritide group (8.2 mm Hg) than in the nitroglycerin group (6.3 mm Hg), but no significant difference was noted in dyspnea and only modest improvement in global clinical status.

78. Sackner-Bernstein JD, et al. Short-term risk of death after treatment with nesiritide for decompensated heart failure: a pooled analysis of randomized controlled trials. *JAMA* 2005;293:1900–1905.

The authors reviewed the primary reports of completed clinical trials (as of December 2004), which predominantly compared nesiritide to diuretics or vasodilators. Data came from the sponsor (Scios Inc.), the FDA, PubMed, and scientific meetings manuals. The final study included 3 of 12 (862 patients total) randomized trials identified, as the remainder did not meet inclusion criteria of randomized, double-blinded trials in patients with acutely decompensated HF. Overall, all-cause mortality at 30 days trended to be higher in the nesiritide group (7.2% vs. 4.0%; RR, 1.74; p = 0.059). The meta-analysis signaled the possible harm caused by routine infusion of nesiritide for acutely decompensated HF.

79. O'Connor CM, et al.; The ASCEND-HF trial. Effect of nesiritide in patients with acute decompensated heart failure. *N Engl J Med* 2011;365:32–43.

Design: Prospective, international, multicenter, double-blind, placebo-controlled, randomized trial. The coprimary end points were change in dyspnea scores at 6 and 24 hours, and composite clinical end point of HF hospitalization or death at 30 days.

Purpose: To assess the safety of nesiritide in patients with acute HF, and its efficacy at improving dyspnea.

Population: 7,141 patients with acute HF including both symptoms, and at least 1 objective sign (this included radiography, laboratory, or echocardiographic criteria).

Exclusion Criteria: High risk of hypotension or concurrent treatment with inotropic agents.

Treatment: Nesiritide infusion or placebo infusion for 24 to 168 hours.

Results: Self-reported dyspnea scores improved more commonly in patients assigned to nesiritide versus placebo at 6 hours (44.5% vs. 42.1%; p = 0.03) and at 24 hours (68.2% vs. 66.1%; p = 0.007); however, these did not meet the prespecified levels for statistical significance ($p \leq 0.005$ for both or $p \leq 0.0025$ for both). Rates of HF hospitalization or death were 9.4% in the nesiritide group versus 10.1% for placebo (p = 0.31). Rates of worsening renal function were similar; however, significant hypotension developed more commonly in the nesiritide group (26.6% vs. 15.3%; $p < 0.001$).

Comments: This study provided some reassurance that nesiritide was not associated with increased mortality within 30 days of its use; nevertheless, the authors concluded that it has a limited role in the care of HF patients, owing to its marginal benefits and side effect profile.

80. Chen HH, et al. Low-dose dopamine or low-dose nesiritide in acute heart failure with renal dysfunction: the ROSE acute heart failure randomized trial. *JAMA* 2013;310:2533–2543.

Design: Prospective, multicenter, double-randomized, placebo-controlled clinical trial. The coprimary end points were cumulative urine volume and change in serum cystatin C, both at 72 hours.

Purpose: To assess the utility of adding either low-dose dopamine or nesiritide to usual diuretic treatment of acute HF.

Population: 360 patients hospitalized within 24 hours for acute HF complicated by renal dysfunction.

Treatment: Patients were first open randomized (1:1) to either the dopamine (n = 177) or nesiritide (n = 183) arms. Subsequently, they were blindly randomized to either active treatment or placebo (2:1 favoring active treatment).

Results: Neither dopamine nor nesiritide had significant effect on cumulative urine volume, and neither had effects on 72-hour change in cystatin C levels. Additional analyses did not yield any significant benefits to either agent, over placebo, for congestion, renal function, or clinical outcomes.

AMIODARONE

81. Doval HC, et al.; Grupo de Estudio de la Sobrevida en la Insuficiencia Cardiaca en Argentina (GESICA). Randomized trial of low-dose amiodarone in severe HF. *Lancet* 1994;344:493–498.

Design: Prospective, randomized, open, parallel-group, multicenter study. Follow-up period was 2 years. The primary end point was total mortality.

Purpose: To evaluate the effect of low-dose amiodarone on mortality in patients with severe HF without symptomatic ventricular arrhythmias.

Population: 516 NYHA class II to IV patients with stable functional capacity and not requiring antiarrhythmic therapy.

Exclusion Criteria: Amiodarone treatment during the prior 3 months; MI, HF onset, or syncope in the prior 3 months; and history of sustained VT or VF.

Treatment: Amiodarone, 500 mg/day for 14 days, and then 300 mg once daily for 2 years; or standard therapy (diuretics, digoxin, ACE inhibitors).

Results: Amiodarone group had 28% RR in mortality at 2 years (33.5% vs. 41.4%; $p = 0.024$) and 31% RR in hospitalization due to worsening HF (45.8% vs. 58.2%; $p = 0.0024$). Reductions were seen in both sudden death (27% RR; $p = 0.16$) and death due to progressive HF (23% risk reduction; $p = 0.16$). These benefits were present in all examined subgroups and were independent of the presence of nonsustained VT. Side effects were reported in 17 (6.1%) amiodarone patients, of whom 12 discontinued therapy.

Comments: The study was blinded only to coordination center personnel, had a unique population (10% with Chagas disease), and was terminated at the two-thirds point.

82. Singh SN, et al.; Survival Trial of Antiarrhythmic Therapy in HF (HF-STAT). Amiodarone in patients with congestive heart failure and asymptomatic ventricular arrhythmia. N *Engl J Med* 1995;333:77–82 (editorial, 121–122).

Design: Prospective, randomized, double-blind, placebo-controlled, multicenter study. The primary end point was overall mortality and sudden death from cardiac causes. Follow-up period was 45 months.

Purpose: To evaluate the effect of antiarrhythmic therapy on mortality in patients with HF and asymptomatic ventricular arrhythmia.

Population: 674 patients with symptoms of HF, cardiac enlargement, fewer than 10 premature ventricular contractions, and EF of 40% or less.

Exclusion Criteria: MI in the prior 3 months, history of cardiac arrest or sustained VT, need for antiarrhythmic therapy, and SBP <90 mm Hg.

Treatment: Amiodarone, 800 mg/day for 14 days, 400 mg/day for 50 weeks, and then 300 mg/day; or placebo. Other therapy consisted of vasodilators (all patients), with or without digoxin or diuretics.

Results: No significant differences were found in mortality or sudden death [30.6% (amiodarone) vs. 29.2%; 15% vs. 19%; $p = 0.43$]. However, amiodarone was associated with a trend toward lower mortality in the subgroup of patients with nonischemic cardiomyopathy ($p = 0.07$). The amiodarone group also had better suppression of ventricular arrhythmias and a greater increase in EF at 2 years (+10.5% vs. + 4.1%).

Comments: This VA-based trial had notable differences compared with GESICA—older patients (+6 years), more men (GESICA, 48% lower mortality in females vs. 26% in men), and healthier patients with higher EFs. However, subgroup analysis showed that the greatest benefits in HF-STAT occurred in NYHA class II patients.

INOTROPIC AND OTHER AGENTS

83. DiBianco R, et al. A comparison of oral milrinone, digoxin and their combination in the treatment of patients with chronic heart failure. N Engl J Med 1989;320:677–683.

This prospective, randomized trial was composed of 230 patients comparing 12 weeks of digoxin, milrinone, and their combination. Both agents alone improved exercise tolerance (+64 seconds vs. +82 seconds) and lowered frequency of decompensation [15% and 34% vs. 47% (placebo)]. Overall, no significant difference was found between the effects of the two drugs. Milrinone and digoxin were no better than digoxin alone.

84. Packer M, et al.; Prospective Randomized Milrinone Survival Evaluation (PROMISE). Effect of oral milrinone on mortality in severe chronic heart failure. N Engl J Med 1991;325:1468–1475.

Design: Prospective, randomized, double-blind, placebo-controlled, multicenter study. Mean follow-up period was 6.1 months. The primary end point was all-cause mortality.

Purpose: To evaluate the effect of oral administration of the phosphodiesterase milrinone on mortality in patients with severe HF.

Population: 1,088 NYHA class III or IV patients and EF <35%.

Exclusion Criteria: Obstructive valvular disease; history of serious ventricular arrhythmia; MI in prior 3 months; SBP <85 mm Hg; and requirement for β-blockers, calcium channel blockers, and antiarrhythmic drugs.

Treatment: Milrinone, 40 mg/day orally, or placebo. All patients were on digoxin, diuretics, and ACE inhibitors.

Results: Study was terminated early. Milrinone was associated with significantly higher all-cause mortality (30% vs. 24%; $p = 0.038$) and CV mortality rates (29.4% vs. 22.6%; $p = 0.016$). The milrinone group had a 69% increased risk of sudden cardiac deaths ($p = 0.005$), whereas no increased risk of death was found because of progressive HF. Adverse effects were worst among class IV patients (53% higher mortality; $p = 0.006$).

85. Cohn JN, et al.; for the Vesnarinone Trial Investigators. A dose-dependent increase in mortality with vesnarinone among patients with severe heart failure. N Engl J Med 1998;339:1801–1806.

This prospective, randomized, double-blind, placebo-controlled, multicenter study enrolled 3,833 patients with NYHA class III or IV HF and an LVEF 30% or less despite optimal treatment (any regimen of diuretics, vasodilators, ACE inhibitor, and digitalis). Patients received vesnarinone (30 or 60 mg) or placebo once daily. At follow-up (mean, 286 days), the placebo group had significantly fewer deaths than did the 60-mg vesnarinone group (18.9% vs. 22.9%; $p = 0.02$). Increased mortality with vesnarinone was mostly owing to increased sudden death rate (12.3% vs. 9.1%). QOL (assessed by Minnesota Living with Heart Failure Questionnaire) improved significantly more in the 60-mg vesnarinone group than in the placebo group at 8 weeks ($p < 0.001$) and 16 weeks ($p = 0.003$), but by 26 weeks, the differences were no longer significant. Agranulocytosis occurred in 1.2% and 0.2% of those given vesnarinone, 60 and 30 mg/day, respectively.

86. Packer M, et al. Comparison of omapatrilat and enalapril in patients with chronic heart failure: the Omapatrilat Versus Enalapril Randomized Trial of Utility in Reducing Events (OVERTURE). Circulation 2002;106:920–926.

Design: Prospective, randomized, placebo-controlled, blinded, parallel-group, multicenter trial. The primary end point was all-cause mortality or hospitalization for HF. Average follow-up, 15 months.

Purpose: To prove superiority or noninferiority of the vasopeptidase inhibitor omapatrilat compared to enalapril in patients with HF.

Population: 5,770 patients with NYHA class II to IV HF for more than 2 months due to ischemic or nonischemic heart disease, EF <30%, hospitalized for HF in the past year, and receiving diuretics at the time of enrollment.

Exclusion Criteria: Included reversible cause(s) of HF, no HF admission in the previous 48 hours, probable cardiac transplant or LVAD candidate, acute coronary syndrome in the previous month, coronary revascularization or an acute cerebral ischemic event in the previous 3 months, and history of VT, VF, or sudden death (unless ICD had been placed and had not fired in the previous 2 months).

Treatment: Omapatrilat, 40 mg/day, or enalapril, 20 mg/day.

Results: A nonsignificant trend was found toward a lower incidence of death or hospitalization for HF in the omapatrilat group compared with the enalapril group (32% vs. 34%; p = 0.19). All-cause mortality rates were not significantly different (17% vs. 18%). The trend was strong enough to show that omapatrilat was not inferior to enalapril.

87. Cuffe MS, et al.; for the Outcomes of a Prospective Trial of Intravenous Milrinone for Exacerbations of Chronic Heart Failure (OPTIME-HF) Investigators. Short-term intravenous milrinone for acute exacerbation of chronic heart failure: a randomized controlled trial. JAMA 2002;287:1541–1547.

This trial randomized 951 patients with exacerbation of chronic HF not requiring intravenous inotropic support to 48 hours of milrinone or placebo. A total of the median number of days hospitalized for CV causes within 60 days after randomization did not differ significantly between patients given milrinone (6 days) compared with placebo (7 days; p = 0.71). Sustained hypotension requiring intervention (10.7% vs. 3.2%; p < 0.001) and new atrial arrhythmias (4.6% vs. 1.5%; p = 0.004) occurred more frequently in patients who received milrinone. The milrinone and placebo groups did not differ significantly in in-hospital mortality (3.8% vs. 2.3%; p = 0.19) or 60-day mortality (10.3% vs. 8.9%).

88. Ghali JK, et al. Efficacy and safety of oral conivaptan: a V1A/V2 vasopressin receptor antagonist, assessed in a randomized, placebo-controlled trial in patients with euvolemic or hypervolemic hyponatremia. J Clin Endocrinol Metab 2006;91:2145–2152.

In this early, pivotal trial of vasopressin antagonists, investigators randomly assigned 74 patients with euvolemic or hypervolemic hyponatremia to either conivaptan or placebo. They assessed change in serum sodium from baseline (measured by area under the curve) after 5 days. Conivaptan led to faster and more significant improvement in serum sodium, compared to placebo, at the expense of increased rates of headache, hypotension, nausea, and constipation.

89. Schrier RW, et al.; The SALT-1 and SALT-2 Trials. Tolvaptan, a selective oral vasopressin V2-receptor antagonist, for hyponatremia. N Engl J Med 2006;355:2099–2112.

Design: Two, prospective, randomized, placebo-controlled, double-blinded, multicenter trials. The two primary end points were change in average daily sodium (area under the curve) at 4 days and at 30 days.

Purpose: To assess the safety and efficacy of tolvaptan for treatment of hyponatremia due to cirrhosis or HF.

Population: 448 patients with euvolemic or hypervolemic hyponatremia; approximately 30% of patients overall had hyponatremia due to HF and mean baseline serum sodium was approximately 129.

Key Exclusion Criteria: Hypovolemia, or relative hypotension; serum sodium <120 mmol/L in association with neurologic sequelae.

Treatment: Tolvaptan (15 mg) or placebo; tolvaptan dose was subsequently increased to 30 mg and 60 mg daily, if necessary.

Results: Increase in sodium concentration was significantly higher in the tolvaptan group, versus placebo, at both 4 days ($p < 0.001$) and 30 days ($p < 0.001$). There was a rebound effect in the tolvaptan group after day 30, however.

90. Gheorghiade M, et al. Short-term clinical effects of tolvaptan, an oral vasopressin antagonist, in patients hospitalized for heart failure: the EVEREST Clinical Status Trials. JAMA 2007;297:1332–1343.

Design: Two identical prospective, multicenter, international, double-blind, placebo-controlled, randomized trial. The primary end point was a composite of changes in global clinical status and body weight at day 7 (or discharge).

Purpose: To assess the acute treatment effects of tolvaptan in patients hospitalized with HF.

Population: Two cohorts of patients hospitalized for HF with LVEF ≤40%; 2,048 patients in trial A and 2,085 patients in trial B.

Key Exclusion Criteria: Relative hypotension or severe renal dysfunction.

Treatment: Tolvaptan (30 mg daily) or placebo.

Results: Tolvaptan resulted in improvement in the composite primary outcome, as well as more significant weight loss when compared to placebo at 7 days (trial A, 3.35 kg lost vs. 2.73 kg for placebo, $p < 0.001$; and trial B, 3.77 kg lost vs. 2.79 kg for placebo, $p < 0.001$). While more patients noted improved dyspnea on tolvaptan (trial A, 76.7% vs. 70.6%; trial B, 72.1% vs. 65.3%; $p < 0.001$ for both), there was no difference in global clinical status between tolvaptan and placebo.

91. Konstam MA, et al. Effects of oral tolvaptan in patients hospitalized for worsening heart failure: the EVEREST Outcome Trial. JAMA 2007;297:1319–1331.

The EVEREST Outcome trial was the culmination of the above EVEREST Clinical Status Trials to assess the effect of tolvaptan on hard, clinical end points. In the overall 4,133-patient population, the dual primary end points were all-cause mortality and cardiovascular death or HF hospitalization. After a median of 9.9 months follow-up, tolvaptan had no effect on all-cause mortality (25.9% vs. 26.3%, $p = 0.68$) nor on cardiovascular morbidity (42% vs. 40.2%, $p = 0.55$).

MECHANICAL ASSIST DEVICES AND SURGICAL OPTIONS

92. Mancini D, et al. Comparison of exercise performance in patients with chronic severe heart failure versus left ventricular assist devices. Circulation 1998;98:1178–1183.

Metabolic exercise testing was performed in 65 HF and 20 LVAD patients. Peak oxygen consumption was significantly higher in the LVAD group (15.9 mL/kg/min vs. 12.0 mL/kg/min; $p < 0.001$). At peak exercise, the LVAD group also had a significantly higher HR, BP, and cardiac output, whereas PCWP was lower (14 mm Hg vs. 31 mm Hg; $p < 0.001$). LVAD patients also had better hemodynamic measurements at rest, including higher cardiac output and lower PCWP.

93. Mancini DM, et al. Low incidence of myocardial recovery after left ventricular assist device implantation in patients with chronic heart failure. Circulation 1998;98:2383–2389.

A retrospective chart review of 111 LVAD recipients identified only 5 successfully explanted patients. A prospective attempt to identify explantable patients by using exercise testing was then undertaken on 39 consecutive patients, of whom 15 were able to exercise with maximal device support. Peak average oxygen consumption was 14.5 mL/kg/min, and Fick cardiac output 11.4 L/min. Seven patients remained normotensive while exercising at 20 cycles/min, and their peak oxygen consumption decreased from 17.3 to 13.0 mL/kg/min. In one of these patients, the LVAD was successfully explanted.

94. Rose EA, et al.; Randomized Evaluation of Mechanical Assistance for the Treatment of Congestive Heart Failure (REMATCH) Study Group. Long-term mechanical left ventricular assistance for end-stage heart failure. *N Engl J Med* 2001;345:1435–1443.

Design: Prospective, randomized, multicenter trial. The primary end point was all-cause mortality or hospitalization for HF. Average follow-up, 14.5 months.

Purpose: To prove superiority of the implantable LVAD compared with standard therapy in patients with end-stage HF.

Population: 129 patients with end-stage HF who were ineligible for cardiac transplantation.

Exclusion Criteria: Included eligibility for cardiac transplantation, absence of symptoms of NYHA class IV in the previous 90 days, EF 25% or less, or a peak oxygen consumption of more than 14 mL/kg/min.

Treatment: A vented electric LVAD or optimal medical therapy. Patients could continue β-blockers if they had been administered for at least 60 of the 90 days before randomization.

Results: The LVAD group had a 48% reduction in mortality compared with the medical therapy group ($p = 0.001$). At 1 year, survival rates were 52% in the LVAD group and 25% in the medical therapy group ($p = 0.002$), whereas the rates at 2 years were 23% and 8% ($p = 0.09$), respectively. The frequency of serious adverse events in the LVAD was 2.35 times that in the medical therapy group (95% CI, 1.86 to 2.95), with a predominance of infection, bleeding, and malfunction of the device. The QOL was significantly improved at 1 year in the LVAD group.

Comments: Because fewer than 25% of LVAD patients were alive at 2 years, these results may not be of sufficient magnitude to convince the medical community and insurance companies that this technology (or at least this particular device) can be considered a good alternative to transplantation.

95. Slaughter MS, et al. Advanced heart failure treated with continuous-flow left ventricular assist device. *N Engl J Med* 2009;361:2241–2251.

Design: Randomized trial. Primary composite end point was survival free from disabling stroke and repair or replacement of the device at 2 years.

Purpose: To compare continuous-flow LVAD to older pulsatile-flow LVAD and the effect on long-term outcomes.

Population: A total of 200 patients were randomly assigned (in 2:1 ratio) to undergo implantation of a continuous-flow LVAD (134 patients) or a pulsatile-flow LVAD (66 patients). Previously, 60% had undergone CRT, and by the time of surgery, roughly 80% were receiving intravenous inotropes and 20% had an intra-aortic balloon pump.

Results: The continuous-flow device demonstrated better primary end point achievement at 2 years, compared to the pulsatile-flow device (46% vs. 11%; $p < 0.001$), and patients with continuous-flow devices had better survival rates at 2 years (58% vs. 24%; $p = 0.008$). For secondary end points, the continuous-flow device proved superior in terms of reduced adverse events and device replacement and improved QOL and functional capacity.

Comments: The 1-year survival of only 68% in the continuous-flow device group was attributed to early deaths in this patient population due to the advanced nature of their disease at the time of device implantation. Future studies will likely evaluate the benefit of implantation in patients with less-advanced disease.

96. Aaronson KD, et al. Use of an intrapericardial, continuous-flow, centrifugal pump in patients awaiting heart transplantation. *Circulation* 2012;125:3191–3200.

This was one of the first trials to demonstrate the safety and feasibility of a new LVAD device, the HeartWare pump, in patients requiring mechanical circulatory support awaiting transplant. The HeartWare was designed to be smaller, to fit in the pericardium, and with less metal-on-metal wear and tear (for durability). The investigators implanted to new device in 140 patients and compared their outcomes to 499 patients contemporaneously treated with an approved LVAD at the time. The investigational pump was successfully implanted in 90.7% of patients (vs. 09.1% of controls, $p < 0.001$ for noninferiority). They noted improvements in functional capacity and quality of life commensurate with the contemporaneous pump, with good short-term safety results.

97. Hernandez AF, et al. Long-term outcomes and costs of ventricular assist devices among Medicare beneficiaries. JAMA 2008;300:2398–2406.

As the burden of HF increases and the availability of LVADs has become more widespread, their use increased dramatically. This has been particularly true among older patients, who may not be candidates for cardiac transplantation. This landmark analysis looked at the use and outcomes of LVADs in nearly 3,000 US Medicare beneficiaries. They noted significant mortality (30% to 50% at 1 year) and morbidity (rehospitalization up to 50% within 6 months) for these patients, as well as the consequent financial costs. This analysis highlights the risks and costs of deploying a novel technology across broader populations of patients with disease.

98. Jones RH, et al.; STICH Hypothesis 2 Investigators. Coronary bypass surgery with or without surgical ventricular reconstruction. N Engl J Med 2009;360:1705–1717.

Design: A multicenter, nonblinded, randomized trial at 127 clinical sites in 26 countries. The primary outcome was the time to death from any cause or hospitalization for cardiac causes. Secondary outcomes included death from any cause at 30 days, and hospitalization for any cause and for cardiovascular causes, MI, and stroke.

Purpose: The trial included two major components. Patients in the Hypothesis 1 component were randomly assigned to receive either medical therapy alone or medical therapy plus CABG. The Hypothesis 1 component of the trial is reported below. Patients in the Hypothesis 2 component were randomly assigned to receive either medical therapy plus CABG or medical therapy plus CABG and SVR. The results of the Hypothesis 2 component are described herein.

Population: Patients were eligible for enrollment if they had surgically appropriate CAD and a LV EF of ≤35%.

Results: SVR reduced the ESV index by 19%, as compared with a reduction of 6% with CABG alone. Cardiac symptoms and exercise capacity improved similarly in the two groups. However, no significant difference was observed in the primary outcome, death, or cardiac rehospitalization (59% in the CABG-alone group vs. 58% for CABG plus SVR group, $p = 0.90$).

99. Velazquez EJ, et al. Coronary-artery bypass surgery in patients with left ventricular dysfunction. N Engl J Med 2011;364:1607–1616.

In these results of the Hypothesis 1 cohort, 1,212 patients with LVEF ≤35% with CAD were randomized to either CABG or medical therapy alone. The primary outcome of all-cause mortality at a median follow-up of 56 months was not different in the 2 groups (36% for CABG vs. 41% for medical therapy, $p = 0.12$). However, there was a trend toward lower cardiovascular mortality in the CABG group (28% vs. 33%, $p = 0.05$). Nevertheless, this has led to reevaluation of the uniform use of surgical revascularization in patients with severe CAD and LV dysfunction.

100. Acker MA, et al. Mitral-valve repair versus replacement for severe ischemic mitral regurgitation. N Engl J Med 2014;370:23–32.

As part of the Cardiothoracic Surgical Trials Network, the investigators randomized 251 patients with severe ischemic MR to undergo mitral-vale repair or chordal-sparing mitral valve replacement. Roughly three-quarters underwent concomitant CABG surgery, and the primary end point was LV ESV index at 12 months. Valve replacement provided a more durable improvement in regurgitation (moderate/severe MR at 12 months: 2.3% vs. 32.6%, $p < 0.00$), and there was no difference in LVESVI between the cohorts.

INVASIVE THERAPY

101. Binanay C, et al. Evaluation study of congestive heart failure and pulmonary artery catheterization effectiveness: the ESCAPE trial. JAMA 2005;294:1625–1633.

Design: Multicenter, randomized controlled trial. The primary end point was days alive out of the hospital during the first 6 months.

Purpose: To determine whether PAC is safe and effective for improving outcomes in hospitalized patients with severe HF.

Population: 433 patients hospitalized for HF, meeting one of the three severity criteria: (1) HF hospitalization within the previous year; (2) urgent visit to the ED; or (3) treatment during the previous month with more than 160 mg of furosemide daily (or equivalent). Additionally, patients had to have had at least 3 months of symptoms despite ACE inhibitors and diuretics, EF ≤30%, systolic BP ≤125 mm Hg, and at least one sign and one symptom of congestion.

Treatment: HF management guided by PAC placement or by clinical assessment. For both groups, target PCWP was 15 mm Hg and target right atrial pressure was 8 mm Hg.

Results: There was no significant difference in the primary outcome, between the two groups (133 days for the PAC group vs. 135 days for clinical assessment; $p = 0.99$). Mortality and days in the hospital were also not different. However, patients in the PAC group did have higher incidence of in-hospital complications (21.9% vs. 25; $p = 0.04$).

Comments: There was a trend toward improved outcomes at centers in the trial with higher enrollment and greater experience with PA catheters, suggesting that PA catheters may be beneficial if monitored closely by an experienced clinical team and if the data are acted upon quickly and appropriately.

102. Constanza MR, et al.; for the UNLOAD Trial Investigators. Ultrafiltration versus intravenous diuretics for patients hospitalized for acute decompensated heart failure. J Am Coll Cardiol 2007;49:675–683.

The investigators randomized 200 patients with acute, hypervolemic, decompensated HF to either standard intravenous diuretic therapy or intravenous ultrafiltration for fluid and sodium removal. None of the patients was in cardiogenic shock, and all had baseline serum creatinine levels of <3.0 mg/dL. Patients in the ultrafiltration group had greater overall average weight loss at 48 hours, the primary end point (5.0 kg vs. 3.1 kg; $p = 0.001$). There were no differences in acute renal failure, hypotension, or adverse events between the groups. Additionally, while there were improvements in subjective dyspnea similarly in both groups, patients' report of improvement did *not* correlate with amount of fluid removed (in either group). Notably, patients in the ultrafiltration group had significantly lower rates of rehospitalization and rehospitalization days at 90 days. Additionally, those in the ultrafiltration group required lower doses of oral diuretic at discharge than did those in the standard intravenous diuretic group, suggesting that ultrafiltration may have a "sparing" effect on the kidney.

103. Klersy C, et al. A meta-analysis of remote monitoring of heart failure patients. J Am Coll Cardiol 2009;54:1683–1694.

The authors reviewed and combined 20 randomized controlled trials and 12 cohort studies of remote patient monitoring for chronic HF. The combined populations included 6,258 and 2,354 patients, respectively, over follow-up of 6 to 12 months. These included in-person remote follow-up (by telephone), as well as technology-based remote monitoring. The authors noted that both randomized trials and cohort studies consistently found that remote monitoring was associated with significantly lower mortality (RR, 0.83; p = 0.006 for randomized trials; RR, 0.53; p < 0.001 for cohorts) and hospitalizations (RR, 0.93; p = 0.03 for randomized trials; RR, 0.52; p < 0.001 for cohorts). They conclude that remote monitoring conveys a consistent and significant reduction in HF morbidity and mortality.

104. Abraham WT, et al.; The CHAMPION Trial. Wireless pulmonary artery haemodynamic monitoring in chronic heart failure: a randomised controlled trial. *Lancet* 2011;377:658–666.

In this proof-of-concept study, investigators at 64 US centers implanted wireless implantable hemodynamic monitoring systems in 550 patients with NYHA III HF (irrespective of LVEF). Patients were blinded and randomly assigned to either usual care (control) or active monitoring whereby their physician would have access to daily hemodynamic monitoring. After 6 months of follow-up, HF hospitalizations were significantly reduced in the active monitoring group (0.32 vs. 0.44; HR, 0.72; p = 0.0002). Of the overall cohort, eight patients experienced device failure or complication.

ADDITIONAL THERAPEUTIC CONSIDERATIONS

105. Rich MW, et al. A multidisciplinary intervention to prevent the readmission of elderly patients with congestive heart failure. *N Engl J Med* 1995;333:1190–1195.

This prospective, randomized trial was composed of 282 high-risk patients aged 70 years or older hospitalized with HF. Patients were assigned to standard care (control group) or nurse-directed, multidisciplinary care, consisting of comprehensive education of the patient and family, a prescribed diet, social service consultation, medication review, and intensive follow-up. A trend was noted toward improved survival without readmission (primary end point) in the multidisciplinary intervention group (64.1% vs. 53.6%; p = 0.09). The total number of hospital admissions was significantly lower in the multidisciplinary intervention group (53 vs. 94; p = 0.02), including 56% fewer HF-related admissions (24 vs. 54; p = 0.04). The intervention group had an overall lower cost of care ($460 less per patient). Finally, in a subgroup of 126 patients, QOL scores at 90 days improved significantly more in the intervention patients (p = 0.001).

106. Riegel B, et al. State of the science: promoting self-care in persons with heart failure: a scientific statement from the American Heart Association. *Circulation* 2009;120:1141–1163.

This statement from the AHA provided background and support to aspects of HF management that begin with the patient. The authors call attention to the many patient-based interventions, often known as "lifestyle modifications," that may improve outcomes in HF, as well as paradigms for maintenance and management of patient self care.

Anticoagulation

107. Massie BM, et al. Randomized trial of warfarin, aspirin, and clopidogrel in patients with chronic heart failure: the Warfarin and Antiplatelet Therapy in Chronic Heart Failure (WATCH) trial. *Circulation* 2009;119(12):1616–1624.

Design: Prospective, randomized, clinical trial. The primary outcome was the time to first occurrence of death, nonfatal MI, or nonfatal stroke.

Purpose: To determine the optimal antithrombotic agent for HF patients with reduced EFs who are in sinus rhythm.

Population: 1,587 men and women ≥18 years of age with symptomatic HF for at least 3 months who were in sinus rhythm and had LVEF of ≤35%.

Treatment: Patients were assigned to one of the following three treatment arms—blinded aspirin 162 mg, blinded clopidogrel 75 mg daily, or open-label warfarin (target INR of 2.5 to 3.0 with a designated acceptable range of 2.0 to 3.5). There was no loading dose for either clopidogrel or aspirin.

Results: There was no difference between groups for the primary end point of death, nonfatal MI, or nonfatal stroke (HR 0.98 for warfarin vs. aspirin, 1.08 for clopidogrel vs. aspirin, and 0.89 for warfarin vs. clopidogrel; all p = NS). Rates of hospitalization for HF were significantly higher in the aspirin group than in the warfarin group (p = 0.02), and there were fewer strokes in the warfarin group, compared with either aspirin or clopidogrel. More bleeding occurred in the warfarin group, compared to clopidogrel [p = 0.01 (p = 0.22 for warfarin vs. aspirin)].

108. Homma S, et al.; The WARCEF Trial. Warfarin and aspirin in patients with heart failure and sinus rhythm. N Engl J Med 2012;366(20):1859–1869.

Design: Prospective, international, multicenter, double-blind, randomized controlled trial. The primary end point was first occurrence of ischemic stroke, intracerebral hemorrhage, or all-cause death at a mean follow-up of 3.5 years.

Purpose: To assess whether aspirin or warfarin anticoagulation was superior for patients with HF, in sinus rhythm.

Population: 2,305 patients with HFrEF (LVEF ≤ 35%) in sinus rhythm; approximately 43% had ischemic cardiomyopathy.

Key Exclusion Criteria: Any other indication for chronic anticoagulation therapy.

Treatment: Aspirin 325 mg daily or dose-adjusted warfarin (titrated to target INR 2 to 3.5).

Results: Rates of the primary outcome were not different between the two groups (7.47 events per 100 patient-years for warfarin vs. 7.93 for aspirin; HR for warfarin, 0.93; p = 0.4). While ischemic stroke was lower in the warfarin group (HR, 0.52; p = 0.005), major bleeding was also higher. Rates of intracranial hemorrhage were not significantly different (0.27 for warfarin vs. 0.22 with aspirin; p = 0.82).

Comments: The authors conclude that the decision between aspirin and warfarin should be patient specific (and likely modulated by prior atherosclerotic cardiovascular events and future stroke risk).

Exercise

109. Wilson JR, et al. Circulatory status and response to cardiac rehabilitation in patients with heart failure. Circulation 1996;94:1567–1572.

This study showed that only some patients respond well to exercise and offered insights into the pathophysiology of nonresponders. Thirty-two patients underwent maximal exercise treadmill testing and then rehabilitation for 3 months. Twenty-one had a normal cardiac output response to exercise, of whom 43% responded to the rehabilitation regimen (more than 10% increase in peak oxygen consumption and anaerobic threshold). Of the other 11 patients, 3 stopped rehabilitation (because of exhaustion) and 1 responded (9%; p < 0.04). The former group was likely limited by deconditioning, whereas the latter group was impaired by circulatory failures.

110. Hambrecht R, et al. Regular physical exercise corrects endothelial dysfunction and improves exercise capacity in patients with chronic heart failure. Circulation 1998;98:2709–2715.

This small prospective randomized study of 20 patients showed that exercise training resulted in increased peak oxygen uptake (+26% at 6 weeks; p < 0.01). This increase correlated with endothelium-dependent changes in peripheral blood flow (r = 0.64; p < 0.005), suggesting that improved endothelial function contributes modestly to increased exercise capacity.

111. O'Connor CM, et al. Efficacy and safety of exercise training in patients with chronic heart failure: HF-ACTION randomized controlled trial. JAMA 2009;301:1439–1450.

Design: Prospective, international, multicenter, randomized, controlled trial. The primary end point was a composite of all-cause mortality or hospitalization.

Purpose: To assess the benefit, if any, to a supervised, controlled exercise regimen in patients with stable HF.

Population: 2,331 outpatients with HFrEF (LVEF ≤35%) who were deemed medically stable (NYHA II-IV).

Treatment: Usual care or usual care plus 36 supervised aerobic exercise training sessions.

Results: In the protocol-specific analysis, exercise training was not associated with a significant reduction in the primary end point (65% for exercise vs. 68% for usual care; $p = 0.13$). However, after multivariable adjustment, exercise was found to be associated with reductions in the primary end point (adjusted HR, 0.89; $p = 0.03$), as well as the composite of cardiovascular death or hospitalization (adjusted HR, 0.85; $p = 0.03$). Importantly, there was not a surfeit of adverse events in HF patient assigned to regimented aerobic exercise programs.

112. Flynn KE, et al. Effects of exercise training on health status in patients with chronic heart failure: HF-ACTION randomized controlled trial. JAMA 2009;301:1451–1459.

The primary results of the HF-ACTION trial are described above. The authors also assessed the effect of aerobic exercise intervention on patient-reported outcomes in HF. Using the Kansas City Cardiomyopathy Questionnaire over a median of 2.5 years of follow-up, they found that supervised exercise was associated with greater improvement in overall scores (mean 5.21 vs. 3.28; $p < 0.001$). However, this was an early and persistent effect, as there was little change in either group after 3 months.

chapter 6

Arrhythmias

Benjamin A. Steinberg and Christopher P. Cannon

ATRIAL ARRHYTHMIAS

Epidemiology

Atrial fibrillation (AF) remains by far the most common sustained arrhythmia in the US population with a lifetime risk for people over the age of 40 of approximately 25% (2) and leads to more hospitalizations than does any other arrhythmia. AF prevalence is highest in those with clinical cardiovascular disease and occurs most commonly among older age groups and those with concomitant heart failure (HF) (2,4). The average age at onset is 70 to 74 years (age 65 years for lone AF); women tend to present at an older age than do men. The presence of AF is a significant risk factor for stroke, and a substantial proportion of strokes have been attributed to AF. Furthermore, AF patients appear to have higher adjusted mortality rates than do those without AF (3). Atrial flutter, a related but more organized and less common rhythm, also is associated with a modestly higher stroke risk than that for individuals in normal sinus rhythm (NSR) (11; *Am J Cardiol* 1997;79:1043–1047). The current consensus is that active atrial flutter should be treated similarly to AF, in terms of thromboembolic risk and prophylaxis. Other aspects of care for atrial flutter, and much less common atrial arrhythmias, may vary considerably; however, there remains little, robust evidence to guide these clinical decisions, and thus, we will focus primarily on AF.

Natural History

The clinical course of AF is heterogeneous: some patients have only self-terminating paroxysms that occur with variable frequency (but last <7 days), whereas others always require intervention to terminate episodes. Spontaneous conversion rates are variable (<15% to as high as 78%) and depend on the population studied. Higher rates of spontaneous conversion are associated with shorter AF duration (<12 hours), younger age, and lack of associated heart disease.

In general, patients who are older, have more structural heart disease, and have a longer history of symptoms tend to progress toward more persistent and chronic AF, sometimes despite aggressive management. Among patients with persistent (non–self-terminating within 7 days) AF, normal sinus rhythm (SR) can be restored in most, but 50% or more will have recurrences within 1 year.

Etiologies and Risk Factors

Many new cases of AF do not have a single clear etiology. From 3% to 11% of AF patients have structurally normal hearts. Conversely, new-onset AF often occurs in the setting of acute cardiac or noncardiac illness. Common examples include pneumonia, pulmonary embolism, and other acute pulmonary conditions; sepsis; acute myocardial infarction (MI); and major surgery. In these cases, treatment of the underlying illness is of primary importance. Cardiac surgery is associated with a distinct and high risk of postoperative AF, which occurs in 30% to 40% of patients undergoing coronary artery bypass graft (CABG) or valve surgery; however, it often is temporary. Other acute precipitants of AF include alcohol intoxication ("holiday heart syndrome"), pericarditis, myocarditis, and thyroid disease. AF also may be triggered by other primary arrhythmias that are curable by radiofrequency (RF) catheter ablation.

A variety of chronic cardiac conditions are associated with the development of AF; most common among these are hypertension and congestive heart failure (CHF). In a classic multivariable model based on subjects followed up for 38 years in the Framingham Heart Study, odds ratios (ORs) for the development of AF were highest for CHF (men, 4.5; women, 5.9), followed by valve disease (1.8, 3.4), hypertension (1.5, 1.4), and diabetes mellitus (1.4, 1.6). Prior MI was an independent risk factor for men (OR, 1.4) but not women. Rheumatic heart disease (specifically, mitral stenosis) has a strong association with AF, but because of its declining prevalence in developed nations, the valvular lesion more commonly associated with AF is mitral regurgitation. Nevertheless, patients with AF in the setting of rheumatic disease (termed *valvular* AF) are a particularly high risk of stroke. AF is likely a sequela of these conditions as a result of atrial dilation inducing myocardial fibrosis and subsequent electrical remodeling. Other cardiopulmonary conditions associated with AF include hypertrophic, dilated, and restrictive cardiomyopathies; atrial septal defect and other congenital abnormalities; and sleep apnea syndromes (obstructive and central). In addition, many older patients with AF have concomitant sinus node dysfunction, known as the tachycardia–bradycardia syndrome. In those patients, both arrhythmias appear related to underlying degeneration and fibrosis of normal atrial tissue.

Although the definitive pathophysiologic mechanisms have not been described, the following is a list of contributors to the development of AF classified by prevalence:

1. Major contributors: age, hypertension, CHF, ischemic heart disease, and postcardiac surgery.
2. Common contributors: alcohol intoxication, pulmonary disease, valvular heart disease, rheumatic heart disease, cardiomyopathy, and thyrotoxicosis.

3. Less common contributors: pericarditis, infiltrative cardiac disease (e.g., sarcoidosis), atrial myxoma, autonomic dysfunction, ventricular/atrial septal defect, and pulmonary embolism.
4. There is increasing evidence of heritability of AF risk, and several genetic loci have been linked to increased risk of developing AF (7).

Stroke Risk Factors

Data from the Framingham Heart Study initially documented the roughly five-fold increased incidence of stroke among AF patients compared with age, sex, and hypertensive-matched contemporaries without AF and highlighted the remarkably high rates of stroke in patients with AF due to rheumatic heart disease (relative risk, 17.6). Predictors of stroke were further evaluated in a meta-analysis of pooled control group patients from five major anticoagulation trials (8). Among clinical variables, independent risk factors for stroke (with associated ORs) included previous stroke or transient ischemic attack (TIA) (2.5), hypertension (1.6), CHF (1.4), age (1.4 per decade), and diabetes mellitus (1.7). In patients with nonvalvular AF, transesophageal echocardiography (TEE) identification of thrombus, spontaneous echo contrast or reduced flow velocity in the LA appendage, and complex atherosclerotic plaque in the aorta have been shown to be risk factors for stroke. These data culminated in the development of the $CHADS_2$ risk score, derived from a National Registry of Atrial Fibrillation (NRAF) cohort, to assess risk of stroke in patients with AF not on anticoagulation (12). This score was widely used to identify patients who would benefit from anticoagulation (see below) but had poor discriminatory power for patients with score of 0–1. Subsequently, the CHA_2DS_2-VASc score was developed from data in the Euro Heart Survey (13), incorporating additional cutoffs for age, and additionally points for female sex and the presence of atherosclerotic cardiovascular disease (coronary, peripheral, or aortic plague) (**Table 6.1**). Both of these scores have been validated multiple times across multiple cohorts, and while they appear to provide predictive power across a wide range of populations and disease states, several studies have also demonstrated that each risk factor varies in significance depending on the population (14).

Treatment

The American College of Cardiology (ACC), American Heart Association (AHA), and Heart Rhythm Society (HRS) published comprehensive guidelines in 2014, as a revision to their 2001 and 2006 guidelines on the management of AF (1). The following will briefly cover key aspects of management; the reader is referred to the guidelines for a more detailed review of these topics.

RATE VERSUS RHYTHM CONTROL

Some patients are unstable or severely symptomatic with AF due to hypotension, CHF, and/or angina. In such cases, cardioversion must be performed promptly and in some occasions as an emergency. Often, however, the symptoms due to AF can be eliminated or at least minimized by controlling the

Table 6.1		Risk of Stroke in the Euro Heart Survey, Stratified by CHA_2DS_2-VASc Score		
CHA_2 DS_2-VASc Score	**No.**	**Number of TE Events**	**TE Rate During 1 y (95% CI)**	**TE Rate During 1 y, Adjusted for Aspirin Prescription, %[a]**
0	103	0	0 and (0–0)	0
1	162	1	0.6% (0.0–3.4)	0.7
2	184	3	1.6% (0.3–4.7)	1.9
3	203	8	3.9% (1.7–7.6)	4.7
4	2.8	4	1.9% (0.5–4.9)	2.3
5	95	3	3.2% (0.7–9.0)	3.9
6	57	2	3.6% (0.4–12.3)	4.5
7	25	2	8.0% (1.0–26.0)	10.1
8	9	1	11.1% (0.3–48.3)	14.2
9	1	1	100% (2.5–100)	100
Total	1,084	25	p value for trend 0.003	

[a]Theoretical TE rates without therapy; corrected for the percent of patients receiving aspirin within each group, assuming that aspirin provides a 22% reduction in TE risk.

CHA_2DS_2-VASc score is calculated by adding one point for each of the following conditions—CHF, hypertension, age 65–74 y, vascular disease, or diabetes mellitus—and adding two points for having had a prior stroke or transient ischemic attack or age ≥75 years. CI indicates confidence interval.

Data from Lip GY, et al. Refining clinical risk stratification for predicting stroke and thromboembolism in atrial fibrillation using a novel risk factor-based approach: the euro heart survey on atrial fibrillation. *Chest* 2010;137:263–272.

rate of ventricular response. When AF becomes persistent, practitioners and patients then face a choice between rate control (allowing AF with an acceptable ventricular rate) and rhythm control (attempting to maintain SR) as alternative long-term strategies. Beyond the elimination of AF-related symptoms, advocates of rhythm control have hypothesized that maintenance of SR will reduce the rates of stroke and potentially death, compared with a rate-control approach. These hypotheses were partially tested in the North American AFFIRM and European RACE randomized trials (15,16). In both trials, rhythm control failed to lower the incidence of stroke or death as compared to rate control with anticoagulation.

However, these trials were limited and the debate continues as further studies, such as the "on-treatment" analysis of AFFIRM and substudies of the DIAMOND trial, suggested that SR is associated with a lower risk of death. But an AFFIRM subgroup analysis also confirmed that antiarrhythmic drugs are associated with an increased risk of death when controlling for the presence of SR. This means that in practice, the beneficial effects of maintaining SR with antiarrhythmics may be negated by their underlying proarrhythmic and noncardiac toxicities (17–19). Therefore, the prospect of interventional therapies to maintain SR, such as catheter ablation, remains appealing. To date, catheter ablation has been largely reserved for patients failing medical therapy (e.g., antiarrhythmic drugs); however, its safety and efficacy continue to improve earlier in the AF disease process.

When deciding which management strategy to pursue, it is important to assess the severity of symptoms, exercise tolerance, and patient preference. Though further studies are needed, it appears that patients on a pharmacologic rhythm-control regimen continue to be at risk for thromboembolism (possibly through asymptomatic recurrence of AF or other, poorly described mechanisms). Thus, it is imperative that chronic anticoagulation therapy be addressed to prevent thromboembolism in high-risk individuals regardless of the choice of rhythm versus rate control (1).

Among patients managed with rate control only, there has been extensive debate regarding the appropriate target heart rate (HR). It has been well described that chronic, elevated HR can lead to left ventricular dysfunction; however, the extent of rate control required to avoid such sequelae has not been shown definitely. The RACE II trial was specifically designed to address this question—they randomized 614 patients with AF to "strict" (<80 bpm) versus "lenient" (<110 bpm) rate control and did not demonstrate a difference in the primary outcome of a composite of cardiovascular death, HF hospitalization, stroke, systemic embolism, bleeding, or life-threatening arrhythmias (20). Nevertheless, the trial had shortcomings and critics remain vocal that it did not conclusively answer the question—in referencing these data, the guidelines also acknowledge the well-known dangers of persistent tachycardia.

PHARMACOLOGIC AGENTS FOR CONTROL OF THE VENTRICULAR RATE

1. β-Blockers: Multiple studies have been done comparing the efficacy of β-blockers to placebo, and these have shown their efficacy to be agent-specific. In the AFFIRM study, they were also found to be more effective than calcium channel blockers with 70% of patients on *β-blockers* reaching their target HR compared to 54% of patients on calcium channel blockers (15). Atenolol (21), metoprolol (22), timolol, pindolol, and nadolol have all been shown to be more effective than placebo both at rest and with exercise. Studies looking at xamoterol (23) showed good exertional HR control but were inconsistent at rest, while labetalol was shown to be ineffective at rest (24). Carvedilol is often recommended for use in HF, but there are no trials that have compared its efficacy to placebo for use in rate control. For acute rate control, intravenous (IV) metoprolol or esmolol in continuous infusion is commonly prescribed. However, β-blockers should not be used in patients with severe bronchospasm and should be used with caution in the presence of severe left ventricular (LV) dysfunction, particularly if decompensated.
2. Calcium channel blockers: The nondihydropyridine calcium channel blockers diltiazem and verapamil have been shown in several randomized trials to be more effective than either placebo or digoxin at reducing the ventricular rate both at rest and during exercise in patients with AF (22). When

compared head-to-head, diltiazem and verapamil were shown to have equal efficacy. However, they should be used very cautiously in patients with HF or LV dysfunction, owing to their significant negative inotropic properties.

3. Digoxin, a cardiac glycoside, is felt to act by increasing vagal tone and not through direct myocardial effects. It is most effective for chronic AF, not paroxysmal AF, and it takes hours to achieve maximal effect, so it is not effective for acute rate control. It also works poorly if high sympathetic tone is present, and studies have shown it to be ineffective during exercise (21). Historically, digoxin has been favored in patients with HF, as it may improve symptoms and reduce hospitalization events; however, more recent data have called into question the safety of digoxin among several different populations.

PHARMACOLOGIC AGENTS FOR THE ACUTE CONVERSION OF ATRIAL FIBRILLATION

Antiarrhythmic drugs have complex pharmacologic and physiologic actions, and all carry some potential for side effects, including both noncardiac toxicity and proarrhythmic activity (i.e., the induction of potentially dangerous rhythms). These risks are modified by a number of factors, including renal function, gender, LV systolic function, LV hypertrophy, and the presence of ischemic heart disease. Understanding these risks is essential to maximize the therapeutic index of any treatment decision. When choosing to proceed with pharmacologic conversion, it is important to note that pharmacologic conversion is most effective when started within 7 days of the initiation of an episode of AF.

Intravenous Agents

1. Amiodarone: Amiodarone is one of the most widely used antiarrhythmic medication, and it has Class I, II, III, and IV antiarrhythmic properties. The data for amiodarone in the acute cardioversion of AF are mixed, but they overall favor the use of amiodarone for acute cardioversion (1). In some trials, amiodarone showed little to no efficacy at acute cardioversion, while several meta-analyses have demonstrated that amiodarone has similar efficacy to other Class Ic agents, though it is slower to convert patients to NSR (25–28). It is generally more effective for AF of <7 days' duration but also demonstrated moderate efficacy compared to placebo when converting persistent AF (28,29). Overall, it is generally well tolerated even in critically ill patients and in those with structural heart disease and/or HF. In these patients, it is considered first-line treatment for acute conversion. Adverse effects may include hypotension, sinus bradycardia, phlebitis, gastrointestinal upset, hepatic dysfunction, thyroid disorders (both hypo and hyper), pulmonary toxicity, and, very rarely, torsade de pointes. When used chronically, it is imperative to monitor for ocular, pulmonary, thyroid, and hepatic toxicities.

2. Ibutilide: Initial studies of this Class III agent showed modest to high conversion rates with AF, particularly when administered within a few weeks of the onset of AF (35,47), but the data are insufficient to establish its efficacy for conversion of persistent AF of longer duration. Studies have also shown ibutilide to be slightly

more effective at converting atrial flutter than AF, compared both to itself and to other antiarrhythmics (35). Addition of beta blockade or magnesium to an ibutilide infusion may increase the conversion rate of both AF and flutter (36; see also *Pacing Clin Electrophysiol* 2007;30:1331–1335). Given ibutilide's propensity to prolong the QTc, there is an approximately 2% to 4% risk of sustained polymorphic ventricular tachycardia (VT) and torsade de pointes (highest incidence in women) (47). Administering 4 g of IV magnesium sulfate in concert with ibutilide was shown to decrease the QTc in one trial (37), though there are no studies showing that this decreases rate of torsade de pointes. In contrast, the coadministration of esmolol with ibutilide reduced the rate of torsade de pointes from 6.5% to zero in one study (36). Overall, given this propensity for ventricular arrhythmia, it is recommended that ibutilide be avoided in patients with low ejection fractions.

3. Procainamide: Hypotension occurs in 10% to 15% of patients, and QT prolongation and torsade de pointes are known risks. A few studies have shown procainamide to be more effective than placebo (38), but the studies of comparative effectiveness are mixed. One showed better effectiveness than propafenone, but most show poorer effectiveness compared to other antiarrhythmics in the conversion of acute-onset AF (<48 hours) (35,38). It is unclear if procainamide is effective terminating persistent AF of >48 hours. Procainamide is primarily recommended for treatment of rapid AF in the setting of preexcitation (Wolff-Parkinson-White syndrome) in the 2014 AHA/ACC/HRS guidelines (1).

4. Intravenous versions of flecainide and propafenone are available outside but not within the United States. Both are considered Class I recommendations for conversion of AF (1). Direct comparison of IV to oral flecainide showed similar efficacy but shorter onset of action with IV flecainide (39). In comparative effectiveness studies, IV flecainide is similar in efficacy to IV ibutilide (40) and direct comparison of IV propafenone to IV ibutilide has suggested that ibutilide is more effective (41). When comparing IV and oral propafenone, IV propafenone was shown to have similar efficacy to oral propafenone but a faster onset of action. Intravenous sotalol also is available outside the United States but is not recommended for acute conversion of AF (see section below on "Oral Agents").

Oral Agents

1. Amiodarone: Amiodarone is also available in an oral formulation, though most studies of acute cardioversion of AF were done using the IV form. Because of its large volume of distribution, oral amiodarone is much slower to take effect than are other agents when used for acute conversion, though it has a very low incidence of proarrhythmia. One study found oral amiodarone to be more effective than placebo for the cardioversion of chronic AF (34% vs. 0%) (see *J Cardiovasc Pharmacol Ther* 2000;6:341–350). Because of the limited number of trials available, oral amiodarone has a Class IIa recommendation for cardioversion of AF (1).

2. Flecainide: Flecainide is a type Ic antiarrhythmic that has been shown to have similar efficacy at cardioversion in both the IV and oral forms and has a Class I recommendation for the acute cardioversion of AF (1). A single oral loading dose of flecainide has been shown to be more effective than placebo at converting AF of <7 days' duration. Those trials also showed flecainide has equal efficacy with oral propafenone, but it was more effective than oral amiodarone at both 3 and 8 hours postmedication administration. Direct comparison of IV to oral flecainide showed similar efficacy but shorter onset of action with IV flecainide (39). Overall, the effectiveness of flecainide for AF of >7 days' duration has not been adequately studied. However, it was studied as an "as-needed" outpatient regimen (along with propafenone), the "pill-in-the-pocket" approach, to good effect in selected patients (42). This approach, combined with an AV nodal blocking agent, is included as a IIa recommendation in the guidelines (1). Side effects including transient hypotension, QRS widening, and conversion to atrial flutter with rapid ventricular response have occurred. This agent is contraindicated in patients with ischemic heart disease or LV dysfunction (1).

3. Propafenone: This type Ic medication has been studied extensively in the literature and has a Class I recommendation for the cardioversion of AF in the AHA/ACC/HRS guidelines (1). A meta-analysis looking at 11 studies of oral propafenone loading—usually 600 mg given in a single dose—for recent-onset AF (<7 to 14 days) estimated success rates between 56% and 83% (43). Its rate of conversion was also comparable to that of oral flecainide. Comparisons to placebo, oral amiodarone, and oral quinidine with AF of <7 days found superior rates of conversion with propafenone during the first 8 hours after drug administration. There are few data to support its use in AF of >7 days in duration. As with flecainide, transient arrhythmias around the time of cardioversion can occur, and the drug should be avoided in patients with impaired LV function or coronary disease. There are few data on its safety in those with structural heart disease.

4. Quinidine: Most trials of quinidine were done with digoxin administered concurrently and in a quinidine load with repeated doses given every 2 to 3 hours until cardioversion or a total dose of 600 to 1,500 mg was achieved. Most studies compared quinidine plus digoxin to oral propafenone and placebo. They found that quinidine plus digoxin was less effective than propafenone until 24 hours postadministration, at which point the proportion of patient in normal SR is comparable between all three groups (44). One study comparing quinidine/digoxin to oral sotalol found better efficacy with quinidine/digoxin. Quinidine can cause QT prolongation and torsade de pointes. Its vagolytic properties can increase the ventricular response; thus, coadministration of a rate-controlling agent is recommended (45).

5. Dofetilide: This newer Class III agent has a Class I recommendation for the cardioversion of AF, with the caveat that it should not be initiated out of hospital (1). Its efficacy in the conversion of AF/flutter to normal SR was established in two randomized, placebo-controlled trials: European

and Australian Multicenter Evaluative Research on Atrial Fibrillation Dofetilide (EMERALD) and Symptomatic Atrial Fibrillation Investigation and Randomized Evaluation of Dofetilide (SAFIRE-D). Short-term conversion rates were approximately 10% for the 250 μg b.i.d. dose and approximately 30% for the 500 μg b.i.d. dose, compared with 1% for placebo. The SAFIRE-D study specifically looked at chronic AF and showed that dofetilide is more effective at converting chronic AF at doses of 500 μg b.i.d. with most conversions occurring in the first 36 hours (50). QT prolongation and torsade de pointes can occur and have led to requirements for inpatient drug initiation. Unlike that of most other agents, however, the safety of dofetilide has been established in patients with LV dysfunction and coronary disease.

Given concerns over the use of antiarrhythmic drugs in patients with structural heart disease, additional safety studies were conducted. Dofetilide was compared with placebo in 1,518 subjects hospitalized with new or worsening CHF and LV dysfunction (DIAMOND-CHF) and 1,510 subjects with severe LV dysfunction after MI (DIAMOND-MI). In patients with AF at baseline, dofetilide was much more effective than placebo at restoring SR (44% vs. 13% at 1 year; p <0.001) and maintaining SR (hazard ratio, 0.35; p < 0.001). Furthermore, patients in SR at baseline were less likely to develop new AF with dofetilide than with placebo (2.0% vs. 6.6%; p < 0.001). No difference in total mortality was found in either trial. Torsade de pointes was seen in 3.3% of dofetilide patients in DIAMOND-CHF, but after adjustments in the dosing algorithm, this was reduced to 0.9% in DIAMOND-MI. Dofetilide thus appears safe in the CHF/post-MI populations, but initiation of therapy must take place in hospital with careful dose calculation (based on creatinine clearance) and QT interval monitoring (48,49).

6. Other: Sotalol and digoxin are not recommended for the acute conversion of AF (1). Both IV and oral digoxin have been shown to have no efficacy in converting AF to SR in several studies (51). Studies with sotalol have been mixed, with SAFE-T demonstrating similar efficacy to amiodarone with acute cardioversion (29). Calcium channel blockers and disopyramide either have not been adequately studied or appear ineffective for the acute conversion of AF.

PHARMACOLOGIC AGENTS FOR LONG-TERM MAINTENANCE OF SINUS RHYTHM

With exceptions, the same oral agents reviewed earlier for immediate conversion also are used for maintenance of SR. Because of findings of increased mortality in specific clinical trials (CAST, SWORD), the Class Ia and Ic drugs are generally recommended only for patients without structural or ischemic heart disease. Brief additional comments are as follows.

1. Amiodarone. In addition to its well-documented safety in the presence of coronary artery disease (CAD) and LV dysfunction, amiodarone appears to be the most effective agent for long-term maintenance of SR when compared

to pure Ic agents as shown in CTAF, AFFIRM, and SAFE-T (17,29,52). Despite its increased efficacy, the potential for noncardiac toxicity (liver, lung, thyroid) and other side effects (ophthalmologic, skin discoloration) requires consideration, particularly in younger patients. For this reason, the AHA/ACC/HRS guidelines recommend that amiodarone be reserved for first-line maintenance therapy only in those with contraindications to other agents and even then only with careful consideration of risks and benefits. It may be used as second-line therapy for all other patients whose AF is refractory to other medications.

2. Dofetilide. Dofetilide is the only antiarrhythmic drug other than amiodarone with good safety data in CHF and CAD (48,49). Both the DIAMOND and SAFIRE-D studies showed that dofetilide was more effective than placebo in the maintenance of SR and prevention of new AF (18,48–50). Dofetilide should be avoided in patients with severe renal impairment or those with significant LV hypertrophy (>1.5 cm). It also has a number of important drug-to-drug interactions. Initiation of this medicine should take place in an inpatient setting due to proarrhythmia.

3. Sotalol. It is a type III antiarrhythmic with additional type II β-blocker effects. In several studies, sotalol was shown to be better than placebo for the maintenance of NSR (29,53) and similar in efficacy to quinidine (54). Some studies comparing sotalol to propafenone demonstrated equal efficacy at <1 year (55), while other long-term studies showed propafenone to have better long-term efficacy after 6 months (56). In comparison to amiodarone, the CTAF and SAFE-T studies showed sotalol to be less effective than amiodarone at maintaining NSR (29,52). Sotalol is renally excreted and prolongs the QT interval. It is not recommended for use in HF, severe renal dysfunction, or in patients with marked LV hypertrophy (>1.5 cm in the most recent guidelines).

4. Dronedarone is a multiclass antiarrhythmic with similar electrophysiologic properties to amiodarone, but without the iodine moiety that has been thought to cause amiodarone's thyroid, liver, and lung toxicities. Several randomized trials have shown dronedarone to have no proarrhythmic, thyroid, or pulmonary toxicities and to be more effective than placebo at preventing recurrent AF (30). This safety profile was confirmed in the large ATHENA trial that also found dronedarone to be associated with a reduced risk of death and cardiovascular hospitalization compared to placebo in patients with AF or flutter (31). When comparing dronedarone directly to amiodarone, the DIONYSOS trial showed that amiodarone was associated with less AF recurrence but had more side effects compared to dronedarone (33). However, dronedarone should be avoided in patients with HF or permanent AF. The ANDROMEDA trial found a doubling in the rate of death among patients with severe HF taking dronedarone (32). Furthermore, the most recent PALLAS trial demonstrated increased rates of incident HF, stroke, and cardiovascular death in patients with permanent AF treated with dronedarone, compared with placebo (34).

5. Flecainide. A type Ic antiarrhythmic that is better than placebo for maintenance of SR. In comparison to other antiarrhythmics, flecainide has similar efficacy to both quinidine and propafenone (57), but patients were less likely to have side effects and more likely to stay on flecainide. Its use should be targeted to patients with no structural heart disease.

6. Propafenone. A type Ic antiarrhythmic that is better than placebo for maintenance of normal SR (58). Higher doses result in increased efficacy but were also shown to result in increased side effects (58). Propafenone is similar in efficacy to flecainide (57) but possibly better than quinidine. Some studies comparing sotalol to propafenone demonstrated equal efficacy at <1 year (55), while other long-term studies showed propafenone to have better long-term efficacy after 6 months (56). A few studies have compared amiodarone to propafenone, with two showing superior efficacy (52; *Pacing Clin Electrophysiol* 2000;23:1883–1887) and one showing equal efficacy (59). It carries the same adverse effects and warnings as other Class Ic antiarrhythmics.

7. Class Ia agents (disopyramide, quinidine, procainamide). As a group, the Ia agents have fewer data supporting their efficacy than do either the Ic or Class III agents, although quinidine has been studied more than the others (45). Each of these agents is associated with QT prolongation and potentially important noncardiac adverse effects. Their use for maintenance of SR has been steadily declining, relative to other agents, and they do not appear in the most recent guidelines.

CATHETER AND SURGICAL ABLATION
Catheter Ablation

The use of catheter-based interventions for AF has grown dramatically with their increasing safety and effectiveness. The primary approach continues to be the electrical isolation of the pulmonary veins, where most AF activity is detected (60). Initially, the approach was studied mainly in relatively young patients with structurally normal hearts and appeared to improve or eliminate AF episodes in 50% to 70% of subjects; generally, it is found to be more successful when AF is paroxysmal rather than persistent (see *Circulation* 2002;105:1077). Nevertheless, emerging data on trials of catheter ablation, as well as meta-analyses, have led to support for the procedure in the latest ACC/AHA/HRS guidelines—it is a Class I recommendation for patients with symptomatic paroxysmal AF who have failed at least 1 antiarrhythmic drug and is a Class IIa recommendation as an initial approach (1). These recommendations are based on several trials, most looking at radiofrequency (RF) catheter ablation as second-line therapy for patients who failed antiarrhythmic drug therapy alone, and limited to performing ablation with the objective of reducing symptoms of AF (61–66). A subsequent meta-analysis identified significant benefit in freedom from AF at 1 year following the procedure (67). Additional randomized, controlled trials have examined RF catheter ablation as first-line therapy for paroxysmal AF in patients not previously treated with antiarrhythmic medications and found RF catheter ablation to be superior to antiarrhythmic drug therapy at maintaining NSR even out to 2 years (68,69).

The approach to catheter ablation of AF has also continued to evolve and may include dramatically different techniques in the future. There is evidence to support a much more targeted approach to AF ablation, using proprietary algorithms to identify specific electrical phenomena ("rotors") for more effective ablation (70). Furthermore, alternative ablative technologies to radiofrequency, including cryoablation ("freezing" tissue), have proven effective and potentially safer (71). Importantly, catheter ablation for AF has not been demonstrated to improve hard clinical end points, such as stroke or mortality—upcoming trials are powered to answer this question.

Surgical Ablation

Cox and other investigators developed surgical approaches to compartmentalize the atria to alter the underlying substrate for AF. This procedure (the Cox maze) has undergone many revisions and a number of similar methods using ablative energy sources rather than incisions have been developed. These interventions are typically performed adjunctively with mitral valve (MV) or other cardiac surgery, though occasionally, they are used independently in patients with significant, symptomatic, persistent AF who have been refractory to all other interventions. Most studies of patients undergoing this procedure are of small sample size and without blinding, though several meta-analyses have confirmed that the maze procedures can result in the restoration of NSR in 60% to 90% of patients (72,73). Surgical pulmonary vein isolation (PVI) by RF ablation has been shown to be as effective as the modified Cox maze procedure at restoring NSR in patients with chronic AF and MV disease (74,75).

ELECTRICAL CARDIOVERSION

Electrical cardioversion is favored for immediate management of unstable patients and appears to have greater efficacy (approximately 70% to 90%) than do drugs for the elective conversion of AF of short- to medium-term duration. Unfortunately, recurrence soon or late after cardioversion is common, with some studies showing a recurrence rate as high as 50%. Aside from minor skin irritation, adverse events are relatively rare and may include the unmasking of significant sinus bradycardia. The most significant potential risk related to cardioversion is thromboembolism, and specific guidelines regarding pericardioversion anticoagulation exist and are reviewed later (1).

Type and Amount of Energy

Although traditional teaching dictates starting cardioversion attempts at low energies (50 to 100 J), a randomized study using monophasic waveform devices found a significantly higher success rate at higher energies. Success rates were 14%, 39%, and 95%, respectively, with initial energies of 100, 200, and 360 J. Patients treated with higher initial energies received fewer shocks and lower cumulative energy, and no patient had detectable myocardial injury by troponin testing (see *Am J Cardiol* 2000;86:348–350). External defibrillators with biphasic waveforms have now become standard of care. Studies using these defibrillators, compared with older monophasic devices, have shown equivalent or increased efficacy (76; see also *Am J Cardiol* 2004;93:1495–1499) at relatively lower energies and have been used successfully in patients for whom previous attempts with monophasic defibrillators failed [see *Am J Cardiol* 2002;90(3):331–332]. Another study showed decreased cutaneous burns due to the lower energy used (see *Resuscitation* 2006;71(3):293–300. Epub 2006 Sep 20). Several studies have looked into how much energy should be applied to biphasic cardioversion. In two studies, longer duration of AF (77) and body mass index (BMI) of >25 (78) were both correlated with increased energy requirement to achieve cardioversion, and both concluded that starting with higher energy results in fever shocks. As such, the guidelines support this approach.

Anticoagulation Before and After Cardioversion

It has been noted since the 1920s that cardioversion (either pharmacologic or electrical) is associated with a transient increase above the already elevated baseline risk of thromboembolism in AF. This is related in part to the release of already-formed clot in the left atria, as well as the delayed recovery of atrial mechanical function postcardioversion, resulting in de novo clots (also known as "stunning"). There is a lack of randomized, controlled trials on the use of anticoagulation during cardioversion, but given the long-observed risk in observation studies of thromboembolism with AF, specific recommendations regarding pericardioversion anticoagulation have been developed. The following summarizes the recommendations for antithrombotic therapy in patients undergoing cardioversion (see AHA/ACC/HRS guidelines for further details):

1. Patients with AF <48 hours in duration may be cardioverted without prior anticoagulation, but anticoagulation should be given during cardioversion and for 4 weeks following cardioversion in patients at high risk of stroke (Class I); in those at low risk of stroke, it may be reasonable to omit anticoagulation altogether (Class IIa). More recent observational data support a more aggressive approach to postcardioversion anticoagulation (83).
2. Patients with hemodynamically unstable AF of recent onset should be cardioverted as an emergency without preceding anticoagulation but should be given heparin concurrently if possible and treated afterward with warfarin [international normalized ratio (INR), 2 to 3] for 3 to 4 weeks.
3. Patients with AF of longer than 48 hours or unknown duration should be given anticoagulation for at least 3 weeks before and 4 weeks after cardioversion (Class I).
4. Documenting the absence of thrombus in the LA appendage by TEE is an acceptable alternative to the 3 weeks of anticoagulation preceding cardioversion (Class I). The safety of this approach has been established through both nonrandomized and randomized studies (79,80).

The potential role of low molecular weight heparin or non–vitamin K oral anticoagulants (NOACs; see below) compounds as a substitute for IV heparin or warfarin around the time of cardioversion is reasonable. One randomized study reported data suggesting the noninferiority of enoxaparin for this indication (92), but this is difficult to prove, given the generally low rate of embolic events during this short time. Data on the use of NOACs in this setting are largely limited to subgroup analyses from the major, randomized clinical trials (see *Circulation* 2011;123:131–136, *J Am Coll Cardiol* 2013;61:1998–2006, and *J Am Coll Cardiol* 2014;63:1082–1087).

PREVENTION OF THROMBOEMBOLISM

Long-Term Anticoagulation

Thromboembolic stroke is the most serious complication of AF, and many studies have been done to characterize this risk. In a meta-analysis of major trials of anticoagulation for stroke prevention in AF, anticoagulation with warfarin reduced stroke risk by roughly 60% versus placebo, compared with approximately 20% reduction with aspirin (95). When anticoagulation is used, a target INR of 2.0 to 3.0 should be targeted (91), as the SPAF III trial (92) showed an increased rate of ischemic stroke and embolic complications with lower INR (**Table 6.2**). The ACTIVE-W trial showed superiority of warfarin over dual antiplatelet therapy with aspirin and clopidogrel (95). Despite the clear benefit of anticoagulation with regard to the stroke risk, anticoagulation carries clear risks of hemorrhagic complications. In order to balance these risks, several guidelines have attempted to define risk stratification schemes for patients with AF. The CHADS2 score is one of the most validated and integrates aspects of the AFI and SPAF algorithms (see **Table 6.2**). However, the latest guidelines have moved to use primarily the next generation of the $CHADS_2$ score, the CHA_2DS_2-VASc score.

Recommendations for long-term anticoagulation based on the AHA/ACC/HRS guidelines are listed as follows and apply mainly to patients with nonvalvular AF and no additional indications for anticoagulation (e.g., mechanical heart valves):

1. If the patient has lone AF, a CHA_2DS_2-VASc score of 0, antithrombotic therapy is not necessary, as the baseline stroke risk of this cohort is low.
2. If the patient has CHA_2DS_2-VASc score of 1, it is reasonable to use any of the three strategies: no antithrombotic therapy, antiplatelet therapy only (i.e., aspirin), or long-term oral anticoagulation (Class IIb).
3. Patients with nonvalvular AF and a CHA_2DS_2-VASc score of 2 or more should receive long-term oral anticoagulation with either vitamin K antagonism or NOAC.
4. The optimal duration of warfarin treatment after cardioversion is not known, although 4 weeks is recommended by the AHA/ACC/HRS guidelines (1). Thus far, no study has clearly demonstrated that a strategy of SR maintenance reduces the risk of stroke to the extent that anticoagulation can be

Table 6.2 Major Randomized Trials of Warfarin for Prevention of Thromboembolism in Nonvalvular Atrial Fibrillation

Annual Event Rate (%) Study	Primary End Point(s)	Target INR	Warfarin	Control	Value
AFASAK (78)	Stroke, TIA, embolic complications to viscera and extremities	2.8–4.2	2.0	5.5[a]	<0.05
BAATAF (79)	Ischemic stroke	1.5–2.7	0.4	3.0[b]	0.002
SPAF I (80)	Ischemic stroke, systemic emboli	2.0–3.5	2.3	7.4[a]	0.01
CAFA (81)	Nonlacunar stroke, non-CNS embolic event, ICH, other fatal hemorrhage	2.0–3.0	3.5	5.2[a]	NS
SPINAF (82)	Cerebral infarction	1.4–2.8	0.9	4.3	0.001
EAFT (83)	Vascular death, any stroke, MI, recent stroke/ TIA, systemic embolism	2.5–4.0	8.0	15.0[a]	0.001
SPAF II (84)	Ischemic stroke, systemic emboli	2.0–4.5	1.9	1.7[c]	0.15
SPAF III (86)	Ischemic stroke, systemic emboli	2.0–3.0	1.9	7.9[d]	<0.0001
AFASAK II (87)	Stroke, systemic emboli	2.0–3.0	2.8	3.6[c]	NS

[a]Placebo group.
[b]No treatment but aspirin allowed.
[c]Aspirin.
[d]Aspirin and fixed low-dose warfarin (mean INR, 1.3).
[e]Low-dose warfarin.

CAFA, Canadian atrial fibrillation anticoagulation; SPAF, stroke prevention in atrial fibrillation; INR, international normalized ratio; ICH, intracranial hemorrhage; MI, myocardial infarction; TIA, transient ischemic attack; CNS, central nervous system; NS, not significant.

discontinued. Additionally, several bleeding scores have also been developed to identify patients at high risk of major bleeding in the setting of oral anticoagulation. However, net clinical benefit analyses have consistently favored oral anticoagulation in all but highest bleeding risk patients (98). There has been no prospective trial demonstrating benefit to withholding anticoagulation on the bases of a bleeding risk score.

Non–Vitamin K Oral Anticoagulants

One of the major advances in the care of patients with AF over the last decade has been the development of several NOACs as alternatives to warfarin for the prevention of stroke or systemic embolism. They do not require the coagulation monitoring or dosage titrations inherent in vitamin K antagonism. The first dabigatran, is an oral direct thrombin inhibitor. It demonstrated favorable results in the RE-LY trial where high- and low-dose dabigatran were compared to standard warfarin therapy for use in AF. Low-dose dabigatran (110 mg twice daily) was noninferior to warfarin at the prevention of thromboembolic events, but with a lower risk of bleeding events. High-dose dabigatran (150 mg twice daily) had decreased thromboembolic events compared to warfarin therapy and an equal risk of bleeding events (99). Subsequently, several oral factor Xa inhibitors were developed, including rivaroxaban, apixaban, and edoxaban.

The Rivaroxaban Once Daily Oral Direct Factor Xa Inhibition Compared with Vitamin K Antagonism for Prevention of Stroke and Embolism (ROCKET AF) trial demonstrated that once-daily rivaroxaban was noninferior to dose-adjusted warfarin for the prevention of stroke or systemic embolism in a relatively high-risk population of patients with AF (100).

Apixaban was tested in two major, phase three trials. The first, the Apixaban Versus Acetylsalicylic Acid (ASA) to Prevent Stroke in Atrial Fibrillation Patients Who Have Failed or Are Unsuitable for Vitamin K Antagonist Treatment (AVERROES) trial was a landmark study that enrolled patients who could not tolerate or did not want warfarin therapy (101). The investigators demonstrated that the apixaban was superior to aspirin for prevention of thromboembolism, *without* a significantly increased risk of bleeding (though bleeding was numerically higher in patients assigned to apixaban vs. aspirin). Apixaban was then compared to warfarin in the Apixaban for Reduction in Stroke and Other Thromboembolic Events in Atrial Fibrillation (ARISTOTLE) trial, demonstrating significant reductions in both thromboembolism and all-cause mortality, compared with dose-adjusted warfarin (102).

The third oral factor Xa inhibitor for stroke prevention in AF, edoxaban, was compared to dose-adjusted warfarin in the Effective Anticoagulation with Factor Xa Next Generation in Atrial Fibrillation–Thrombolysis in Myocardial Infarction 48 (ENGAGE AF-TIMI 48) trial (103). The trial tested two once-daily dosing regimens of edoxaban and demonstrated equivalent rates of stroke or systemic embolism, with significantly lower rates of major bleeding and cardiovascular death for each dose compared with warfarin.

The four major trials above, comparing an NOAC to dose-adjusted warfarin, were combined in a major meta-analysis (104). The study demonstrates consistent and significant overall reductions in stroke and systemic embolism, as well as all-cause mortality and intracranial hemorrhage, for the group of patients assigned to NOAC versus dose-adjusted warfarin. Importantly, there may be significant heterogeneity around the risks of other major bleeding and GI bleeding, depending on the NOAC studied.

Other Strategies to Prevent Thromboembolism

While oral anticoagulation is highly effective at reducing the risk of stroke in patients with AF at high risk, it is not without risk. A significant minority of patients cannot tolerate these drugs due to bleeding risk, and some will experience stroke despite adequate therapy. Therefore, alternative strategies for stroke prevention in AF have been explored and have largely centered around the mechanical "isolation" or "exclusion" of the left atrial appendage (LAA), a nidus of thrombus that is thought to contribute significantly to stroke risk in AF patients. Several devices have proceeded through advanced clinical trial and include the Watchman LAA occlusion device, which is delivered endovascularly (105), and the LARIAT exclusion device, which "snares" the LAA via pericardial access (106). Each is now FDA approved for use.

OTHER TREATMENT MEASURES
Atrial Pacemakers

Pacing the right atrium from two sites and implanting pacemakers with automated atrial overdrive algorithms are two novel pacemaker-based interventions for reducing the "burden" of AF. These are reviewed separately (see the section "Cardiac Pacing Studies").

Atrioventricular Junction Ablation with Permanent Pacemaker Implantation

In patients for whom maintenance of SR is no longer feasible or desired, but who still have significant symptoms with AF, benefits have been demonstrated with the combination of atrioventricular junction (AVJ) ablation and implantation of a ventricular pacemaker. This provides the ultimate form of rate control and eliminates the irregular ventricular response that in some patients contributes to symptoms, even at moderate rates. However, given that the atria remain in AF, symptoms may persist and the risk for clot and thromboembolism remains; thus, this strategy does not change the requirement for anticoagulation.

ATRIAL FIBRILLATION PREVENTION AFTER CARDIAC SURGERY

Postoperative AF is especially common after cardiac operations, occurring in approximately 25% of patients. Postoperative AF occurs most frequently on postoperative days 2 to 3. Several studies have shown that its occurrence is associated with higher morbidity. Among cardiac surgery patients, one study found that postoperative AF was associated with increased mortality at 1 and 6 months. Postoperative AF also results in an extended length of hospital stay.

The use of β-blockers after surgery has been consistently shown to reduce the incidence of AF and has become standard practice (107). In one meta-analysis of 24 randomized studies, β-blocker therapy reduced post-CABG AF by 77% (107). Preoperative initiation of β-blockers also was found to be more effective than postoperative initiation.

Several randomized, controlled studies have evaluated the prophylactic use of IV or oral amiodarone (108). Although amiodarone typically reduced the incidence of in-hospital AF, these reductions translated into a significantly shorter hospital stay in only one trial, when oral amiodarone was started 7 days preoperatively (108). One randomized study has compared amiodarone with a β-blocker (propranolol; see *Am Heart J* 2001;142:811). Amiodarone was associated with a lower incidence of postoperative AF, but no difference in length of hospital stay was found. The most recent guidelines support β-blocker use for postoperative treatment of AF (Class I) and amiodarone as an option for preoperative prophylaxis (Class IIa) (1). Additionally, recommendations are largely consistent with those for patients with nonoperative AF, with limited evidence. Other trials have evaluated agents such as oral sotalol (no advantage over other β-blockers with increased risk of torsade de pointes), dofetilide (more effective than placebo) (109), procainamide (not effective), and verapamil (not effective).

VENTRICULAR ARRHYTHMIAS

It is estimated that approximately 420,000 out-of-hospital cardiac arrests occur each year in the United States. Previous studies estimated that sudden cardiac death (SCD) accounts for fatalities in more than 250,000 of these events, the majority attributable to unstable ventricular arrhythmias.

Immediate Therapy: Automated External Defibrillators

Because most patients with witnessed cardiac arrest have "shockable" ventricular tachyarrhythmias just after collapse, and survival rates are critically related to the rapidity of defibrillation, substantial effort has been expended in developing and deploying automated external defibrillators (AEDs) in public areas. These devices, which require little to no training to operate, were originally shown to improve survival to hospital discharge among cardiac arrest victims when supplied to first-responder firefighters, as compared with waiting slightly longer for paramedics (111). Given both their ease of use and clear survival advantage, studies have been done to look at their effectiveness when deployed broadly in the community. Pilot studies of AED use in casinos (112) and commercial airplanes (113) demonstrated excellent performance of both AED rhythm diagnostics and shocking efficacy, leading to rates of survival to hospital discharge of 40% to 50% for victims of ventricular fibrillation (VF). These led to the large PAD study that looked at the use of AEDs by trained laypersons (19,000 volunteers) across multiple public venues in North America. The PAD study found a significant advantage in survival to hospital discharge when AEDs were used compared to cardiopulmonary resuscitation (CPR) alone (23.4% vs. 14%) (114). Though AEDs are now being placed in more and more locations, the evidence to date does not support their widespread deployment in private homes (115), particularly given that more arrests due to ventricular arrhythmias occur in public places and not the home (116).

Immediate Therapy: Intravenous Amiodarone

Two important trials, ARREST and ALIVE, provided more robust data than did smaller prior studies on the immediate resuscitation of cardiac arrest (100,101). These trials demonstrated that a bolus of IV amiodarone, when given to patients with pulseless VT or VF refractory to initial attempts at defibrillation, results in improved survival to hospital admission compared with either placebo or IV lidocaine. However, the ARREST and ALIVE studies were not large enough to demonstrate improvement in more pertinent end points, such as survival to hospital discharge, but nonetheless solidified the role of IV amiodarone as the first-choice antiarrhythmic drug therapy for VT/VF in Advanced Cardiac Life Support (ACLS) guidelines.

Secondary Prevention Trials: Drugs versus Implantable Cardioverter–Defibrillators

Three important randomized trials comparing implantable cardioverter–defibrillators (ICDs) with antiarrhythmic drugs for survivors of cardiac arrest or hemodynamically significant ventricular arrhythmias were completed in the 1990s: CASH, CIDS, and AVID (**Table 6.3**). Subsequently, there was an explosion of data supporting the implantation of such devices in various populations. Device technology continues to be in a phase of rapid evolution, and concurrent with execution of the trials, perspectives on drug therapy changed as well.

The CASH study randomized cardiac arrest survivors to amiodarone, metoprolol, ICD, or propafenone (119). The propafenone group was terminated early because of excess mortality compared with the ICD group. At long-term follow-up, a nonsignificant trend toward lower all-cause mortality favored the ICD group versus the combined amiodarone and metoprolol groups. CIDS was a "purer" comparison of ICDs versus amiodarone for survivors of cardiac arrest and documented unstable VT (120). As with CASH, a trend emerged in favor of ICDs for the end points of total and arrhythmic mortality but again did not reach statistical significance. The AVID trial was the largest and most definitive of the three trials, randomizing more than 1,000 patients to ICD or antiarrhythmic drug (96% amiodarone) (121). AVID showed significantly better 2-year survival in the ICD group (75% vs. 64%; $p < 0.02$), leading many observers to conclude that CASH and CIDS were simply underpowered. Thus, in aggregate, the trials indicate that ICDs are superior to drug therapy. As a result, ICDs now

Table 6.3 Survival Trials of ICD Therapy Versus Conventional Medical Management

	AVID (104)	Cash (102)	CIDS (103)	MADIT I (113)	MADIT II (115)	DINAMIT (116)	SCD-HeFT (117)	IRIS (118)	AMIOVIRT (120)	Definite (121)
Pt population/entry criteria	Primary VF; VT with syncope, or VT with EF ≤40% and significant symptoms	SCD survivors w/ documented ventricular arrhythmias	VF; cardiac arrest, sustained VT (poorly tolerated or EF ≤35%), or syncope with spontaneous or inducible VT	Prior MI + EF ≤35% NYHA Class I-III + NSVT on EPS	Prior MI, EF ≤30%, NYHA Class I-III	6-40 d post-MI, EF <35%, weakened cardiac autonomic function	NYHA Class II or III CHF and an EF of ≤35% recurrent VT	5-31 d post-MI, EF <35%, at least 1 predictor of NSVT	Stable, NIDCM, EF <35%, and asymptomatic complexes or NSVT	NIDCM, EF <36%, and premature ventricular
Treatment	ICD vs. amiodarone or sotalol	ICD, amiodarone, metoprolol, or propafenone	ICD or amiodarone	ICD or conventional medical therapy	ICD or conventional medical therapy	ICD or conventional medical therapy	Amiodarone, ICD, or conventional medical therapy	ICD or conventional medical therapy	ICD or amiodarone	ICD or conventional medical therapy

(Continued)

Table 6.3 Survival Trials of ICD Therapy Versus Conventional Medical Management (*Continued*)

	AVID (104)	Cash (102)	CIDS (103)	MADIT I (113)	MADIT II (115)	DINAMIT (116)	SCD-HeFT (117)	IRIS (118)	AMIOVIRT (120)	Definite (121)
Primary end point	All-cause mortality	All-cause mortality	All-cause mortality	All-cause mortality	All-cause mortality	All-cause mortality	All-cause mortality	All-cause mortality	All-cause mortality	All-cause mortality
Results	39% lower mortality for ICD patients (at 3 y, 24.6% vs. 35.9%; $p < 0.02$)	38% lower mortality for ICD patients vs. amiodarone and meto-prolol (36% vs. 44%; $p = 0.08$)a	20% lower mortality for ICD patients vs. amiodarone (8.2% per y vs. 10.2% per y; $p = 0.14$)	54% lower mortality for ICD patients (17% vs. 39%; $p = 0.009$)	28% lower mortality for ICD patients (at 20 mo, 14.2% vs. 19.8%)	No benefit for mortality (reduced arrhythmia death offset by nonar-rhythmia death)	23% lower mortality (hazard ratio for ICD patients offset by nonarrhyth-mia death)	No benefit for mortality (reduced arrhythmia death of follow-up)	Stopped early for futility (no effect at 1 or 3 y)	35% reduction in mortality hazard for ICD patients

aEnrollment in the propafenone arm was stopped in 1992 because of a high mortality rate.

EF, ejection fraction; ICD, implantable cardioverter defibrillator; VF, ventricular fibrillation; VT, ventricular tachycardia; NYHA, New York Heart Association.

carry a Class I indication for first-line treatment in the secondary prevention population, after the exclusion of reversible causes of cardiac arrest (144).

Primary Prevention Trials: Antiarrhythmic Drugs

In the 1970s and early 1980s, a high incidence of sudden death was observed in survivors of acute MI, and several methods of predicting increased risk for future arrhythmic events were identified, including depressed ejection fraction, complex ventricular ectopy/nonsustained VT (NSVT) on ambulatory electrocardiogram (ECG) monitoring, the presence of late potentials on signal-averaged ECG, and the induction of sustained tachycardias with invasive electrophysiologic study (EPS). These insights led to primary prevention trials in MI survivors, initially with antiarrhythmic drugs. Unfortunately, these trials demonstrated that with the exception of amiodarone, antiarrhythmic drugs appear to *increase* mortality in this patient population. In particular, Vaughan-Williams Class I agents propafenone, encainide, flecainide (122), and moricizine (123) all demonstrated excess mortality compared with control groups in randomized studies of post-MI patients. In contrast, oral amiodarone appeared to reduce arrhythmic events and sudden death in several trials enrolling post-MI and CHF patients (125–128), although consistent improvements in all-cause mortality were not observed. This was confirmed in the amiodarone arm of the SCD-HeFT trial where all-cause mortality was not improved by amiodarone as compared to placebo (134). A meta-analysis of amiodarone trials (129) suggested a small advantage in overall survival compared with placebo or alternative antiarrhythmic drugs. The Class III antiarrhythmic drug dofetilide had a neutral effect on mortality in post-MI and CHF patients but is currently approved for use only in AF (see the section "Pharmacologic Agents for the Acute Conversion of Atrial Fibrillation"). Generally, the most recent ACC/AHA/ESC guidelines recommend against the routine use of antiarrhythmic drugs for the chronic treatment or prevention of SCD (109).

Primary Prevention Trials: Drugs versus Implantable Cardioverter–Defibrillators

After the disappointing results of antiarrhythmic drug trials, primary prevention trials involving ICDs were completed. The ICD trials again focused on the post-MI population known to be at high risk for SCD, and the first two major trials—MADIT and MUSTT (130,131)—selected patients with low ejection fractions, NSVT, and inducible VT at EPS. As with the secondary prevention trials, a clear advantage emerged in favor of ICDs compared with medical therapy with or without antiarrhythmic drugs.

Subsequently, the results of the MADIT II trial, which selected coronary patients >30 days post-MI on the basis of low ejection fraction alone (30% or less), demonstrated a statistically significant 28% relative reduction in mortality with prophylactic ICD implantation (132; see **Table 6.3**). These results were confirmed in the SCD-HeFT trial that found a 23% reduction in mortality with prophylactic ICD implantation when compared to both placebo and amioda-rone in patients with a low ejection fraction (35% or less) and NYHA Class II or III HF (134).

Given the impressive results of the primary prevention ICD trials in ischemic cardiomyopathy, two trials looked into primary prevention ICD placement in patients <30 to 40 days out from an MI. The DINAMIT and IRIS trials enrolled patients with decreased ejection fractions, elevated resting HRs, and recent MIs (<40 and <30 days, respectively). Both found no decrease in all-cause mortality in the ICD arms compared to placebo, despite the fact that the IRIS study showed a decreased rate of SCD in the ICD arm (which was balanced by an increase in non-SCDs in that arm) (133,135). Based on the DINAMIT results (which were later confirmed in IRIS), the most recent ACC/AHA/HRS guidelines (144) consider a Class I recommendation ICD therapy for patients with LVEF <35% and NYHA Class II or III HF [or left ventricular ejection fraction (LVEF) <30% for NYHA Class I HF] at least 40 days post-MI and 3 months after coronary revascularization therapy.

Primary Prevention Trials: Nonischemic Cardiomyopathy Patients

In contrast to the progress in sudden death prevention in coronary disease patients, the question of whether antiarrhythmic drugs or ICDs provide additional mortality benefit for nonischemic cardiomyopathy patients beyond that provided by optimal medical therapy has been more difficult to answer. Two small early studies showed no benefit of ICD in nonischemic dilated cardiomyopathy (NIDCM) compared to either placebo [Cardiomyopathy Trial (CAT)] or amiodarone (AMIOVIRT). The CAT compared ICD with control in only NIDCM patients (LVEF <30%) and was terminated early due to lower than expected rates (136). This resulted in underpowered results, with a mortality difference between the two groups of 26% (ICD) versus 31.5%; p = NS. AMIOVIRT compared amiodarone alone to amiodarone plus ICD treatment in NIDCM (LVEF <35%) and found no difference in survival between treatment groups (137). These studies were followed up with the larger DEFINITE and SCD-HeFT trials. DEFINITE enrolled patients with dilated cardiomyopathy (DCM) (LVEF <35%), frequent premature ventricular contractions (PVCs), or NSVT and compared ICD to standard medical therapy. It found that the ICD arm was associated with a statistically significant reduction in the risk of SCD from arrhythmias, but there was only a trend toward statistical significance in the reduction of all-cause mortality (the primary end point) in the ICD arm compared to standard treatment (138). This was likely due to a lower than expected mortality rate in the standard medical treatment arm leaving the study underpowered. The SCD-HeFT trial, which enrolled both ischemic and NIDCM patients, was the first trial to find a statistically significant reduction in all-cause mortality with ICD use in NIDCM (134). Based on this study, the 2008 AHA/ACC/HRS guidelines give prophylactic ICD placement a Class I recommendation for patients with NIDCM and NYHA Class II or III HF (144).

Studies of Emerging Tachyarrhythmia Therapies

The development of the transvenous ICD was a significant advance in the treatment of patients with life-threatening arrhythmias; however, there are limitations to this approach and it may not be feasible in all patients (e.g., patients receiving dialysis with challenging vascular access). For these patients, the development of a subcutaneous ICD (S-ICD) has represented another major advance. The S-ICD was first demonstrated to be feasible in a small, 78-patient study for both primary and secondary prevention (139). Based on the lead configurations in these patients, larger studies were performed (140,141), and the device was subsequently FDA approved. However, it should be noted that this device is primarily for defibrillation of ventricular arrhythmias—it cannot provide backup pacing (as a transvenous ICD can), nor can it administer antitachycardia pacing for treatment of ventricular arrhythmias.

Another shortcoming of conventionally programmed ICDs is the occurrence of shocks for non–life-threatening arrhythmias (inappropriate shocks). Several studies have shown they may occur in up to one-third of patients receiving an ICD and are associated with both significant stress and anxiety, as well as worse clinical outcomes. In an effort to avoid such events, two landmark trials were conducted testing alternative ICD programming strategies to reduce inappropriate shocks while preserving the benefit of ICDs. Both the PREPARE and MADIT-RIT randomized trials showed that more conservative ICD programming (withholding therapy for a set time period or up to a higher HR) not only reduced inappropriate shocks but also reduced all-cause mortality as well (142,143). Although the guidelines have yet to incorporate these findings, electrophysiologists have embraced such strategies.

CARDIAC PACING STUDIES

Traditionally, permanent pacemakers have been used for the treatment of bradyarrhythmias. However, evolving pacemaker technologies have shown utility in the management of tachyarrhythmias, CHF, and, to a limited extent, vasovagal syncope.

Pacemaker Mode Selection Trials

In clinical practice, most cardiologists implant dual-chamber pacemakers in patients with bradyarrhythmias, except those with chronic AF. Despite the sound rationale for physiologic dual-chamber pacing—including maintenance of AV synchrony, avoidance of retrograde ventriculoatrial (VA) conduction, and preservation of normal HR response in patients with intact sinus node function—objective benefits of dual-chamber pacing have proved difficult to quantify prospectively. Several clinical trials have shown that atrial or dual-chamber pacing, when compared with single-chamber ventricular (VVI) pacing, prevents pacemaker syndrome and is associated with a lower incidence of new or permanent AF, particularly among patients with sinus node dysfunction. However, improvements in "harder" end points, such as stroke or death, were seen in one preliminary study but not confirmed in larger, later trials [CTOPP, MOST (146,147)]. Furthermore, in the Dual Chamber and VVI Implantable Defibrillator (DAVID) Trial Investigators, dual-chamber pacing was compared with ventricular backup pacing in 506 patients with an implantable defibrillator and EF of 40% or less, and the backup pacing group had a better 1-year survival free of death or hospitalization for CHF (83.9% vs. 73.3%; relative hazard, 1.61; 95% CI, 1.06 to 2.44) (148), suggesting unnecessary pacing, which might desynchronize the two ventricles and may be harmful. Investigators in the PACE trial further demonstrated such detrimental effects that chronic right ventricle (RV) pacing can have on the LV (149).

Pacing for Vasovagal Syncope

Therapy for patients with frequent episodes of vasovagal syncope is challenging and generally unsatisfactory. Nonrandomized data previously suggested that a subset of vasovagal syncope patients with pronounced cardioinhibitory (bradycardia) physiology benefits from permanent pacing. To this end, pacemakers were developed that automatically pace at high rates when triggered by prespecified decreases in intrinsic HR (rate-drop response). Early randomized trials showing significant benefits of rate-drop response [such as the Vasovagal Pacemaker Study (VPS)] were unblinded, leaving suspect their results (150,151). These were followed by the Second Vasovagal Pacemaker Study (VPS II) and SYNPACE, which were fully blinded studies of highly symptomatic patients with bradycardia during tilt-table testing. Contrary to the results of the unblinded studies, VPS II showed only a modest, nonstatistically significant benefit (152), while SYNPACE was terminated early due to the inability of pacing to show a statistically significant reduction in syncopal events at the interim analysis (153). It should be noted, especially given the VPS II results, that both studies were underpowered to see a modest effect with pacing. More recently, the Third International Study on Syncope of Uncertain Etiology (ISSUE-3) trial studied the use of pacemakers in a much more select cohort of patients—they had to have ≥3 syncopal episodes and documented asystolic pauses on an implantable loop recorded (3 seconds with syncope or 6 seconds without) (154). In this cohort with severe cardioinhibitory syncope, use of a pacemaker did effectively reduce the recurrence of syncope. However, the guidelines have yet to reflect these data, and pacing for vasovagal syncope remains an uncommon treatment.

Pacing for Prevention of Atrial Fibrillation

Based on observed benefits of standard right atrial (RA) pacing in preventing AF in susceptible patients, investigators have explored whether the development of specialized pacing software to provide automated atrial overdrive pacing or the implantation of atrial leads at two separate sites can achieve even better suppression of AF than standard dual-chamber pacing. Overdrive RA pacing appears to reduce the "burden" of AF somewhat (155), but the superiority of dual-site versus single-site pacing has not been clearly established. Statistically, significant findings for particular end points and/or in specific subgroups have been reported with these approaches, but the magnitude of benefit, the clinical relevance of the end points, and the future of these forms of therapy remain uncertain (156,157).

Resynchronization Therapy for Congestive Heart Failure

Of patients with chronic CHF due to systolic ventricular dysfunction, 30% or more have electrical conduction defects (bundle branch block or intraventricular conduction delay) that cause delayed activation of portions of the ventricular myocardium. The resulting electrical dyssynchrony within or between ventricles appears to impair further the mechanical efficiency of the heart, contributing to HF symptoms and possibly mortality. To address this, pacing systems incorporate leads delivered through the coronary sinus system that provide early stimulation to the epicardial surface of the posterolateral LV, the site typically activated latest in these patients. These systems allow for LV or biventricular (BiV) pacing, known as cardiac "resynchronization" therapy (CRT).

Early studies of CRT demonstrated immediate hemodynamic benefits from BiV pacing (see review: *J Am Coll Cardiol* 2002;39:194), as well as improvements in various subjective and objective measures of HF severity, including New York Heart Association functional class, 6-minute walk test, peak oxygen consumption, and quality of life (QOL) (158–160). In the MIRACLE study, 453 NYHA Class III or IV patients with EF <35% who underwent BiV pacing system placement were randomized to active pacing (atrially synchronized BiV pacing) or no pacing for 6 months (160). The active-pacing group had significant improvement in all measured parameters, including EF and hospitalization for worsening HF.

Subsequent studies with longer follow-up showed a significant *survival* advantage in addition to the symptom improvements seen with CRT treatment both with (CRT-D) and without ICD (CRT-P) compared to standard medical management (161). The COMPANION trial enrolled 1,520 patients with Class III or IV CHF with QRS <120 ms and found death and hospitalization were significantly reduced with BiV pacing and BiV pacing plus ICD (CRT-D). In addition, the CRT-D group had a highly significant 36% mortality reduction compared to optimal drug therapy (162). This was further confirmed in the CARE-HF trial that looked at 813 patients with Class II or IV HF and with a QRD >120 ms and an LVEF of <35%. Again, the CRT arm was associated with a decreased rate of the primary end point of death or hospitalization (39% CRT vs. 55% medical therapy; $p < 0.001$), but in this trial, there was also a significant reduction in mortality in the CRT group (20% CRT vs. 30% medical therapy; $p < 0.002$) (164). These findings were in addition to the QOL and objective improvements that were also seen in the prior studies (161,164). The

MADIT-CRT trial further broadened the potential impact of CRT to include patients with milder symptoms of CHF, NYHA Class I or II, and demonstrated benefit of CRT-D therapy in this population (163). Given the high cost of these devices, criteria for optimal patient selection are extremely important.

These data, particularly the survival data, resulted in a Class Ia recommendation in the 2008 ACC/AHA/HRS guidelines (144). However, this recommendation was refined in the 2012 guidelines update to more precisely specify groups most likely to benefit (145). Recommendations for CRT are thus stratified by underlying rhythm, NYHA class, ECG pattern (LBBB vs. non-LBBB), and QRS duration.

Importantly, the guidelines also acknowledge the likely benefit of CRT in patients with depressed EF who also required consistent ventricular pacing. These patients essentially constitute a cohort with LBBB and significantly prolonged QRS duration. Coupled with evidence that chronic RV pacing will lead to LV dysfunction in a subset of patients with *normal* EF, many investigators speculated that any patient requiring pacing who was at risk of LV dysfunction should receive a CRT device. This hypothesis was tested in the landmark Biventricular versus Right Ventricular Pacing in Heart Failure Patients with Atrioventricular Block (BLOCK HF) trial (165). The investigators implanted CRT devices in 691 patients with NYHA I–III, EF ≤50%, and an indication for chronic pacemaker therapy; the patients were then randomized to either RV pacing or BiV pacing. At a mean follow-up of 3 years, the BiV pacing group had a significantly lower rate of primary outcome events (death, acute HF, or increase in LV size; 45.8% vs. 55.6%; HR 0.74; 95% CI interval, 0.60 to 0.90).

REFERENCES

Atrial Fibrillation

GUIDELINES

1. **January CT, et al.** 2014 AHA/ACC/HRS Guideline for the Management of Patients With Atrial Fibrillation: a report of the American College of Cardiology/American Heart Association Task Force on Practice Guidelines and the Heart Rhythm Society. *Circulation* 2014;130:e199–e267.

This major update incorporated newer risk stratification algorithms for stroke (i.e., CHA_2DS_2-VASc), NOACs, broader use of ablation, among others.

EPIDEMIOLOGY

2. **Lloyd-Jones DM, et al.** Lifetime risk for development of atrial fibrillation: the Framingham Heart Study. *Circulation* 2004;110(9):1042–1046.

A population-based study done in Framingham, MA, between 1968 and 1999 that included 3,999 men and 4,726 women. It found a lifetime risk for the development of AF in patients over the age of 40 to be 26% for men and 23% for women. Excluding patients with CHF and prior MI, the lifetime risk for AF was approximately 16%.

3. **Benjamin EJ.** Impact of atrial fibrillation on the risk of death: the Framingham Heart Study. *Circulation* 1998;98(10):946–952.

A population-based study done in Framingham, MA. After 40 years of follow-up, AF was associated with an OR for death of 1.5 (95% CI, 1.2 to 1.8) in men and 1.9 (95% CI, 1.5 to 2.2) in women after adjusting for age, hypertension, smoking, diabetes, LV hypertrophy, MI, CHF, valvular heart disease, and stroke. AF was also noted to diminish the female advantage in survival.

4. Go AS. Prevalence of diagnosed atrial fibrillation in adults: national implications for rhythm management and stroke prevention: the AnTicoagulation and Risk Factors in Atrial Fibrillation (ATRIA) Study. *JAMA* 2001;285(18):2370–2375.

A large cross-sectional study of adults aged 20 and older in an HMO population. The prevalence of AF was noted to be 0.95% (1.1% in men vs. 0.8% in women). Prevalence of AF increased with age from 0.1% in adults <55 years of age to 9% in adults over the age of 80. Given this prevalence, they estimated that approximately 2.3 million US adults currently have AF, which is projected to increase 2.5-fold to more than 5.6 million by the year 2050, with more than 50% of affected individuals aged 80 years or older.

5. Kopecky SL, et al. The natural history of lone atrial fibrillation. *N Engl J Med* 1987;317:669–674.

In this population-based study of Olmstead County, MN, residents between 1950 and 1980, 3,623 persons were found to have AF, of whom 97 (2.7%) were younger than 60 years (mean age, 44 years at diagnosis) and had no overt cardiovascular disease or precipitating illness. Among these lone AF patients, 21% had an isolated episode, 58% had recurrent AF, and 22% had chronic AF. At 15-year follow-up, only 1.3% of patients had a stroke on a cumulative actuarial basis, and no difference was found in survival or stroke-free survival among patients with the three types of lone AF. Based on these findings, the authors suggest that routine anticoagulation may not be indicated in individuals with lone AF.

6. Chen YH, et al. KCNQ1 gain-of-function mutation in familial atrial fibrillation. *Science* 2003;299:251–254.

This seminal paper brought genetics and AF to the forefront, as the investigators identified potassium channel mutations involved in the causative pathway of the development of hereditary, persistent AF. This demonstrated the possibilities for genetic sciences to help elucidate mechanisms of disease.

7. Tsai CT, et al. Molecular genetics of atrial fibrillation. *J Am Coll Cardiol* 2008;52(4):241–250.

Many studies have identified genetic markers associated with subsequent development of AF. This review highlights several of the most important genetic loci, as well as their downstream effects. The authors call attention to the fact that loci coding for ion channels, calcium handling, fibrosis, and inflammation appear to all be related to the development of AF.

RISK STRATIFICATION

8. Atrial Fibrillation Investigators. Risk factors for stroke and efficacy of antithrombotic therapy in atrial fibrillation: an analysis of pooled data from 5 randomized controlled trials (AFASAK, SPAF, BAATAF, SPINAF, CAFA). *Arch Intern Med* 1994;154:1449–1457.

Pooled data from these five trials showed that warfarin use was associated with a 68% reduction in stroke risk (to 1.4% per year) and 33% lower all-cause mortality. This significant benefit of warfarin also was present in patients with paroxysmal/intermittent AF [1.7% per year (warfarin) vs. 5.7% per year (placebo)]. Risk factors for thromboembolism were history of hypertension, prior stroke or TIA, diabetes, and age older than 65 years. A nonsignificant increase was seen in the frequency of major bleeding. Two of these five trials randomized patients to an aspirin group; the pooled risk reduction versus placebo was 36%.

9. Benjamin EJ, et al. Left atrial size and the risk of stroke and death: the Framingham Heart Study. *Circulation* 1995;92:835–841.

This analysis focused on 3,099 patients aged 50 years or older. For each 1-cm increase in LA size, the relative risk of stroke was 2.4 in men and 1.4 in women, and for death, 1.3 and 1.4 in men and women, respectively.

10. Benjamin EJ, et al. Impact of atrial fibrillation on the risk of death. *Circulation* 1998;98:946–952.

Of 5,209 Framingham Study participants, in 296 men and 325 women, AF developed during 40 years of follow-up. AF patients were more likely (at baseline) to smoke and have hypertension, LV hypertrophy on ECG, history of MI, CHF, valvular disease, and stroke or TIA. AF was associated with an adjusted OR for death of 1.5 (95% CI, 1.2 to 1.8) in men and 1.9 (95% CI, 1.5 to 2.2) in women. The presence of AF increased the risk of dying at all ages. Most of the excess mortality was seen in the first 30 days after AF developed.

11. Seidl K, et al. Risk of thromboembolic events in patients with atrial flutter. *Am J Cardiol* 1998;82:580–583.

This retrospective analysis focused on 191 consecutive patients with atrial flutter. At an average follow-up of 26 months, embolic events had occurred in 11 (7%) patients. Acute (<48 hours) embolism occurred in four patients (three after DC cardioversion, one after catheter ablation). In multivariate analysis, the only independent predictor of embolic events was hypertension (OR, 6.5; 95% CI, 1.5 to 45).

12. Gage BF, et al. Validation of clinical classification schemes for predicting stroke: results from the National Registry of Atrial Fibrillation. *JAMA* 2001;285:2864–2870.

The investigators combined data from 1733 US Medicare beneficiaries to create the NRAF. Through 2,121 patient-years of follow-up, 94 patients experienced ischemic stroke, and a risk prediction model was developed based on these events. This gave rise to the $CHADS_2$ score—one point is assigned for each of CHF, hypertension, age $\geq$75 years, and diabetes mellitus, and two points are assigned for a history of prior stroke or TIA. The risk score was widely adopted as a benchmark for clinical trials of anticoagulation in AF and remained part of the guidelines until 2014.

13. Lip GY, et al. Refining clinical risk stratification for predicting stroke and thrombo-embolism in atrial fibrillation using a novel risk factor-based approach: the euro heart survey on atrial fibrillation. *Chest* 2010;137:263–272.

Investigators from the Euro Heart Survey acknowledged the poor risk discrimination of the $CHADS_2$ score for patients at the lower-end spectrum ($CHADS_2$ score $\leq$1). They therefore conducted this analysis in 1,084 European patients (with 25 stroke events), deriving the CHA_2DS_2-VASc score—it built on the $CHADS_2$ score, whereby patients with age 65 to 74 received 1 point (2 points for $\geq$75), and additional points were given for female sex (1 point) or a history of vascular disease (1 point). They demonstrated a 0% event rate in patients with a CHA_2DS_2-VASc score of 0 and a 0.6% event rate in those with a score of 1. This system has since been adopted in some form in the US and European AF guidelines.

14. Olesen JB, et al. Validation of risk stratification schemes for predicting stroke and thromboembolism in patients with atrial fibrillation: nationwide cohort study. *BMJ* 2011;342:d124.

The authors analyze data from 121,280 patients with nonvalvular AF in Denmark to compare the utility of the $CHADS_2$ and CHA_2DS_2-VASc scores. They demonstrated improved discrimination with the CHA_2DS_2-VASc score (c-statistic 0.888) versus the

CHADS$_2$ score (0.812) when assessing event rates out to 10 years. More importantly, they highlight a differential effect for each of the components of the risk scores—not all risk factors are equivalent. For example, at 1-year follow-up, female sex conferred a significant risk of hospitalization or death from thromboembolism (adjusted HR 1.6; p = 0.04) whereas vascular disease did not (adjusted HR 0.96; p = 0.96); however, at 10-year follow-up, female sex was no longer a significant risk factor (adjusted HR 1.24; p = 0.08), but vascular disease was highly significant (adjusted HR 2.22; p < 0.0001).

RATE VERSUS RHYTHM CONTROL

15. Wyse G; for the Atrial Fibrillation Follow-up Investigation of Rhythm Management (AFFIRM) Investigators. A comparison of rate control and rhythm control in patients with atrial fibrillation. N Engl J Med 2002;347:1825–1833.

This prospective, randomized, multicenter study enrolled 4,060 patients with AF more than 6 hours but <6 months in duration. Eligible patients were aged 65 years or older or had one or more risk factors for stroke, could not have failed cardioversion, and had to be willing to accept randomization to rate versus rhythm control. Patients were randomized to rhythm control with electrical cardioversion and antiarrhythmic drugs (initially 39% amiodarone, 33% sotalol, and 15% IC agents) or to rate control with standard agents. Amiodarone was ultimately given to 60% of patients. Warfarin was continued indefinitely in the rate-control arm but could be discontinued at the local physicians' discretion in the rhythm-control arm if SR was maintained for 1 month. At follow-up (average 3.5 years), no significant differences were found between the two groups in all-cause mortality (primary end point) and other major secondary end points including stroke [7.3% (rhythm control) vs. 5.7%; p = NS]. However, many have argued that the AFFIRM trial is too broadly applied and that young patients with paroxysmal AF may still benefit from a rhythm-control strategy.

16. Van Gelder IC, et al. A comparison of rate control and rhythm control in patients with recurrent persistent atrial fibrillation (RACE). N Engl J Med 2002;347:1834–1840.

This smaller trial had a general structure similar to that of the AFFIRM, enrolling 256 patients in the rate-control group and 266 patients in the rhythm-control group. Discontinuation of warfarin after a period of SR was mandated by the study for the rhythm-control group. At 3 years, no statistically significant difference was seen between the groups in the primary composite end point of cardiovascular death, HF hospitalization, embolic events, severe bleeding, pacemaker implantation, or severe drug side effects [17.2% (rate control) vs. 22.0%]. Trends toward more embolic events, HF, and adverse drug events were seen in the rhythm-control arm. Event rates were higher in hypertensive patients.

17. Corley SD, et al.; AFFIRM Investigators. Relationships between sinus rhythm, treatment, and survival in the Atrial Fibrillation Follow-up Investigation of Rhythm Management (AFFIRM) Study. Circulation 2004;109:1509–1513.

An "on-treatment" reanalysis of the AFFIRM study looking at the relationship to survival of cardiac rhythm status and antiarrhythmic drug use independently of each other. In this analysis, both the presence of NSR and warfarin use were associated with a lower risk of death. After adjusting for NSR, antiarrhythmic drug use was associated with increased mortality. They concluded that NSR was either a determinate of survival or a marker of an unknown factor that was associated with survival. Increased mortality associated with antiarrhythmic drugs was likely negated by the survival benefit of NSR resulting in the similar mortality rate with rate control seen in the original AFFIRM analysis.

18. Pederson OD, et al. Efficacy of dofetilide in the treatment of atrial fibrillation–flutter in patients with reduced left ventricular function. A Danish Investigations of Arrhythmia and Mortality ON Dofetilide (DIAMOND) Substudy. Circulation 2001;104:292–296.

The subgroup analysis of the two DIAMOND studies (DIAMOND-CHF, DIAMOND-MI) that looked at the effect of NSR and dofetilide on the mortality and hospitalization rate of patients with AF and atrial flutter. Dofetilide was shown to be more effective than placebo at the maintenance of NSR (79% vs. 42%; $p < 0.001$), but dofetilide had no effect on all-cause mortality. When pooling patients from both treatment groups who achieved NSR and comparing them to those that did not, NSR was associated with a significantly lower mortality (see Ref. 46 for more details on the DIAMOND trial).

19. Roy D, et al.; for the Atrial Fibrillation and Congestive Heart Failure (AF-CHF) Investigators. Rhythm control versus rate control for atrial fibrillation and heart failure. N Engl J Med 2008;358:2667–2677.

Design: Randomized, international, multicenter trial; the primary end point was time to cardiovascular death over mean follow-up of 37 months.

Purpose: To compare the strategy of rate control to that of rhythm control in patients with AF and concomitant CHF.

Population: 1,376 patients with AF and symptomatic CHF with EF ≤35%.

Treatment: Aggressive rhythm control with electrical cardioversion (repeat, if needed) if pharmacologic cardioversion failed, compared with pharmacologic rate control predominantly with β-blockers and digitalis.

Results: Cardiovascular mortality was similar between the two groups at 37 months (27% of rhythm-control group vs. 25% in rate-control group; $p = 0.59$). Notably, secondary outcomes including worsening HF were similar between the two groups and subgroup analyses did not reveal any preferential effects.

20. Van Gelder IC, et al. Lenient versus strict rate control in patients with atrial fibrillation. N Engl J Med 2010;362:1363–1373.

Design: Prospective, open-label, randomized trial. The primary end point was a composite of cardiovascular death, HF hospitalization, stroke, systemic embolism, bleeding, or life-threatening arrhythmia at 3 years.

Purpose: To determine the benefit, if any, of a "strict" rate-control strategy (<80 bpm) versus "lenient" rate control (<110 bpm) for AF

Population: 614 patients with permanent AF

Treatment: One or more AV nodal blocking agents (β-blockers, nondihydropyridine calcium channel blockers, and/or digoxin) were administered to achieve the randomly assigned HR goal (as measured by resting HR in clinic).

Results: A primary end point event occurred in 12.9% patients in the lenient group, versus 14.9% in the strict rate-control group ($p < 0.0001$ for noninferiority).

Comments: While this trial failed to demonstrate the superiority of a strict rate-control strategy, there were limitations. Attainment of target rate was different in each group (only 67% of patients in the strict group achieved goal HR vs. 98% in the lenient group), and some would argue that *how* rate control is achieved matters (e.g., there is emerging evidence that digoxin may be higher risk).

DRUG TRIALS FOR RATE AND RHYTHM CONTROL IN ATRIAL FIBRILLATION

21. Farshi R, et al. Ventricular rate control in chronic atrial fibrillation during daily activity and programmed exercise: a crossover open-label study of five drug regimens. J Am Coll Cardiol 1999;33:304–310.

The investigators compared five pharmacologic therapies for exercise-induced rapid ventricular rates in 12 patients with chronic AF. These included oral digoxin, diltiazem, atenolol, digoxin plus diltiazem, or digoxin plus atenolol; primary end point was variability in 24-hour ventricular rate monitoring. When compared to diltiazem alone and atenolol alone, the ventricular rate with the digoxin plus atenolol combination was significantly lower and proved to be the most effective therapy at suppressing diurnal fluctuations in rate.

22. Ahuja RC, et al. Digoxin or verapamil or metoprolol for heart rate control in patients with mitral stenosis—a randomised cross-over study. *Int J Cardiol* 1989;25:325–331.

An open-label, randomized, crossover study comparing digoxin (0.25 to 0.5 mg daily), metoprolol (50 to 100 mg twice daily), and verapamil (40 to 80 mg three times daily). In the AF arm (10 patients), 80% of patients on verapamil, 40% on metoprolol, and 30% on digoxin reported a >50% subjective improvement in HR control. When treadmill testing was performed, the total work done by the patients was 555 ± 232 kpm (no medications), 1,379 ± 553 kpm on verapamil, 1,251 ± 575 kpm on metoprolol, and 716 ± 340 kpm on digoxin.

23. Lawson-Matthew PJ, et al. Xamoterol improves the control of chronic atrial fibrillation in elderly patients. *Age Ageing* 1995;24:321–325.

A double-blind, crossover study comparing xamoterol (200 mg twice daily) plus placebo or digoxin. When xamoterol or digoxin was used alone, there was no difference in the daytime maximal HR (132 bpm with xamoterol vs. 122 bpm with digoxin; $p > 0.05$), while the nocturnal minimum HR was significantly higher with xamoterol (85 bpm compared to 62 bpm; $p < 0.0001$). When xamoterol was combined with digoxin, the nocturnal minimum HR was significantly raised (68 bpm; $p < 0.05$), and the daytime maximal HR was lowered (115 bpm; $p < 0.05$). There were fewer pauses of >1.5 seconds with xamoterol alone.

24. Wong CK, et al. Usefulness of labetalol in chronic atrial fibrillation. *Am J Cardiol* 1990;66:1212–1215.

A randomized, crossover trial comparing labetalol to digoxin, digoxin plus labetalol, and placebo. There was no difference in the exercise tolerance between any groups. Digoxin showed no decrease in the maximal exercise HR compared to placebo (177 bpm digoxin vs. 175 bpm placebo; $p > 0.05$). Labetalol either with or without digoxin was shown to be more effective than placebo at reducing maximal exercise HR (156 bpm labetalol alone, 154 bpm labetalol plus digoxin, 177 bpm placebo; $p < 0.01$).

25. Hilleman DE, et al. Conversion of recent-onset atrial fibrillation with intravenous amiodarone: a meta-analysis of randomized controlled trials. *Pharmacotherapy* 2002;22:66–74.

A meta-analysis of 18 randomized controlled trials looking at a total of 550 patients receiving IV amiodarone, 451 patients receiving other antiarrhythmic therapy, and 202 patients receiving placebo. The pooled unadjusted rate of conversion to NSR was 76% for IV amiodarone, 72% for other antiarrhythmics, and 60% for placebo. When looking just at the placebo-controlled trials, the conversion rates were 82.4% for IV amiodarone compared to 59.7% placebo ($p = 0.003$). There was no difference between IV amiodarone and the other antiarrhythmics in the antiarrhythmic controlled trials (72.1% vs. 71.9%; $p = 0.84$). Safety was similar in amiodarone and the other antiarrhythmics with 17% versus 14% adverse events including infusion phlebitis, bradycardia, and hypotension.

26. Chevalier P, et al. Amiodarone versus placebo and classic drugs for cardioversion of recent-onset atrial fibrillation: a meta-analysis. *J Am Coll Cardiol* 2003;41:255–262.

A meta-analysis of six studies with 595 patients comparing amiodarone to placebo and seven studies with 579 patients comparing amiodarone to Class Ic antiarrhythmics. Statistical significance comparing amiodarone to placebo was not reached until 6 to 8 hours after infusion (RR, 1.23; $p = 0.022$) and continued through 24 hours (RR, 1.44;

p < 0.001). Amiodarone was inferior to Class Ic antiarrhythmics up to 8 hours postinfusion (RR, 0.67; *p* < 0.00), but no difference was seen after 24 hours (RR, 0.95, *p* = 0.50).

27. Letelier LM, et al. Effectiveness of amiodarone for conversion of atrial fibrillation to sinus rhythm: a meta-analysis. *Arch Intern Med* 2003;163:777–785.

A meta-analysis of 21 studies that compared amiodarone to placebo, digoxin, or calcium channel blockers for the conversion of AF to SR. The relative risk for achieving SR with amiodarone compared to placebo, digoxin, or calcium channel blocker was 1.4 in AF of <48 hours in duration (95% confidence interval of 1.25 to 1.57) compared to 4.33 in AF of >48 hours in duration (95% confidence interval of 2.76 to 6.77).

28. Doyle JF, et al. Benefits and risks of long-term amiodarone therapy for persistent atrial fibrillation: a meta-analysis. *Mayo Clin Proc* 2009;84:234–242.

A meta-analysis of 12 randomized controlled trials that involved 5,060 patients with persistent AF comparing amiodarone to either placebo or another rate-control drug. The rate of conversion was higher in amiodarone compared to placebo or rate-control drug (RR, 3.2; 95% CI, 1.9 to 5.5). No defense was seen in long-term mortality (RR, 0.95; 95% confidence interval, 0.8 to 1.1; *p* = 0.51). Discontinuation of therapy due to adverse effects was more common with amiodarone (RR, 3.0; 95% confidence interval, 1.4 to 6.2).

29. Singh BN, et al.; for the Sotalol Amiodarone Atrial Fibrillation Efficacy Trial (SAFE-T) Investigators. Amiodarone versus sotalol for atrial fibrillation. *N Engl J Med* 2005;352:1861–1872.

A double-blind, placebo-controlled trial of 665 patients with persistent AF comparing amiodarone, sotalol, and placebo. Patients were given oral preparations and were then followed for conversion to NSR. If no conversion was achieved by 28 days, the patients then underwent electrical cardioversion. The primary end point was time to recurrence of AF. Pharmacologic cardioversion in the first 28 days occurred in 27.1% of patients on amiodarone, 24.2% on sotalol, and 0.8% on placebo (*p* = 0.45 amiodarone vs. sotalol, *p* < 0.001 placebo vs. either sotalol or amiodarone). There was no statistical difference in the rate of conversion with electrical cardioversion for those who failed pharmacologic cardioversion at 28 days (72.3% on amiodarone, 73.5% on sotalol, and 67.9% on placebo; *p* = 0.54). The median time to recurrence of AF was 487 days with amiodarone, 74 days with sotalol, and 6 days with placebo in the intention-to-treat analysis, showing amiodarone to be superior to both sotalol and placebo (*p* < 0.001) and sotalol to be superior to placebo (*p* < 0.001). In a subgroup analysis looking at ischemic heart disease, there was no difference between sotalol or amiodarone and maintenance of NSR (median time to recurrence 428 days with sotalol, 569 days with amiodarone; *p* = 0.53).

30. Singh BN, et al. Dronedarone for maintenance of sinus rhythm in atrial fibrillation or flutter. *N Engl J Med* 2007;357(10):987–999.

A report of two double-blind, randomized, controlled trials enrolling 1,237 patients with paroxysmal AF to compare dronedarone (400 mg twice daily) to placebo in the maintenance of normal SR. In both trials, the mean time to recurrence was shorter in the dronedarone arm than the placebo arm (41 and 39 days with dronedarone vs. 96 and 158 days with placebo; *p* = 0.01 and 0.002 for dronedarone vs. placebo). There was no significant difference in the rate of pulmonary, thyroid, or liver toxicities between dronedarone and placebo.

31. Hohnloser SH, et al. Effect of dronedarone on cardiovascular events in atrial fibrillation. *N Engl J Med* 2009;360(7):668–678.

The **ATHENA** trial. A double-blinded, randomized, controlled trial of 4,628 patients with paroxysmal or persistent AF/atrial flutter comparing dronedarone (400 g twice daily) to placebo. Dronedarone was associated with a reduced risk of both the primary combined end point of death or cardiovascular hospitalization compared to placebo (31.9%

dronedarone vs. 39.4 placebo; $p < 0.001$) and the secondary end point of cardiovascular death alone (2.7% dronedarone vs. 3.9% placebo; $p = 0.03$). The principal side effects were gastrointestinal disturbances, bradycardia, QT prolongation, and serum creatinine increase.

32. Kober L, et al. **Increased mortality after dronedarone therapy for severe heart failure.** N Engl J Med 2008;358(25):2678–2687.

The **ANDROMEDA** trial. A double-blind, randomized, placebo-controlled trial of 627 patients with severe LV systolic dysfunction (NYHA Class III or IV) comparing dronedarone (400 mg twice daily) to placebo. The trial was stopped early due to safety reasons due to an increased risk of death in the dronedarone group (8.1% dronedarone vs. 3.8% placebo; $p = 0.03$). The deaths were principally due to worsening HF and not proarrhythmia.

33. Le Heuzey JY, et al. **A short-term, randomized, double-blind, parallel-group study to evaluate the efficacy and safety of dronedarone versus amiodarone in patients with persistent atrial fibrillation: the DIONYSOS study.** J Cardiovasc Electrophysiol 2010;21:597–605.

DIONYSOS trial compared amiodarone 600 mg daily to dronedarone 400 mg twice a day in the maintenance of normal SR postelectrical cardioversion done in 504 patients with persistent AF. There was a lower rate of AF recurrence in the amiodarone arm compared to the dronedarone arm (24.3% amiodarone vs. 36.5% dronedarone; $p < 0.001$). There were less thyroid toxicities, bradycardia, and premature study drug discontinuation in the dronedarone arm, but there were also more frequent gastrointestinal side effects in patients taking dronedarone.

34. Connolly SJ, et al.; The (Permanent Atrial Fibrillation Outcome Study Using Dronedarone on Top of Standard Therapy) PALLAS Study. Dronedarone in high-risk permanent atrial fibrillation. N Engl J Med 2011;365:2268–2276.

Design: Prospective, randomized, double-blinded, placebo-controlled clinical trial. The first coprimary end point was the composite of stroke, MI, systemic embolism, or cardiovascular death. The second coprimary end point was the composite of unplanned cardiovascular hospitalization or all-cause death.

Purpose: The investigators hypothesized that dronedarone would reduce cardiovascular events in a high-risk AF population.

Population: 3,236 patients with cardiovascular risk factors and permanent AF for at least 6 months.

Treatment: Dronedarone, 400 mg twice daily, or placebo

Results: The trial was terminated early due to a signal of significantly increased risk of the first coprimary end point in the dronedarone group (43 events vs. 19; HR, 2.29; $p = 0.0002$). There was a consistent effect across the components of the coprimary end points, including higher risk of cardiovascular death (HR, 2.11; $p = 0.046$), arrhythmic death (HR, 3.26; $p = 0.03$), and stroke (HR, 2.32; $p = 0.02$).

Comments: It was partly on the basis of this trial that dronedarone now carries a boxed warning against its use in patients with permanent AF.

35. Stambler BS, et al. **Antiarrhythmic actions of intravenous ibutilide compared with procainamide during human atrial flutter and fibrillation: electrophysiological determinants of enhanced conversion efficacy.** Circulation 1997;96:4298–4306.

A randomized, partially blinded (ibutilide arm only), placebo-controlled study looking at ibutilide compared to procainamide in AF and atrial flutter. Ibutilide appeared to be more effective at cardioversion of AF than procainamide (32% vs. 5%; p value not stated) or placebo (0%). With atrial flutter, cardioversion occurred in 64% of patients on ibutilide, compared to 0% on procainamide or placebo (p value not stated). The difference in conversion rates between AF and atrial flutter with ibutilide did reach statistical significance at 32% versus 64% ($p < 0.05$).

36. Fragakis N, et al. Acute beta-adrenoceptor blockade improves efficacy of ibutilide in conversion of atrial fibrillation with a rapid ventricular rate. *Europace* 2009;11:70–74.

An open-label, randomized, controlled trial in 90 patients comparing ibutilide alone to ibutilide plus esmolol infusion in the conversion of AF. When esmolol was combined with ibutilide, 67% converted to normal SR compared to 46% of patients given ibutilide alone (p 0.04). It was also noted that the slower the HR was at the time of ibutilide administration, the higher the likelihood of cardioversion ($p = 0.015$). The addition of esmolol had the added effect of shortening the QTc (433 ms with esmolol, 501 ms without; $p = 0.003$). This may have attributed to the lower rates of proarrhythmia when comparing the esmolol infusion group (0%) to the ibutilide-alone group (6.5%, one case of sustained polymorphic VT, three of NSVT). Though there were no VT episodes in the esmolol group, there were two cases of severe bradycardia in that group.

37. Caron MF, et al. The effects of intravenous magnesium sulfate on the QT interval in patients receiving ibutilide. *Pharmacotherapy* 2003;23:296–300.

A double-blinded, randomized, placebo-controlled trial comparing adjunctive IV magnesium to placebo in 20 patients with AF and atrial flutter undergoing chemical cardioversion with ibutilide. A total of 4 g of magnesium sulfate was given to the patients in this study (2 g prior to ibutilide and 2 g after). In the placebo group, the QTc increased 18% from baseline 30 minutes after the administration of ibutilide (p 0.007) compared to 4.4% with magnesium (not statistically significant difference from baseline) (no magnesium vs. magnesium; $p = 0.04$). No torsade de pointes occurred in either group.

38. Kochiadakis GE, et al. A comparative study of the efficacy and safety of procainamide versus propafenone versus amiodarone for the conversion of recent-onset atrial fibrillation. *Am J Cardiol* 2007;99(12):1721–1725.

A single-blinded, placebo-controlled study in 362 patients with recent-onset AF comparing procainamide, propafenone, amiodarone, and placebo. Success was any conversion to normal SR within 24 hours of drug administration. The rates of conversion were 68.53% of patients on procainamide, 80.21% on propafenone, 89.13% on amiodarone, and 61.11% on placebo, with all medication groups being more effective than placebo ($p < 0.05$). Amiodarone and propafenone were also more effective than procainamide ($p < 0.05$). The time to cardioversion was faster for procainamide (median time 3 hours) and propafenone (medical time 1 hour) than amiodarone (median time 9 hours) or placebo (median time 17 hours) (log-rank $p < 0.001$).

39. Alp NJ, et al. Randomised double blind trial of oral versus intravenous flecainide for the cardioversion of acute atrial fibrillation. *Heart* 2000;84:37–40.

A randomized, double-blind, placebo-controlled trial of 79 patients comparing IV flecainide to liquid oral flecainide. There was no difference between the conversion rate of oral and IV flecainide. Two hours after drug administration, 64% of patients on IV flecainide and 68% of patients on oral flecainide converted to normal SR ($p = 0.74$). This improved to 72% and 75%, respectively, at 8 hours ($p = 0.76$). There was a difference in the mean time to cardioversion, with IV flecainide achieving cardioversion at a mean of 52 minutes postadministration compared to a mean of 110 minutes with oral flecainide ($p = 0.002$).

40. Reisinger J, et al. Flecainide versus ibutilide for immediate cardioversion of atrial fibrillation of recent onset. *Eur Heart J* 2004;25(15):1318–1324.

A single-blinded, randomized, controlled trial compared IV flecainide to IV ibutilide in 207 patients with recent-onset AF (<48 hours). Success was any cardiovascular (CV) within 90 minutes of drug infusion. There was no difference between the conversion rate of IV flecainide (56.4%) and IV ibutilide (50.0%) ($p = 0.34$).

41. Zhang N, et al. Comparison of intravenous ibutilide vs. propafenone for rapid termination of recent onset atrial fibrillation. *Int J Clin Pract* 2005;59(12):1395–1400.

A single-blinded, randomized, controlled trial of 82 patients with AF comparing IV ibutilide and IV propafenone. Success was any cardioversion within 90 minutes of drug infusion. Ibutilide was more effective at cardioversion than was propafenone (70.73% with ibutilide vs. 48.78% with propafenone; $p = 0.043$).

42. Alboni P, et al. Outpatient treatment of recent-onset atrial fibrillation with the "pill-in-the-pocket" approach. *N Engl J Med* 2004;351:2384–2391.

In an effort to study the feasibility of outpatient self-administration of flecainide or propafenone for paroxysmal AF, the investigators enrolled 210 patients with recent, successful pharmacologic cardioversion with either agent (patients with adverse effects were excluded). They were given oral versions of either drug, to be self-administered with the onset of symptoms; in all, 165 patients had 618 episodes of arrhythmia over mean follow-up of 15 months. Attempted treatment of 569 episodes was successful in 534 (94%), with symptom resolution at mean 113 minutes. Health facility utilization (emergency room visits and hospitalizations) was significantly lower during the study period than the year prior to enrollment ($p < 0.001$ for both measures).

43. Khan IA. Single oral loading dose of propafenone for pharmacological cardioversion of recent-onset atrial fibrillation. *J Am Coll Cardiol* 2001;37(2):542–547.

A meta-analysis of 11 studies looking at a single oral loading dose of propafenone 600 mg for the conversion of AF. The published success rates ranged from 56% to 83% and depended on the duration of AF. The single oral loading dose regimen was significantly more effective than placebo only in the first 8 hours. After 24 hours, it was no different than placebo. The conversion time varied from 110 to 287 minutes. Comparing IV to oral formulations, the IV form was more effective only in the first 2 hours, but after that, both forms had equal effectiveness. Adverse effects were transient arrhythmia, transient QRS widening, and hypotension. The transient arrhythmias were principally at the time of conversion and included bradycardia, atrial flutter, and junctional rhythms.

44. Capucci A, et al. Safety of oral propafenone in the conversion of recent onset atrial fibrillation to sinus rhythm: a prospective parallel placebo-controlled multicentre study. *Int J Cardiol* 1999;68:187–196.

A randomized placebo control trial in 246 patients with recent-onset AF (<48 hours) comparing oral quinidine (1,100 mg) plus digoxin (0.75 to 1 mg IV), oral propafenone (450 to 600 mg), oral propafenone (450 to 600 mg) plus digoxin (0.75 to 1 mg IV), and placebo. At 3 hours, both propafenone groups (with and without digoxin) were more effective than quinidine plus digoxin and placebo ($p < 0.05$), but by 24 hours, there was no statistical difference between treatment groups or placebo. The mean time to conversion was 4.0 ± 4.1 hours for the propafenone group, 5.0 ± 8.6 hours for propafenone plus digoxin, 5.4 ± 4.5 hours for quinidine plus digoxin, and 7.8 ± 7.2 hours for the placebo ($p < 0.01$ propafenone vs. placebo).

45. Coplen SE, et al. Efficacy and safety of quinidine therapy for maintenance of sinus rhythm after cardioversion: a meta-analysis of randomized controlled trials. *Circulation* 1990;82:1106–1116.

This analysis focused on six trials with 808 patients. Quinidine use was associated with less AF recurrence. At 3, 6, and 12 months, 69%, 58%, and 50% of quinidine-treated patients were in normal SR versus 45%, 33%, and 25% of controls. Despite the lower recurrence rates, the quinidine group had a higher all-cause mortality rate (2.9% vs. 0.8%; $p < 0.05$).

46. Gosselink TM, et al. Low-dose amiodarone for maintenance of sinus rhythm after cardioversion of atrial fibrillation or flutter. *JAMA* 1992;267:3289–3293.

This study was composed of 89 AF patients for whom previous therapy failed. A loading dose of amiodarone (600 mg over a 4-week period) was followed by an average daily dose of 204 mg. Fifteen (16%) patients converted to normal SR during loading; 90% were in SR after cardioversion, and 53% remained in normal SR at 3-year follow-up. No proarrhythmia was documented.

47. Stambler BS, et al. Efficacy and safety for repeated intravenous doses of ibutilide for rapid conversion of atrial flutter of fibrillation. Circulation 1996;94:1613–1621.

This randomized trial was composed of 266 patients with sustained (3 hours to 45 days) AF or flutter. Patients received one or two 10-minute infusions of ibutilide, separated by 10 minutes (1.0 mg + 0.5 mg or 1 mg + 1 mg), or placebo. Ibutilide converted 47% of patients overall (vs. 2% with placebo), with better success in atrial flutter than in AF (63% vs. 31%). The average time to termination was 27 minutes. No significant differences were seen between dosing regimens. Polymorphic VT occurred in 8.3% but was sustained in 1.7%.

48. Torp-Pedersen C, et al.; for the Danish Investigations of Arrhythmia and Mortality on Dofetilide (DIAMOND-CHF) Study Group. Dofetilide in patients with congestive heart failure and left ventricular dysfunction. N Engl J Med 1999;341:857–865.

Design: Multicenter, randomized, double-blinded, placebo-controlled trial. Primary end point was death from any cause at median follow-up of 18 months.

Purpose: To assess the safety of dofetilide, a novel antiarrhythmic, in patients with CHF, with severe LV dysfunction.

Population: 1,518 patients with symptomatic CHF and severe LV dysfunction.

Treatment: Dofetilide (500 μg for patients in AF, 250 μg for those in SR; doses were subsequently based on renal function) or placebo.

Results: As an assessment of safety, the primary end point of all-cause mortality was not different in the two groups (41% for dofetilide vs. 42% for placebo). Yet, there was a higher incidence of torsade de pointes in the dofetilide group (3.3% vs. 0%). However, patients in the dofetilide group were less likely to be hospitalized for worsening HF; for those in AF, they were more likely to be converted to SR (12% vs. 1%), and for those in the dofetilide group, they were more likely to stay in SR.

49. Kober L, et al.; for the Danish Investigations of Arrhythmia and Mortality on Dofetilide (DIAMOND-MI) Study Group. Effect of dofetilide in patients with recent myocardial infarction and left-ventricular dysfunction: a randomised trial. Lancet 2000;356:2052–2058.

Design: Multicenter, randomized, double-blinded, placebo-controlled trial. Primary end point was all-cause mortality, with secondary endpoints of cardiac and arrhythmic death.

Purpose: To assess the safety of dofetilide in patients with recent MI and severe LV dysfunction.

Population: 1,510 patients with severe LV dysfunction and recent MI within 7 days; at baseline, 8% of patients had AF or atrial flutter.

Treatment: Dofetilide or placebo.

Results: There was no significant difference in outcomes between the two groups—all-cause mortality (31% for dofetilide vs. 32% for placebo), cardiac mortality (26% vs. 28%), and arrhythmic mortality (17% vs. 18%) were all similar. Patients in the dofetilide group with AF or flutter were more likely to convert to SR (42% vs. 13%; $p = 0.002$); however, all seven cases of torsade de pointes were in the dofetilide group.

50. Singh S, et al. Efficacy and safety of oral dofetilide in converting to and maintaining sinus rhythm in patients with chronic atrial fibrillation or atrial flutter: the

symptomatic atrial fibrillation investigative research on dofetilide (SAFIRE-D) study. *Circulation* 2000;102:2385–2390.

A double-blind, placebo-controlled trial of 325 patients with AF and atrial flutter comparing dofetilide (125, 250, or 500 µg) to placebo. Conversion rates for dofetilide were 6.1% with 125 µg, 9.8% with 250 µg, and 29.9% with 500 µg compared to 1.2% with placebo [dofetilide vs. placebo was significant at 250 µg ($p = 0.015$) and 500 µg ($p < 0.001$)]. For those who were successfully cardioverted, the probability of remaining in normal SR at 1 year was 0.4 at 125 µg, 0.37 at 250 µg, and 0.58 at 500 µg compared to 0.25 with placebo (500 µg vs. placebo was significant at $p = 0.001$). Two patients (0.8%) on dofetilide experienced an episode of torsade de pointes between days 1 and 2 of treatment, and one patient (0.4%) experienced SCD on day 8.

51. The Digitalis in Acute Atrial Fibrillation (DAAF) Trial Group. Intravenous digoxin in acute atrial fibrillation. Results of a randomized, placebo-controlled multicentre trial in 239 patients. *Eur Heart J* 1997;18:649–654.

A double-blind, randomized, placebo-controlled trial of 239 patients with recent-onset AF (<7 days) comparing IV digoxin (variable weight-based dosing given at 3 to 4 time points) and placebo. At 16 hours, 51% of patients on digoxin and 46% of patients on placebo were converted to normal SR ($p = $ NS). Digoxin was associated with a lower HR at 2 hours compared to placebo (104.6 ± 20.9 bpm compared to 116.8 ± 22.5 bpm; $p = 0.0001$).

52. Roy D, et al.; for the Canadian Trial of Atrial Fibrillation (CTAF) Investigators. Amiodarone to prevent recurrence of atrial fibrillation. *N Engl J Med* 2000;342: 913–920.

Design: Prospective, randomized, multicenter trial. Mean follow-up of 16 months.

Purpose: To evaluate the efficacy of amiodarone in preventing recurrent AF.

Population: 403 patients with symptomatic AF.

Treatment: Amiodarone, sotalol, or propafenone (average daily doses at 1 year were 194, 231, and 554 mg, respectively).

Results: Only 35% of amiodarone patients had a documented recurrence of AF compared with 63% taking the other antiarrhythmics. Discontinuation of study drug due to adverse effects occurred in 18% of amiodarone patients and 11% of sotalol/propafenone patients ($p = 0.06$).

53. Benditt DG, et al.; D,L-Sotalol Atrial Fibrillation/Flutter Study Group. Maintenance of sinus rhythm with oral D,L-sotalol therapy in patients with symptomatic atrial fibrillation and/or atrial flutter. *Am J Cardiol* 1999;84:270–277.

A double-blind, randomized, placebo-controlled trial of 253 patients with AF or atrial flutter comparing the SR maintenance efficacy of sotalol (at 80, 120, or 160 mg twice daily) to placebo. All patients were in SR at the initiation of treatment and they were followed for 12 months. The median time to recurrence on placebo was 27 days. With sotalol, it was 106 days at 80 mg ($p = 0.066$ vs. placebo), 229 days at 120 mg (p 0.004 vs. placebo), and 175 days at 160 mg ($p = 0.102$). The 160-mg dose was associated with more side effects and dropouts. No cases of torsade de pointes, sustained VT, or VF were reported.

54. de Paola AA, et al.; SOCESP Investigators. Efficacy and safety of sotalol versus quinidine for the maintenance of sinus rhythm after conversion of atrial fibrillation. *Am J Cardiol* 1999;84:1033–1037.

A randomized controlled trial of 121 patients postcardioversion for AF (<6 months) comparing sotalol (160 to 320 mg/day) and quinidine (600 to 800 mg/day). At 6 months, 74% of patients on sotalol and 68% on quinidine were still in normal SR ($p = $ NS). For those who had recurrences, the mean time to occurrence was longer in the sotalol group than with the quinidine group (69 days vs. 10 days; $p < 0.05$) and the average HR was lower in the sotalol group ($p < 0.05$). Interestingly, sotalol was more effective than quinidine for patients who had been in AF <72 hours prior to cardioversion (93% with sotalol vs. 64% with quinidine; $p = 0.01$), while patients in AF > 72 hours prior to cardioversion had better success on quinidine (68% on quinidine vs. 33% on sotalol; $p < 0.05$). 5% of patients in the sotalol group and 2% in the quinidine group experienced proarrhythmic events.

55. Bellandi F, et al. Long-term efficacy and safety of propafenone and sotalol for the maintenance of sinus rhythm after conversion of recurrent symptomatic atrial fibrillation. *Am J Cardiol* 2001;88(6):640–645.

A double-blind, placebo-controlled trial in 300 patients with AF comparing propafenone, sotalol, and placebo at the maintenance of normal SR postcardioversion. At 1-year postcardioversion, 63% of patients on propafenone and 73% on sotalol were in normal SR compared to 35% on placebo (placebo vs. either drug; $p = 0.001$). The dropout due to side effects was equal in the propafenone and sotalol groups (9% and 10%, respectively). The likelihood of remaining in SR was higher for younger patients with smaller LA size and without heart disease.

56. Kochiadakis GE, et al. Sotalol versus propafenone for long-term maintenance of normal sinus rhythm in patients with recurrent symptomatic atrial fibrillation. *Am J Cardiol* 2004;94(12):1563–1566.

A single-blind, prospective, randomized, controlled trial in 254 patients with AF comparing sotalol (480 mg/day) to propafenone (150 mg three times daily) in the maintenance of normal SR. 81% of patients on sotalol, 52% on propafenone, and 87% on placebo experienced recurrence of AF ($p < 0.001$ for propafenone vs. sotalol or placebo). The mean period to recurrence was also greater with propafenone at 26 months compared to 18 months with sotalol and 11 months with placebo.

57. Chimienti M, et al. Safety of long-term flecainide and propafenone in the management of patients with symptomatic paroxysmal atrial fibrillation: report from the Flecainide and Propafenone Italian Study (FAPIS) Investigators. *Am J Cardiol* 1996;77:60A–65A.

A randomized, open-label trial of 200 patients with paroxysmal AF comparing flecainide (200 to 300 mg daily) with propafenone (450 to 900 mg daily). Efficacy was measured indirectly by the number of patients who completed the study at 12 months. 77% of flecainide-treated patients completed the study compared to 75% of propafenone-treated patients ($p = 0.72$). 11% and 13% of patients dropped out due to lack of efficacy, respectively. There was no significant difference in the number of adverse events between groups.

58. Pritchett EL, et al.; Rythmol Atrial Fibrillation Trial (RAFT) Investigators. Efficacy and safety of sustained-release propafenone (propafenone SR) for patients with atrial fibrillation. *Am J Cardiol* 2003;92:941–946.

A double-blind, randomized, controlled trial of 523 patients with paroxysmal AF comparing propafenone SR (225, 325, or 425 mg twice daily) to placebo in the maintenance of normal SR. The median time to recurrence with propafenone SR was 112 days with 225 mg, 291 days with 325 mg, and >300 days with 425 mg compared to 41 days with placebo ($p < 0.001$ for 325 and 425 mg vs. placebo, and $p = 0.014$ for 225 mg vs. placebo). There were more adverse events leading to withdrawal in the 425-mg group (25% with 425 mg vs. 12.7% and 14.1% with 225 and 325 mg, respectively; p not reported).

59. Kochiadakis GE, et al. Long-term maintenance of normal sinus rhythm in patients with current symptomatic atrial fibrillation: amiodarone vs. propafenone, both in low doses. *Chest* 2004;125:377–383.

In this trial, the investigators randomized 146 patients with refractory AF, in a prospective, single-blinded manner, to amiodarone (200 mg/day) or propafenone (450 mg/day) after cardioversion and followed them for AF recurrence or side effects over approximately 20 months of follow-up. AF recurred in 25 of the 72 patients in the amiodarone group at a mean of 9.8 months, versus 33 of 74 patients in the propafenone group at an average of 3.8 months. However, 12 patients in the amiodarone group, compared with 2 in the propafenone group, reported side effects necessitating the withdrawal of study drug (while still in SR).

CATHETER AND SURGICAL ABLATION

Catheter Ablation

60. Haissaguerre M, et al. Spontaneous initiation of atrial fibrillation by ectopic beats originating in the pulmonary veins. N Engl J Med 1998;339:659–666.

This seminal paper by Haissaguerre was one of the first to ascribe the fibrillatory waves of AF to the pulmonary veins, which formed the basis of all subsequent catheter-based therapies for AF.

61. Stabile G, et al. Catheter ablation treatment in patients with drug-refractory atrial fibrillation: a prospective, multi-centre, randomized, controlled study (Catheter Ablation for the Cure Of Atrial Fibrillation Study). Eur Heart J 2006;27:216–221.

This multicenter, randomized, controlled trial studied ablation therapy for patients with paroxysmal AF, in whom antiarrhythmic therapy had failed. These 137 patients enrolled and received either antiarrhythmic therapy alone or antiarrhythmic therapy plus cavotricuspid, left inferior pulmonary vein–mitral isthmus, and circumferential pulmonary vein ablation (CPVA). The primary end point, recurrence of AF (for >30 seconds) at 1 year, occurred in 63 of 69 patients in the control group (91.3%), versus 30 of 68 patients (including 4 who had atrial flutter recur) in the ablation cohort (44.1%; $p < 0.001$ for the comparison).

62. Pappone C, et al. A randomized trial of circumferential pulmonary vein ablation versus antiarrhythmic drug therapy in paroxysmal atrial fibrillation: the APAF Study. J Am Coll Cardiol 2006;48:2340–2347.

198 patients with paroxysmal AF resistant to routine drug therapy were randomized to maximum antiarrhythmic drug therapy (with flecainide, sotalol, or amiodarone) or to CPVA. At 1 year, 93% of patients in the ablation group were free of atrial tachyarrhythmias, compared with 35% in the drug therapy group. Adverse events in the ablation group included one TIA and one pericardial effusion.

63. Oral H, et al. Circumferential pulmonary-vein ablation for chronic atrial fibrillation. N Engl J Med 2006;354:934–941.

This randomized, controlled trial of CPVA included 146 patients with chronic AF and assigned them to amiodarone and two cardioversions alone or in addition to CVPA. Cardiac rhythm was followed daily by telephonic monitoring for 1 year. Intention-to-treat analysis showed 74% of patients in the CVPA group versus 58% in the control group were free from AF and without antiarrhythmic drug therapy ($p = 0.05$). However, there was significant crossover (77% of the control group), and 26% of patients initially assigned to CVPA required repeat ablation for AF. They did observe a beneficial effect of SR on LA diameter.

64. Jaïs P, et al. Catheter ablation versus antiarrhythmic drugs for atrial fibrillation: the A4 study. Circulation 2008;118(24):2498–2505.

This was a randomized, multicenter, prospective trial of CVPA in 112 patients with paroxysmal AF; they were assigned to either CVPA or "new" antiarrhythmic drug therapy (alone or a combination of agents). Freedom from recurrence of AF was observed in 13 of 55 (23%) patients in the drug group, versus 46 of 52 patients (89%) in the ablation group at 1 year. Crossover, once again, was significant in the drug, as 63% (37 of 55) went on to undergo ablation.

65. Wilber DJ, et al.; for the ThermoCool AF Trial Investigators. Comparison of antiarrhythmic drug therapy and radiofrequency catheter ablation in patients with paroxysmal atrial fibrillation: a randomized controlled trial. JAMA 2010;303(4):333–340.

One hundred and sixty-seven patients with paroxysmal AF (who had failed one antiarrhythmic drug) were randomized in a 2:1, unblinded fashion to either PVI or antiarrhythmic drug therapy (dofetilide, flecainide, propafenone, sotalol, or quinidine). Over 9 months of follow-up, freedom from AF persisted in 66% of patients in the ablation group, versus 16% of those in the drug therapy group ($p < 0.001$ for hazard ratio of 0.30 for ablation). Adverse consequences of treatment were recorded in 8.8% of those in the drug therapy group and 4.9% of those in the ablation group.

66. Wilber DJ, et al. Comparison of antiarrhythmic drug therapy and radiofrequency catheter ablation in patients with paroxysmal atrial fibrillation: a randomized controlled trial. JAMA 2010;303(4):333–340.

Design: Prospective, multicenter, open-label, randomized trial of catheter ablation for AF. The primary end point was a protocol-defined treatment failure: documented, symptomatic, paroxysmal AF within 9 months. The investigators also assessed treatment-related adverse events within 30 days.

Purpose: To determine if catheter ablation was superior to antiarrhythmic drug therapy for the management of paroxysmal AF.

Population: 167 patients with paroxysmal AF who had failed at least 1 antiarrhythmic drug and had 3 or more AF episodes within 6 months

Treatment: Catheter ablation versus antiarrhythmic drug therapy (2:1 assignment).

Results: Patients undergoing catheter ablation were significantly more likely to remain arrhythmia-free at 9 months (65% vs. 16%; $p < 0.0010$), though they experienced numerically more adverse events within 30 days (8.8% vs. 4.9%).

Comments: This was one of several, important trials that has supported the use of catheter ablation of AF to reduce symptomatic recurrence in patients with paroxysmal AF who have failed antiarrhythmic drug therapy.

67. Piccini JP, et al. Pulmonary vein isolation for the maintenance of sinus rhythm in patients with atrial fibrillation: a meta-analysis of randomized, controlled trials. *Circ Arrhythm Electrophysiol* 2009;2(6):626–633.

The authors pooled data on 693 patients from 6 randomized trials comparing catheter ablation of AF to medical therapy (antiarrhythmic drugs). They identified a significant benefit in freedom from AF at 12 months in patients assigned to undergo catheter ablation (77% vs. 29%; OR, 9.74). They also demonstrated that ablation was associated with reduced cardiovascular hospitalization (14 vs. 93 per 100 person-years; rate ratio, 0.15). Major complications occurred in 2.6% of patients in the ablation group.

68. Wazni OM, et al. Radiofrequency ablation vs. antiarrhythmic drugs as first-line treatment of symptomatic atrial fibrillation: a randomized trial. JAMA 2005;293:2634–2640.

In order to assess the use of PVI as first-line therapy for symptomatic, paroxysmal AF, the investigators randomized 70 patients to either PVI with RF ablation or antiarrhythmic drug therapy and followed for 1 year for the recurrence of AF. Such treatment failures occurred in 22 of 35 patients (63%) who received drug therapy, versus 4 of 32 patients (13%) who underwent PVI. QOL at 6 months improved significantly more for patients in the PVI group, and patients in this group had significantly fewer hospitalizations during the 1-year follow-up period (9% vs. 54% for drug therapy; $p < 0.001$).

69. Morillo CA, et al. Radiofrequency Ablation vs Antiarrhythmic Drugs as First-Line Treatment of Paroxysmal Atrial Fibrillation (RAAFT-2). JAMA 2014;311(7):692.

Design: Prospective, international, multicenter, randomized trial of catheter ablation for AF. The primary end point was time to recurrence of any atrial tachyarrhythmia of ≥30 seconds (symptomatic or asymptomatic) out to 2 years.

Purpose: To assess the benefit of catheter ablation as first-line therapy for paroxysmal AF.

Population: 127 patients with paroxysmal AF, naïve to any rhythm-controlling therapies.

Treatment: Patients were randomized to undergo catheter ablation or to be treated with antiarrhythmic drug therapy.

Results: The primary end point, recurrence of atrial tachyarrhythmia, occurred significantly more frequently in the antiarrhythmic arm compared to those assigned to catheter ablation (72% vs. 54%; $p = 0.02$). Symptomatic recurrence was also more common in the antiarrhythmic group (59% vs. 47%; $p = 0.03$). There were no deaths or strokes in the study group, and 4 ablation procedures were complicated by cardiac tamponade.

Comments: This was one of the first studies to demonstrate the feasibility of catheter ablation as a first-line approach to patients with paroxysmal AF.

70. Narayan SM, et al. Direct or Coincidental Elimination of Stable Rotors or Focal Sources May Explain Successful Atrial Fibrillation Ablation: On-Treatment Analysis of the CONFIRM Trial (Conventional Ablation for AF With or Without Focal Impulse and Rotor Modulation). J Am Coll Cardiol 2013;62(2):138–147.

The study was one of the first to test a novel, proprietary approach to AF ablation, Focal Impulse and Rotor Modulation (FIRM). Such rotors were identified in 98 of 101 patients (during 107 ablation procedures), and those patients were randomly assigned (2:1) to receive or not receive FIRM ablation at the time of conventional ablation. At a mean follow-up of 273 days, 80% of patients who had complete rotor ablation were free of AF, compared with 18% of patients with incomplete rotor ablation ($p < 0.001$). This continues to be an exciting and evolving potential approach to AF ablation (see also *J Am Coll Cardiol* 2012;60(7):628–636).

71. Packer DL, et al. Cryoballoon Ablation of Pulmonary Veins for Paroxysmal Atrial Fibrillation: First Results of the North American Arctic Front (STOP AF) Pivotal Trial. J Am Coll Cardiol 2013;61(16):1713–1723.

The STOP AF trial was a pivotal, early study of an alternative ablative technology to radiofrequency—cryotherapy. One hundred and sixty-three patients with paroxysmal AF who had failed ≥1 antiarrhythmic therapy were randomized (2:1) to either cryoballoon ablation or antiarrhythmic drug therapy. At 12 months, 70% of cryoballoon patients achieved treatment success, compared with 7.3% of antiarrhythmic drug patients ($p < 0.001$).

Surgical Ablation

72. Barnett SD, et al. Surgical ablation as treatment for the elimination of atrial fibrillation: a meta-analysis. J Thorac Cardiovasc Surg 2006;131:1029–1035.

The authors review the evidence for use of the modified Maze procedure [to include biatrial (BA) ablation, compared with traditional LA modification, for the treatment of AF, through use of MEDLINE search]. In all, 69 studies were included and captured outcomes in 5,885 patients with survival data up to 3 years. While patients receiving BA procedures did not demonstrate a survival advantage, they did remain free from recurrence of AF longer and in greater numbers at each time point.

73. Reston JT, et al. Meta-analysis of clinical outcomes of maze-related surgical procedures for medically refractory atrial fibrillation. Eur J Cardiothorac Surg 2005;28:724–730.

The authors pooled data from four randomized studies and six retrospective comparisons of MV surgery patients with paroxysmal AF undergoing valve repair alone or with simultaneous maze procedure. However, the authors included different studies for the assessment of different end points, with the total population culminating in 905 patients. There was no significant difference in mortality between the two groups; however, restoration of SR favored the maze group (80.7% vs. 17.3%; $p < 0.000001$), as did the rate of stroke (0% vs. 5.8%; $p = 0.008$). The study offers weak evidence in favor of the maze procedure but also highlights the dearth of sound clinical data on which to evaluate it.

74. Albrecht A, et al. Randomized study of surgical isolation of the pulmonary veins for correction of permanent atrial fibrillation associated with mitral valve disease. *J Thorac Cardiovasc Surg* 2009;138:454–459.

The authors sought to evaluate the efficacy of surgical PVI, compared with maze procedure, for the treatment of chronic, permanent AF. In a total of 60 patients, they randomized 20 to each procedure (as well as a control group, which received no AF procedure with their MV correction); all had concomitant MV disease that was also corrected. Relative risk for AF late postoperatively was 0.07 in the PVI group ($p < 0.001$ vs. control) and 1.195 in the maze group ($p = 0.002$ vs. control). There was no statistical difference between the two interventions (RR, 0.358; $p = 0.215$). The study provides support to these surgical techniques for the correction of AF in the setting of MV disease.

75. Srivastava V, et al. Efficacy of three different ablative procedures to treat atrial fibrillation in patients with valvular heart disease: a randomised trial. *Heart Lung Circ* 2008;17(3):232–240.

In patients undergoing surgical correction of rheumatic heart disease, the authors randomized 160 patients with concomitant AF to one of the following four strategies: BA ablation (Cox maze), LA portion of the Cox maze, PVI, and a control group (no maze). Ablation was performed with RF microbipolar coagulation and cryoablation. SR was restored in 6.25% of patients in the BA maze group, 57.5% in the LA maze, 67.5% of the PVI group, and 20% of patients in the control group. This suggested that the long bypass and cross-clamp times of the traditional Cox maze procedure may not be required to achieve SR in patients undergoing surgery for concomitant rheumatic valve disease.

ELECTRICAL CARDIOVERSION AND PERICARDIOVERSION ANTICOAGULATION

76. Kawabata VS, et al. Monophasic versus biphasic waveform shocks for atrial fibrillation cardioversion in patients with concomitant amiodarone therapy. *Europace* 2007;9:143–146.

The investigators at one center randomized 154 patients with AF and receiving amiodarone to serial biphasic or serial monophasic (using twice as much energy as the biphasic group) shocks for DC cardioversion of AF. Patients converted to SR on the first shock in similar proportions between the two groups; success with serial shocks was also similar. The number of shocks required was similar in the two groups as well.

77. Wozakowska-Kaplon B, et al. Efficacy of biphasic shock for transthoracic cardioversion of persistent atrial fibrillation: can we predict energy requirements? *Pacing Clin Electrophysiol* 2004;27:764–768.

In 94 patients referred for biphasic cardioversion for AF, the authors achieved a success rate of 89% in a stepwise increase in energy, as required. However, a mean of 2.2 shocks was required, with energy of 217 J; by comparison, success of cardioversion using either 50 J or 50 J then 100 J was only a combined 51%. Duration of AF was the only predictor of lower energy requirement, and thus, it is recommended to start at 200 J for the vast majority of patients.

78. Glover BM, et al. Biphasic energy selection for transthoracic cardioversion of atrial fibrillation. The BEST AF Trial. *Heart* 2008;94:884–887.

The investigators prospectively randomized 380 patients with AF to either escalating biphasic energy (100, 150, 200, 200 J) or nonescalating biphasic energy (200, 200, 200 J) for cardioversion. Success of first shock was significantly higher in the nonescalating group (71% vs. 48%; $p < 0.01$) and for patients with a higher BMI. In patients with normal BMI (≤ 25 kg/m^2), there were no significant differences in the rate of success on the first shock, for subsequent shocks, or overall.

79. Manning WJ, et al. Cardioversion from atrial fibrillation without prolonged antico-agulation with the use of transesophageal echocardiography to exclude the presence of atrial thrombi. N *Engl J Med* 1993;328:750–755.

This study was composed of 94 patients with AF of more than 2 days' duration (average, 4.5 weeks). Eighty patients received heparin before cardioversion; 14 thrombi were seen by TEE versus only 2 of 14 seen on transthoracic echocardiography (2 of these patients died suddenly, whereas the other 10 were cardioverted after prolonged oral anticoagula-tion). No embolic events occurred in the other patients [78 of 82 successfully cardioverted (47 by drugs)].

80. Klein AL, et al.; for the Assessment of Cardioversion Using Transesophageal Echocardiography (ACUTE) Investigators. Use of transesophageal echocardiography to guide cardioversion in patients with atrial fibrillation. N *Engl J Med* 2001;344: 1411–1420.

Design: Prospective, randomized, open, multicenter study. Primary end point was embolic events.

Purpose: To evaluate the safety and efficacy of TEE-guided cardioversion in patients with AF.

Population: 1,222 patients with AF of more than 48 hours' duration.

Exclusion Criteria: Included atrial flutter (and no history of AF), long-term warfarin therapy, hemodynamic instability, and contraindications to TEE.

Treatment: Cardioversion after 3 or more weeks of warfarin or TEE-guided cardioversion. All received a minimum of 4 weeks of warfarin after cardioversion.

Results: No difference between the groups was found in the incidence of embolic events [0.5% (TEE-guided) vs. 0.8%]. The TEE approach was associated with lower rates of hemorrhage, mostly minor (2.9% vs. 5.5%; $p = 0.03$). The TEE group had a higher initial successful cardioversion rate (71.1% vs. 65.2%; $p = 0.03$); however, SR rates were similar at 8 weeks.

81. Page RL, et al. Biphasic versus monophasic shock waveform for conversion of atrial fibrillation: the results of an international randomized, double-blind multicenter trial. *J Am Coll Cardiol* 2002;39:1956–1963.

This prospective, randomized, double-blind, multicenter trial compared the effective-ness of monophasic versus biphasic shocks for the cardioversion of AF. The 203 patients were randomized to monophasic or biphasic shocking waveforms, and received successive shocks, as needed, at three shared energies (100, 150, and 200 J), and then maximum output for the respective devices (200 J biphasic, 360 J monophasic) and, if necessary, a final crossover shock at maximum output of the alternate waveform. The success rate was higher for biphasic than for monophasic shocks at each of the three shared energy levels (100 J, 60% vs. 22%; 150 J, 77% vs. 44%; 200 J, 90% vs. 53%; $p < 0.0001$). On average, biphasic patients required fewer shocks (1.7 vs. 2.8; $p < 0.0001$) and lower total energy (217 J vs. 548 J; $p < 0.0001$) for successful conversion. The biphasic shock waveform also was associated with a lower frequency of dermal injury (17% vs. 41%; $p < 0.0001$).

82. Stellbrink C, et al. Safety and efficacy of enoxaparin compared with unfractionated heparin and oral anticoagulants for prevention of thromboembolic complications in cardioversion of nonvalvular atrial fibrillation: the Anticoagulation in Cardioversion using Enoxaparin (ACE) trial. *Circulation* 2004;109:997–1003.

This European study included 496 patients with nonvalvular AF scheduled to undergo elective cardioversion. Subjects were randomized to IV unfractionated heparin followed by phenprocoumon or to enoxaparin, 1 mg/kg twice daily for 3 to 8 days followed by 40 or 60 mg b.i.d. Most (86%) of the cardioversions were TEE guided. The primary composite end point of all-cause mortality, neurologic events, embolic events, and major bleeding occurred (in intention-to-treat analysis) in 4.8% of unfractionated heparin patients and 2.8% of enoxaparin patients ($p_{noninferiority}$ = 0.013). Investigators concluded that enoxaparin was not inferior.

83. Airaksinen KE, et al. Thromboembolic complications after cardioversion of acute atrial fibrillation: the FinCV (Finnish CardioVersion) study. *J Am Coll Cardiol* 2013;62(13):1187–1192.

The investigators used administrative data in Finland to assess the risk of stroke following cardioversion for AF <48h, in the absence of anticoagulation. There were 2,481 patients studied, and they experienced 38 thromboembolic events within 30 days of cardioversion. The events increased dramatically with additional $CHADS_2$ risk factors, such as HF (OR, 2.9; 95% CI, 1.1 to 7.2) and diabetes (OR, 2.3; 95% CI, 1.1 to 4.9). These data call into question a uniform approach of withholding anticoagulation in the setting of cardioversion for acute (<48 h) AF.

LONG-TERM ANTICOAGULATION

84. Peterson P, et al. Atrial Fibrillation, Aspirin, Anticoagulation (AFASAK) study. Placebo-controlled, randomized trial of warfarin and aspirin for prevention of thromboembolic complications in chronic atrial fibrillation. *Lancet* 1989;333:175–178.

Design: Prospective, randomized, partially open (warfarin), partially blinded (aspirin vs. placebo) study. Follow-up period was 2 years. Primary end point was thromboembolic complications (TIA, minor stroke, nondisabling stroke, fatal stroke, or embolism to viscera or extremities).

Purpose: To assess the efficacy of low-dose warfarin in preventing strokes in patients with nonrheumatic AF.

Population: 1,007 patients aged 18 years with chronic AF.

Exclusion Criteria: Prior anticoagulation for 6 months, cerebrovascular events in the prior 1 month, and blood pressure (BP) >180/100 mm Hg.

Treatment: Low-dose warfarin [target prothrombin time (PT), 1.2 to 1.5 times control (approximate INR, 2.8 to 4.2)]; aspirin, 75 mg/day; or placebo.

Results: The warfarin group had significantly fewer thromboembolic complications [1.5% vs. 6.0% (aspirin) and 6.3% (placebo)]. Vascular death occurred in 0.9%, 3.6%, and 4.5% of the warfarin, aspirin, and placebo groups (p < 0.02), respectively. Warfarin patients had more frequent nonfatal bleeding (6.3% vs. 0.6% and none of aspirin and placebo patients).

85. Boston Area Anticoagulation Trial for Atrial Fibrillation (BAATAF). The effect of low-dose warfarin on the risk of stroke in patients with non-rheumatic atrial fibrillation. *N Engl J Med* 1990;323:1505–1511.

Design: Prospective, randomized, open, controlled, multicenter study. Mean follow-up period was 2.2 years. Primary end point was ischemic stroke.

Purpose: To assess the efficacy of low-dose warfarin in preventing strokes in patients with nonrheumatic AF.

Population: 420 patients (mean age, 63 years) with chronic or intermittent AF.

Exclusion Criteria: Prosthetic valves, severe HF, stroke in the prior 6 months, and contraindications to or requirement for aspirin or warfarin therapy.

Treatment: Warfarin [target PT, 1.2 to 1.5 times normal (achieved in 83%)]; aspirin was allowed in the control group.

Results: Trial was terminated early because of strong evidence in favor of warfarin. The warfarin group had 86% fewer strokes [0.41% per year vs. 2.98% per year (control group); $p = 0.002$] and a 62% lower death rate (2.25% per year vs. 5.97% per year; $p = 0.005$). The warfarin group had more minor hemorrhages (38 patients vs. 21 patients).

86. SPAF Investigators. Stroke Prevention in Atrial Fibrillation Study: final results. *Circulation* 1991;84:527–539.

Design: Prospective, randomized, partially open (warfarin), partially blind (aspirin vs. placebo), multicenter study. Primary events were ischemic stroke and systemic embolism. Mean follow-up was 1.3 years.

Purpose: To determine the efficacy and safety of warfarin and aspirin compared with placebo for the prevention of ischemic stroke and systemic embolism in patients with nonrheumatic AF.

Population: 1,330 patients with chronic or intermittent AF.

Exclusion Criteria: Prosthetic valves, mitral stenosis, MI in the prior 3 months, and stroke or TIA in the prior 2 years.

Treatment: Group 1 [627 patients (most 75 years or younger)]: warfarin (target PT, 1.3 to 1.8 times normal (approximate INR, 2.0 to 4.5)]; aspirin, 325 mg/day; or placebo. Group 2 (703 nonanticoagulation candidates): aspirin or placebo.

Results: Aspirin-treated patients had 67% fewer primary events than did placebo patients (3.6% per year vs. 6.3% per year; $p = 0.02$). In the warfarin-eligible patients, warfarin reduced the risk of primary events by 67% compared with placebo (2.3% per year vs. 7.4% per year; $p = 0.01$). Primary events or death were reduced 58% by warfarin ($p = 0.01$) and 32% by aspirin ($p = 0.02$). Disabling stroke or vascular death was reduced 54% by warfarin and a nonsignificant 22% by aspirin ($p = 0.33$). Significant bleeding rates were similar in all three groups (1.4% to 1.6% per year). Significant risk factors for stroke were (a) prior cerebrovascular accident, (b) CHF within preceding 100 days, (c) hypertension and among the echocardiographically assessed features, (d) left atrium more than 5 cm, and (e) LV dysfunction. If one clinical factor was present, the risk of stroke was 7% per year; if two or all three factors were present, the risk was 18% per year. The group without any risk factors (26%) had an event rate of only 1% per year.

Comments: Placebo arm of group 1 was discontinued in late 1989 because of the strong evidence of superiority of both warfarin and aspirin over placebo.

87. Connolly SJ, et al. Canadian Atrial Fibrillation Anticoagulation study (CAFA). *J Am Coll Cardiol* 1991;18:349–355 (editorial, 301–302).

Design: Prospective, randomized, double-blind, placebo-controlled, multicenter study. Primary end points were nonlacunar ischemic stroke, other systemic embolism, and intracranial or fatal hemorrhage.

Purpose: To evaluate the effectiveness and safety of warfarin in AF patients.

Population: 378 patients with recurrent paroxysmal or chronic AF.

Exclusion Criteria: Clear indications or contraindications to anticoagulation, stroke, or TIA in the prior year, MI in the prior month, use of antiplatelet drug(s), and uncontrolled hypertension.

Treatment: Warfarin (target INR, 2 to 3) or placebo.

Results: Target INR was achieved with only 44% frequency (subtherapeutic values in 39.6%). The warfarin group had a nonsignificant 37% risk reduction in primary outcome events (3.5% per year vs. 5.2% per year; p = 0.26). Major/fatal and minor bleeding events were common with warfarin use (2.5% per year vs. 0.5% per year and 16% per year vs. 9.4% per year).

Comments: Trial was terminated early because of the AFASAK and SPAF results.

88. Ezekowitz MD, et al.; VA Stroke Prevention in Non-rheumatic Atrial Fibrillation (SPINAF). Warfarin in the prevention of stroke associated with non-rheumatic atrial fibrillation. N Engl J Med 1992;327:1406–1412.

Design: Prospective, randomized, double-blind, placebo-controlled, multicenter study. Average follow-up period was 1.8 years. Primary end point was cerebral infarction.

Purpose: To evaluate whether low-intensity anticoagulation will decrease the risk of stroke in patients with nonrheumatic AF.

Population: 571 men, 46 with prior stroke, without echocardiographic evidence of rheumatic heart disease and AF on two ECG tracings 4 weeks apart.

Exclusion Criteria: Contraindications to or requirement for anticoagulation, BP >180/105 mmHg, and use of nonsteroidal anti-inflammatory drugs.

Treatment: Warfarin (target INR, 1.4 to 2.8) or placebo.

Results: A 79% risk reduction was observed among patients without a history of stroke (0.9% per year vs. 4.3% per year; p = 0.001). Significant benefit also was seen in patients older than 70 years (0.9% per year vs. 4.8% per year; p = 0.02) and with a history of prior stroke (6.1% per year vs. 9.3% per year). Major hemorrhage rates were similar [1.3% per year (warfarin) vs. 0.9% per year]. Cerebral infarction occurred more frequently among patients with a history of cerebral infarction [9.3% per year (placebo group) and 6.1% per year (warfarin group)].

Comments: An analysis of 516 evaluable admission computed tomography (CT) scans showed that 14.7% had one silent infarct. Strokes during the study were not predicted by infarct on admission CT scan but rather by active angina [placebo group, 15% (angina) vs. 5%].

89. European Atrial Fibrillation Trial (EAFT) Study Group. Secondary prevention in non-rheumatic fibrillation after transient ischemic attack or minor stroke. Lancet 1993;342:1255–1262.

Design: Prospective, randomized, partially open (anticoagulant therapy), double-blind aspirin treatment, placebo-controlled, multicenter study. Primary end points were death from vascular disease, any stroke, MI, and systemic embolism. Mean follow-up period was 2.3 years.

Purpose: To evaluate and compare the effectiveness of oral anticoagulation and aspirin in AF patients with recent minor cerebrovascular events.

Population: 1,007 patients with nonrheumatic AF and minor stroke or TIA in the previous 3 months.

Exclusion Criteria: Use of nonsteroidal anti-inflammatory or other antiplatelet drugs, MI in the prior 3 months, and scheduled coronary surgery or carotid endarterectomy within next 3 months.

Treatment: Group 1 (669 patients): warfarin (target INR, 2.5 to 4.0), or aspirin, 300 mg daily, or placebo. Group 2: contraindications to anticoagulation; 338 patients.

Results: Anticoagulation was more effective than aspirin and placebo—8% versus 15% and 17% annual rates of primary outcome events; risk of stroke was especially lower in warfarin-treated patients [4% per year vs. 12% per year (placebo)]. Overall, warfarin use was associated with 90 fewer vascular events per 1,000 patient-years (vs. 40 with aspirin). Bleeding events were common in warfarin-treated patients [2.8% per year vs. 0.9% per year (aspirin patients)]. Analysis of group 2 patients showed that the optimal INR range was 2.0 to 3.9, with most bleeding complications occurring when the INR was >5.0, and no significant treatment effect was seen if INR was <2.0.

90. SPAF II. Warfarin versus aspirin for prevention of thromboembolism in atrial fibrillation. *Lancet* 1994;43:687–691.

Design: Prospective, randomized, open, parallel-group, multicenter study. Primary events were stroke and systemic embolism. Mean follow-up period was 2.3 years.

Purpose: To define the long-term benefits and risks associated with warfarin compared with aspirin, according to age and risk of thromboembolism.

Population: 1,100 patients, 715 patients aged 75 years or younger and 385 older than 75 years, with AF in the prior 12 months.

Exclusion Criteria: Lone AF if younger than 60 years and stroke or TIA in the prior 2 years.

Treatment: Warfarin (target INR, 2.0 to 4.5) or aspirin 325 mg daily.

Results: No significant difference was observed between groups. However, 12 of 28 events in the warfarin group occurred while patients were not taking warfarin. Thus, a 50% difference in favor of warfarin is evident if these events are excluded. Event rates per year for patients aged 75 years or younger were 1.3% versus 1.9% ($p = 0.24$) and older than 75 years, 3.6% versus 4.8% ($p = 0.39$). Low-risk younger patients (no hypertension, recent HF, or prior thromboembolism) had a low 0.5% per year primary event rate. Among older patients, stroke rates were similar in the two treatment groups (aspirin, 4.3% per year; warfarin, 4.6% per year). Among warfarin-treated patients, the intracranial hemorrhage was significantly higher in older versus younger patients (1.6% vs. 4.2%; $p = 0.04$).

Comments: Randomization was performed separately for the two age groups.

91. Hylek EM, et al. An analysis of the lowest effective intensity of prophylactic anticoagulation for patients with non-rheumatic atrial fibrillation. *N Engl J Med* 1996;335:540–546.

This retrospective, case–control analysis focused on 74 consecutive patients with ischemic strokes taking warfarin (INR measured at admission) and 222 controls (INR measured closest to admission day of case patient). The risk of stroke increased significantly at INRs <2.0; the adjusted OR for stroke was 2.0 if the INR was 1.7 to 2.0, 3.3 if the INR was 1.5 to 2.0, and 6.0 if the INR was 1.3 to 2.0. Other independent risk factors were prior stroke (OR, 10.4), diabetes (OR, 2.9), hypertension (OR, 2.5), and smoking (OR, 5.7).

92. SPAF III. Adjusted-dose warfarin vs. low-intensity, fixed-dose warfarin and aspirin for high-risk patients with atrial fibrillation: SPAF III randomised clinical trial. *Lancet* 1996;348:633–638.

Design: Prospective, randomized, partially open, multicenter study. Primary events were ischemic stroke and systemic embolism. Mean follow-up period was 1.1 years.

Purpose: To compare the safety and effectiveness of a combination of low-intensity, fixed-dose warfarin plus aspirin with adjusted-dose warfarin in AF patients at high risk of stroke.

Population: 1,044 AF patients with one of the following: CHF or EF 25% or less, prior thromboembolism, systolic blood pressure (SBP) >160 mm Hg, or woman older than 75 years.

Exclusion Criteria: Conditions requiring standard anticoagulation therapy and contraindications to aspirin or warfarin.

Treatment: Fixed-dose warfarin [initial INR, 1.2 to 1.5 (mean, 1.3)] and aspirin (325 mg/day) or adjusted-dose warfarin [INR, 2 to 3 (mean, 2.4)].

Results: Trial was terminated early. The low-INR group had four times more ischemic strokes and systemic emboli (7.9% per year vs. 1.9% per year; $p < 0.0001$). Rates of disabling stroke (5.6% per year vs. 1.7% per year; $p = 0.0007$) and of primary or vascular death (11.8% per year vs. 6.4% per year; $p = 0.002$) also were higher with combination therapy. Bleeding rates were similar. The greatest benefits of standard adjusted-dose warfarin were seen in patients with prior thromboembolism.

93. Gullov AL, et al. AFASAK II. Fixed minidose warfarin, aspirin alone and in combination, versus adjusted-dose warfarin for stroke prevention in atrial fibrillation. *Arch Intern Med* 1998;158:1513–1521 (editorial, 1487–1491).

Design: Prospective, randomized, controlled, single-center study. Primary end points were stroke and systemic thromboembolic events.

Purpose: To investigate the effects of minidose warfarin alone and in combination with aspirin in chronic AF patients.

Population: 677 patients (median age, 74 years) with chronic AF documented by ECG tracings at least 1 month apart.

Exclusion Criteria: Lone AF in patients 60 years or younger, SBP more than 180 mm Hg, diastolic BP more than 100 mm Hg, and stroke or TIA in the prior 6 months.

Treatment: Warfarin, 1.25 mg/day; warfarin, 1.25 mg/day; aspirin, 300 mg/day; aspirin alone; or warfarin alone (target INR, 2 to 3).

Results: Trial was terminated early because of SPAF III results. One-year cumulative primary event rates were as follows: minidose warfarin, 5.8%; warfarin plus aspirin, 7.2%; aspirin alone, 3.6%; and adjusted-dose warfarin, 2.8% ($p = 0.67$). No significant differences were seen at 3 years. Major bleeding events were rare.

94. Hart RG, et al. Antithrombotic therapy to prevent stroke in patients with atrial fibrillation: a meta-analysis. *Ann Intern Med* 1999;131:492–501.

The investigators combined data from 16 randomized trials of warfarin or aspirin in 9,874 patients with AF, for the prevention of stroke. Compared to placebo, warfarin reduced stroke by 62% (2.7% per year for primary prevention, 8.4% per year for secondary prevention), whereas aspirin reduced stroke by 22% (1.5% per year for primary prevention, 2.5% per year for secondary prevention). In head-to-head comparison, warfarin was better than aspirin at stroke prevention [relative risk reduction (RRR), 36%; 95% CI, 14% to 52%].

95. Hart RG, et al. Meta-analysis: antithrombotic therapy to prevent stroke in patients who have nonvalvular atrial fibrillation. *Ann Intern Med* 2007;146(12):857–867.

This updated meta-analysis combined the results of 29 trials comparing dose-adjusted warfarin, antiplatelet therapy, and controls, for stroke prevention in AF. Overall, 2,900 patients were included in 6 trials of warfarin versus control, 4876 patients were included in 8 trials of antiplatelets versus control, and 12,962 patients in 12 trials compared warfarin to antiplatelet therapy (several randomized comparisons were inconclusive). They demonstrate a significant 64% reduction in stroke with warfarin (95% CI, 49% to 74%), 22% reduction in stroke for antiplatelet agents (95% CI, 6% to 35%), and an RRR of 39% for warfarin over antiplatelet therapies (95% CI, 22% to 52%). They also highlight that absolute increases in intracranial bleeding (approximately 0.3% per year) were less than the absolute reductions in stroke.

96. The ACTIVE Investigators. Clopidogrel plus aspirin versus oral anticoagulation for atrial fibrillation in the Atrial fibrillation Clopidogrel Trial with Irbesartan for prevention of Vascular Events (ACTIVE W): a randomised controlled trial. *Lancet* 2006 367:1903–1912.

Design: Prospective, randomized, controlled trial. Treatment assignment was open, but end point adjudication was blinded. The primary end point was a composite of stroke, non-CNS systemic embolism, MI, or vascular death.

Purpose: To assess the efficacy of aspirin plus clopidogrel, versus warfarin, for stroke prevention in patients with AF.

Population: 6,706 patients with AF and at least one additional risk factor for stroke.

Major Exclusion Criteria: Mitral stenosis

Treatment: Aspirin (75 to 100 mg daily) plus clopidogrel (75 mg daily) or dose-adjusted warfarin (target INR 2.0 to 3.0).

Results: After median follow-up of 1.28 years, the trial was terminated early due to clear superiority of warfarin, with the annual rate of primary end points of 3.93% for anticoagulation, versus 5.6% for dual antiplatelet therapy ($p = 0.0003$). Total bleeding rates favored oral anticoagulation, also (13.2% vs. 15.4%; $p = 0.001$).

97. The ACTIVE Investigators. Effect of Clopidogrel Added to Aspirin in Patients with Atrial Fibrillation (ACTIVE A). *N Engl J Med* 2009;360:2066–2078.

Design: Prospective, randomized, double-blinded, controlled trial. The primary end point was a composite of stroke, non-CNS systemic embolism, MI, or vascular death at a median of 3.6 years of follow-up.

Purpose: To assess the safety and efficacy of adding clopidogrel to aspirin, for the prevention of stroke in patients with AF.

Population: 7,554 patients with AF and additional risk for stroke, who could not receive oral anticoagulation.

Treatment: Clopidogrel (75 mg daily) or placebo, in addition to aspirin (75 to 100 mg daily).

Results: Rates of the primary end point were 6.8% for patients receiving clopidogrel, versus 7.6% for those receiving placebo ($p = 0.01$). There was a significantly higher risk of bleeding in the clopidogrel group (2.0% vs. 1.3%; $p < 0.001$).

Comments: Importantly, there were a variety of reasons cited for patients not being eligible for warfarin, principally that a physician judged oral anticoagulation to be appropriate (50%) or patient preference (the sole reason in 26%).

98. Singer DE, et al. The net clinical benefit of warfarin anticoagulation in atrial fibrillation. *Ann Intern Med* 2009;151:297–305.

In an effort to assess the net clinical benefit of warfarin anticoagulation in AF, the authors pooled data on 13,559 adults, over 66,000 person-years of follow-up in an integrated health care delivery system. They balanced ischemic (presumed thromboembolic) stroke events against hemorrhagic events with an impact weight factor applied (hemorrhagic events counted 1.5× more than ischemic ones). After stratifying patients by $CHADS_2$ score, investigators found an overall 0.68% net clinical benefit in favor of warfarin; however, this varied greatly across the spectrum of $CHADS_2$ score. Those with a $CHADS_2$ of 0 or 1 had essentially no clinical benefit, while those with a score of 4 to 6 derived a 2.22% yearly net clinical benefit. Notably, there was a significant net clinical benefit in older patients (those over 84 years) of 2.34%.

NON–VITAMIN K ORAL ANTICOAGULANTS

99. Connolly SJ, et al.; the RE-LY Steering Committee and Investigators. Dabigatran versus warfarin in patients with atrial fibrillation. *N Engl J Med* 2009;361:1139–1151.

Design: Prospective, multicenter, international, open-label, randomized trial. The primary end point was stroke or systemic embolism at mean follow-up of 2 years.

Purpose: To evaluate the efficacy and safety of the oral direct thrombin inhibitor dabigatran for stroke prevention in AF.

Population: 18,113 patients with nonvalvular AF and increased risk of stroke.

Key Exclusion Criteria: Valvular AF, mechanical heart valves, other indications for oral anticoagulation, or severe renal dysfunction.

Treatment: Dose-adjusted warfarin, dabigatran 110 mg b.i.d., dabigatran 150 mg b.i.d.

Results: Primary end point events occurred at 1.69% per year in the warfarin group versus 1.53% per year in the dabigatran 110-mg group and 1.11% in the 150-mg dabigatran group. Major bleeding occurred at 3.36% per year in the warfarin group, versus 2.71% per year in the dabigatran 110 mg group, and 3.11% per year in the dabigatran 150-mg group. Hemorrhagic stroke rates also favored dabigatran: 0.38% per year for warfarin, versus 0.12% and 0.10% for the 110- and 150-mg dabigatran groups, respectively. All of these margins met the statistical test for noninferiority except the bleeding comparison of warfarin and dabigatran 150 mg. There were no differences in the mortality rates among the groups.

Comments: This trial led to the approval of dabigatran in the United States at only the 150 mg dose, and it is the only NOAC to demonstrate reduced *ischemic stroke* compared to warfarin. However, roughly 10% of patients experienced dyspepsia as a side effect. Dabigatran is also approved at a 75-mg twice-daily dosing for patients with significant renal dysfunction; however, this was not studied in the RE-LY trial.

100. Patel MR, et al.; The ROCKET AF Trial. Rivaroxaban versus warfarin in nonvalvular atrial fibrillation. *N Engl J Med* 2011;365:883–891.

Design: Prospective, multicenter, international, double-blinded, active-controlled, randomized trial. The primary end point was stroke or systemic embolism at a median follow-up of 707 days.

Purpose: To assess the efficacy and safety of the oral factor Xa inhibitor rivaroxaban for stroke prevention in AF.

Population: 14,264 patients with nonvalvular AF at high risk of stroke (mean $CHADS_2$ score of 3.5).

Key Exclusion Criteria: Valvular AF, mechanical valve replacement, other indication for oral anticoagulation, severe renal dysfunction.

Treatment: Dose-adjusted warfarin or rivaroxaban 20 mg daily (15 mg daily for patients with creatinine clearance of 30 to 49 mL/min).

Results: The per-protocol analysis was an on-treatment assessment of the primary end point and demonstrated noninferiority of rivaroxaban (1.7% per year) versus warfarin (2.2% per year; HR for rivaroxaban, 0.79; $p < 0.001$). Similar results were observed in the intention-to-treat analysis. There was no significant difference in the rates of major or nonmajor clinically relevant bleeding between rivaroxaban (14.9% per year) and warfarin (14.5% per year; hazard for rivaroxaban, 1.03; $p = 0.44$); however, patients assigned rivaroxaban had significantly lower rates of ICH compared with warfarin (0.5% vs. 0.7%; $p = 0.02$).

Comments: This trial led to the approval of rivaroxaban for stroke prevention in AF. It should be noted that the time-in-therapeutic range for warfarin patients in the trial was lower than many hoped (55%); also, there was an increase in stroke rate at study end in patients in the rivaroxaban due to a lag in time to therapeutic INR during the transition to open-label warfarin. Lastly, subsequent analyses demonstrated a significantly higher rate of gastrointestinal bleeding in the rivaroxaban group (see *J Am Coll Cardiol* 2014;63:891–900).

101. Connolly SJ, et al.; The AVERROES Trial. Apixaban in patients with atrial fibrillation. N Engl J Med 2011;364:806–817.

Design: Prospective, international, multicenter, double-blinded, double-dummy, randomized trial. The primary end point was stroke or systemic embolism at mean follow-up of 1.1 years.

Purpose: To assess the efficacy and safety of the oral factor Xa inhibitor apixaban for stroke prevention in patients with AF not candidates for warfarin.

Population: 5,599 patients with nonvalvular AF at increased risk of stroke, but unsuitable candidates for warfarin.

Key Exclusion Criteria: Valvular disease requiring surgery or other indications for oral anticoagulation.

Treatment: Aspirin 81 to 243 mg daily versus apixaban 5 mg twice daily.

Results: The trial was terminated early due to overwhelming evidence of benefit in the apixaban group—1.6% per year primary event rate versus 3.7% for aspirin (HR for apixaban, 0.45; $p < 0.001$). Annual rates of mortality (3.5% for apixaban vs. 4.4% for aspirin; $p = 0.07$), major bleeding (1.4% for apixaban vs. 1.2% for aspirin; $p = 0.6$), and numbers of intracranial hemorrhage events (11 for apixaban, 13 for aspirin) were all statistically similar.

Comments: This was a landmark trial highlighting the bleeding risks of aspirin therapy and potential role for an NOAC in this patients. It should be noted that 40% of patients in AVERROES had prior warfarin therapy, and roughly 40%y overall were not candidates for warfarin due to difficulty or expected difficulty in maintaining INR in the appropriate range (as opposed to high bleeding risk).

102. Granger CB, et al.; The ARISTOTLE Trial. Apixaban versus warfarin in patients with atrial fibrillation. N Engl J Med 2011;365:981–992.

Design: Prospective, international, multicenter, double-blinded, double-dummy, randomized study. The primary end point was stroke or systemic embolism at mean follow-up of 1.8 years.

Purpose: To assess the efficacy and safety of the oral factor Xa inhibitor apixaban for stroke prevention in AF.

Population: 18,201 patients with nonvalvular AF at increased risk for stroke.

Key Exclusion Criteria: Significant mitral stenosis, other indication for oral anticoagulation, or severe renal dysfunction.

Treatment: Dose-adjusted warfarin or apixaban 5 mg twice daily; 2.5 mg twice daily was used in patients with ≥2 of the following risk factors: age ≥80 years, weight ≤60 kg, and/or serum creatinine ≥1.5 mg/dL.

Results: Rates of the primary end point were 1.27% for apixaban versus 1.60% for warfarin (HR for apixaban, 0.79; $p < 0.001$ for noninferiority, $p = 0.01$ for superiority). Major bleeding was significantly lower for apixaban (2.13% per year vs. 3.09% per year, HR for apixaban, 0.69; $p < 0.001$), as were rates of intracranial hemorrhage (0.24% vs. 047%; HR for apixaban, 0.51; $p < 0.001$).

Comments: Apixaban was subsequently approved based on this trial, and it was the only individual study to demonstrate significantly lower mortality with an NOAC versus warfarin (though a trend was observed in the others and confirmed in meta-analyses).

103. Giugliano RP, et al.; The ENGAGE AF- TIMI 48 Trial. Edoxaban versus warfarin in patients with atrial fibrillation. N Engl J Med 2013;369:2093–104.

Design: Prospective, international, multicenter, double-blinded, double-dummy, randomized trial. The primary end point was stroke or systemic embolism at median follow-up of 2.8 years.

Purpose: To assess the efficacy and safety of the oral factor Xa inhibitor edoxaban for stroke prevention in AF.

Population: 21,105 patients with nonvalvular AF at increased risk for stroke.

Key Exclusion Criteria: Significant mitral stenosis, other indication for oral anticoagulation, high risk of bleeding due to dual antiplatelet therapy, or severe renal dysfunction.

Treatment: Dose-adjusted warfarin, edoxaban 60 mg daily, or edoxaban 30 mg daily; edoxaban dosing was halved for patients with any of the following: estimated creatinine clearance 30 to 50 mL/min, body weight ≤60 kg, or concomitant use of verapamil, dronedarone, or quinidine (potent P-glycoprotein inhibitors).

Results: Annual rates of the primary end point were 1.5% for warfarin, versus 1.18% for high-dose edoxaban (HR, 0.79; p < 0.001 for noninferiority), and 1.61% for low-dose edoxaban (HR, 1.07; p = 0.005 for noninferiority). Annual major bleeding rates were 3.43% for warfarin, versus 2.75% for high-dose edoxaban (HR, 0.80; p < 0.001), and 1.61% for low-dose edoxaban (HR, 0.47; p < 0.001). Cardiovascular death was significantly lower for high-dose edoxaban (2.74% per year; HR, 0.86; p = 0.01) and low-dose edoxaban (2.71% per year; HR, 0.85; p = 0.008), compared with warfarin (3.17% per year). Rates of intracranial hemorrhage were also lower in both edoxaban groups (0.39% and 0.26% per year) versus warfarin (0.85% per year; p < 0.001 for each comparison with warfarin).

Comments: The ENGAGE AF-TIMI 48 trial demonstrated consistent findings with other trials of factor Xa inhibitors for stroke prevention, but with an additional dosing strategy.

104. Ruff CT, et al. Comparison of the efficacy and safety of new oral anticoagulants with warfarin in patients with atrial fibrillation: a meta-analysis of randomised trials. *Lancet* 2014;383:955–962.

The authors combined the results of the above four phase three trials comparing NOACs to warfarin for stroke prevention in AF. This included 41,411 patients assigned to NOACs and 29,272 to warfarin. They demonstrated several consistent findings across trials, such as lower risks of stroke or systemic embolism (RR, 0.81; p < 0.000), intracranial hemorrhage (RR, 0.48; p < 0.000), and all-cause mortality (RR, 0.90; p = 0.0003). However, as hazards in the individual trials varied, there was significant heterogeneity around the end point of major bleeding (RR, 0.86; p = 0.06), which varied depending on the local warfarin control; NOACs overall were associated with increased GI bleeding (RR, 1.25; p = 0.04) (**Fig. 6.1**). Of note, these primary results included only the high-dose arms of the two studies with multiple dosing levels (RE-LY, ENGAGE AF-TIMI 48).

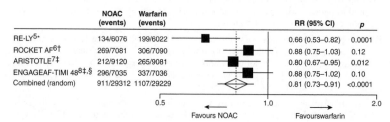

Figure 6.1 • Stroke or systemic embolic events. Data are n/N, unless otherwise indicated. Heterogeneity: I^2 = 47%; p = 0.13. NOAC, new oral anticoagulant; RR, risk ratio. [*]Dabigatran 150 mg twice daily. [†]Rivaroxaban 20 mg once daily. [‡]Apixaban 5 mg twice daily. [§]Edoxaban 60 mg once daily. (From **Ruff CT, et al.** Comparison of the efficacy and safety of new oral anticoagulants with warfarin in patients with atrial fibrillation: a meta-analysis of randomised trials. *Lancet* 2014;383:955–962.)

NONPHARMACOLOGIC STROKE PREVENTION IN AF

105. Reddy VY, et al. Percutaneous Left Atrial Appendage Closure for Stroke Prophylaxis in Patients With Atrial Fibrillation: 2.3-Year Follow-up of the PROTECT AF (Watchman Left Atrial Appendage System for Embolic Protection in Patients With Atrial Fibrillation) Trial. *Circulation* 2013;127(6):720–729.

In this long-term follow-up of the PROTECT AF trial, the authors assessed the safety and efficacy of this interventional approach to stroke prevention in AF in 707 patients with nonvalvular AF and at least 1 risk factor for stroke. Patients were randomized 2:1 to Watchman or continued warfarin; those assigned to Watchman discontinued warfarin roughly 45 days after the procedure and maintained dual antiplatelet therapy for 4.5 months (with indefinite aspirin). After a mean of 2.3 years of follow-up, rates of stroke, systemic embolism, and cardiovascular death were 3.0% in the Watchman group versus 4.3% in the warfarin group (RR, 0.71; probability of noninferiority >0.999). Not only did this demonstrate the feasibility of the Watchman device, but also it provided some of the strongest support implicating the LAA in the pathogenesis of stroke for patients with AF.

106. Bartus K, et al. Percutaneous left atrial appendage suture ligation using the LARIAT device in patients with atrial fibrillation: initial clinical experience. *J Am Coll Cardiol* 2013;62(2):108–118.

The LARIAT is a ligation device deployed around the LAA via the pericardium, to exclude it from the circulation. This prospective cohort study looked long-term outcomes of LARIAT placement in 89 patients at high risk of stroke due to nonvalvular AF, who were not candidates for anticoagulation. The device was successfully deployed in 96%, and rates of complete appendage occlusion were 95% at 1 and 3 months and 98% at 1 year (though 1-year follow-up was only available for 65 patients).

Atrial Fibrillation Prevention After Surgery

107. Andrews TC, et al. Prevention of supraventricular arrhythmias after coronary artery bypass surgery: a meta-analysis of randomized controlled trials. *Circulation* 1991;84(5 suppl):III236.

This meta-analysis included 1,549 patients from 24 randomized, controlled studies. Patients were excluded if they had an LVEF <30%, insulin-dependent diabetes, AV block, and sick sinus syndrome, and those undergoing noncardiac operations. The initiation of preoperative β-blockers was found to be more effective than postoperative initiation, and beta-blocker therapy reduced post-CABG AF by 77%.

108. Daoud EG, et al. Preoperative amiodarone as prophylaxis against atrial fibrillation after heart surgery. *N Engl J Med* 1997;337:1785.

This prospective, randomized, double-blind study enrolled 124 patients scheduled to undergo elective cardiac surgery. Patients were randomized at least a week before surgery to oral amiodarone (600 mg/day for 7 days and then 200 mg/day until hospital discharge) or placebo. Postoperative AF occurred significantly less in the amiodarone group (25% vs. 53%; p = 0.003). Amiodarone patients had a shorter and less costly hospital stay compared with placebo patients (6.5 days vs. 7.9 days, p = 0.04; $18,375 vs. $26,491, p = 0.03). No significant differences were seen between the groups in nonfatal and fatal postoperative complications.

109. Serafimovski N, et al. Usefulness of dofetilide for the prevention of atrial tachyarrhythmias (atrial fibrillation or flutter) after coronary artery bypass grafting. *Am J Cardiol* 2008;101:1574–1579.

In a randomized, double-blinded fashion, the investigators assigned 133 patients undergoing CABG, with or without valve surgery, to either dofetilide or placebo just prior to surgery. The primary end point of postoperative atrial tachyarrhythmias occurred in 36% of patients receiving placebo versus 18% of those receiving dofetilide (absolute RR, 18%; $p < 0.017$). In those patients on dofetilide who did develop an atrial tachyarrhythmia, their length of stay was still a day less than those in the placebo arm. There was no occurrence of torsade de pointes in either group.

Ventricular Arrhythmias

GUIDELINES

110. Zipes DP, et al. ACC/AHA/ESC 2006 guidelines for management of patients with ventricular arrhythmias and the prevention of sudden cardiac death: a report of the American College of Cardiology/American Heart Association Task Force and the European Society of Cardiology Committee for Practice Guidelines (Writing Committee to Develop Guidelines for Management of Patients With Ventricular Arrhythmias and the Prevention of Sudden Cardiac Death). *J Am Coll Cardiol* 2006;48:e247–e346.

IMMEDIATE THERAPY: AUTOMATED EXTERNAL DEFIBRILLATORS

111. Weaver WD, et al. Use of the automatic external defibrillator in the management of out-of-hospital cardiac arrest. N Engl J Med 1988;319:661–666.

This prospective study of 1,287 consecutive cardiac arrest victims compared outcomes of defibrillation performed by first-responder firefighters using automatic external defibrillators with paramedics, who on average arrive on scene slightly later. Among patients for whom defibrillation was attempted, survival to hospital discharge was better when administered by firefighters (30%) than when waiting slightly longer for paramedics (19%; $p < 0.001$).

112. Valenzuela TD, et al. Outcomes of rapid defibrillation by security officers after cardiac arrest in casinos. N Engl J Med 2000;343:1206–1209.

This study tracked outcomes of treating cardiac arrest victims at a number of casinos with AEDs operated by (minimally) trained security officers. Of 105 subjects whose initial rhythm was VF, 53% survived to hospital discharge. Survival was better for witnessed than for unwitnessed arrests and when defibrillation was performed in less than versus more than 3 minutes (74% vs. 49%). These results suggest that use of AEDs by nonmedical personnel is feasible and effective.

113. Page RL, et al. Automated external defibrillator use aboard a domestic airline. N Engl J Med 2000;343:1210–1216.

In this pilot study, AEDs were furnished aboard aircraft of one domestic US carrier. The 200 AED uses were reported, 99 of them for unconscious patients. Shocks were advised and delivered by the AEDs in 14 of 14 patients with VF and in no patients with other rhythms (sensitivity and specificity of ECG diagnostics, both 100%). Survival to hospital discharge was 40% in the VF patients. Again, the use of AEDs by nonmedical personnel was supported.

114. Hallstrom AP, et al.; for the Public Access Defibrillation (PAD) Trial Investigators. Public-access defibrillation and survival after out-of-hospital cardiac arrest. N Engl J Med 2004;351:637–646.

The investigators randomly assigned various community centers (malls, apartment complexes, etc.) to emergency response systems including layperson training of CPR or CPR plus use of AED. This included roughly 19,000 volunteers from across North America, and the primary end point was survival to hospital discharge of out-of-hospital arrest victims. Among 128 arrests in the AED group, 30 survived to hospital discharge, compared to 15 of the 107 arrest victims in the CPR-only group (p = 0.03). There were no inappropriate shocks delivered, and functional status at discharge was not different between the two groups.

115. Bardy GH, et al.; for the HAT Investigators. Home use of automated external defibrillators for sudden cardiac arrest. N Engl J Med 2008;358:1793–1804.

In 7,001 patients at high risk of SCD, namely, those with recent anterior wall MI (but not candidates for internal defibrillator implants), investigators randomly assigned half to receive an AED for their home. For the primary end point of all-cause mortality over a median follow-up of 37.3 months, there was no difference in the two groups (6.4% in the AED group vs. 6.5% in the control; p = 0.77). However, only 35.6% of all deaths were considered to be of sudden, tachyarrhythmic etiology.

116. Weisfeldt ML, et al. Ventricular tachyarrhythmias after cardiac arrest in public versus at home. N Engl J Med 2011;364:313–321.

This was a cohort study of 12,930 out-of-hospital cardiac arrests in 10 American sites from 2005 to 2007. Though 9,564 arrests occurred in the home, the odds of having a "shockable" rhythm (VF or pulseless VT) were significantly higher for arrests in public (adjusted OR, 4.48; p < 0.0001) for bystander-witnessed arrests where an AED was applied. Concordantly, survival to hospital discharge for arrests in public using an AED was significantly higher (35%) than those occurring at home (12%; p = 0.04). This study called into question the strategy of routinely distributing AEDs for home use.

IMMEDIATE THERAPY: INTRAVENOUS AMIODARONE

117. Kudenchuk PJ, et al. Amiodarone for resuscitation after out-of hospital cardiac arrest due to ventricular fibrillation. N Engl J Med 1999;341:871–878.

Design: Prospective, randomized, placebo-controlled, double-blind, single-center trial. Primary end point was survival to hospital admission. Patients were followed up to hospital discharge.

Purpose: To determine whether IV amiodarone, compared with placebo, improved survival to hospital admission in shock-refractory VT/VF.

Population: 504 adult subjects with nontraumatic out-of-hospital cardiac arrest with ongoing pulseless VT or VF after three defibrillations.

Treatment: Epinephrine, 1 mg IV, followed by amiodarone, 300 mg given as an IV push, or placebo, followed by standard ACLS-guided resuscitative measures.

Results: Amiodarone group had a significantly higher survival to admission compared with the placebo group (44% vs. 33%; p = 0.03). Amiodarone was associated with higher frequency of hypotension (59% vs. 48%; p = 0.04) and bradycardia (41% vs. 25%; p = 0.004) compared with placebo.

118. Dorian P, et al. (ALIVE). Amiodarone as compared with lidocaine for shock-resistant ventricular fibrillation. N Engl J Med 2002;346:884–890.

Design: Prospective, randomized, double-blind, controlled, single-center study. Primary end point was survival to hospital admission.

Purpose: To compare IV amiodarone with lidocaine for shock-refractory VT/VF.

Population: 347 adult subjects with nontraumatic out-of-hospital cardiac arrest with ongoing pulseless VF after three defibrillations, IV epinephrine and a fourth defibrillation, or recurrent VF after initially successful defibrillation.

Treatment: Amiodarone, 5 mg/kg IV push plus lidocaine placebo, or lidocaine, 1.5 mg/kg IV push plus amiodarone placebo, followed by standard ACLS-guided resuscitative measures. A second dose of the same study drug (2.5 mg/kg amiodarone or 1.5 mg/kg lidocaine) could be given if VF persisted.

Results: Survival to hospital admission was better with IV amiodarone than with lidocaine (22.8% vs. 12.0%; p = 0.009). Patients treated early (less than the median of 24 minutes from ambulance dispatch to study drug administration) had better survival than those treated late, but within this subgroup, survival remained better with amiodarone (27.7% vs. 15.3%; p = 0.05).

SECONDARY PREVENTION TRIALS: DRUGS VERSUS IMPLANTABLE CARDIOVERTER–DEFIBRILLATORS

119. Kuck KH, et al. Randomized comparison of antiarrhythmic drug therapy with implantable defibrillators in patients resuscitated from cardiac arrest: the Cardiac Arrest Study Hamburg (CASH). *Circulation* 2000;102:748–754 (also see *Am Heart J* 1994;127:1139).

This prospective study, initiated in 1987, initially randomized survivors of SCD in 3:1 fashion to treatment with oral propafenone, amiodarone, or metoprolol or to ICD implantation without concomitant antiarrhythmic drugs. The propafenone arm (56 patients) was terminated in 1992 after interim analysis revealed increased all-cause mortality and sudden death (12% vs. none; p < 0.05) with propafenone compared with ICD over an average follow-up of only 11 months. The remaining three arms of the study enrolled a total of 288 subjects: 99 ICD, 92 amiodarone, and 97 metoprolol. Final analysis at a mean follow-up of 57 months revealed a nonsignificant reduction in all-cause mortality favoring the ICD group over the combination of the amiodarone and metoprolol arms (36% vs. 44%; one-tailed p value 0.08). The relative improvement in survival with ICD compared with amiodarone/metoprolol was greatest at 1 year (42%) and progressively declined as the duration of follow-up lengthened.

120. Connolly SJ, et al. Canadian implantable defibrillator study (CIDS): a randomized trial of the implantable cardioverter defibrillator against amiodarone. *Circulation* 2000;101:1297–1302.

This prospective, randomized study enrolled patients with documented VF or out-of-hospital cardiac arrest without a reversible cause, VT that was poorly tolerated or occurred in the presence of LVEF <35%, or syncope with spontaneous or inducible VT. Patients were randomized to oral amiodarone (n = 331; mean dose, 255 mg/day at 5 years) or ICD implantation (n = 328); 90% of ICD implants were transvenous. A moderate (21% to 28%) degree of crossover between groups occurred, and sotalol and β-blockers were more frequently used by ICD patients. Reductions in total mortality (8.2% vs. 10.2% per year; p = 0.14) and arrhythmic death (3.0% vs. 4.5% per year; p = 0.09) favored the ICD arm but did not reach statistical significance. The trend toward improved survival with ICDs was viewed as consistent with the AVID trial, in which the survival benefit did reach statistical significance.

121. The Antiarrhythmics versus Implantable Defibrillators (AVID) Investigators. A comparison of antiarrhythmic-drug therapy with implantable defibrillators in patients resuscitated from near-fatal ventricular arrhythmias. *N Engl J Med* 1997;337:1576–1583.

Design: Prospective, randomized, open, multicenter study. Primary end point was all-cause mortality.

Purpose: To compare the efficacy of antiarrhythmic drugs (primarily amiodarone) with ICDs for secondary prevention of SCD.

Population: 1,016 subjects resuscitated from VF (45%) or hemodynamically unstable VT (55%) not due to a transient or correctable cause, with LVEF of 40% or less. Most (81%) had a clinical history of CAD.

Exclusion Criteria: Contraindication to amiodarone or ICD implantation.

Treatment: Patients were randomly assigned to antiarrhythmic drug treatment (96% amiodarone) or ICD implantation. Nearly all ICD implants were transvenous, with many pectoral. Crossover was approximately 10% in both groups. Beta-blocker use was three- to fourfold higher among ICD versus amiodarone patients.

Results: Mortality was significantly lower in the ICD group than in the antiarrhythmic drug arm at 1 year (10.7% vs. 17.7%), 2 years (18.4% vs. 25.3%), and 3 years (24.6% vs. 35.9%; $p < 0.02$).

Comments: The study was criticized for the imbalance in beta-blocker use, but the core conclusion of ICD superiority remains generally accepted.

PRIMARY PREVENTION TRIALS: ANTIARRHYTHMIC DRUGS

122. The Cardiac Arrhythmia Suppression Trial (CAST) Investigators. Preliminary report: effect of encainide and flecainide on mortality in a randomized trial of arrhythmia suppression after myocardial infarction. N Engl J Med 1989;321:406–412 (see also Chapter 4).

In 1,727 post-MI patients, encainide and flecainide led to a significantly higher mortality rate through 10 months of follow-up (7.7% vs. 3.0% for placebo; relative risk, 2.5; 95% CI, 1.6 to 4.5). Arrhythmic death also was higher with the IC agents than with placebo (4.5% vs. 1.2%).

123. The Cardiac Arrhythmia Suppression Trial II (CAST II) Investigators. Effect of the antiarrhythmic agent moricizine on survival after myocardial infarction. N Engl J Med 1992;327:227–233.

CAST-II enrolled 2,699 subjects 6 to 90 days after MI with an EF of 40% or less and 6 or more PVCs/hour. Patients were randomized to placebo or the Class Ic agent moricizine in the short-term (2 weeks; $n = 1,325$) and long-term (mean, 18 months; $n = 1,374$) protocols. The study was terminated early because of increased mortality associated with moricizine use in the 14-day protocol (2.6% vs. 0.5%; adjusted $p < 0.01$). Incidence of long-term deaths was similar (15% vs. 12%). The authors concluded that the use of moricizine after MI was not only ineffective but also harmful.

124. Waldo AL, et al.; Survival With Oral D-Sotalol (SWORD) Investigators. Effect of D-sotalol on mortality in patients with left ventricular dysfunction after recent and remote myocardial infarction. Lancet 1996;348:7–12.

The 3,121 post-MI patients with an EF of 40% or less and NYHA Class II to III HF were randomized to D-sotalol (100 to 200 mg, b.i.d.) or placebo. The D-sotalol arm exhibited higher all-cause mortality (5.0% vs. 3.1%), cardiac mortality (4.7% vs. 2.9%), and presumed arrhythmic deaths (3.6% vs. 2.0%) at a mean follow-up of 148 days (all p values <0.01).

125. Doval HC, et al.; for the Grupo de Estudio de la Sobrevida en la Insuficiencia Cardiaca en Argentina (GESICA) Investigators. Randomised trial of low-dose amiodarone in severe congestive heart failure. Lancet 1994;344:493–498.

This trial randomized 516 Argentinean patients with CHF to amiodarone, 300 mg/day, or placebo. A significant proportion of patients had Chagas disease or alcoholism as the etiologies of their LV dysfunction. The trial found a nonsignificant 27% reduction in sudden death ($p = 0.16$) and a significant reduction in total mortality (33.5% vs. 41.4%; $p = 0.02$) in favor of amiodarone.

126. Singh SN, et al.; for the Survival Trial of Antiarrhythmic Therapy in Congestive Heart Failure (CHF-STAT) Investigators. Amiodarone in patients with congestive heart failure and asymptomatic ventricular arrhythmia. N Engl J Med 1995;333:377–382.

Entry criteria for CHF-STAT were symptomatic CHF, EF <40%, more than 10 PVCs/hour, and cardiac enlargement. The majority (70%) of subjects had ischemic cardiomyopathy. The 674 subjects were randomized to amiodarone (maintenance dose, 300 mg/day) or placebo and followed up for a median of 45 months. Amiodarone showed no benefit in terms of overall mortality or SCD.

127. Julian DG, et al. Randomised trial of effect of amiodarone on mortality in patients with left ventricular dysfunction after recent myocardial infarction: EMIAT. *Lancet* 1997;349:667–674.

In 1,486 post-MI patients with an EF of 40% or less, all-cause mortality was similar for amiodarone versus placebo, but a 35% risk reduction ($p = 0.05$) occurred in arrhythmic deaths. The authors concluded that the systematic prophylactic use of amiodarone after MI (with low EF) was not indicated, but the lack of proarrhythmia supports the use of amiodarone in patients for whom antiarrhythmic therapy is indicated for other reasons.

128. Cairns JA, et al. Randomised trial of outcome after myocardial infarction in patients with frequent or repetitive ventricular premature depolarisations CAMIAT. *Lancet* 1997;349:675–682.

CAMIAT randomized 1,202 postinfarct patients with frequent ventricular ectopy (>10 premature ventricular depolarizations per hour) or NSVT to amiodarone or placebo. At a mean follow-up of 1.8 years, a reduction in combined resuscitated VF or arrhythmic death was found with amiodarone (4.5% vs. 6.9%; $p = 0.03$), but no significant difference was seen in all-cause mortality.

129. Sim I, et al. Quantitative overview of randomized trials of amiodarone to prevent sudden cardiac death. *Circulation* 1997;96:2823–2829.

This meta-analysis pooled the results of all trials randomizing subjects to amiodarone or alternative nondevice therapy (including placebo) for the prevention of sudden death, including a minority of subjects in secondary prevention studies. Across trials, amiodarone reduced total mortality by 19% when compared with active control or "usual care" but only 10% when compared with placebo. The treatment effect of amiodarone, when pooled, appeared to be independent of the clinical population studied (post-MI, CHF, or SCD survivors).

PRIMARY PREVENTION TRIALS: DRUGS VERSUS IMPLANTABLE CARDIOVERTER–DEFIBRILLATORS

130. Moss AJ, et al.; for the Multicenter Automated Defibrillator Implantation Trial (MADIT) Investigators. Improved survival with an implanted defibrillator in patients with coronary disease at high risk for ventricular arrhythmia. *N Engl J Med* 1996;335:1933–1940.

Design: Prospective, randomized, open, multicenter trial. The primary end point was all-cause mortality. Average follow-up was 27 months.

Purpose: To compare the efficacy of ICDs with standard medical therapy (generally including antiarrhythmic drugs) for primary prevention of SCD in coronary patients at high risk for SCD.

Population: 196 adult patients with prior MI, documented NSVT, EF of 35% or less, and inducible VT or VF at EPS, not suppressible with IV procainamide.

Exclusion Criteria: Included previous cardiac arrest or VT with syncope, symptomatic hypotension, MI within 3 weeks, CABG surgery within 2 months, or PTCA within 3 months.

Treatment: Patients were randomly assigned to ICD implantation (50% transthoracic, 50% transvenous) or standard medical therapy. In the standard therapy group, 74% received amiodarone, 10% received type I antiarrhythmic drugs, and 7% received sotalol.

Results: Study enrollment was terminated prematurely when interim analysis passed pre-specified stopping criteria. At follow-up, the mortality rate was 17% in the defibrillator group versus 39% in the conventional therapy group, a 54% reduction ($p = 0.009$).

131. Buxton AE, et al.; for the Multicenter Unsustained Tachycardia Trial (MUSTT) Investigators. A randomized study of the prevention of sudden death in patients with coronary artery disease. *N Engl J Med* 1999;341:1882–1890.

Design: Prospective, randomized, open, multicenter trial. Primary end point was cardiac arrest or death from arrhythmia. Median follow-up duration was 39 months.

Purpose: To compare the efficacy of electrophysiologically guided therapy (antiarrhythmic drugs or ICDs if drugs failed) with standard medical therapy (not including antiarrhythmic drugs) for primary prevention of SCD in coronary patients at high risk for SCD.

Population: Adult patients with prior MI, documented NSVT, EF of 40% or less, and inducible VT or VF at EPS. Noninducible patients were followed up in a voluntary registry. The 704 inducible patients were randomized.

Exclusion Criteria: Syncope, sustained VT, or VF more than 48 hours after an acute MI; untreated exercise-induced ischemia.

Treatment: Standard medical therapy (not including antiarrhythmic drugs) or therapy based on serial electrophysiology (EP) testing, which consisted of an antiarrhythmic drug that suppressed VT inducibility, amiodarone (if two previous drug trials failed), or an ICD. Initially, ICDs were reserved for patients with three or more unsuccessful drug trials, but halfway through enrollment, this was relaxed to one or more. Ultimately, 46% of the EP-guided patients were discharged with ICDs, and 45% were treated with drugs: 26% Class I, 10% amiodarone, and 9% sotalol.

Results: Overall, the EP group showed a lower rate of cardiac arrest or arrhythmic death ($p = 0.04$) and lower total mortality (hazard ratio, 0.80; $p = 0.06$). However, all the benefit was achieved among patients who had received an ICD (total mortality, 24% at 5 years), whereas patients treated with EP-guided antiarrhythmic drug therapy had a slightly higher mortality rate (55% at 5 years) compared with standard medical therapy without antiarrhythmic drugs (48%).

132. Moss AJ, et al.; for The Multicenter Automatic Defibrillator Implantation Trial II (MADIT II) Investigators. Prophylactic implantation of a defibrillator in patients with myocardial infarction and reduced ejection fraction. *N Engl J Med* 2002;346:877–883.

Design: Prospective, randomized, open, multicenter trial. Primary end point was all-cause mortality. Average follow-up was 20 months.

Purpose: To compare the efficacy of ICDs with conventional medical therapy (primarily without antiarrhythmic drugs) for primary prevention of SCD in coronary patients at high risk for SCD.

Population: Adult patients with prior MI and EF of 30% or less.

Exclusion Criteria: FDA-approved indication for ICD implantation, NYHA Class IV CHF, MI within 1 month, coronary revascularization procedure within 3 months, or other life-threatening condition.

Treatment: Patients were randomly assigned in 3:2 ratio to ICD implantation (all trans-venous) or standard medical therapy. Amiodarone was used by 13% of ICD subjects and 10% of conventional therapy subjects at last study contact. Use of other cardiac medications, including beta-blockers and ACE inhibitors, was well balanced between groups.

Results: Total mortality was 19.8% in the conventional therapy group and 14.2% in the ICD group (hazard ratio, 0.69; $p = 0.016$). Benefits were consistent across all subgroups. A trend toward an increased rate of hospitalization for CHF was seen in the ICD group

(19.9% vs. 14.9%; $p = 0.09$); this finding may be related to ventricular pacing worsening CHF by creating dyssynchrony in the heart (also, see DAVID results; Ref. 125).

Comments: Based on these results, the updated ACC/AHA Guidelines include ICD implantation in post-MI patients with LVEF 30% or less as a Class IIa recommendation.

133. Hohnloser SH, et al.; for the Defibrillator in Acute Myocardial Infarction (DINAMIT) Investigators. Prophylactic use of an implantable cardioverter-defibrillator after acute myocardial infarction. *N Engl J Med* 2004;351:2481–2488.

Design: Prospective, randomized trial; primary end point was all-cause mortality at mean follow-up of 30 months.

Purpose: To identify the benefit, if any, of ICD implantation early (6 to 40 days) after acute MI.

Population: 674 patients 6 to 40 days following acute MI; they also had reduced EF ($\leq35\%$) and weakened cardiac autonomic function (either depressed pulse variability or elevated 24-hour pulse rate).

Treatment: Placement of single-lead ICD programmed to shock for VT or VF, and for backup pacing at 40 bpm, as well as antitachycardia pacing for certain VT rates, or no device.

Results: Overall mortality did not differ between the two groups, as 62 of 322 patients in the ICD group died, versus 58 of 342 in the non-ICD group (hazard ratio for ICD group, 1.08; $p = 0.66$). Prespecified outcome of death from arrhythmia was significantly reduced, at 12 versus 29 in the ICD and non-ICD groups, respectively (hazard ratio for ICD group, 0.42; $p = 0.009$). This was offset by increased nonarrhythmia death in the ICD group.

134. Bardy GH, et al.; for the Sudden Cardiac Death in Heart Failure Trial (SCD-HeFT) Investigators. Amiodarone or an implantable cardioverter-defibrillator for congestive heart failure. *N Engl J Med* 2005;352:225–237.

Design: Prospective, randomized trial; primary end point was all-cause mortality at median follow-up of 45.5 months.

Purpose: To identify best prevention of SCD for patients with CHF.

Population: 2,521 patients with NYHA Class II or III CHF and an EF of $\leq35\%$.

Treatment: Standard CHF therapy plus placebo, standard therapy plus amiodarone, or standard therapy plus single-lead, shock-only ICD. The amiodarone versus placebo drug branches were double-blinded.

Results: Overall, 70% of patients enrolled for NYHA Class II, with roughly half ischemic in etiology. In the placebo group, there were 244 deaths (29%), versus 240 (28%) in the amiodarone group (hazard ratio, 1.06 for amiodarone vs. placebo; $p = 0.53$) and 182 (22%) in the ICD group (hazard ratio, 0.77 for ICD vs. placebo; $p = 0.007$). Results did not differ based on etiology of CHF (ischemic vs. other). Of note, drug was discontinued in 22% and 32% of patients in the placebo and amiodarone groups, respectively; 14% of patients in the ICD group received open-label amiodarone at some point.

135. Steinbeck G, et al.; for the IRIS Investigators. Defibrillator implantation early after myocardial infarction. *N Engl J Med* 2009;361:1427–1436.

Design: Prospective, randomized trial; primary end point was all-cause mortality at mean follow-up of 37 months.

Purpose: To test the hypothesis that patients at increased risk of ventricular arrhythmia would benefit from ICD placement early after MI.

Population: 898 patients within 5 to 31 days after acute MI with reduced EF ($\leq35\%$) and at least one of the following—HR ≥90 on the first available ECG (602 patients) or NSVT (≥150 bpm) on Holter (208 patients); 88 patients fulfilled both the HR and VT criteria.

Treatment: Single-chamber ICD placement or no device.

Results: There was no significant difference in mortality between those who received ICDs and those who did not (116 of 445 vs. 117 of 453, respectively; hazard ratio, 1.04; p = 0.78). However, incidence of SCD was lower in the ICD group (27 vs. 60; hazard ratio, 0.55; p = 0.049), with, once again, more nonsudden death events in the ICD group. There were no differences in outcomes among patients who fulfilled the different inclusion criteria.

PRIMARY PREVENTION TRIALS: NONISCHEMIC CARDIOMYOPATHY PATIENTS

136. Bansch D, et al.; for the Cardiomyopathy Trial (CAT) Investigators. Primary prevention of sudden cardiac death in idiopathic dilated cardiomyopathy. *Circulation* 2002;105:1453–1458.

This prospective, randomized, multicenter trial enrolled 104 patients with recent onset of DCM (9 months or less), LVEF 30% or less, and in NYHA Class II or III. CAD had to be excluded by angiography. Other exclusion criteria included history of MI, symptomatic bradycardia, VT, or VF. Patients were randomized to ICD or control. Trial was terminated early because 1-year mortality did not reach 30% in the control group. At mean follow-up of 5.5 years, no significant difference in mortality rates was found between the two groups (26.0% vs. 31.5%). The only predictor of mortality was impaired LVEF.

137. Strickberger SA, et al. Amiodarone versus implantable cardioverter-defibrillator: randomized trial in patients with non-ischemic dilated cardiomyopathy and asymptomatic nonsustained ventricular tachycardia—AMIOVIRT. *J Am Coll Cardiol* 2003;41:1707–1712.

Design: Prospective, multicenter, randomized trial; primary end point was all-cause mortality at 3 years.

Purpose: To identify the benefit, if any, of ICD placement versus amiodarone in patients with NIDCM and a history of NSVT.

Population: 103 patients with NIDCM, EF ≤35%, and asymptomatic NSVT.

Treatment: Treatment with amiodarone or placement of an ICD.

Results: The study was stopped by the data safety and monitoring board (DSMB), as it met the prespecified stopping rule for futility. There were no differences in survival between the two groups at 1 or 3 years of follow-up (90% vs. 96% at 1 year, 88% vs. 87% at 3 years amiodarone and ICD, respectively; p = 0.8). Reported trends of improved arrhythmia-free survival and lower overall costs in the ICD group are difficult to interpret in the setting of stoppage for futility and a relatively small sample size.

138. Kadish A, et al.; for the Defibrillators in Non-Ischemic Cardiomyopathy Treatment Evaluation (DEFINITE) Investigators. Prophylactic defibrillator implantation in patients with non-ischemic dilated cardiomyopathy. *N Engl J Med* 2004;350:2151–2158.

Design: Prospective, randomized trial; primary end point was all-cause mortality at mean follow-up of 29 months.

Purpose: To identify the benefit, if any, of ICD placement in patients with NIDCM.

Population: 458 patients with NIDCM, EF <36%, and premature ventricular complexes or NSVT.

Treatment: Placement of a single-chamber ICD (with backup pacing rate of 40 bpm) with standard medical therapy or standard medical therapy alone. Standard medical therapy was a contemporary regimen including ACE inhibitors and beta-blockers.

Results: There were 28 deaths in the ICD group versus 40 in the medical therapy group (hazard ratio, 0.65; *p* = 0.08) and a significant reduction of sudden death from arrhythmia in the ICD group (3 vs. 17; hazard ratio, 0.20; *p* = 0.006). At 2 years, the mortality rate was 7.9% in the ICD group versus 14.1% in the medical therapy group.

STUDIES OF EMERGING TACHYARRHYTHMIA THERAPIES

139. Bardy GH, et al. An entirely subcutaneous implantable cardioverter-defibrillator. N Engl J Med 2010;363:36–44.

This landmark publication introduced providers to the novel, S-ICD, and early experiences within. The manuscript describes the design, positioning, and configuration of the S-ICD, whereby a single coil is positioned just lateral to the sternum, with the generator implanted on the left lateral side. They evaluated several different temporary device configurations in a total of 78 patients eligible for a standard ICD. Ventricular fibrillation was successfully detected and terminated in 100% of the 137 induced episodes.

140. Weiss R, et al. Safety and efficacy of a totally subcutaneous implantable-cardioverter defibrillator. Circulation 2013;128:944–953.

This was a prospective cohort study of 330 patients who met standard criteria for a conventional ICD, did not require pacing, and had not demonstrated pace-terminable VT. S-ICD placement was attempted in 321 and succeeded in 314. Over a mean follow-up of 11 months, there were 38 discrete arrhythmia episodes in 21 patients—all were defibrillated successfully. Inappropriate shocks were delivered in 41 patients (13.1%).

141. Aziz S, et al. The Subcutaneous defibrillator—a review of the literature. J Am Coll Cardiol 2014;63:1473–1479.

The authors review the design and configuration of the first, approved S-ICD, as well as the data supporting its use. Major advantages and disadvantages of the technology are also discussed, in an effort to assist clinicians in identifying appropriate candidates for its use.

142. Wilkoff BL, et al. Strategic programming of detection and therapy parameters in implantable cardioverter-defibrillators reduces shocks in primary prevention patients: results from the PREPARE (Primary Prevention Parameters Evaluation) study. J Am Coll Cardiol 2008;52:541–550.

Using a case-controlled design, the investigators enrolled 700 patients with primary prevention ICDs from 38 centers and followed them for 1 year. These cases were programmed more conservatively, with delayed detection of VT, antitachycardia pacing programmed aggressively, and SVT discrimination for rhythms below 200 bpm. The 689 control patients were derived from prior ICD trials (EMPIRIC and MIRACLE ICD), and their programming was not controlled. Though not powered for mortality, there was a significantly lower, unadjusted death rate in the treatment group versus control (4.9% vs. 8.7%; *p* < 0.01; adjusted HR 0.57; *p* = 0.10). There were also lower rates of all shocks (8.5% vs. 16.9%; *p* < 0.01), shocks for VT/VF (5.4% vs. 9.4%; *p* < 0.01), and shocks for other arrhythmias (3.6% vs. 7.5%; *p* < 0.01). The investigators identified 10 syncopal events in the treatment group that they attributed to the PREPARE programming strategy.

143. Moss AJ, et al. Reduction in inappropriate therapy and mortality through ICD programming. N Engl J Med 2012;367:2275–2283.

Design: Prospective, multicenter, international, single-blinded, randomized trial. The primary end point was the occurrence of first inappropriate arrhythmia therapy (shock or antitachycardia pacing) at a mean follow-up of 1.4 years.

Purpose: To determine the safety and efficacy of conservative ICD programming to reduce inappropriate ICD therapies.

Population: 1,500 patients undergoing de novo ICD or CRT-D implantation for primary prevention.

Treatment: Following device implantation, patients were randomized to be programmed to one of three strategies: (1) high-rate therapy ($\geq$200 bpm); (2) long-delay therapy (60 seconds for 170 to 199 bpm, 12 seconds for 200 to 249 bpm, and 2.5 seconds for $\geq$250 bpm); or (3) conventional therapy (2.5-second delay at 170 to 199 bpm and 1.0-second delay at $\geq$200 bpm).

Results: Both the high-rate (HR 0.21; $p < 0.001$) and long-delay (0.24; $p < 0.001$) groups demonstrated significantly lower risk of the primary end point compared to conventional programming. More importantly, all-cause mortality was reduced in each of the intervention groups, as well (HR for high rate vs. conventional, 0.45; $p = 0.01$; HR for long delay vs. conventional 0.56; $p = 0.06$).

Comments: Following up on the PREPARE study (above), this trial confirmed the findings and signaled a potential major paradigm shift in the programming of ICDs. The trial also supported the mounting evidence that inappropriate shocks can be harmful and are associated with adverse long-term outcomes.

Cardiac Pacing Studies

GUIDELINES

144. Epstein AE, et al. ACC/AHA/HRS 2008 guidelines for device-based therapy of cardiac rhythm abnormalities: a report of the American College of Cardiology/American Heart Association Task Force on Practice Guidelines (Writing Committee to Revise the ACC/AHA/NASPE 2002 Guideline Update for Implantation of Cardiac Pacemakers and Antiarrhythmic Devices). *J Am Coll Cardiol* 2008;51:e1–e62.

145. Tracy CM, et al. 2012 ACCF/AHA/HRS focused update of the 2008 guidelines for device-based therapy of cardiac rhythm abnormalities: a report of the American College of Cardiology Foundation/American Heart Association Task Force on Practice Guidelines. *Circulation* 2012;126:1784–1800.

MODE SELECTION TRIALS

146. Connolly SJ, et al.; for Canadian Trial of Physiologic Pacing (CTOPP) Investigators. Effects of physiologic pacing versus ventricular pacing on the risk of stroke and death due to cardiovascular causes. *N Engl J Med* 2000;342:1385–1391.

Design: Prospective, randomized, multicenter trial. Primary end point was stroke or cardiovascular death.

Purpose: To determine the benefits of physiologic (atrial or dual-chamber) pacing compared with ventricular pacing in patients with symptomatic bradycardia.

Population: 2,568 patients undergoing initial implantation of a permanent pacemaker for symptomatic bradycardia. Approximately 60% of patients had AV block, and 40% had sinus node dysfunction.

Exclusion Criteria: Chronic/persistent AF, prior AV junction ablation, and limited life expectancy.

Treatment: Implantation of physiologic (atrial or dual-chamber) or ventricular pacing system.

Results: At 3 years, no significant difference was found in the primary end point of stroke or cardiovascular death between physiologic and ventricular pacing groups (4.9% vs. 5.5%). No significant differences in total mortality or CHF admission rates were seen. Physiologic pacing was associated with an 18% reduction in the incidence of AF (5.3% per year vs. 6.6% per year; $p = 0.05$).

147. Lamas GA, et al.; for the Mode Selection Trial in Sinus-node Dysfunction (MOST) Investigators. Ventricular pacing or dual-chamber pacing for sinus-node dysfunction. N Engl J Med 2002;346:1854–1862.

Design: Prospective, randomized, multicenter study. Primary end point was death or non-fatal stroke.

Purpose: To determine the benefits of dual-chamber pacing compared with ventricular pacing in patients with sinus node dysfunction.

Population: 2,010 patients undergoing initial implantation of a dual-chamber pacemaker for sinus node dysfunction. Patients were required to be in SR at the time of randomization, but 45% had a history of AF.

Exclusion Criteria: Serious concurrent illness.

Treatment: All patients had dual-chamber pacemakers implanted and then were randomized to dual-chamber (DDD) or ventricular (VVI) pacing modes.

Results: No difference was found between study groups in the incidence of death or nonfatal stroke. In adjusted analyses, small benefits favoring dual-chamber pacing were found for the secondary end points of hospitalization for HF (hazard ratio, 0.73; $p = 0.02$) and death, stroke, or hospitalization for HF (hazard ratio, 0.85; $p = 0.05$). Dual-chamber pacing was also associated with a lower incidence of any AF (hazard ratio, 0.79; $p = 0.008$) and progression to chronic AF (15% vs. 27% of those who had any AF; $p < 0.001$) and greater improvements in several QOL measures than with ventricular pacing. At the last follow-up, 31% of subjects originally assigned to ventricular pacing had crossed over to dual chamber, about half of them for strictly defined pacemaker syndrome.

Comments: A subsequent secondary analysis revealed, as in MOST, a reduction not only in the incidence of AF with dual-chamber pacing but also in the progression to chronic AF (2.8% per year vs. 3.8% per year with VVI pacing; $p = 0.016$) (see J Am Coll Cardiol 2001;38:167).

148. Wilkoff BL, et al.; Dual Chamber and VVI Implantable Defibrillator (DAVID) Trial Investigators. Dual-chamber pacing or ventricular backup pacing in patients with an implantable defibrillator: the Dual Chamber and VVI Implantable Defibrillator (DAVID) Trial. JAMA 2002;288:3115–3123.

Design: Prospective, randomized, single-blind, parallel-group, multicenter trial. Primary end point was composite of death or first hospitalization for CHF.

Purpose: To determine the efficacy of dual-chamber pacing compared with backup ventricular pacing in patients with standard indications for ICD implantation but without indications for antibradycardia pacing.

Population: 506 patients with LVEF of 40% or less, no indication for antibradycardia pacemaker therapy, and no persistent atrial arrhythmias.

Treatment: All had an ICD with dual-chamber rate-responsive pacing capability implanted. ICDs programmed to ventricular backup pacing at 40 per minute (VVI-40) or dual-chamber rate-responsive pacing at 70 per minute (DDDR-70).

Results: The VVI-40 group had a better 1-year survival free of composite end point [83.9% vs. 73.3% (for patients with DDDR-70); relative hazard, 1.61; 95% CI, 1.06 to 2.44]. A trend toward lower mortality in the VVI-40 group was noted (6.5% vs. 10.1%; relative hazard, 1.61; 95% CI, 0.84 to 3.09).

149. Yu C-M, et al.; The Pacing to Avoid Cardiac Enlargement (PACE) Trial. Biventricular pacing in patients with bradycardia and normal ejection fraction. N Engl J Med 2009;361:2123–2134.

The investigators enrolled 177 patients with normal EF, bradycardia (due to either sinus node dysfunction or high-grade AV block), and an already-placed BiV pacemaker. They then randomized them to either BiV pacing or right ventricular apex pacing and followed EF and end-systolic volume at 12 months. At follow-up, EF was significantly lower in the RV pacing group (54% vs. 62%; $p < 0.001$), and LV end-systolic volume was higher in the RV pacing group (35.7 mL vs. 27.6 mL; $p < 0.001$). Average ventricular pacing was 98% in the BiV group and 97% in the RV pacing group ($p = 0.95$). Several issues were raised by this trial, particularly the persistent practice of the RV in patients with sinus node dysfunction (as compared to dual-chamber pacing in an effort to spare the dyssynchrony induced by RV pacing). Investigators cite this as standard of care in China, where the trial was conducted; yet, the vast majority of such patients in the United States would receive dual-chamber devices, in an attempt to minimize dependence on RV pacing (for precisely the reasons demonstrated in the trial).

PACING FOR VASOVAGAL SYNCOPE

150. Connolly SJ, et al.; for the North American Vasovagal Pacemaker Study (VPS) Investigators. A randomized trial of permanent cardiac pacing for the prevention of vasovagal syncope. *J Am Coll Cardiol* 1999;33:16–20.

Design: Prospective, randomized, open, multicenter study. Primary end point was time to first recurrence of syncope.

Purpose: To determine whether permanent pacemakers with rate-drop algorithms can reduce the frequency of vasovagal syncope.

Population: 54 patients with 6 or more prior syncopal episodes and a positive head-up tilt-table test, with syncope or presyncope and "relative bradycardia" (definition differed depending on whether test was performed with isoproterenol).

Treatment: Pacemaker implantation or continuation of medical therapy (not standardized).

Results: Study was terminated prematurely at first interim data analysis when a large treatment effect favoring pacemaker implantation was observed. Syncope had occurred in 19 (70%) of 27 no-pacemaker patients and only 6 (22%) of 27 pacemaker patients ($p < 0.001$). Time to first recurrence was 54 days in the no-pacemaker group and 112 days in the pacemaker group. Additional reductions in the rate of presyncopal events were seen in the pacemaker group but were not statistically significant.

151. Ammirati F, et al.; Syncope Diagnosis and Treatment Study Investigators. Permanent cardiac pacing versus medical treatment for the prevention of recurrent vasovagal syncope: a multicenter, randomized, controlled trial. *Circulation* 2001;104: 52–57.

Design: Prospective, randomized, multicenter study. Primary end point was the first recurrence of syncope.

Purpose: To compare permanent dual-chamber pacemaker with pharmacologic therapy for recurrent vasovagal syncope.

Population: 93 patients with recurrent vasovagal syncope.

Treatment: Dual-chamber, permanent pacemaker implantation with setting of DDD (and a rate-drop response function), or pharmacologic therapy with the beta-blocker atenolol.

Results: Enrollment was terminated at the first interim analysis, as it demonstrated a significant effect favoring the pacemaker group (4.3% recurrence vs. 25.5%; $p = 0.004$) at a median of 135 days.

152. Connolly SJ, et al.; for the Second North American Vasovagal Pacemaker Study Investigators (VPS-II). Pacemaker therapy for prevention of syncope in patients with recurrent severe vasovagal syncope. *JAMA* 2003;289:2224–2229.

Design: Prospective, randomized, double-blind, multicenter study. Primary end point was time to first recurrence of syncope.

Purpose: To determine if pacing therapy reduces the risk of syncope in patients with vasovagal syncope.

Population: 100 patients with 6 or more prior syncopal episodes or ≥3 in prior 2 years and a positive tilt-table test.

Treatment: Dual-chamber pacing (DDD) with rate-drop response or ODO.

Results: At 6 months, the cumulative risk of syncope was 40% for the ODO group and 31% for the DDD group. There was a nonsignificant 30% RRR in time to syncope with DDD pacing ($p = 0.14$). Lead dislodgement or repositioning occurred in seven patients.

153. Raviele A, et al.; Vasovagal Syncope and Pacing Trial Investigators. A randomized, double-blind, placebo-controlled study of permanent cardiac pacing for the treatment of recurrent tilt-induced vasovagal syncope. The vasovagal syncope and pacing trial (SYNPACE). *Eur Heart J* 2004;25:1741–1748.

Design: Prospective, randomized, double-blind, placebo-controlled, multicenter study. Primary end point was time to first recurrence of syncope at median follow-up of 715 days.

Purpose: To determine if *blinded* pacing therapy reduces the risk of recurrent syncope in patients with vasovagal syncope.

Population: 29 patients with history of recurrent syncope and positive head-up tilt testing with asystolic or mixed response.

Treatment: All patients underwent permanent pacemaker implantation; they were then randomized to pacemaker ON or pacemaker OFF.

Results: At follow-up, recurrent syncope occurred in 50% of patients with pacemaker ON and 38% of patients with pacemaker OFF ($p = $ NS); however, time to recurrence tended to be longer in the pacemaker ON group (median 97 days vs. 20 days; $p = 0.38$). These outcomes did not differ among patients with different responses to tilt testing.

Comments: The study highlights the importance of doing blinded, placebo-controlled trials to definitively resolve a hypothesis. While the study size is small, this trial very much put into question the results of earlier, unblinded trials of permanent pacemakers for syncope.

154. Brignole M, et al. Pacemaker therapy in patients with neurally mediated syncope and documented asystole: Third International Study on Syncope of Uncertain Etiology (ISSUE-3): a randomized trial. *Circulation* 2012;125:2566–2571.

Design: Prospective, multicenter, randomized, double-blinded, placebo-controlled trial. The primary end point was syncope recurrence out to 24 months of follow-up.

Purpose: To assess the utility of dual-chamber pacemaker implantation for patients with severe cardioinhibitory syncope

Population: 89 patients with multiple syncopal episodes and documented asystole on implantable loop recorded of ≥3 seconds with syncope or ≥6 seconds without syncope

Key Exclusion Criteria: Syncope without documented asystolic pauses on implantable device.

Treatment: 77 or the 89 patients were randomized to pacemaker implantation with active pacing (including rate-drop response).

Results: Syncope recurrent was significantly reduced in patients assigned to active-pacing mode (25% vs. 57%; $p = 0.039$). This represented a significant relative reduction in syncope of 57%.

Comments: While most trials of permanent pacemakers for vasovagal syncope have yielded disappointing results, this study appears to have identified a small but significant subgroup of patients with severe cardioinhibitory response, who may benefit from pacemaker implantation.

PACING FOR PREVENTION OF ATRIAL FIBRILLATION

155. Carlson MD, et al. A new pacemaker algorithm for the treatment of atrial fibrillation: results of the Atrial Dynamic Overdrive Pacing Trial (ADOPT). *J Am Coll Cardiol* 2003;42:627–633.

This study tested a specific pacing algorithm designed to pace the atrium above patients' intrinsic sinus rates to suppress AF, which is often triggered by atrial ectopic beats. Patients with sinus node dysfunction and two or more episodes of AF in the preceding month were randomized to dual-chamber pacing with or without this algorithm. Investigators reported an approximately 25% reduction in the "burden of AF."

156. Fan K, et al. Effects of biatrial pacing in prevention of postoperative atrial fibrillation after coronary artery bypass surgery. *Circulation* 2000;102:755–760.

In a cohort of 132 patients undergoing CABG surgery at a single center, patients were randomized to RA pacing, LA pacing, BA pacing, or no pacing after surgery. Overdrive pacing at 90 or 10 bpm above the intrinsic rate up to 120 bpm was performed for 5 days in the active-pacing arms. Rates of AF lasting 10 or more minutes or requiring intervention were 12.5% in the BA group and 36%, 33%, and 42% in the LA, RA, and no-pacing groups, respectively ($p < 0.05$ for all comparisons). Total length of stay was reduced about 2 days in the BA-pacing group, compared with the no-pacing group.

157. Saksena S, et al. Improved suppression of recurrent atrial fibrillation with dual-site right atrial pacing and antiarrhythmic drug therapy (Dual-site Atrial Pacing for Prevention of Atrial Fibrillation, DAPPAF). *J Am Coll Cardiol* 2002;40:1140–1150.

This prospective, randomized, single-blind, crossover study enrolled patients who had dual-chamber pacemakers implanted, with two atrial leads: one in the traditional high-RA position and one in the low RA, outside the ostium of the coronary sinus. Patients were then assigned to one of the following three pacing modes—high-RA overdrive, dual-site RA overdrive, or "support" (DDI or VDI at suggested rate of 50 bpm) for 6 months—and then crossed over in random sequence to each of the other modes. Dislodgement of the "extra" low-RA lead was infrequent (1.7%). As expected, the "support" mode of pacing did the worst in terms of tolerability and rate of recurrent AF. Patients in the dual-site RA group were somewhat less likely to cross over because of mode intolerance than were patients in the high-RA group (time to crossover, 5.8 months vs. 4.7 months; $p < 0.01$) but had a similar proportion of mode-related adverse events. For the entire cohort, no significant difference was found between the dual-site and high-RA pacing groups for freedom from symptomatic AF or time to AF recurrence. Post hoc subgroup analysis did suggest the superiority of dual-site over high-RA pacing for AF suppression in patients with one or more AF episodes per week (hazard ratio, 0.62; $p = 0.006$), whereas a trend was seen only for patients taking antiarrhythmic drugs (hazard ratio, 0.67; $p = 0.06$).

RESYNCHRONIZATION THERAPY FOR CONGESTIVE HEART FAILURE

158. Auricchio A, et al. Effect of pacing chamber and atrioventricular delay on acute systolic function of paced patients with congestive heart failure: the Pacing Therapies for Congestive Heart Failure (PATH-CHF) Study Group. *Circulation* 1999;99: 2993–3001.

This single-blind study enrolled 42 patients with NYHA Class III to IV CHF, EF <35%, and QRS durations >120 ms, mostly due to left bundle branch block. All patients received BiV systems with the LV lead placed via limited thoracotomy. After implantation, the immediate hemodynamic performances of three different pacing modes (RV, LV, and BiV) were compared: LV pacing alone appeared most favorable. Patients then entered a 3-month crossover phase to select the optimal mode for the long-term phase, followed by a 12-month period of active pacing. At 12 months, BiV and LV pacing, compared with baseline, were associated with statistically significant improvements in 6-minute walk (446 m vs. 357 m; $p < 0.001$), peak oxygen consumption (1.19 L/min vs. 0.97 L/min; $p = 0.019$), anaerobic threshold (0.91 L/min vs. 0.76 L/min; $p = 0.018$), NYHA class (1.90 vs. 3.05; $p < 0.001$), and QOL (20 vs. 49; $p < 0.001$).

159. Cazeau S, et al.; for the Multisite Stimulation in Cardiomyopathies (MUSTIC) Study Investigators. Effects of multisite biventricular pacing in patients with heart failure and intraventricular conduction delay. N Engl J Med 2001;344:873–880.

Design: Prospective, randomized, single-blind, crossover, multicenter study. Primary end point was the 6-minute walk test.

Purpose: To assess the clinical benefits of BiV pacing (compared with no pacing) in HF patients with electrical conduction delays.

Population: 67 patients in SR with persistent NYHA Class III symptoms despite optimal medical therapy, EF <35%, LVEDD more than 60 mm, QRS duration of >150 ms, and no other indication for pacemaker implantation. Nine patients withdrew before randomization, and 10 failed to complete both study phases.

Exclusion Criteria: Included hypertrophic or restrictive cardiomyopathy, treatable valve disease, acute myocarditis, recent acute coronary syndrome or revascularization procedure, and approved indication for ICD implantation.

Treatment: All patients had full transvenous BiV pacing systems implanted, with RA and RV endocardial leads and LV leads introduced via coronary sinus branches. Two weeks after implant, patients were randomized to consecutive 3-month periods of "inactive" pacing (VVI at 40 bpm) or "active" pacing in a crossover design. Optimal AV delay for active pacing was determined by echocardiographic evaluation at the time of implant.

Results: Initial implantation success rate was 92%. Early lead dislodgement occurred in eight patients and was corrected in all but three. Active pacing, as compared with "inactive," resulted in significant improvement in the average distance walked in 6 minutes (399 m vs. 325 m; $p < 0.001$). Active pacing also was associated with a 32% improvement in the QOL score ($p < 0.001$), and an 8% increase in maximal oxygen consumption ($p < 0.03$).

Comments: Similar benefits with BiV pacing were seen in 64 patients with chronic AF (see *Circulation* 2000;102:3349A).

160. Abraham WT, et al.; for the Multicenter InSync Randomized Clinical Evaluation (MIRACLE) Study Group. Cardiac resynchronization in chronic heart failure. N Engl J Med 2002;346:1845–1853.

Design: Prospective, randomized, double-blind, controlled, multicenter trial. Primary end points were 6-minute walk, NYHA class, and QOL score.

Purpose: To assess the safety and efficacy of BiV pacing, compared with no pacing, in CHF patients with intraventricular conduction delay.

Population: 453 NYHA Class III to IV patients with EF of 35% or less, LVEDD 55 mm or more, QRS duration of 130 ms or more, and 6-minute walking distance of 450 m or less.

Treatment: All received transvenous BiV pacing systems and then were randomized to active pacing (atrially synchronized BiV pacing) or no pacing for 6 months.

Results: Initial implantation success rate was approximately 92%; 30 patients required subsequent repositioning or replacement of the LV pacing lead. Compared with the control group, patients successfully treated with BiV pacing had significantly greater improvements in 6-minute walking distance (+39 m vs. +10 m; p = 0.005), peak oxygen consumption (+1.1 mL/kg/min vs. +0.2 mL/kg/min; p = 0.009), QOL (−18 points vs. −9 points; p = 0.001), time on treadmill (+81 seconds vs. +19 seconds; p = 0.001), and EF (+4.6% vs. −0.2%; p < 0.001). In addition, a significantly larger proportion of BiV patients improved one or more NYHA classes (68% vs. 38%; p < 0.001) and significantly fewer were hospitalized for worsening HF (hazard ratio, 0.50; p = 0.02).

161. Young JB, et al. Combined cardiac resynchronization and implantable cardioversion defibrillation in advanced chronic heart failure. The MIRACLE ICD trial. JAMA 2003;289:2685–2694.

Design: Prospective, randomized, double-blind, parallel-controlled, multicenter trial. Primary end points were changes between baseline and 6 months in QOL, functional class, and 6-minute walk distance.

Purpose: To examine the efficacy and safety of combined CRT and ICD therapy in patients with NYHA Class III or IV CHF despite appropriate medical therapy.

Population: 369 patients with LVEF 35% or less, QRS duration of 130 ms, at high risk of life-threatening ventricular arrhythmias, and in NYHA Class III or IV.

Treatment: All with ICD activated. Control group with CRT off.

Results: CRT group had a greater improvement in median QOL score (p = 0.02) and functional class (p = 0.007) compared to control group, but there was no significant difference in change in 6-minute walk distance (55 m vs. 53 m; p = 0.36). CRT group did have a significant increase in peak oxygen consumption [+1.1 mL/kg/min vs. 0.1 (controls) mL/kg/min; p = 0.04].

162. Bristow MR, et al.; for the Comparison of Medical Therapy, Pacing, and Defibrillation in Heart Failure (COMPANION) Investigators. Cardiac-resynchronization therapy with or without an implantable defibrillator in advanced chronic heart failure. N Engl J Med 2004;350:2140–2150.

This prospective, randomized, multicenter trial enrolled 1,520 patients with moderate or severe HF (HYHA Class III or IV) due to ischemic or nonischemic causes with QRS >120 ms and PR interval >150 ms. Patients were assigned in 1:2:2 fashion to optimal medical therapy, optimal drugs plus CRT, or optimal drugs plus CRT with ICD (CRT-D). The primary end point was a reduction in death or hospitalization for any cause. At 1 year, the risk of the combined end point was reduced by 34% in the CRT group (p < 0.002) and 40% in the CRT-D group (p < 0.001). CRT-D significantly reduced the risk of death alone by 36% (p = 0.003); CTR alone was not significant at 24% (p = 0.059). The CRT-D mortality benefit was similar in those with ischemic and nonischemic etiologies.

163. Moss AJ, et al.; for the MADIT-CRT Trial Investigators. Cardiac-resynchronization therapy for the prevention of heart-failure events. N Engl J Med 2009;361: 1329–1338.

Design: Prospective, randomized, controlled trial. Primary end point was death from any cause or first nonfatal HF event over 2.4 years of follow-up.

Purpose: To identify the benefit, if any, of cardiac resynchronization on morbidity and mortality in patients with NYHA Class I or II HF and ECG evidence of dyssynchrony.

Population: 1,820 patients with ischemic or nonischemic cardiomyopathy, EF ≤30%, QRS duration >130 ms on ECG, and NYHA I or II symptoms.

Treatment: Conventional ICD placement or ICD placement with CRT, randomized in a 3:2 ratio favoring CRT.

Results: Treatment with CRT significantly reduced incidence of the primary end point when compared with ICD therapy alone (17.2% vs. 25.3%; p = 0.001). There was no difference between the ischemic or nonischemic groups; however, the composite primary end point was driven by a reduction in clinical HF events (13.9% for CRT-ICD vs. 22.8% for ICD only; $p < 0.001$), without differences in mortality rates (3.3% for CRT-ICD vs. 2.5% in the ICD-only group). Total deaths, including those which occurred after an HF event, also were similar (6.8% for CRT-ICD vs. 7.3% for ICD only; $p = 0.99$).

164. Cleland JG, et al.; for the Cardiac Resynchronization—Heart Failure (CARE-HF) Study Investigators. The effect of cardiac resynchronization on morbidity and mortality in heart failure. N Engl J Med 2005;352:1539–1549.

Design: Prospective, randomized, controlled trial. Primary end point was death from any cause or unplanned hospitalization for cardiovascular event over a mean follow-up period of 29.4 months.

Purpose: To identify the effects of CRT on morbidity and mortality in patients with NYHA Class III or IV HF.

Population: 813 patients with LV systolic dysfunction, NYHA III or IV symptoms, and cardiac dyssynchrony.

Treatment: Standard medical therapy alone or with CRT.

Results: Primary end points were significantly reduced in the CRT group (39% vs. 55%; $p < 0.001$), and the effect was not just on morbidity, but mortality was significantly reduced in the CRT group as well (20% vs. 30%; $p < 0.002$). Additionally, CRT significantly improved several echocardiographic measures of LV function and efficiency.

165. Curtis AB, et al. Biventricular pacing for atrioventricular block and systolic dysfunction. N Engl J Med 2013;368:1585–1593.

Design: Prospective, multicenter, double-blinded, active-control randomized trial. The primary end point was a composite increased LV end-systolic volume index (by 15%), urgent IV HF therapy, or all-cause mortality at mean follow-up of 37 months.

Purpose: To assess the benefit, if any, to BiV pacing in patients requiring permanent pacemaker with mild LV dysfunction.

Population: 691 patients with an indication for permanent pacemaker (AV block), NYHA I–III HF, and LVEF ≤50%.

Key Exclusion Criteria: Pre-existing implantable cardiac rhythm device or presence of a guideline-recommended indication for CRT.

Treatment: All patients underwent implantation of a CRT device (either CRT-P or CRT-D, as indicated); they were randomized to be programmed with standard RV pacing or to CRT pacing.

Results: A primary end point event occurred in 56% of the RV pacing group, versus 45.8% of the BiV pacing group (HR 0.74; 95% CI, 0.60 to 0.90). Rate of LV lead placement complication was 6.4%.

Comments: This trial established the benefit of a strategy many electrophysiologists had long believed—that in patients with or at high risk of LV dysfunction, who require a high percentage of pacing, CRT therapy is better than standard RV pacing. It should be noted, however, that the benefit of this primary end point was predominantly driven by changes in LV end-systolic volume index.

166. Ruschitzka F, et al.; The EchoCRT Study. Cardiac-resynchronization therapy in heart failure with a narrow QRS complex. N Engl J Med 2013;369:1395–1405.

Design: Prospective, international, multicenter, double-blinded, randomized controlled trial. The primary end point was first occurrence of HF hospitalization or death at mean follow-up of 19.4 months.

Purpose: To assess the benefit, if any, to CRT in patients with narrow QRS and LV dyssynchrony based on echocardiographic assessment.

Population: 809 patients with NYHA III–IV HF, EF ≤35%, standard indication for an ICD, QRS duration <130 ms, LV end-diastolic diameter of ≥55 mm, and echocardiographic evidence of LV dyssynchrony.

Key Exclusion Criteria: Decompensated or inotrope-dependent HF, AF within the last month, or bradycardia requiring pacing.

Treatment: All patients underwent implantation of a CRT device; those successfully implanted were then randomized to CRT capability on or off.

Results: The trial was stopped due to futility—at the time of closure, the primary outcome had occurred in 28.7% of the CRT group versus 25.5% of control patients (HR 1.2; $p = 0.15$). There was a significantly higher rate of death in the CRT group (11.1% vs. 6.4%; $p = 0.02$).

Comments: The identification and measurement of LV dyssynchrony by echocardiography have become highly refined, leading many to speculate that such patients could benefit from CRT. Though terminated prematurely, this trial demonstrated that such patients would not benefit from CRT.

Trial Index

Subject Index

Note: Page numbers followed by "*f*" indicate figures; and those followed by "*t*" indicate tables.

A

Abciximab
  vs. balloon angioplasty, 225
  comparison with eptifibatide, 122
  in non-ST elevation myocardial infarction, 225
  as restenosis prophylaxis, 129
  in ST elevation myocardial infarction, 280
    comparison with stenting, 280
    with reteplase, 285
  in unstable angina, 225
  use in PCI patients, 118, 121, 122
Ablation
  atrioventricular junction, 444
  catheter-based, in atrial fibrillation, 438
  surgical, in atrial fibrillation, 438
Abrupt closure, PCI-related, 126
ACC. *See* American College of Cardiology (ACC)
ACC/AHA. *See* American College of Cardiology (ACC)/American Heart Association (AHA)
ACE. *See* Angiotensin-converting enzyme (ACE) inhibitors
ACE inhibitor (ACEI) therapy, 87
ACEI. *See* ACE inhibitor (ACEI) therapy
Acetylcysteine, for renal dysfunction, 193
ACS. *See* Acute coronary syndrome (ACS)
Activated partial thromboplastin time (aPTT), 248, 336
Acute coronary syndrome (ACS). *See also* Angina; Unstable angina
  pathophysiology of, 216*f*
  plaque rupture associated with, 215
Adenosine diphosphate (ADP) receptor antagonists, 118–121, 119*f*, 120*f*
  in non-ST elevation myocardial infarction, 220–221
  in unstable angina, 220–221
ADP. *See* Adenosine diphosphate (ADP) receptor antagonists
Adrenergic agents, in congestive heart failure, 379
AED. *See* Automated external defibrillators (AED)
AF. *See* Atrial fibrillation (AF)
Aging, as cardiovascular disease risk factors, 22

AHA. *See* American Heart Association (AHA)
Alcohol
  cardioprotective effects of, 13
  as hypertension cause, 18
Aldosterone antagonism, in ST elevation myocardial infarction, 272
Aldosterone blocker, in congestive heart failure, 385–386. *See also* Eplerenone, in congestive heart failure; Spironolactone, in congestive heart failure
Alirocumab, 52–53
Allergic reactions, to contrast agents, 113, 127
Alteplase, in ST-elevation myocardial infarction treatment, 313, 314, 316, 331, 346
American College of Cardiology (ACC), 111
  atrial fibrillation treatment guidelines of, 430
American College of Cardiology (ACC)/American Heart Association (AHA)
  antiplatelet and anticoagulant therapy guidelines of, 222
  classification of stenosis morphology, 111, 141
  exercise treadmill testing guidelines of, 229
  guideline for heart failure, 3, 4*f*, 375, 391, 392
  NSTEMI guidelines by, 222, 224–225, 226, 228
  STEMI guidelines by, 290, 293
American Diabetes Association, 27
American Heart Association (AHA), 111
  atrial fibrillation treatment guidelines of, 430
  omega-3 fatty acids supplementation recommendation of, 11, 61
Amiodarone
  antiarrhythmic activity, in cardiac disease patients, 449
  in atrial fibrillation, 433–438, 445, 446, 449, 450, 457, 459–467, 470, 481, 483–489
  in congestive heart failure, 387, 418
  in immediate cardiac arrest, 446
  implantable cardioverter defibrillator therapy *vs.*, 446, 447*t*, 448*t*
  postoperative atrial fibrillation prophylaxis, 445